Brief C

Contents

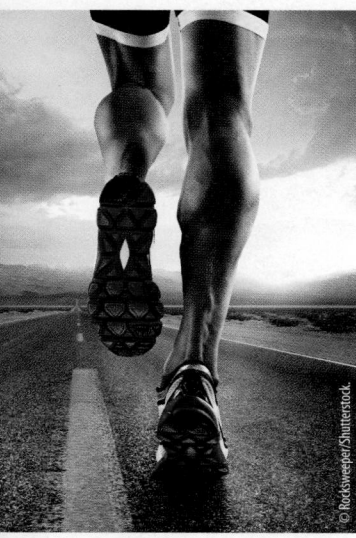

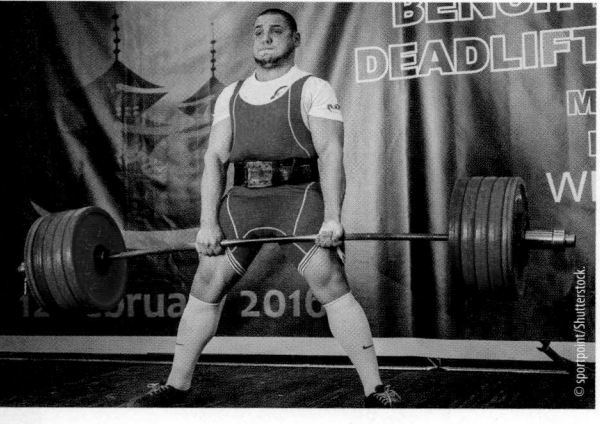

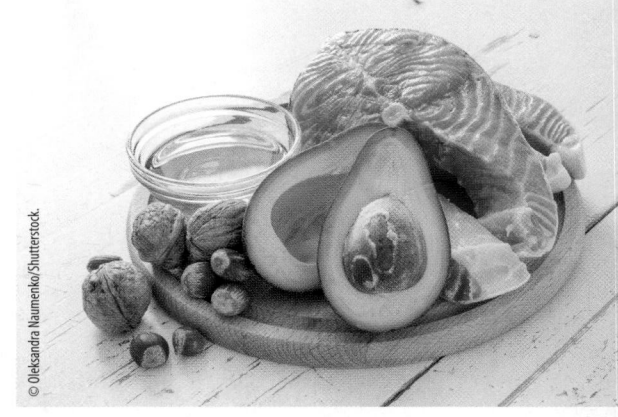

© Oleksandra Naumenko/Shutterstock.

CHAPTER **9**   **Fad Diets and Supplements 177**

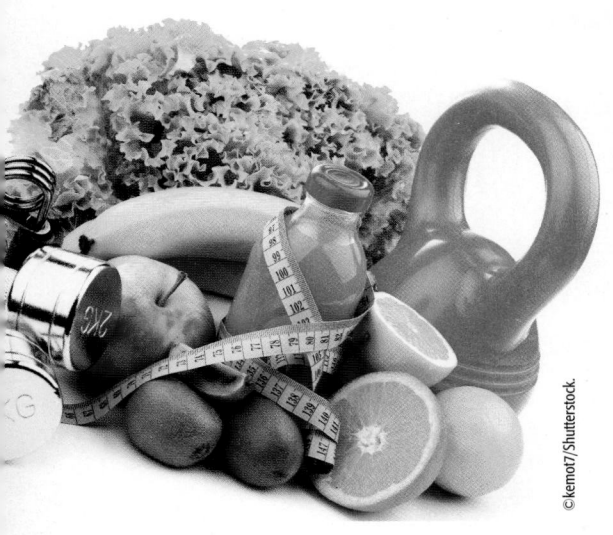

Appendices

©kemot7/Shutterstock.

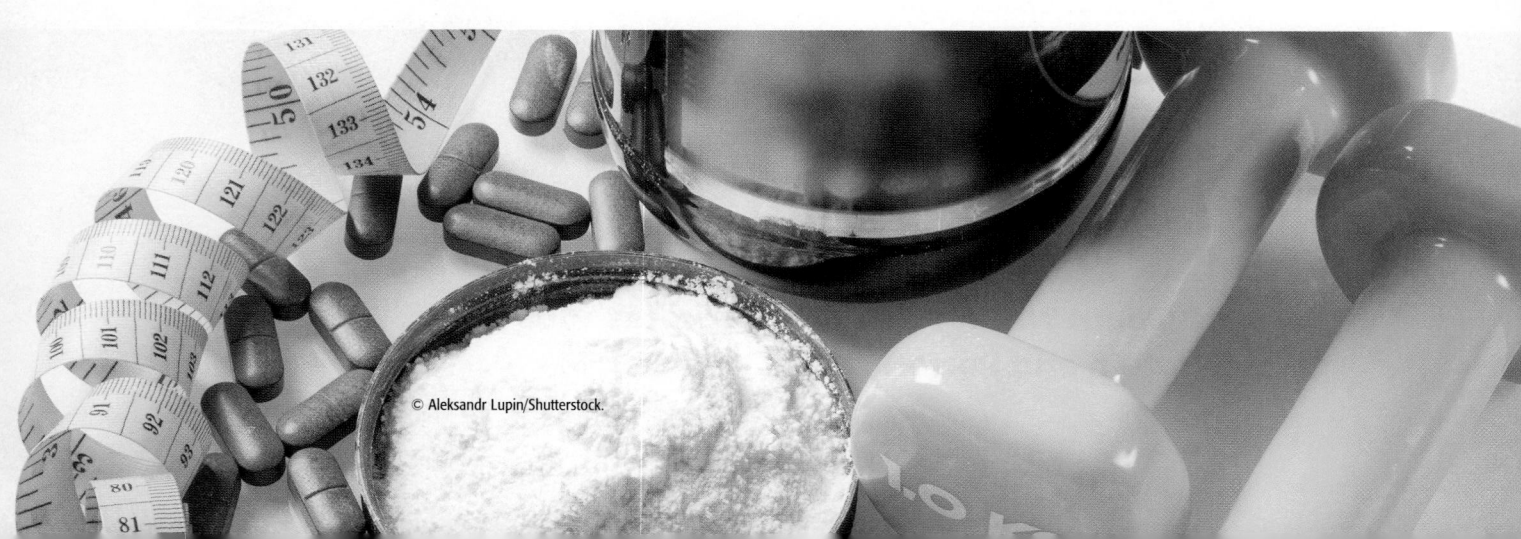

© Aleksandr Lupin/Shutterstock.

A Practical Guide to Personal Conditioning is a concise yet comprehensive resource that connects the science of exercise with real-world applications to sport and human performance. In other words, it provides students with both the "Why?" and the "How?" behind effective exercise prescription and programming.

Although designed as a textbook for undergraduate courses in human performance and/or basic personal conditioning, the information and recommendations provided herein are equally beneficial for exercise enthusiasts interested in "upping their game" or a layperson seeking credible guidance without the need for a personal trainer. The information and concepts presented in the text have been broken down to make them easy to understand and applicable to everyone.

Admittedly, there is a plethora of exercise physiology textbooks and workout guides out there. However, most of the textbooks are lengthy, difficult to read, and fall short in equipping readers with how to develop a personalized exercise and nutrition plan. Additionally, several of the workout guides were written by individuals without formal education in the field of exercise science, but rather, only a fitness certification. Just because someone is certified or is physically fit does not, in itself, make them an expert on fitness!

Much of the information presented in *A Practical Guide to Personal Conditioning* was compiled from numerous exercise physiology texts, peer-reviewed journal articles, and professional seminars and conferences. Even so, most of the information came from the thousands of hours spent by the authors in the gym, on the track, and in the classroom while training their clients, their students, and themselves.

Although this book is written with the intent of being read straight through—as doing so better shows the close relationship between several of the exercise concepts and principles used throughout the text—it is also designed for browsing. The easy-to-use Table of Contents allows students to quickly find information and training recommendations on topics relevant to them.

Finally, *A Practical Guide to Personal Conditioning* is organized in such a way as to facilitate a logical flow of information that maximizes student learning and comprehension. For example, the text includes:

- Dozens of charts, graphs, tables, figures, and photos with the goal of bringing the information and concepts in this book to life.

- Numerous examples and case studies throughout the text aimed at improving student comprehension and retention of the information.

- Several different fitness tests and self-assessments that students can use to evaluate where they are currently compared with where they should be, based on their age and gender.

- End-of-chapter activities and book-end appendices, which allow students the opportunity to develop exercise and nutrition plans personalized to their own specific training goals and needs.

Features of This Text

A Practical Guide to Personal Conditioning includes a range of features to improve retention and engagement with the content.

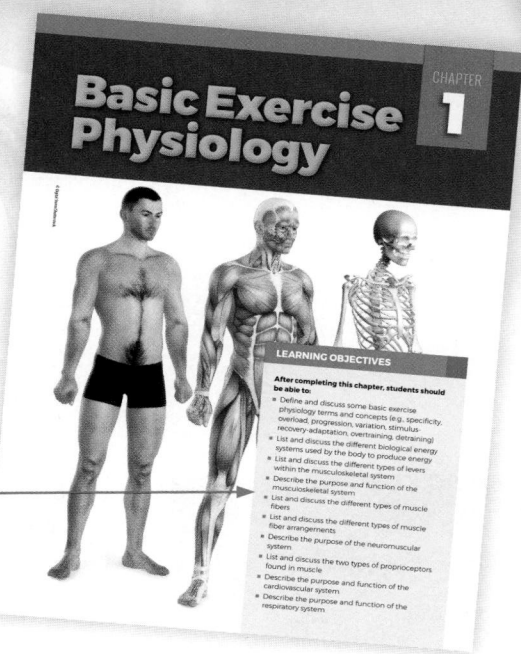

Each chapter begins with **Learning Objectives** highlighting its critical points.

Frequently Asked Questions boxes throughout the text address basic questions about training techniques and nutrition.

Key terms and definitions appear in the margins of the text, enhancing comprehension. In addition, a **Glossary** is included at the end of the text.

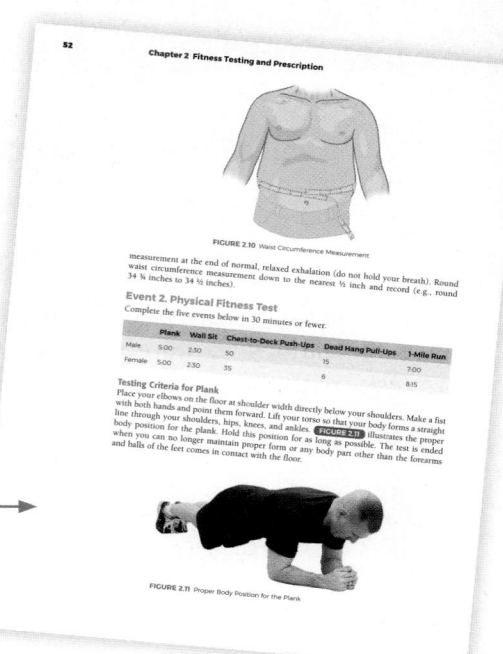

A **comprehensive art package** consisting of color photographs and illustrations ensures that techniques are properly conveyed along with the underlying exercise physiology concepts.

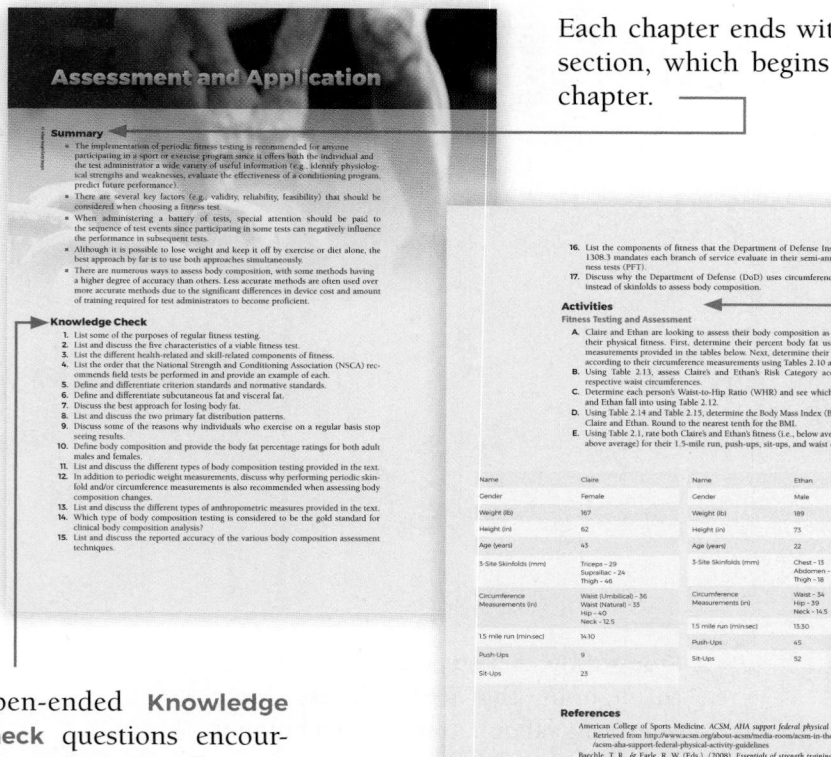

Each chapter ends with an **Assessment and Application** section, which begins with a bulleted **Summary** of the chapter.

End-of-chapter **Activities** provide scenarios in which the reader is asked to consider the chapter content in the context of a person developing his or her own fitness plan.

Open-ended **Knowledge Check** questions encourage readers to reflect on key concepts.

Student Resources

Each new print copy of *A Practical Guide to Personal Conditioning* is accompanied by access to the Navigate Companion Website. Resources on the companion website include the following:

- Practice Quizzes
- Flashcards
- Interactive Glossary
- Crossword Puzzles
- Web Links

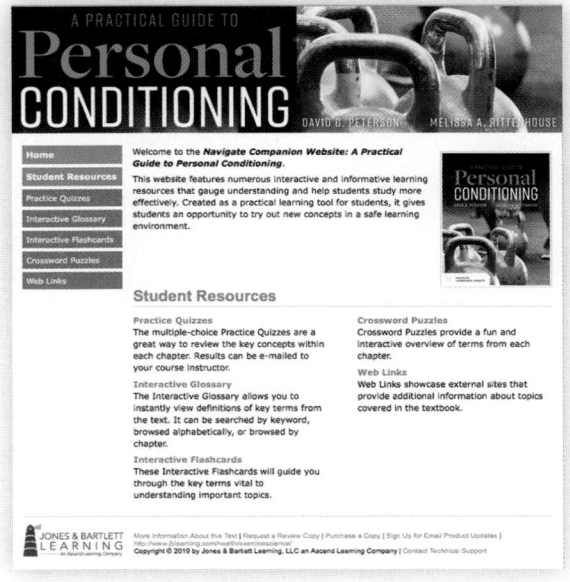

Instructor Resources

Instructors who use *A Practical Guide to Personal Conditioning* in their classroom can receive access to a comprehensive suite of instructor resources. These resources are provided so that they can effectively incorporate the text into their course. The resources include the following:

- Test Bank
- Slides in PowerPoint format
- Image Bank
- Answer Key to End-of-Chapter Activities

I wish I had written this book! Drs. Peterson and Rittenhouse have met a great need—a simple, scientifically based textbook that provides *vital* information for anyone beginning a fitness and/or fat control program. With all of the misinformation available on the Internet and in print, readers will find this accurate, practical textbook a quick source of essential guidance.

–Phil Bishop, EdD
Emeritus Professor of Exercise Science
University of Alabama
Former Marathon and Ultra-Marathon Champion

Information and texts relating to exercise physiology are often presented in standard formats, with a dry, robotic arrangement. With their recent book, *A Practical Guide to Personal Conditioning*, Drs. Peterson and Rittenhouse have incorporated a fresh and innovative method of organizing this challenging topic. This easy-to-use text covers the gamut of topics, including flexibility, strength, and endurance, as well as nutrition and provides succinct guidance for enhancing an individual's health and fitness goals. The authors' direct and streamlined approach will appeal to both novices and experts who are interested in this demanding field of study.

–Vincent K. Ramsey, PhD, CSCS, LMT, EMT-I, DAV
Chair of Sports Exercise Science
United States Sports Academy

A Practical Guide to Personal Conditioning encapsulates the nationally renowned expertise that Drs. Peterson and Rittenhouse have successfully used as a template for developing some of our nation's most elite military fighting forces. The effectiveness of this force is a result of two major components: First, mission-specific training; and second and even more important, the state of readiness of the individual who executes a job, which dictates that he or she must be physically prepared for a wide range of missions. This unique book illuminates a path to prepare and sustain a high level of health and fitness. The authors capitalize on goal-driven program design and performance measurements, using the latest physiology and nutrition research and fitness testing methods. It provides an easily readable yet comprehensive roadmap to achieving and sustaining optimal fitness. I highly recommend this book for those individuals who are interested in gaining the knowledge base for developing a consistently high level of physical performance.

–Professor Carla Criste, PhD
Head Coach, Women's Track and Field
United States Naval Academy

Drs. Peterson and Rittenhouse have put together a great science-based book on fitness that can be used in a classroom setting, by a fitness professional, or by an individual looking to base his or her workout program on science and not on urban legend. This book covers the entire spectrum of fitness topics to build a comprehensive fitness program, covering the science behind resistance training, endurance training, flexibility, and proper nutritional concepts—the complete package!

–Bill McCormack, PhD
Captain (retd), United States Navy
Assistant Professor
Loyola Marymount University

With the myriad of websites, books, mobile apps, and gadgets on the market today, most people have become overwhelmed with the process of taking care of themselves with exercise and proper nutrition. Drs. Peterson and Rittenhouse have written a great guide that provides a straightforward path to fitness. *A Practical Guide to Personal Conditioning* is comprehensive and yet presented in a manner that enables the reader to put the information to immediate use.

–Brian Schilling, PhD, CSCS
Professor and Chair, Kinesiology and Nutrition Sciences
The University of Nevada, Las Vegas

A Practical Guide to Personal Conditioning is my new fitness bible. Being reminded of the science of fitness through easy-to-read sections gives this workout book more than what the average program offers. The recommendations for periodization and the variety of training protocols make this book an invaluable tool for any trainer and/or athlete. I highly recommend reading, taking notes, and performing the workouts described in this book. You will be faster, stronger, and smarter by doing so. My students will be reading this book for sure.

–Stew Smith, CSCS
Fitness Author & Former Navy SEAL
Coach–Special Ops Team, United States Naval Academy

The plan laid out in *A Practical Guide to Personal Conditioning* works! When I first read this book, I was recovering from an injury that resulted in a significant decrease in personal fitness and strength. The easy-to-follow and logical methods presented in the book helped me return to a healthy, active lifestyle. After a few short months, I was back to what I considered my normal strength level. Now, almost a year into the program, I have surpassed all expectations and am regularly increasing the amount of weight I can lift and surprising myself with what I can achieve. In fact, I am now using "big girl" plates for most large muscle group lifts! I highly recommend this book to anyone who wants to see improvement in their personal fitness.

–J. C. Beattie, PhD
Assistant Professor, Department of Physics
United States Naval Academy

David D. Peterson, EdD, CSCS*D, is a retired Naval Aerospace/Operational Physiologist and Certified Strength and Conditioning Specialist (with Distinction) with over 20 years of active duty service experience. He has earned multiple degrees in Exercise Science and is a former competitive powerlifter. He has dedicated his life and career to the study and pursuit of physical fitness and human performance. Having served previously as both the Director of the Human Performance Lab and Deputy Director of the Physical Education Department at the U.S. Naval Academy, Dr. Peterson is now assigned as an Assistant Professor of Kinesiology within the Department of Kinesiology and Allied Health at Cedarville University. Dr. Peterson's military call-sign was the acronym MEAT, standing for "Must Eat All the Time."

Melissa A. Rittenhouse, PhD, RD, CSSD, is a Registered Dietitian and Certified Specialist in Sports Dietetics with a PhD in Exercise Physiology. Dr. Rittenhouse's interest in nutrition and athletic performance intensified as her running career escalated. She competed in the 2004, 2008, and 2012 Olympic Marathon Trials. That is over 12 years of competing at the highest level, which could not have been done without paying special attention to every piece of the puzzle, including proper nutrition, sleep, positive mental health, appropriate training, and recovery. Dr. Rittenhouse enjoys working with highly motivated individuals who challenge themselves to always be better.

© Johner Images/Getty Images.

Denel Bingel, MEd
Professor
Raritan Valley Community College
Branchburg, New Jersey

Kathi Deresinski, MS
Faculty
Health, Sport & Exercise Science
    Department
Triton College
River Grove, Illinois

Ryan R. Fairall, PhD, CSCS, EP-C, CES
Sports Medicine Program Director
Keiser University—Jacksonville
Jacksonville, Florida

Jennifer Fields, MS
Instructor
School of Recreation, Health, and Tourism
George Mason University
Fairfax, Virginia

Jo Sloan, PhD
Assistant Professor
Department of Physical Education
Lane College
Jackson, Tennessee

Martha Swirzinski, EdD
Assistant Professor
Department of Physical Education
Thomas Nelson Community College
Hampton, Virginia

Brandon Yates, MS, CSCS, USAW
Instructor
Quincy College
Quincy, Massachusetts

Seok Yoon, PhD
Associate Professor
Department of Sports Studies and Physical
    Education
Chowan University
Murfreesboro, North Carolina

Patricia Zodda, MS, CPT
Professor and Chair
Department of Exercise and Human
    Performance
Rockland Community College
Suffern, New York

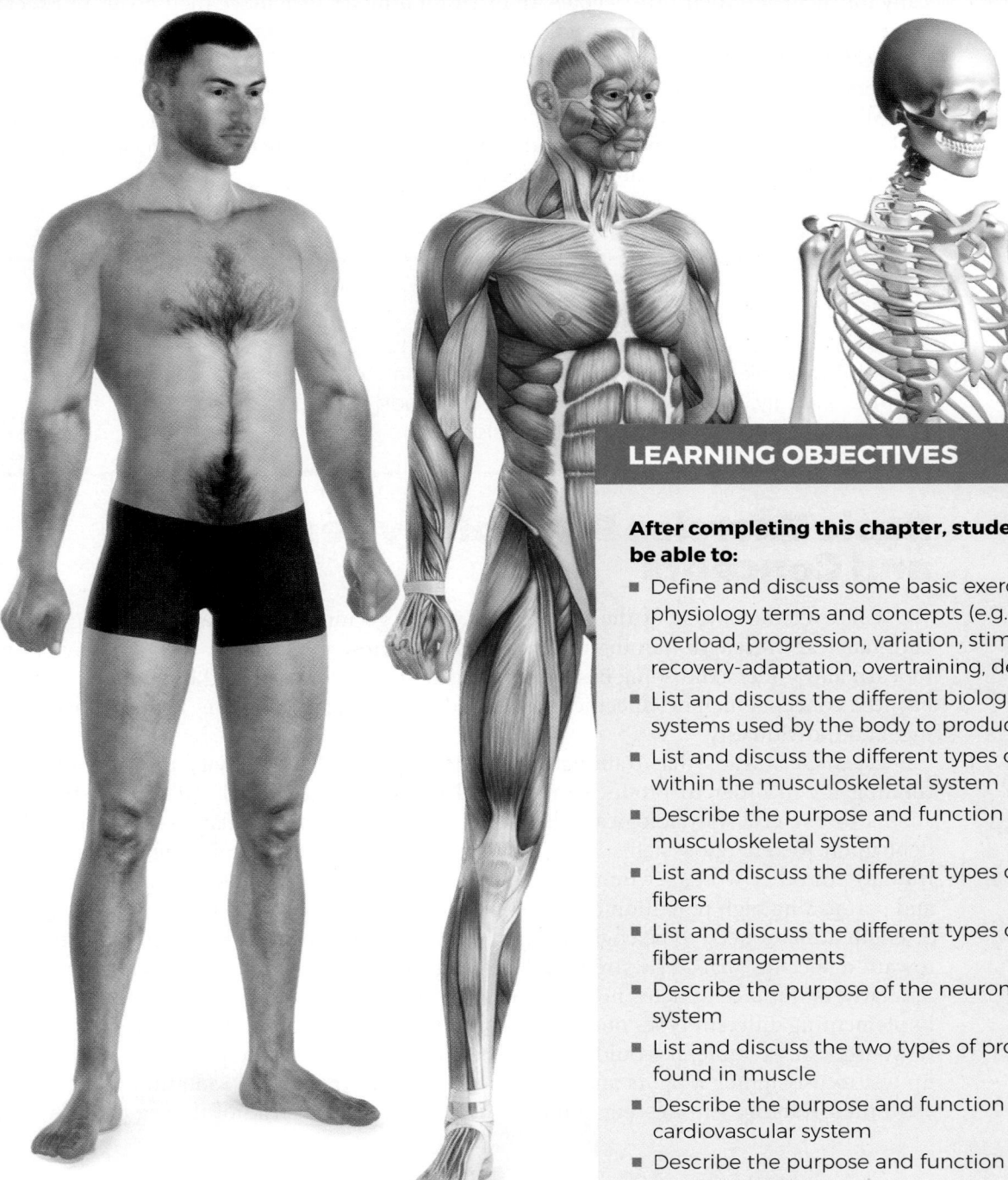

Basic Exercise Physiology

LEARNING OBJECTIVES

After completing this chapter, students should be able to:

- Define and discuss some basic exercise physiology terms and concepts (e.g., specificity, overload, progression, variation, stimulus-recovery-adaptation, overtraining, detraining)
- List and discuss the different biological energy systems used by the body to produce energy
- List and discuss the different types of levers within the musculoskeletal system
- Describe the purpose and function of the musculoskeletal system
- List and discuss the different types of muscle fibers
- List and discuss the different types of muscle fiber arrangements
- Describe the purpose of the neuromuscular system
- List and discuss the two types of proprioceptors found in muscle
- Describe the purpose and function of the cardiovascular system
- Describe the purpose and function of the respiratory system

Introduction

With so many commercial fitness books and exercise programs already available (e.g., Bigger Leaner Stronger, Body for Life, CrossFit, Insanity, P90X, etc.), why bother developing another textbook? Well, unlike most commercial books and programs, *A Practical Guide to Personal Conditioning* provides users with more than just a workout; it provides them with understanding. As the old adage goes:

> *"Give a man a fish and you feed him for a day; teach a man to fish and you feed him for a lifetime."*

The fundamental purpose of this textbook is to provide users with the information and resources necessary to develop an exercise and nutrition plan designed and tailored specifically for them and their fitness goals. In order for athletes to achieve their goals, or excel in their respective sport, they must take into consideration numerous factors, including the physical demands of the event/sport, nutrition, nutrient timing, and the environment (e.g., temperature, altitude, humidity, etc.)

All of the information and recommendations provided herein are supported by science and, therefore, proven to be a safe and effective approach to diet and exercise. Remember, training hard is easy, but training smart can be hard.

FAQ

Why do people exercise?

People exercise for many different reasons: to lose weight, to gain weight, to be healthier, to improve athletic performance, or to make daily life easier. Interestingly, by far (~90%), the most common reason people exercise is to look good when wearing minimal clothing.

Basic Exercise Physiology Terms and Concepts

We will, over the course of the next few chapters, go into great detail, providing specific endurance and strength training recommendations. However, before we do, it is imperative to learn and understand some basic exercise physiology concepts and fundamentals. Some of these concepts include: specificity, overload, progression, variation, recovery, overtraining, and individuality.

Specificity means that training should be relevant to the activity that the athlete is training for in order to produce the desired outcome and should reflect how the body adapts to exercise. Physiological adaptations associated with regular exercise are dependent upon the energy systems, muscle groups, and other biological systems used during training. In other words, swimming on a regular basis will not make you a better runner, and performing high repetition body weight push-ups will not maximize your bench press. Strength athletes need to be cognizant of the load, repetitions, and sets used when training toward a specific goal (e.g., strength, size [aka hypertrophy], power, muscle endurance). Similarly, endurance athletes need to be aware of intensity, duration, and frequency when implementing different types of endurance training in order to produce the desired training response. For example, it would be more beneficial for athletes preparing for a max push-up test to use lighter weights and higher repetitions in the weight room in order to better align their training with testing. Similarly, the back squat, instead of the leg press, may be

Specificity: Training should be relevant to the activity the individual is training for in order to produce the desired training effect.

the preferred exercise during in-season training for lineman since it more closely mimics the stance and body position used in football.

FAQ

What is the difference between exercise and training?

Exercise is, simply, working out. Generally speaking, the main reason people exercise is to improve health and/or to feel/look better. Training, on the other hand, is working out with a specific purpose. Training is structured, deliberate, and geared toward accomplishing pre-determined exercise goals (e.g., run faster, lift more weight, jump higher).

Another factor to consider is whether to incorporate closed kinetic chain or open kinetic chain exercises. A **closed kinetic chain (CKC)** exercise is one in which the terminal joint is fixed and remains in constant contact with either the floor or an immobile surface (e.g., back squat, leg press). In the case of an **open kinetic chain (OKC)** exercise, the terminal joint is free to move and allows for greater concentration of an isolated muscle group (e.g., leg extension, leg curl). As a result, OKC exercises are frequently employed by bodybuilders and athletes who are in rehabilitation. Although CKC exercises offer better joint stability and are considered to be more functional than OKC exercises, most sports incorporate both CKC and OKC movements. The frequent utilization of both has proven to be the best choice for most conditioning programs.

The concept of **overload** means that greater than normal stress is required in order for training adaptations to occur. These adaptations lead to increased athletic performance in terms of speed, strength, power, endurance, etc. Over time, weights should get heavier, number of sets should be increased, and training speeds should become faster in order to facilitate further physiological adaptations. An unfortunate reality is that the degree of adaptation is inversely proportional to training status. This means that the better trained an athlete is, the lesser the degree of physiological adaptation will occur for a given exercise stimulus. Furthermore, once the athlete's **genetic potential** is reached, no further physiological adaptations will occur, even when exposed to a greater training stimulus.

It is necessary to periodically increase training variables (e.g., load, intensity, duration, frequency) in order for improvements to continue over time. This fundamental principle of exercise training and prescription is referred to as **progression**. Most strength and conditioning professionals do not recommend increasing more than one training variable at a time, or increasing any specific training variable by more than 10% per week (e.g., running = mileage; cardio machines = time; strength training = weight). **Variation** means that exercises should be rotated periodically in order to prevent training plateaus and overtraining. Most strength and conditioning professionals recommend that exercises be rotated monthly.

Directed adaptation, on the other hand, means that in order to get better at something, the athlete must perform the exercise repeatedly. From a practical perspective, this means that although most athletes would benefit from alternating their exercises, it may not be the best approach for all sports. For example, Marines should regularly perform pull-ups as it is one of the events in the United States Marine Corps Physical Fitness Test (PFT) and is a perishable skill, if not performed regularly. Similarly, in the case of competitive powerlifting, it is imperative that these athletes regularly perform the bench, squat, and deadlift. However, to promote future gains and prevent training plateaus, it may prove beneficial to periodically employ slight modifications to the core lifts (e.g., changes in stance, grip width, etc.).

Closed kinetic chain (CKC): Exercises where the hand (for arm movement) or foot (for leg movement) are fixed, cannot move, and remains in constant contact with an immobile surface, usually the ground or base of a machine (e.g., leg press).

Open kinetic chain (OKC): Exercises that are performed where the hand or foot are free to move (e.g., dumbbell lateral raises).

Overload: Greater than normal stress (load) is required in order for training adaptations to occur. These adaptations lead to increased athletic performance in terms of speed, strength, power, endurance, etc.

Genetic potential: Theoretical optimum performance capability that an individual could achieve in a specific activity, after an ideal upbringing, nutrition, and training.

Progression: Periodic increases in training variables (e.g., load, intensity, duration, frequency) in order for improvements to continue over time.

Variation: Periodic rotation of exercises in order to prevent training plateaus and/or overtraining.

Directed adaptation: A fundamental principle to exercise programming that states that in order to get better at something, you must train it over and over.

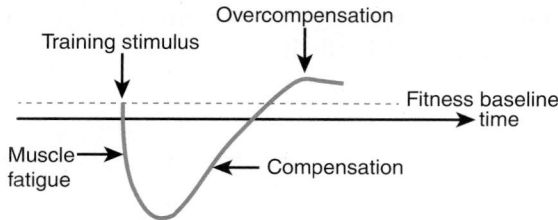

FIGURE 1.1 Stimulus-Recovery-Adaptation

The time required between exercise sessions for the body to repair damaged tissue and replenish depleted energy stores is termed **recovery**. The amount of time required to fully recover depends on the type and intensity of the exercise performed. Insufficient recovery time will limit training adaptations and may lead to overtraining.

The concept of **Stimulus-Recovery-Adaptation (SRA)** states that physiological adaptations associated with exercise take place during recovery and not during training. **FIGURE 1.1** depicts the relationship between training stimulus, recovery and adaptation (CoachR.org, n.d.). In order for physiological adaptations to occur and continue over time, it is important to afford enough rest between training sessions.

Performing another training session too soon can lead to overtraining because the body will not have enough time to repair itself before being exposed to another session. On the other hand, waiting too long between training sessions can lead to no performance improvements or, even, detraining. As a result, training frequency recommendations for each different type of exercise should be based on the amount of time required to recover. Following are the recovery recommendations for various types of conditioning (American College of Sports Medicine, 2011; Centers for Disease Control and Prevention, 2015).

- Moderate endurance training: 24 hours
- Moderate strength / intense endurance training: 48 hours
- Intense strength training: 72–96 hours

It is important to note that these recommendations are not set in stone and may differ from person to person. Several factors can influence one's ability to recover, including age, injury status, and current fitness level. The above recommendations provide basic guidance as to when one should repeat the same workout or train the same muscle group. For example, performing strength training every day is acceptable as long as the same muscle group is not trained back to back on subsequent days (e.g., bench press on Monday followed by a push-up pyramid workout on Tuesday). A better approach to daily strength training would be to perform chest/tricep exercises on Monday, back/bicep exercises on Tuesday, and shoulder/leg exercises on Wednesday, then repeat. The same rules apply to endurance training. Although it may be acceptable to perform long, slow-distance runs every day, it is not recommended to perform sprint training on subsequent days.

Effectively combining strength training and endurance training into one comprehensive training plan without violating recovery recommendations can be challenging. For example, it would not be advisable to perform lower body strength training on Monday and then perform sprints on Tuesday as both workouts target type II (fast twitch) muscle fibers of the lower extremities. Instead, it would be better to conduct both on the same day and then afford 72 hours of recovery, or perform lower body strength training on Monday and then wait to perform sprint training on Wednesday, thereby providing at least 48 hours of recovery.

FIGURE 1.2 depicts the relationship between the timing for (a) improving performance, (b) overtraining, and (c) no performance change or detraining.

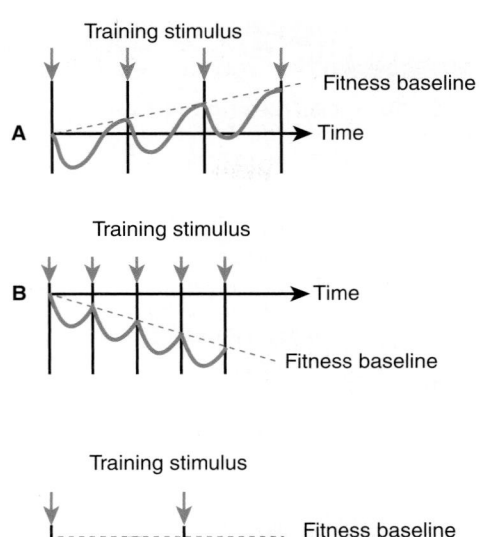

FIGURE 1.2 SRA Curve for **(A)** Improving Performance, **(B)** Overtraining, and **(C)** Training Plateaus and/or Detraining

The principle of **fatigue management** states that recovery becomes incomplete as fatigue accumulates over time. Therefore, after several weeks of hard training, it is recommended to take some time off or reduce both training volume and training intensity. One effective strategy to prevent overtraining is to incorporate a **deload** (aka active rest) week every 4–6 weeks.

Overtraining occurs when an athlete reaches a point in training when there is a decrease in performance and/or plateauing. This is a result of consistently performing at a level or training load that exceeds their recovery capacity. Overtraining can be difficult to diagnose as many of the symptoms are similar to other medical or psychological conditions. Additionally, symptoms may differ from one athlete to the next.

In most cases, overtraining is caused by the lack of rest between intense bouts of exercise. Although high-intensity and high-volume training is often required to initiate certain physiological adaptations (e.g., increased speed, size, power, endurance); it is imperative that athletes incorporate rest and reduced training days to allow the body to adapt and recover. When overtraining occurs, total rest is required. Therefore, it is imperative to identify the signs and symptoms of overtraining early and put into place the necessary corrective actions (e.g., deload week, additional sleep per night, prescribed nutritional strategies). **TABLE 1.1** on the next page depicts some of the signs (aka markers) associated with overtraining (Al-Masri, 2011; Beachle & Earle, 2008; Haff & Triplett, 2016).

It is important to note that the physiological adaptations associated with chronic exercise are not permanent, but rather transient and reversible. In fact, any training adaptation will slowly change to pre-training levels, a process known as **detraining**, if the training stimulus is reduced or eliminated. Significant reductions in both metabolic and work capacity have been documented after only 1–2 weeks of detraining. Some training adaptations are completely lost after several months of detraining. One study showed a 25% decrease in **VO₂max** after 20 days of consecutive bedrest with similar decrements reported in maximal **stroke volume** and **cardiac output** (McCardle, 2015). This equates to roughly a 1% decrease in physiological function per day.

Fatigue management: After several weeks of hard training, recovery becomes incomplete as fatigue accumulates over time, thereby requiring an intentional decrease in training volume and/or intensity.

Deload: A short planned period of recovery. A typical deload period will last a week.

Overtraining: The point where a person displays a decrease in performance and/or plateauing as a result of consistently performing at a level or training load that exceeds their recovery capacity.

Detraining: Physiological adaptations associated with chronic exercise are not permanent. Once the stimulus is reduced or eliminated, the biological system(s) will revert back to pre-training levels.

VO₂max: Maximum amount of oxygen that an individual can utilize during intense or maximal exercise. It is measured as milliliters of oxygen used in one minute per kilogram of body weight (ml/kg/min).

Stroke volume: Amount of blood ejected from the left ventricle in one contraction.

TABLE 1.1 Markers of Overtraining

General Markers	Endurance Training Markers	Strength Training Markers
Inability to Sleep	Decreased Desire to Train	Decreased Desire to Train
Loss of Appetite	Decreased Performance	Decreased Performance
Inability to Lose/Gain Weight	Increased Sympathetic Stress Response	Increased Sympathetic Stress Response
Depression/Irritability	Increased Creatine Kinase	Increased Creatine Kinase
Elevated Resting HR	Increased Muscle Soreness	Increased Muscle Soreness
Continuously Feeling Tired	Decreased Testosterone	–
Poor Mental Focus	Increased Cortisol Release	–
Inability to Finish Workouts	Decreased VO$_2$max	–
Drop in Performance	Decreased Muscle Glycogen	–
Increased Susceptibility to Illness/Infection	Altered Resting Heart Rate and Blood Pressure	–

Data from Al-Masri L., & Bartlett, S. (2011). *100 Questions & answers about sports nutrition and exercise.* Burlington, MA: Jones & Bartlett; Beachle, T. R., & Earle, R. W. (Eds.). (2008). *Essentials of strength training and conditioning.* (3rd ed.). Champaign, IL: Human Kinetics; Haff, G., & Triplett, N. (Eds.). (2016). *Essentials of strength training and conditioning.* (4th ed.). Champaign, IL: Human Kinetics.

Depicted here are some of the anticipated detraining timeframes for several key components of fitness.

- *Aerobic Capacity*: 30 ± 5 days
- *Max Strength*: 30 ± 5 days
- *Anaerobic Capacity*: 18 ± 5 days
- *Muscle Endurance*: 15 ± 5 days
- *Flexibility*: 7 ± 2 days
- *Max Speed*: 5 ± 3 days

Similar to the effects of detraining, the aging process results in decrements in both endurance and strength training performance. The process of age-related loss of skeletal muscle mass and strength is called sarcopenia. Research suggests that decreases in training volume and intensity are likely contributors to these losses, and that remaining active can reduce these effects by as much as 50%. Following are some of the anticipated decrements in performance associated with age.

- *After age 30*: 10–15% decrease in muscle size and strength per decade
- *After age 40*: 0.5% decrease in VO$_2$max per year
- *After age 60*: 2.4% decrease in VO$_2$max per year

The principle of individuality suggests that training adaptations may differ greatly from person to person, and that genetics play a major role in how fast and to what degree an individual will respond to a specific training stimulus. As a result, training programs should be tailored to the individual to account for these differences (e.g., ability, skill, gender, experience, motivation, injury, and training status). Additionally, just because an individual responds well to one type of training stimulus (e.g., strength training), it does not mean that he or she will respond well to all types of training.

Cardiac Output: The amount of blood the heart pumps through the circulatory system in a minute. Stroke volume and the heart rate determine cardiac output.

Sarcopenia: Age-related loss of skeletal muscle mass and strength.

Individuality: Genetics plays a major role in how fast and to what degree one will respond to a particular training program.

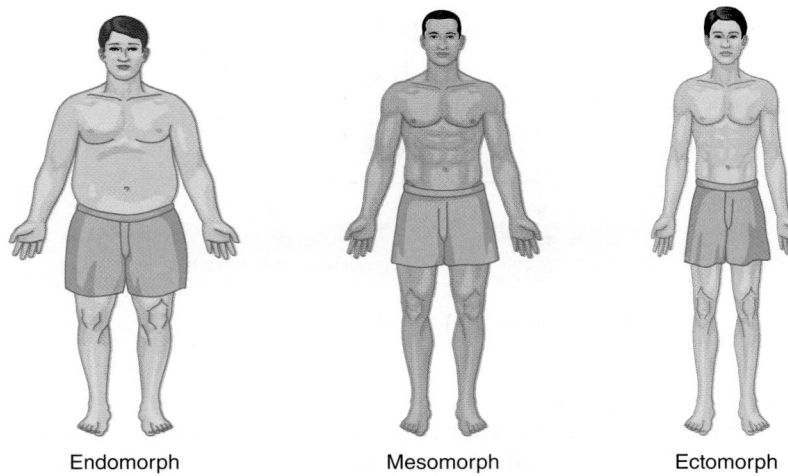

Endomorph   Mesomorph   Ectomorph

FIGURE 1.3 Three Basic Body Types

FIGURE 1.3 illustrates the three basic body types (i.e., endomorph, mesomorph, and ectomorph). Body type tends to influence certain aspects of fitness and sport participation. For example, a mesomorph will likely respond better to strength training in terms of size, strength, and power development than an ectomorph. This is largely due to various genetic differences, such as tendon insertion points and overall fiber type composition (i.e., predominantely more type II [fast twitch] fibers compared with type I [slow twitch]). Conversely, most elite-level long distance runners or duration endurance athletes tend to be ectomorphs.

Biological Energy Systems

The conversion of macronutrients (i.e., carbohydrates, proteins, fats) into useable forms of energy is called **bioenergetics**. **Metabolism** is the combined total of all **exergonic reactions** (releases energy) and **endergonic reactions** (requires energy) within the body. The source of energy for all physiological reactions, especially muscle contraction, that occur within the body is **adenosine triphosphate (ATP)**. The three basic energy systems used to replenish ATP are phosphagen, glycolysis, and oxidative. Exercise duration and intensity determine which system is used to replenish ATP.

The **phosphagen system** provides ATP primarily for short-term, high-intensity activities. However, it is involved at the beginning of all activity regardless of exercise intensity. The phosphagen system provides energy via the breakdown of ATP and **creatine phosphate (CP)**. One of the phosphate groups from CP combines with **adenosine diphosphate (ADP)** to replenish ATP stores. This process continues until exercise stops or the intensity is low enough to allow glycolysis or the oxidative system to take over. During rest, this process is reversed, allowing CP to return to pre-exercise levels.

$$CP + ADP \rightleftharpoons C + ATP$$

It is important to note that CP is stored in the muscle in relatively small amounts, which explains why the phosphagen system can only provide energy for a short period of time (≤ 6 seconds). Type II (fast-twitch) fibers contain more CP than type I (slow-twitch) fibers. This means that individuals with a higher percentage of type II fibers are likely able to replenish ATP at a faster rate. The ability to store more CP is likely part of the reason why some individuals are able to sprint faster and longer than others.

Bioenergetics: Study of the transformation of energy in living organisms.

Metabolism: Metabolism is the total processes (both anabolic and catabolic) used by the body to get or make energy from food.

Exergonic reaction: A reaction that loses energy as a result of the reaction.

Endergonic reaction: A reaction that requires energy to be driven.

Adenosine triphosphate (ATP): Principal molecule for storing and transferring energy in cells.

Phosphagen system: Fastest method to resynthesize ATP used for all-out exercise lasting up to about 10 seconds. However, since there is a limited amount of stored CP and ATP in the muscle, fatigue occurs rapidly.

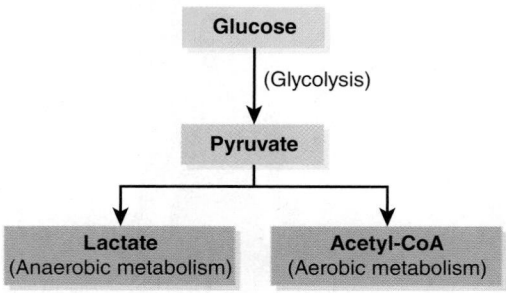

FIGURE 1.4 Two Fates of Pyruvate

Creatine phosphate (CP): A phosphate group found in muscle cells that stores phosphates to provide energy for muscular contraction.

Adenosine diphosphate (ADP): A nucleotide composed of adenosine and two phosphate groups that is formed as an intermediate between ATP and AMP and that is reversibly converted to ATP by the addition of a high-energy phosphate group.

Glycolysis: Process in cell metabolism by which carbohydrates and sugars, especially glucose, are broken down to produce ATP and pyruvic acid.

Sarcoplasm: The colorless material comprising the living cell, excluding the nucleus.

Anaerobic metabolism: Means of producing energy through the combustion of carbohydrates in the absence of oxygen.

Fast glycolysis: Method of providing energy for activities of short duration (i.e., 10-30 seconds), that replenishes very quickly and produces 2 ATP molecules per glucose molecule.

Aerobic metabolism: Means of producing energy through the combustion of carbohydrates, amino acids, and fats in the presence of oxygen.

Glycolysis is the breakdown of carbohydrates, either glycogen or glucose, to resynthesize ATP. The process of glycolysis involves multiple catabolic reactions and is not as rapid as the phosphagen system at producing ATP. However, because there is a greater supply of glycogen and glucose compared with CP, the duration capacity is significantly longer than that of the phosphagen system. Both the phosphagen system and glycolysis occur in the **sarcoplasm** of the muscle cell.

The end result of glycolysis is pyruvate. Depending on exercise intensity and the availability of oxygen, pyruvate will either be converted to lactate or shuttled into the mitochondria of the muscle cell, where it will enter the Krebs cycle (**FIGURE 1.4**). When pyruvate is converted to lactate, a process called **anaerobic metabolism** or **fast glycolysis**, ATP resynthesis occurs at a faster rate but for a shorter duration (6 seconds to 2 minutes). When pyruvate enters the Krebs cycle, a process called **aerobic metabolism** or **slow glycolysis**, ATP resynthesis occurs at a slightly slower rate but for a longer duration (2–3 minutes or longer). It is important to note that both the phosphagen and glycolysis systems fall under the anaerobic metabolism umbrella. Within this umbrella (i.e., the glycolysis system), there are two distinct pathways: fast glycolysis and slow glycolysis. Fast glycolysis is at the left end of the anaerobic metabolism spectrum and functions similar to that of the phosphagen system. Slow glycolysis is at the right end of the anaerobic metabolism spectrum and functions similar to that of the oxidative system. Ultimately, the fate of pyruvate is determined by the energy needs of the muscle cell. If energy must be provided quickly, as with sprinting or strength training, pyruvate is converted into lactate. If the energy demand is not as great and oxygen is available in sufficient quantities, such as when walking or slow jogging, pyruvate is shuttled from the sarcoplasm to the mitochondria, where it is converted to acetyl-CoA before entering the Krebs cycle.

The oxidative system is the primary source of ATP production at rest and during low-intensity activities. Although the oxidative system can metabolize protein, carbohydrates and fats are the preferred substrates. Protein is generally not metabolized in significant amounts unless performing long bouts of exercise (> 90 minutes) or during long periods of starvation (Beachle & Earle, 2008; Haff & Triplett, 2016). At rest, roughly 70% of the ATP produced comes from fats and 30% comes from carbohydrates. However, as exercise intensity increases, there is a shift in substrate preference from fats to carbohydrates. In fact, during high-intensity activity, almost 100% of the ATP produced comes from carbohydrates. During prolonged steady-state activity, both carbohydrates and fats are employed to produce ATP. The actual percentage of contribution from each is based on exercise intensity, duration, and substrate availability.

Also produced during the Krebs cycle are **nicotinamide adenine dinucleotide (NADH)** and **flavin adenine dinucleotide (FADH)** molecules. These molecules transport hydrogen atoms produced during the Krebs cycle to the **electron transport chain (ETC)**, where they are passed down the chain to produce additional energy for ATP production. The oxidative

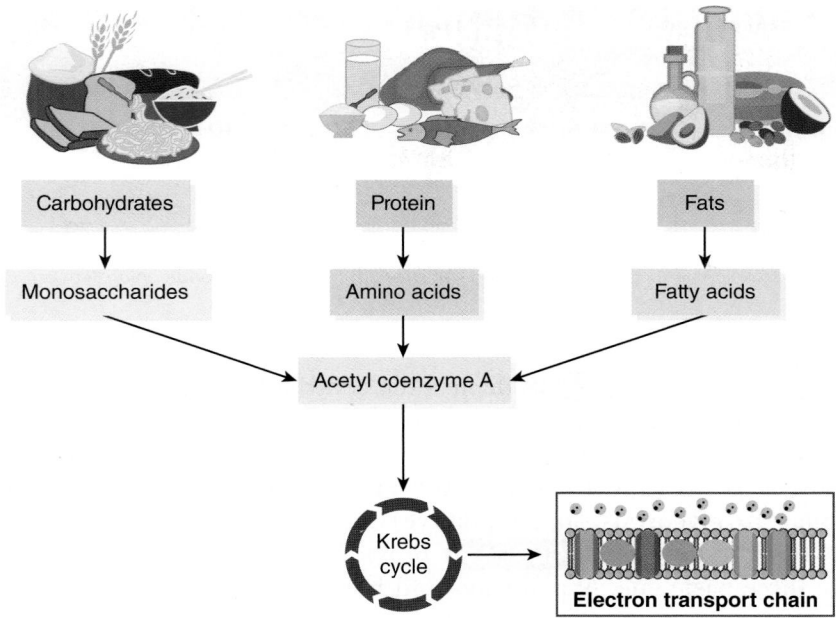

FIGURE 1.5 Substrate Metabolism

system, beginning with glycolysis, yields approximately a total of 38 ATP molecules from one molecule of blood glucose (Beachle & Earle, 2008; Haff & Triplett, 2016). Concersely, the phosphagen system produces only one ATP molecule per CP + ADP reaction, and glycolysis produces only two ATP molecules per molecule of glucose.

As previously discussed, carbohydrates, fats, and proteins can all be used by the oxidative system to produce energy. However, each substrate must first be broken down and converted into Acetyl CoA. For example, the process of breaking down free fatty acids into Acetyl CoA and hydrogen protons is called **beta oxidation**. FIGURE 1.5 provides an abbreviated depiction of substrate metabolism.

Knowing how energy is produced and replenished within the body is important because it helps to provide the how and why to effectively train for specific types of exercise. TABLE 1.2 depicts the differences between the three biological energy systems in terms of exercise duration, intensity, and recommended work-to-rest ratios (Beachle & Earle, 2008;

Slow glycolysis: Method of providing energy for activities of relatively short duration (i.e., 2–3 minutes), that replenishes quickly and produces 2 ATP molecules per glucose molecule.

Nicotinamide adenine dinucleotide (NADH): One of two redox cofactors created during the Krebs cycle that is used during the electron transport chain to produce energy (ATP).

Flavin adenine dinucleotide (FADH): One of two redox cofactors created during the Krebs cycle that is used during the electron transport chain to produce energy (ATP).

Electron transport chain (ETC): A series of complexes that transfer electrons from electron donors to electron acceptors and couples with the transfer of protons across a membrane.

Beta oxidation: Catabolic process by which fatty acid molecules are broken down in the mitochondria to form acetyl-CoA and enter the Krebs cycle.

TABLE 1.2 Exercise Duration and Intensity Specifics for the Various Biological Energy Systems

Energy System	Substrate Source	Exercise Duration	Exercise Intensity	Work-to-Rest Ratio
Phosphagen	Creatine Kinase (CK)	≤ 6 sec	Extremely High	1:20
Phosphagen/Fast Glycolysis	CK/Carbohydrates	6–30 sec	Very High	1:12
Glycolysis	Carbohydrates	30 sec to 2 min	High	1:3 to 1:5
Slow Glycolysis/ Oxidative	Carbohydrates/Fat	2–3 min	Moderate	1:3 to 1:4
Oxidative	Carbohydrates/Fat	> 3 min	Low	1:1 to 1:3

Data from Beachle, T. R., & Earle, R. W. (Eds.). (2008). *Essentials of strength training and conditioning.* (3rd ed.). Champaign, IL: Human Kinetics; Haff, G., & Triplett, N. (Eds.). (2016). *Essentials of strength training and conditioning.* (4th ed). Champaign, IL: Human Kinetics.

TABLE 1.3 Percentage of Anaerobic and Aerobic Metabolism Contribution

% Contribution	0–5 sec	30 sec	60 sec	90 sec	150 sec	200 sec
Anaerobic Metabolism	96	75	50	35	30	22
Aerobic Metabolism	4	25	50	65	70	78

Data from Haff, G., & Triplett, N. (Eds.). (2016). *Essentials of strength training and conditioning.* (4th ed). Champaign, IL: Human Kinetics.

Haff & Triplett, 2016). **TABLE 1.3** depicts the contribution percentage of anaerobic and aerobic metabolism based on exercise duration (Haff & Triplett, 2016).

It is important to note that although exercise duration and intensity depicts which metabolic pathway will provide the greatest contribution, all three pathways (i.e., phosphagen, glycolysis, and oxidative) are still contributing to overall energy production to some degree. **FIGURE 1.6** provides a graphic depiction of the overlap between the three basic energy pathways and how they relate to exercise intensity and duration.

This is an important concept because it explains the body's ability to initiate and sustain activities of various exercise intensities and durations. For example, if the activity lasts less than 10–15 seconds, the body is able to provide and produce enough ATP via the phosphagen system, regardless of exercise intensity. However, after 10–15 seconds, the body has to transition to glycolysis in order to continue producing ATP and providing it to the working muscles. In most cases, this means that the exercise intensity has to be reduced in order for the activity to continue. This explains why athletes are capable of running faster 200-meter split times (which are fueled primarily by the phosphagen system) than 400-meter split times (which are fueled primarily by glycolysis). After roughly 3 minutes of steady-state exercise, the oxidative system takes over and produces the majority of ATP. Since all three pathways (i.e., phosphagen, glycolysis, and oxidative) are in use continually, and in conjunction with each other, it is recommended to train and develop each individually.

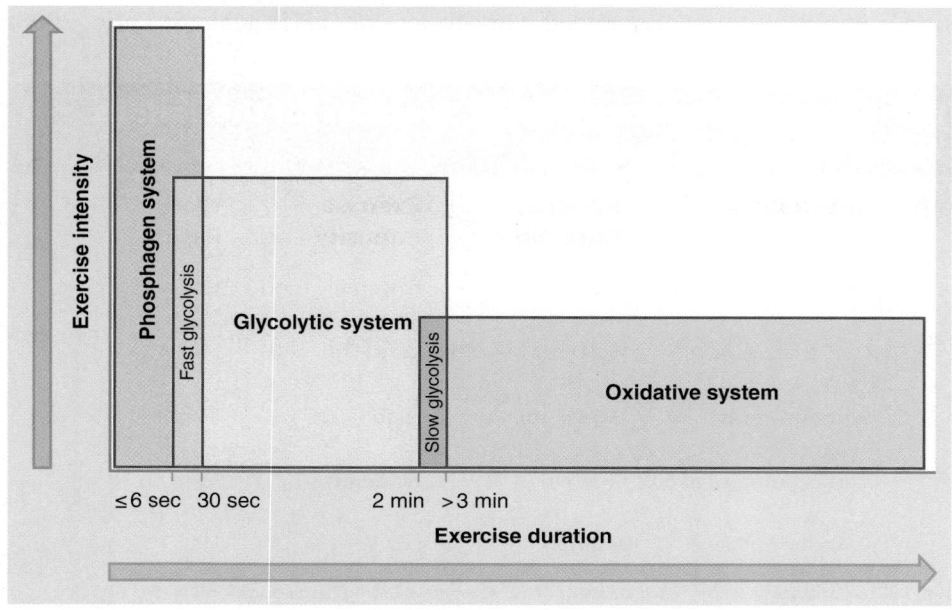

FIGURE 1.6 Contributions of the Various Energy Systems during Exercise

Short-distance sprints (e.g., 40-yard, 100-meter, 200-meter) lasting less than 30 seconds help to develop the phosphagen system; longer distance sprints lasting between 30 seconds to 2–3 minutes (e.g., 200-meter, 400-meter, 800-meter) help to develop the glycolytic system; and steady-state exercises lasting longer than 3 minutes (e.g., 800-meter sprints, mile repeats, long slow distance running) help to develop the oxidative system.

Oxygen Uptake and Endurance Performance

During low-intensity endurance exercise, oxygen consumption increases for the first few minutes until a steady-state is reached. At the start, the body is unable to provide enough energy via the phosphagen and glycolytic energy systems to sustain activity. The difference between the amount of oxygen required for activity and what is available is termed **oxygen deficit**. After exercise, the demand for oxygen remains high and consumption rates remain above pre-exercise levels for a period of time. The extra oxygen needed to "repay" the body's demands is termed **oxygen debt** (aka **excess post-exercise oxygen consumption [EPOC]**), as shown in **FIGURE 1.7**. This figure shows that during low-intensity, steady-state exercise, the body is able to provide enough oxygen to sustain physical activity. In contrast, **FIGURE 1.8** shows that during high-intensity, steady-state exercise, the body is unable to provide enough oxygen, resulting in a reduction of exercise intensity, duration, or both.

The following example illustrates the importance of employing effective pacing strategies and the impact of oxygen uptake on endurance performance. For example, Athlete 1 and Athlete 2 were both training for the 1.5-mile run on a standard 400-meter track (6 laps = 1.5 miles). Prior to the event, both athletes were tested in a lab and determined to have the same VO$_2$max score of 48.6 ml/kg/min. Since there is a strong correlation between 1.5-mile run times and VO$_2$max, both athletes should be able to run 1.5 miles in roughly 10 minutes and 30 seconds (10:30). On race day, Athlete 1 feels good and decides to start off faster than a 7-minute mile pace (7-minute mile pace = 10:30 1.5-mile run time). Athlete 2 also feels good but decides to start off and maintain a 7-minute mile pace. **FIGURE 1.9** on the next page shows the lap split times for both Athlete 1 and Athlete 2.

As shown in the figure, although both athletes have the same level of aerobic fitness (VO$_2$max = 48.6 ml/kg/min) and capacity to run 1.5 miles in 10:30, only Athlete 2 was able to do so. This is because Athlete 1 started off too fast and subsequently was unable to maintain that pace for the duration of the test. After roughly 3 minutes of high-intensity, steady-state exercise, Athlete 1 was no longer able to provide enough oxygen via the oxidative

Oxygen deficit: Difference between the oxygen required and what is actually taken in during a bout of high-intensity exercise.

Oxygen debt: Period of time after high-intensity exercise when the demand for oxygen is greater than the supply.

Excess post-exercise oxygen consumption (EPOC): A measurably increased rate of oxygen intake following strenuous activity intended to erase the body's "oxygen deficit."

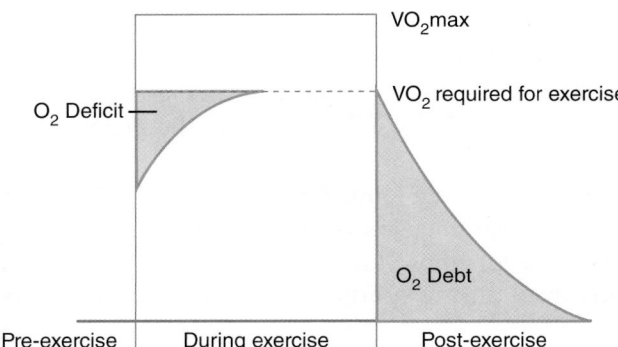

FIGURE 1.7 Low-Intensity, Steady-State Exercise

Data from Haff, G., & Triplett, N. (Eds.). (2016). *Essentials of Strength Training and Conditioning.* (4th ed). Champaign, IL: Human Kinetics.

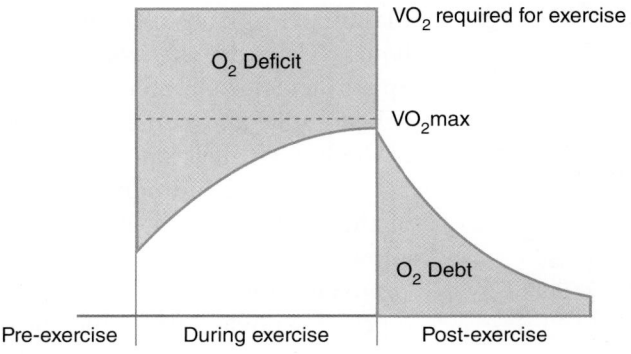

FIGURE 1.8 High-Intensity, Steady-State Exercise

Data from Haff, G., & Triplett, N. (Eds.). (2016). *Essentials of Strength Training and Conditioning.* (4th ed). Champaign, IL: Human Kinetics.

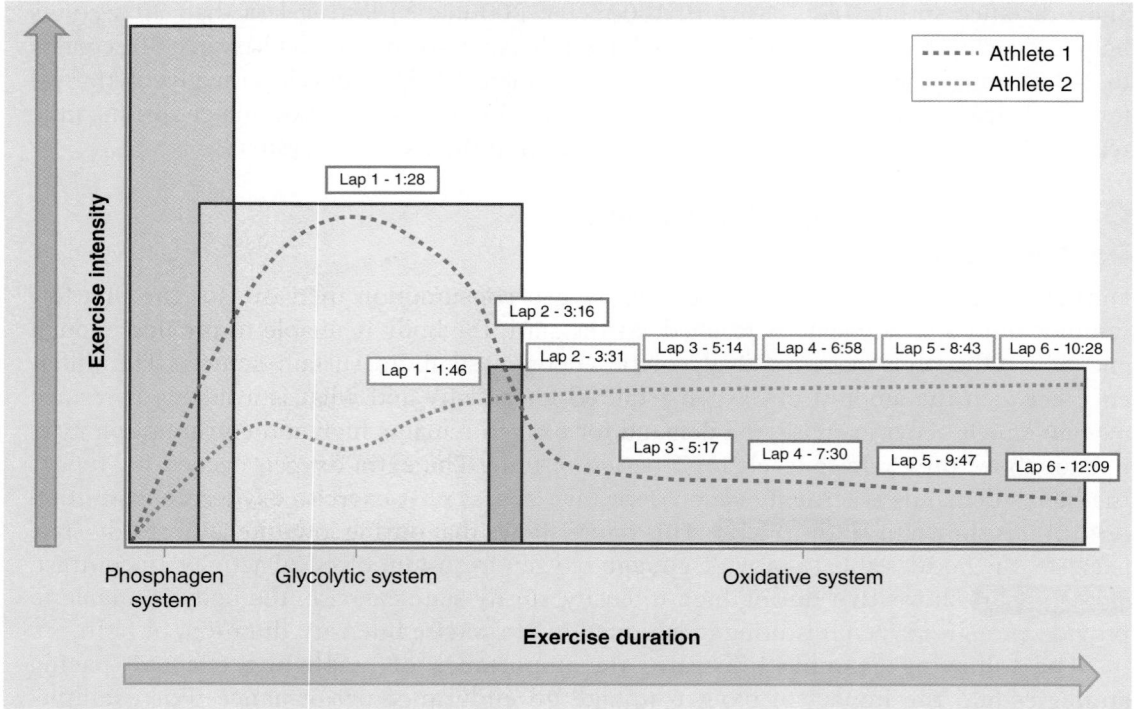

FIGURE 1.9 Effect of Pacing Strategy on Run Performance

Axial skeleton:
Bones that comprise the skull and vertebral column.

Appendicular skeleton: Bones that comprise the limbs as well as shoulder and pelvic girdles.

Joint: Point of articulation between two or more bones.

Fibrous joints: Form of articulation in which bones are connected by a fibrous tissue. Fibrous joints have no joint cavity and movement is minimal or nonexistent.

Cartilaginous joints: Joint covered with cartilage to allow movement between bones.

Synovial joints: Joint that has fibrous capsule surrounding the articulating surfaces of adjoining bones and is filled with synovial fluid.

system to sustain a sub 7-minute mile pace. As a result, Athlete 1 was forced to slow down in order to continue. Additionally, Athlete 1 developed a significant oxygen deficit during the first 800 meters (2 laps), which further impacted the oxidative system's ability to provide enough oxygen. Collectively, this explains why Athlete 1's split times continued to increase (become slower) for laps 3 through 6.

In contrast, Athlete 2, despite also feeling good, consciously decided to start off and stay at a 7-minute mile pace. In doing so, Athlete 2 was able to provide enough oxygen via the oxidative system, did not develop an oxygen deficit and, as a result, was able to maintain a 7-minute mile pace for the duration of the test.

Musculoskeletal System

The purpose of the musculoskeletal system is to provide structural support, allow motion, and protect vital organs. The musculoskeletal system is composed of bones, joints, muscles, tendons (connective tissue that attaches muscle to bone), and ligaments (connective tissue that attaches bone to bone). The human skeleton consists of approximately 206 different bones. The **axial skeleton** consists of the skull, vertebral column, ribs, and sternum. The **appendicular skeleton** consists of the shoulder girdle; bones of the arms, wrists, and hands; pelvic girdle; and bones of the legs, ankles and feet. **FIGURE 1.10** depicts the major bones of the human skeleton.

The connection point between two bones is called a joint. **Fibrous joints** (e.g., sutures of the skull) allow little to no movement; **cartilaginous joints** (e.g., intervertebral disks) allow limited movement; and **synovial joints** (e.g., elbow, knee) allow greater movement. Synovial joints are the joints primarily involved during sports and exercise. There are six types of synovial joints. Specifically:

1. Hinge (e.g., elbow, knee)
2. Ball and socket (e.g., hip, shoulder)
3. Pivot (e.g., neck)

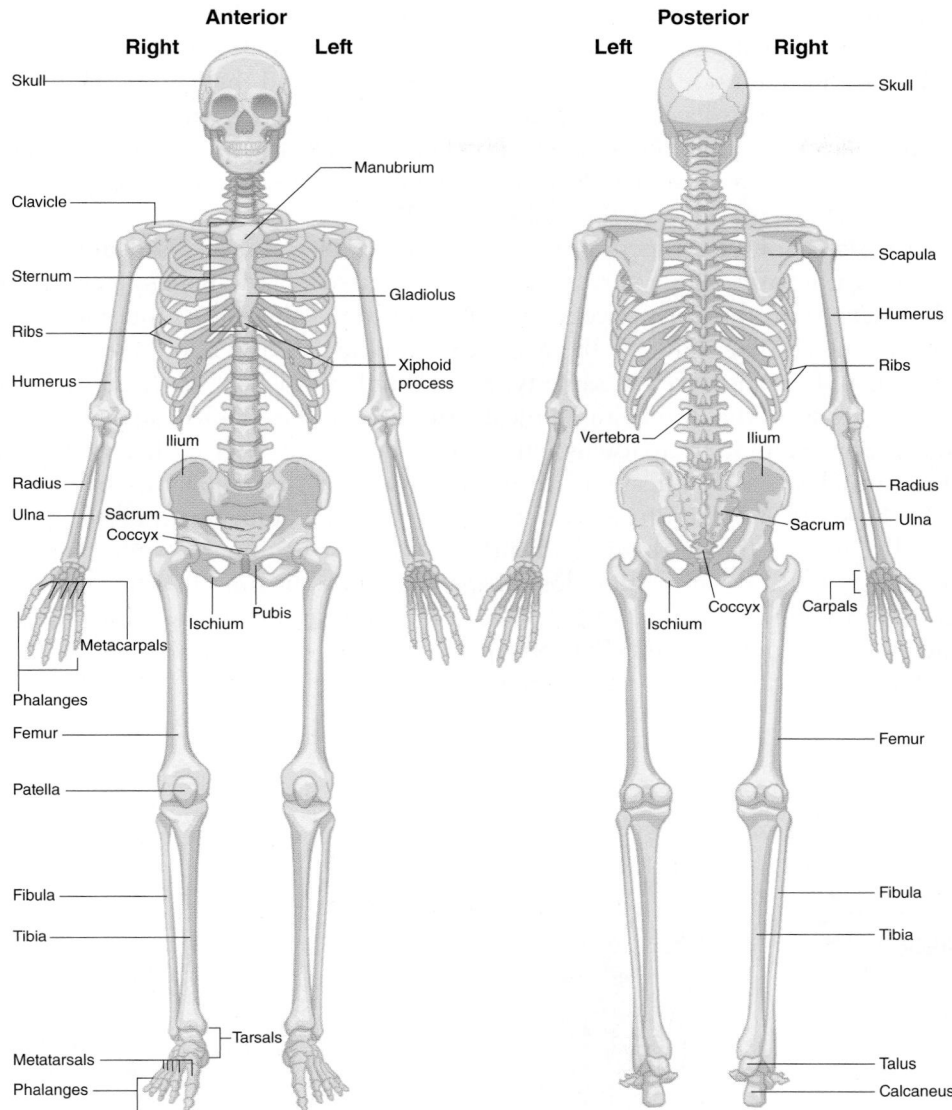

FIGURE 1.10 Major Bones of the Human Skeleton

4. Gliding (e.g., wrist)
5. Saddle (e.g., thumb)
6. Planar (e.g., ankle)

The muscles of the body cannot directly apply force to the ground or external objects. Instead, they pull against the bones, thereby causing them to move about a particular joint or joints, which subsequently results in force being applied to the ground or other external objects. Muscles cannot push; they can only pull. However, through the body's complex system of bony levers, as a muscle contracts, it can exert a pushing force against external objects (Haff & Triplett, 2016).

Levers of the Musculoskeletal System

Movements that occur during exercise and sports are accomplished through a series of bony levers as a result of the muscle's connection and interaction with the bone. There are three types of levers within the body: first-class lever, second-class lever, and third-class lever. Levers are classified by the relative position of the **fulcrum** (pivot point of a lever) to the muscle attachment and load. A **first-class lever** has the fulcrum in the middle with the

Fulcrum: The point on which a level rests or pivots.

First-class lever: A situation when a lever has the fulcrum in the middle with a muscle attachment on one side and the load (resistance) on the other.

Second-class lever:
A situation when a lever has the fulcrum on one side with the muscle attachment on the other side and the load in the middle.

Third-class lever:
A situation when a lever has the fulcrum on one side, the load on the other side and the muscle attachment in the middle.

muscle attachment on one side and the load (resistance) on the other. An example of a first-class lever is tricep push-downs (elbow extension). A **second-class lever** has the fulcrum on one side, with the muscle attachment on the other side, and the load in the middle. An example of a second-class lever is calf extensions (ankle plantarflexion). A **third-class lever** has the fulcrum on one side, the load on the other side, and the muscle attachment in the middle. An example of a third-class lever is bicep curls (elbow flexion). A depiction of the different types of levers is provided in **FIGURE 1.11** .

In most cases, muscles function at a considerable mechanical disadvantage and are exposed to significantly higher forces than those exerted on the hands, feet, ground, or external objects. If not properly accounted for, exposure to these high internal forces may result in acute or chronic injury to the respective muscle and/or tendon.

Although all humans have the same type and number of levers, there are considerable differences in terms of the overall anatomical structure and mechanical advantage between individuals. For example, individuals who have tendons inserted farther away from the joint (fulcrum) have a significant mechanical advantage that allows them to lift more weight. In the sport of powerlifting, which requires the slow movement of heavy weights, this is ideal. However, the mechanical advantage gained by having the tendon farther away from the joint results in a subsequent loss of speed because the muscle is forced to contract more in order to move the joint. In other words, there is an inverse relationship between force and velocity around a joint. For example, in tennis, which requires the quick acceleration of a racquet, this results in a huge mechanical disadvantage.

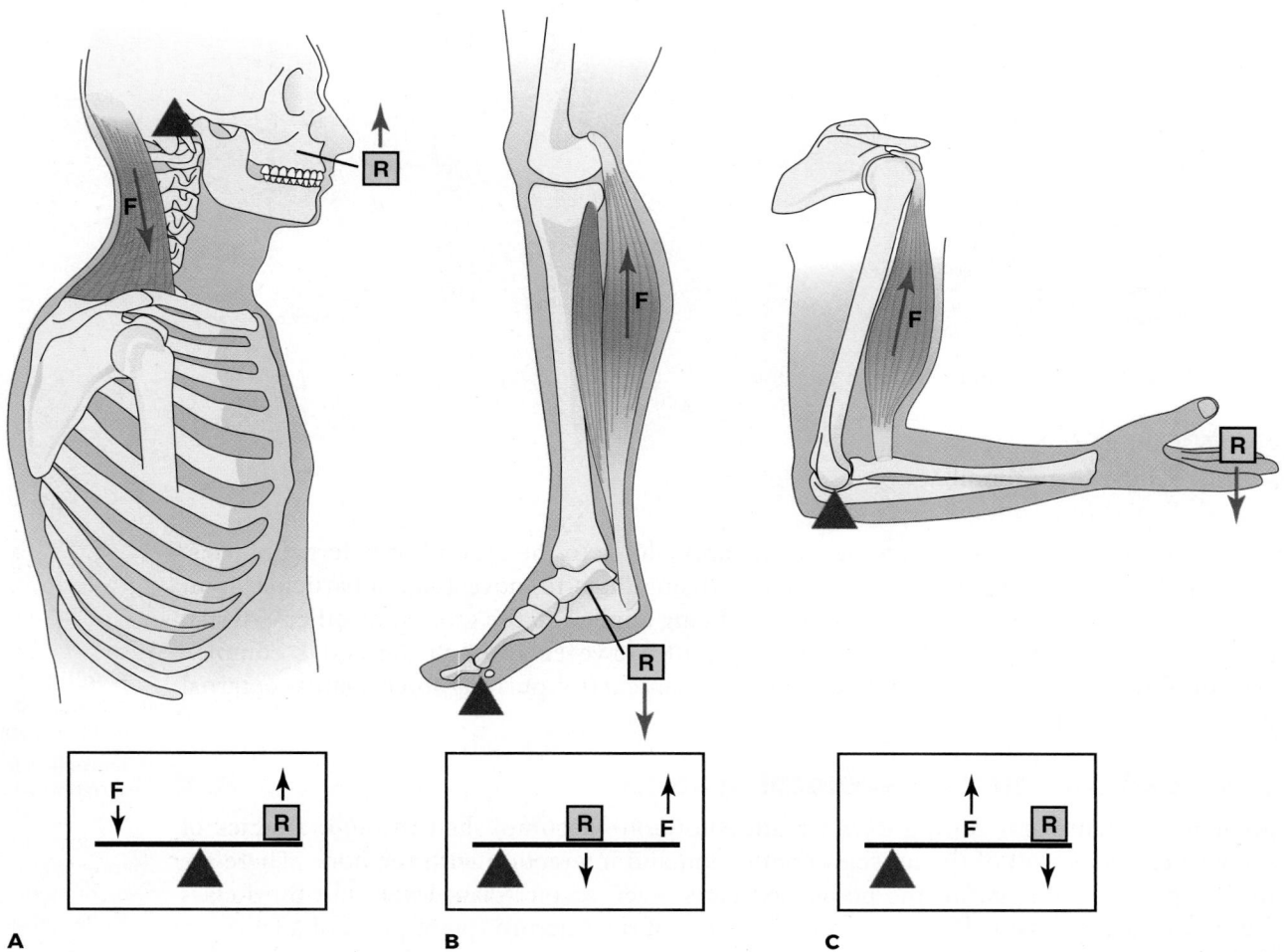

FIGURE 1.11 Different Types of Levers: **A)** First-Class Lever; **B)** Second-Class Lever; **C)** Third-Class Lever; (F = Force; R = Resistance)

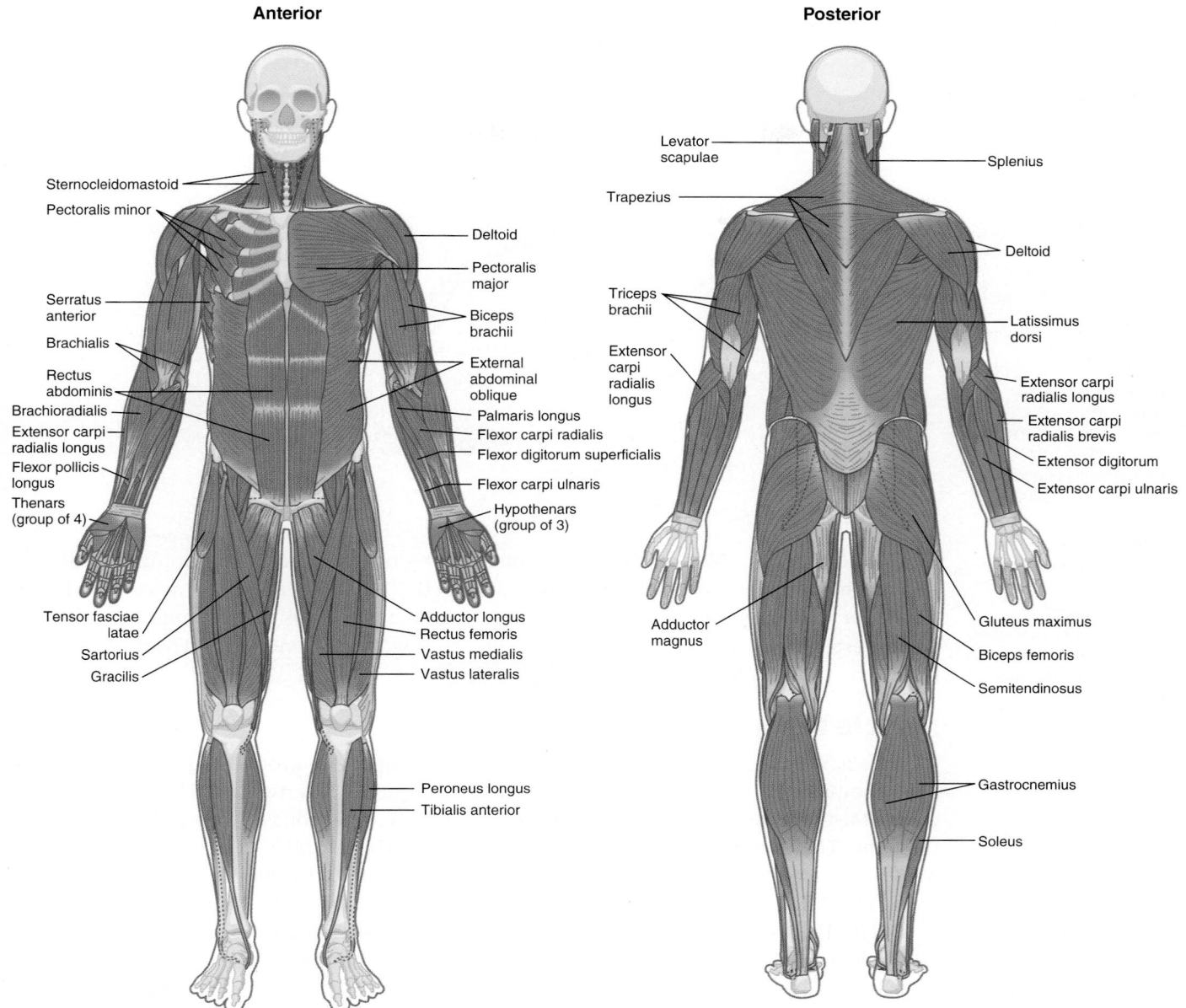

Anterior

Sternocleidomastoid
Pectoralis minor
Serratus anterior
Brachialis
Rectus abdominis
Brachioradialis
Extensor carpi radialis longus
Flexor pollicis longus
Thenars (group of 4)
Tensor fasciae latae
Sartorius
Gracilis

Deltoid
Pectoralis major
Biceps brachii
External abdominal oblique
Palmaris longus
Flexor carpi radialis
Flexor digitorum superficialis
Flexor carpi ulnaris
Hypothenars (group of 3)
Adductor longus
Rectus femoris
Vastus medialis
Vastus lateralis
Peroneus longus
Tibialis anterior

Posterior

Levator scapulae
Trapezius
Triceps brachii
Extensor carpi radialis longus
Adductor magnus

Splenius
Deltoid
Latissimus dorsi
Extensor carpi radialis longus
Extensor carpi radialis brevis
Extensor digitorum
Extensor carpi ulnaris
Gluteus maximus
Biceps femoris
Semitendinosus
Gastrocnemius
Soleus

FIGURE 1.12 Major Muscles of the Human Body

The skeletal muscle is an organ composed of muscle tissue, connective tissue, nerves, and blood vessels. There are more than 430 different skeletal muscles within the human body. **FIGURE 1.12** depicts the major muscles. All skeletal muscles attach to the bone at two attachment points. For limb musculature, the points are referred to as either **proximal attachment** points (closer to the midline of the body) or **distal attachment** points (farther from the midline of the body). For trunk musculature, the points are referred to as either **superior attachment** points (closer to the head) or **inferior attachment** points (closer to the feet).

Muscle fibers, also called muscle cells, are grouped in bundles that can contain as many as 150 individual fibers. Each bundle is surrounded by connective tissue called **perimysium**. All of the connective tissue surrounding the muscle fiber is continuous with the tendon. This allows the tension created in the muscle to be transmitted to the tendon and, in turn, to the bone to which it is attached.

Within each muscle fiber are numerous slender threads of muscle tissue called **myofibrils**, which contain myofilaments (i.e., **myosin** and **actin**) that are responsible for

Proximal attachment: Being situated close to the point of attachment to the body.

Distal attachment: Being situated far from the point of attachment to the body.

Superior attachment: Being situated closer to or towards the head of the body.

Inferior attachment: Being situated closer to or towards the feet.

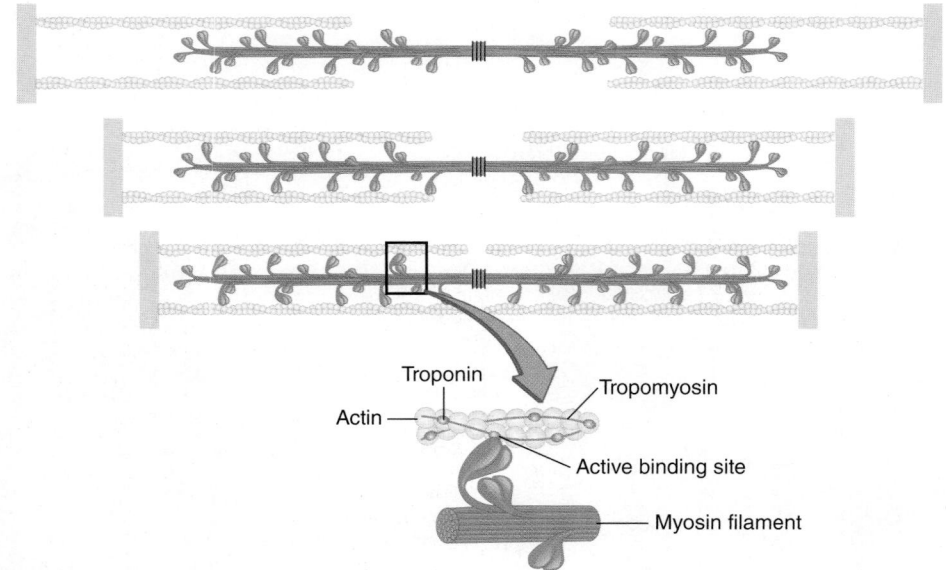

FIGURE 1.13 Sliding-Filament Theory

Perimysium: Thin layer of connective tissue that surrounds each individual muscle fiber.

Myofibril: Long, cylindrical organelle in striated muscle cells, composed mainly of actin and myosin filaments, that run the entire length of the cell.

Myosin: Globulin that combines with actin to form actomyosin (protein complex in muscle fibers that shortens when stimulated and causes muscle contractions).

Actin: A cellular protein found in microfilaments that is active in muscular contraction, cellular movement, and maintenance of cell shape.

Sarcomere: Fundamental unit of muscle structure, comprised of actin and myosin filaments, responsible for muscle contraction.

Sliding-filament theory: Actin (thin) filaments of muscle fibers slide past the myosin (thick) filaments during muscle contraction.

Myosin heavy chain (MHC): Portion of the myosin filament responsible for muscle contraction. There are three types of MHC (i.e., type I, IIa, IIx), each with a different contractile speed. MHC IIx has the fastest contractile speed (and is called fast-twitch), whereas MHC I has the slowest (and is called slow-twitch).

muscle contraction. Myosin filaments consist of a globular head, hinge point, and fibrous tail. Actin filaments consist of two strands arranged in a double helix. The myosin and actin filaments come together to form the smallest contractile unit of skeletal muscle, called the **sarcomere**. The process of the actin filaments sliding inward onto the myosin filaments is called the **sliding-filament theory** (**FIGURE 1.13**).

Muscle Fiber Types

Myosin is a protein complex consisting of four component proteins, two myosin heavy chain complexes, and two myosin light chain complexes intertwined. The **myosin heavy chain (MHC)** portion of the myosin protein complex is responsible for pulling the actin filament. There are three types of MHCs in humans: MHC I, MHC IIa, and MHC IIx. Each MHC type has its own speed of muscle contraction. MHC IIx has the fastest contractile speed and MHC I has the slowest.

MHC IIa and MHC IIx fibers are referred to as **fast-twitch fibers**. MHC I fibers are referred to as **slow-twitch fibers**. Although some fibers may only have one type of MHC, most of the time, they contain a mixture, sometimes referred to as **intermediate fibers (aka fast oxidative-glycolytic fibers)**. Each muscle group (e.g., biceps, chest, quadriceps) contains a certain percentage of each fiber type (sometimes with adjacent fibers being completely different types). The overall percentage of each fiber type will differ from person to person.

Slow-twitch fibers are reddish in appearance, due to their high **myoglobin** (protein that carries and stores oxygen within the muscle) and mitochondria content. As a result, they are very efficient at producing **adenosine triphosphate (ATP)**, via aerobic metabolism, and are extremely fatigue resistant. Fast-twitch fibers are considerably larger than slow-twitch fibers and are whitish in appearance. Although they are able to contract three to four times faster than slow-twitch fibers, they have much lower endurance capability and generate most of their ATP via anaerobic metabolism. As previously discussed, there are two distinct types of fast-twitch fibers: MHC IIa and MHC IIx. MHC IIa fibers have higher blood flow capacity, capillary density, and mitochondrial content than MHC IIx. These fibers are best equipped for activities of moderate-to-high intensity, lasting only a few minutes (e.g., 1-mile run). MHC IIx fibers have very little blood supply, low-capillary density, and low-mitochondrial content. MHC IIx fibers can generate more force than MHC IIa fibers and are better equipped for high-intensity, low-duration activities, such as short distance sprinting. **FIGURE 1.14** depicts the three basic types of muscle fibers.

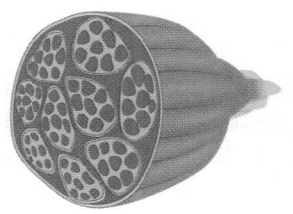
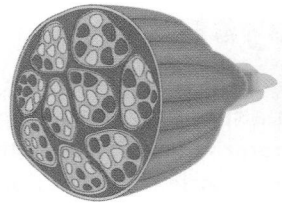
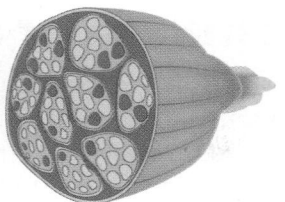

| **Slow-twitch fibers** | **Intermediate fibers** | **Fast-twitch fibers** |
| High mitochondrial content | Medium mitochondrial content | Low mitochondrial content |

FIGURE 1.14 Muscle Fiber Types

Muscle Fiber Arrangement

The degree to which a muscle is able to generate force is largely dependent upon how its fibers are arranged. The **angle of pennation** is the angle formed between the orientation of the muscle fibers and the long axis of its tendon. A **pennate muscle** is one in which the muscle fibers are obliquely aligned with its tendon. This is important because muscles with a greater angle of pennation are able to generate more force than those with a lesser angle of pennation. However, as mentioned previously, there is an inverse relationship between a muscle's ability to generate force and its ability to generate velocity (speed). As a result, muscles with a greater angle of pennation have a lower contraction velocity.

Although most muscles are pennated, few have angles of pennation greater than 15 degrees (Beachle & Earle, 2008; Haff & Triplett, 2016). Additionally, the angle of pennation for a given muscle does not remain constant but increases as the muscle shortens. The angle of pennation may also vary depending on factors such as heredity and training. This may help to explain some of the strength and speed differences between individuals with muscles that are relatively the same size. **FIGURE 1.15** shows the different types of muscle fiber arrangements along with an example of each.

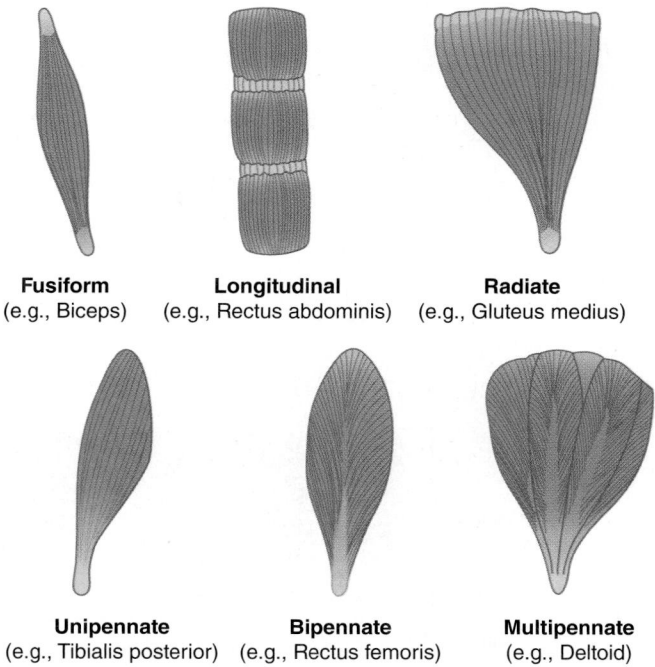

| **Fusiform** | **Longitudinal** | **Radiate** |
| (e.g., Biceps) | (e.g., Rectus abdominis) | (e.g., Gluteus medius) |

| **Unipennate** | **Bipennate** | **Multipennate** |
| (e.g., Tibialis posterior) | (e.g., Rectus femoris) | (e.g., Deltoid) |

FIGURE 1.15 Muscle Fiber Arrangements

Fast-Twitch Fiber: A type of muscle fiber that is composed of strong, rapidly contracting fibers, adapted for high-intensity, low-endurance activities.

Slow-twitch fiber: A type of muscle fiber that develops less tension more slowly than a fast-twitch fiber but is more fatigue resistant due to its high oxygen content and enzyme activity.

Intermediate fibers (aka fast oxidative-glycolytic fibers): Fast twitch muscle fibers that have been converted via endurance training. These fibers are slightly larger in diameter, have more mitochondria, greater blood supply, and more fatigue resistance than typical fast twitch fibers.

Myoglobin: An iron-containing protein found in muscle fibers that combines with oxygen released by red blood cells and transfers it to the mitochondria of muscle cells to produce energy.

Adenosine triphosphate (ATP): Principal molecule for storing and transferring energy in cells.

Angle of pennation: An angle formed between the orientation of the muscle fibers and the long axis of its tendon.

Pennate muscle: Muscle fibers that are obliquely aligned with its tendon.

Neuromuscular System

The purpose of the neuromuscular system is to provide a connection between the brain and the muscles in order to solicit a specific action or response (e.g., muscle contraction). Muscle fibers are innervated by **motor neurons** that transmit electrochemical signals from the brain, via the spinal cord, to the muscle. The junction between a motor neuron and the muscle fiber it innervates is called the **neuromuscular junction**. Although each motor neuron can innervate numerous muscle fibers, each muscle has only one neuromuscular junction. Collectively, a motor neuron and the muscle fibers that it innervates are called a **motor unit**.

The more motor units involved in a muscle contraction, the greater is the force produced. In addition to the number, the size and the firing of the motor units can also influence the magnitude of force production (Haff & Triplett, 2016). Regular participation in sports and exercise can improve neuromuscular control by making the body more efficient at recruiting the number and frequency of the motor units involved. **FIGURE 1.16** provides an abbreviated depiction of a motor unit.

Proprioception

Proprioceptors are specialized sensory receptors located within joints, muscles, and tendons that detect pressure and tension and relay that information to the brain. Most of this information is handled subconsciously and, therefore, does not require conscious thought to process. There are two types of proprioceptors within the muscle: muscle spindles and Golgi tendon organs.

Muscle spindles are located within the belly of the muscle and run parallel to normal muscle fibers. Muscle spindles detect changes and the rate of change in muscle length. When a muscle fiber is stretched, it activates its adjacent muscle spindle, which sends a signal (via a motor neuron) to the central nervous system and brain, which, in turn, causes the muscle to contract.

Golgi tendon organs are located in the tendons near the myotendinous junction (where the muscle and tendon come together). Golgi tendon organs are activated when the tendon

Motor neuron: A nerve cell (neuron) whose cell body is located in the spinal cord and whose fiber (axon) projects outward from the spinal cord to innervate and control muscle cells.

Neuromuscular junction: A chemical synapse (junction) formed by the contact between the presynaptic terminal of a motor neuron and the postsynaptic membrane of a muscle fiber.

Motor unit: Physiological unit composed of a motor neuron and the skeletal muscle fibers innervated by that motor neuron's axonal terminals.

Proprioceptors: Specialized sensory receptors located within joints, muscles, and tendons that detect pressure and tension and relay that information to the brain.

Muscle spindle: A sensory organ located within the muscle that is sensitive to the stretch of the muscle.

Golgi tendon organ: Proprioceptive sensory receptor organ that senses changes in muscle tension.

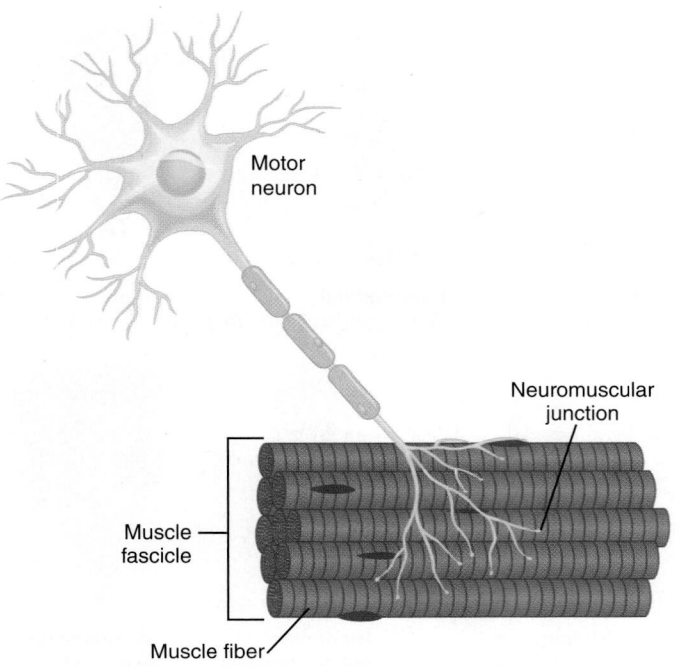

FIGURE 1.16 A Motor Unit

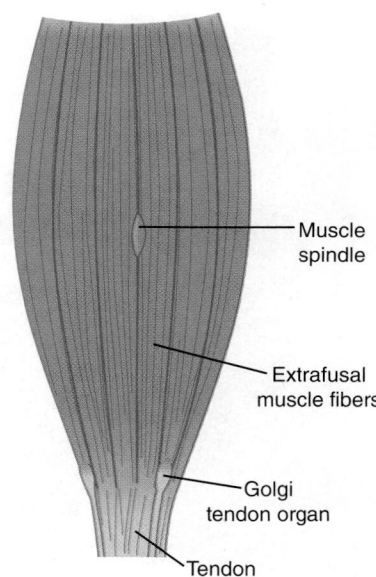

Muscle spindle

Extrafusal muscle fibers

Golgi tendon organ

Tendon

FIGURE 1.17 A Muscle Spindle and Golgi Tendon Organ

attached to an active muscle is stretched. As the tension to the tendon is increased, the Golgi tendon organ sends an inhibitory response (via a motor neuron) to the central nervous system and the brain, which, in turn, causes the muscle to relax. This results in a reduction of tension within both the tendon and muscle. Input from the Golgi tendon organs are minimal when exposed to low levels of tension; however, it increases dramatically when exposed to heavy loads.

Muscle spindles and Golgi tendon organs are natural safeguards built into the musculoskeletal system to protect the body from injury. Whereas the muscle spindles cause the muscle to contract to prevent injury, the Golgi tendon organs cause the muscle to relax. The ability of the brain to override the inhibitory response from the Golgi tendon organs is believed to be one of the primary physiological adaptations of regular (heavy) strength training. **FIGURE 1.17** depicts the appearance and location of muscle spindles and Golgi tendon organs.

Cardiovascular System

The purpose of the cardiovascular system is to transport oxygen and various nutrients to the working tissues of the body. Additionally, it transports waste products (e.g., carbon dioxide) to the lungs via the bloodstream, where they are removed from the body via exhalation. The cardiovascular system is composed of the heart, blood vessels (i.e., arteries, arterioles, veins, venules, capillaries), and blood.

The heart is a four-chambered organ composed of two interconnected but distinct pumps. The right pump pushes blood to the lungs, while the left pump pushes blood to the periphery of the body. Blood enters the heart via the right or left **atrium**, which then delivers blood to the corresponding **ventricle**. Contractions of the right and left ventricles then push the blood to the pulmonary and peripheral circulations, respectively. **FIGURE 1.18** on the next page depicts the structure of the human heart as well as the direction of blood flow.

The primary function of blood is to transport oxygen from the lungs to the tissues and transport carbon dioxide from the tissues to the lungs. The major component of blood is red blood cells. In addition to **hemoglobin** (red protein in the blood responsible for transporting

Atrium: Either of the two upper chambers of the heart that receive blood from the veins and in turn push it into the ventricles.

Ventricle: Either of the two lower chambers of the heart that receive blood from the atria and in turn push it into the arteries.

Hemoglobin: The oxygen-carrying pigment and predominant protein found in red blood cells.

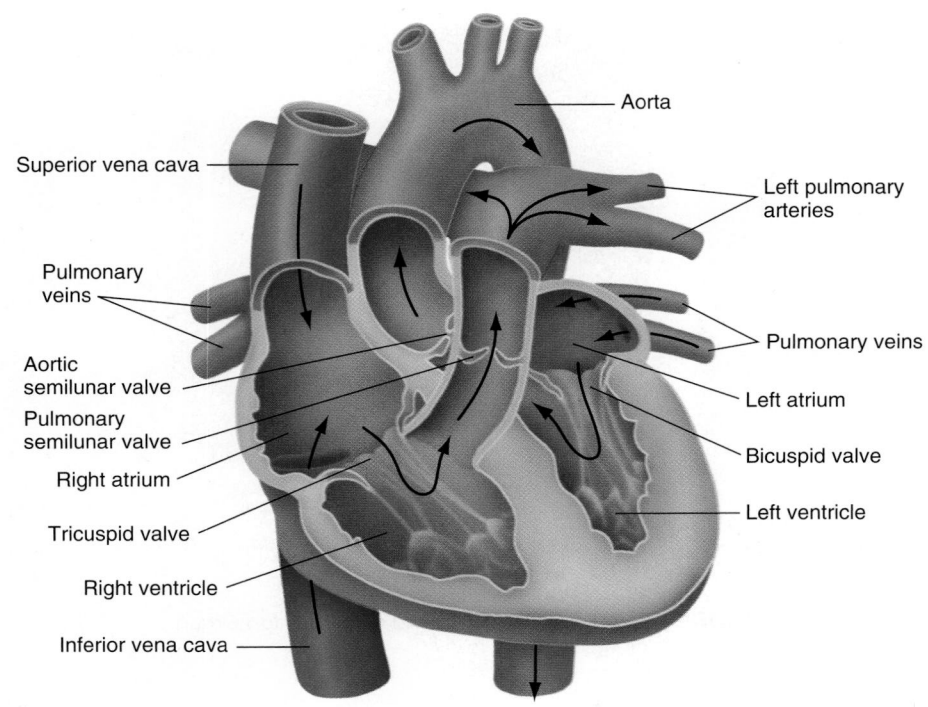

FIGURE 1.18 The Human Heart

Carbonic anhydrase: An enzyme that catalyzes the decomposition of carbonic acid into carbon dioxide and water, facilitating transfer of carbon dioxide from tissues to blood and from blood to alveolar air.

Arterial system: A system of arteries and arterioles that carry oxygenated blood away from the heart.

Artery: A large diameter blood vessel that carries blood from the heart to another part of the body.

Arteriole: A small diameter blood vessel in the microcirculation that extends and branches out from an artery and leads to capillaries.

Venous system: A system composed of veins and venules that returns deoxygenated blood back to the heart.

Vein: A large diameter blood vessel that carries blood low in oxygen content from the body back to the heart.

Venule: A small diameter blood vessel that connects the capillaries to the veins.

Capillary: Any of the minute blood vessels that form networks throughout the tissues and are used to carry oxygen, nutrients, and waste products between the blood and tissues.

oxygen), red blood cells also carry large quantities of **carbonic anhydrase** (enzyme responsible for combining carbon dioxide and water), which helps facilitate the removal of carbon dioxide.

The **arterial system**, which is composed of **arteries** and **arterioles** (small branches of blood vessels that route blood from the arteries to the capillaries), carry oxygenated blood away from the heart. The **venous system**, which is composed of **veins** and **venules** (small branches of blood vessels that collect blood from the capillaries to the veins), returns deoxygenated blood back to the heart. The capillaries connect the arterial and venous systems. The function of **capillaries** is to facilitate the exchange of oxygen, nutrients, hormones, and other substances between the blood and the interstitial fluid (fluid that bathes and surrounds tissue cells) in various tissues of the body. **FIGURE 1.19** provides an abbreviated depiction of the direction of blood flow through the arterial and venous systems.

Respiratory System

The primary function of the respiratory system is the exchange of oxygen and carbon dioxide. Air is taken in and travels from the nasal cavity (and possibly oral cavity) to the lungs through the **trachea**, **bronchi**, **bronchioles**, and **alveoli**. **FIGURE 1.20** shows the basic anatomy of the human respiratory system. During respiration, oxygen diffuses from the alveoli into the blood and carbon dioxide diffuses from the blood into the alveoli. This process of oxygen and carbon dioxide moving in opposite directions through the alveolar capillary membrane is called **diffusion**.

The amount of air moving in and out of the lungs is controlled by the expansion and recoil of the lungs. However, the lungs do not actively expand or recoil themselves but are forced to do so by movement of the diaphragm and ribcage. The muscles that elevate

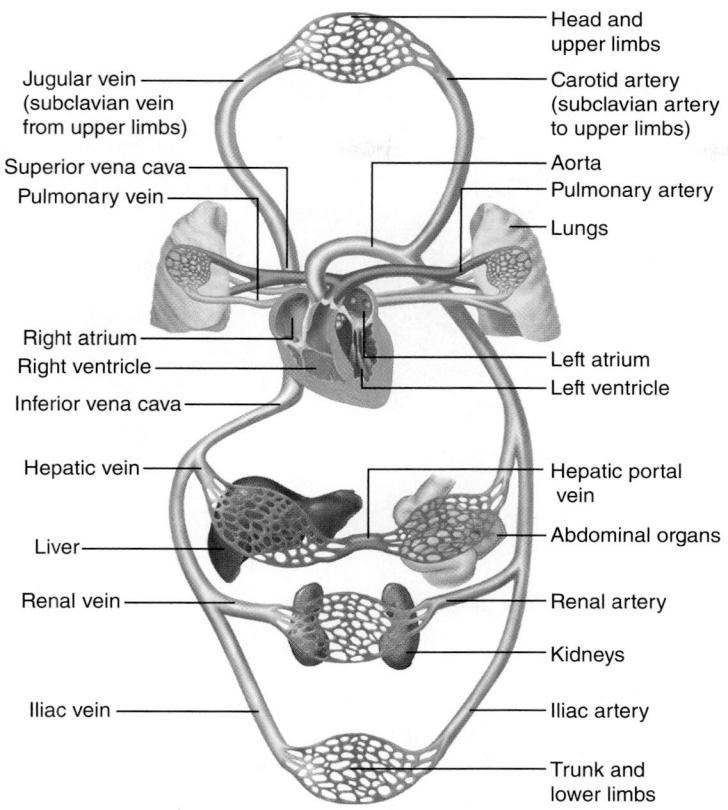

FIGURE 1.19 The Circulatory System

Trachea: A large membranous tube reinforced by rings of cartilage that extends from the larynx to the bronchial tubes and conveys air to and from the lungs.

Bronchi: Either of the two main branches of the trachea leading into the lungs where they divide into smaller branches (bronchioles).

Bronchioles: Tiny branch of air tubes within the lungs that connect the bronchi to the alveoli (air sacs).

Alveoli: The tiny air sacs within the lungs that allow for rapid gaseous exchange.

Diffusion: The passive movement of molecules (e.g., oxygen, carbon dioxide) along a concentration gradient traveling from regions of higher to regions of lower concentration.

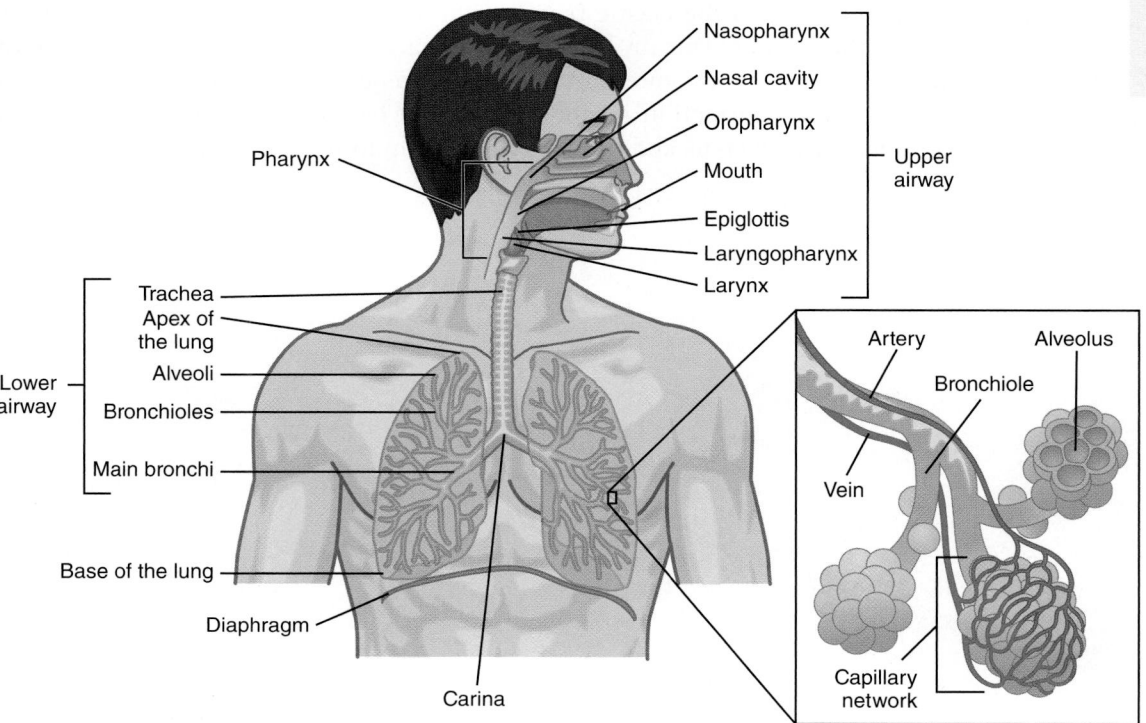

FIGURE 1.20 The Human Respiratory System

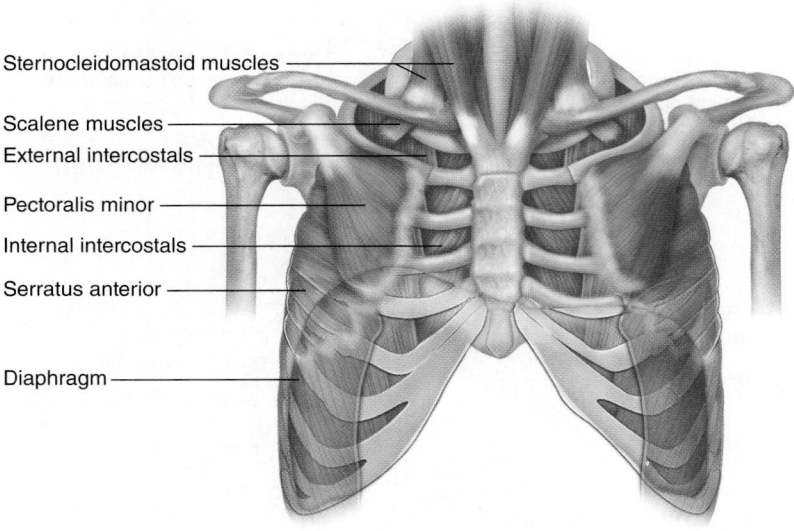

Sternocleidomastoid muscles

Scalene muscles

External intercostals

Pectoralis minor

Internal intercostals

Serratus anterior

Diaphragm

FIGURE 1.21 Muscles of Respiration

Muscles of inspiration: Muscles that elevate the ribcage during inhalation.

Muscles of expiration: Muscles that depress the ribcage during exhalation.

the ribcage during inhalation are called **muscles of inspiration** and include the external intercostals, sternocleidomastoids, anterior serrati, and scaleni. The muscles that depress the ribcage during exhalation are called **muscles of expiration** and include the rectus abdominis, external and internal obliques, transversus abdominis, and internal intercostals. **FIGURE 1.21** shows the different muscles involved in respiration.

During normal (non-exertional) breathing, respiration is accomplished almost entirely by movement of the diaphragm. Inhalation occurs as the diaphragm contracts (creating a negative pressure in the chest cavity) and air is drawn into the lungs. Exhalation occurs as the diaphragm relaxes and the elastic recoil of the lungs and chest cavity compresses the lungs, forcing the air out. During heavy (exertional) breathing, the elastic forces of the lungs and chest cavity are not enough to produce the necessary respiration. The extra force is achieved by the contraction of abdominal muscles (rectus abdominis, external and internal obliques, transversus abdominis), which help to push the diaphragm upward (Haff & Triplett, 2016).

Assessment and Application

Summary

- People exercise for a variety of reasons; however, improving one's appearance is by far the most common.
- In order to effectively prepare for a sport and/or develop a sound exercise plan, individuals should have a basic understanding of exercise physiology terms and concepts.
- Some of the more important concepts include specificity of training, overload principle, exercise progression and variation, stimulus-recovery-adaptation (SRA), overtraining, and detraining.
- There are three biological energy systems that the body uses to fuel activity: phosphagen, glycolytic, and oxidative systems. The two factors that determine which of the three systems is used to fuel activity are exercise intensity and duration.
- The primary purpose of the musculoskeletal system is to provide the body with structural support, allow movement, and protect the internal organs.
- There are three different types of muscle fibers: slow-twitch, intermediate, and fast-twitch fibers. Each type of fiber differs in size, endurance, strength, and fatigue-resistance capacities.
- The primary purpose of the cardiovascular system is to provide oxygen and other nutrients to the various tissues of the body and remove the waste products produced during metabolism.
- The primary purpose of the respiratory system is to allow an exchange of oxygen and carbon dioxide.

Knowledge Check

1. List and discuss some of the different reasons why people exercise.
2. Define specificity and discuss why it is important in terms of exercise prescription and programming.
3. Differentiate between exercise and training.
4. Define overload and discuss why it is important in terms of exercise prescription and programming.
5. Define stimulus-recovery-adaptation and discuss why it is important in terms of exercise prescription and programming.
6. What are some of the signs (aka markers) associated with overtraining? Discuss similarities and differences between endurance and strength training markers.
7. Define sarcopenia and discuss the impact it has on athletic performance.
8. List the anticipated detraining timeframes for aerobic capacity, anaerobic capacity, speed, muscular strength, muscular endurance, and flexibility.
9. Define individuality and discuss why it is important in terms of exercise prescription and programming.
10. List and discuss the three different biological energy systems that the body uses to fuel physical activity.

11. Discuss how a pacing strategy can influence long-distance run times.
12. Discuss the primary purpose of the musculoskeletal system.
13. List and discuss the different types of joints within the body.
14. List and discuss the three types of levers within the musculoskeletal system.
15. Define the sliding-filament theory and discuss the mechanisms responsible for a muscle contraction.
16. List and discuss the different types of muscle fibers.
17. List and discuss the seven different types of muscle fiber arrangements.
18. Discuss the primary purpose of the neuromuscular system.
19. Define a motor neuron and discuss its role in a muscle contraction.
20. Define and differentiate a muscle spindle and Golgi tendon organ.
21. Discuss the primary purpose of the cardiovascular system.
22. Describe the pathway of blood flow through the heart.
23. Discuss the primary purpose of the respiratory system.
24. Discuss the differences between normal (non-exertional) breathing and heavy (exertional) breathing.

Activities

Basic Exercise Physiology

A. Claire and Ethan recently performed metabolic testing at a local university's Human Performance Lab. VO$_2$max scores were measured at 36 ml/kg/min and 38 ml/kg/min, respectively. Two days later, they both participated in a 1.5-mile run for time. Claire's run time was 14:10 and Ethan's run time was 14:22. Explain how Ethan's slower-than-expected run time could have been affected by his pacing strategy.

References

Al-Masri L., & Bartlett, S. (2011). *100 Questions & answers about sports nutrition and exercise*. Burlington, MA: Jones & Bartlett.

American College of Sports Medicine. *ACSM, AHA support federal physical activity guidelines*. Retrieved from http://www.acsm.org/about-acsm/media-room/acsm-in-the-news/2011/08/01/acsm-aha-support-federal-physical-activity-guidelines

Beachle, T. R., & Earle, R. W. (Eds.). (2008). *Essentials of strength training and conditioning* (3rd ed.). Champaign, IL: Human Kinetics.

Centers for Disease Control and Prevention. *The benefits of physical activity*. Retrieved from https://www.cdc.gov/physicalactivity/basics/pa-health/index.htm

Coachr.org. *Training theory*. Retrieved from http://www.coachr.org/training_theory.htm.

Haff, G., & Triplett, N. (Eds.). (2016). *Essentials of strength training and conditioning* (4th ed.). Champaign, IL: Human Kinetics.

McArdle, W., Katch, F., & Katch, V. (2015). *Exercise physiology: Energy nutrition, and human performance* (8th ed.). Philadelphia, PA: Lippincott Williams & Wilkins.

Fitness Testing and Prescription

LEARNING OBJECTIVES

After completing this chapter, students should be able to:

- Discuss the purpose and benefits of regular fitness testing
- List and discuss key factors that should be considered before selecting a fitness test
- List the recommended sequence of events for fitness tests
- List the various modalities used by the military services in their physical fitness tests
- List and discuss the different methods of body composition testing

Introduction

Fitness test: A series of exercises designed to assess fitness (e.g., endurance, strength, agility, etc.).

Field test: A test used to assess ability that is performed away from the laboratory and does not require extensive training or expensive equipment to administer.

A **fitness test** is a series of exercises designed to assess specific components of fitness (e.g., endurance, strength, agility, etc.). A **field test** is a test used to assess a particular component of fitness and is not performed in the laboratory and does not require extensive training or expensive equipment to administer.

A fitness test should be performed before starting any new exercise program and it should be repeated periodically in order to document an individual's initial fitness level and his or her improvements made over time. Regular fitness testing serves the following purposes:

- Identifies physiological strengths and weaknesses
- Ranks individuals for selection purposes
- Predicts future performances
- Evaluates the effectiveness of the training program
- Tracks personnel performance over time
- Assigns training parameters (e.g., recommended % of 1RM)

TABLE 2.1 identifies the minimal required scores for "average fitness" as classified by the American College of Sports Medicine (ACSM) for several different components of fitness (American College of Sports Medicine, 2001). Knowing where you are in terms of your current level of physical fitness can be a powerful motivator to start or continue with an exercise program.

In order for a fitness test to be a viable assessment option it must include the following parameters:

- *Validity*: A test should accurately measure what it is supposed to measure. The 1.5-mile run is a valid test for assessing aerobic fitness. Push-ups, however, are not a valid muscular strength test due to the high number of repetitions required to receive a high score. Instead, push-ups are a valid test for assessing muscular endurance.

TABLE 2.1 Age and Gender Related Scores for Average Fitness

Age (years)	20–29		30–39		40–49		50–59		60+	
Gender	Male	Female	Male	Female	Male	Female	Male	Female	Male	Female
VO$_2$max (ml/kg/min)	45.6	39.5	44.1	37.7	42.4	35.9	39	32.6	35.6	29.7
1.5-mile Run (mm:ss)	11:29	13:24	11:54	14:08	12:24	14:53	13:35	16:35	15:04	18:27
Bench Press Weight Ratio (weight lifted/ body weight)	1.14	0.70	0.98	0.60	0.88	0.54	0.79	0.48	0.72	0.47
Push-Ups*	22	15	17	13	13	11	10	7	8	5
Sit-Ups	42	38	39	29	34	24	28	20	22	11
% Body Fat	14.8	19.8	18.4	21	20.8	23.7	22.3	26.7	23	27.5
Waist Circumference† (inch)	35.5	32	35.5	32	35.5	32	35.5	32	35.5	32
Body Mass Index (weight [kg]/height^2 [m^2])	18.5–24.9	18.5–24.9	18.5–24.9	18.5–24.9	18.5–24.9	18.5–24.9	18.5–24.9	18.5–24.9	18.5–24.9	18.5–24.9

*Females tested in the modified (aka "knee push-up") position
†Measurement taken at the superior border of the iliac crest

Data from American College of Sports Medicine. *ACSM, AHA Support federal physical activity guidelines.* Retrieved from http://www.acsm.org/about-acsm/media-room/acsm-in-the-news/2011/08/01/acsm-aha-support-federal-physical-activity-guidelines.

- *Objectivity*: A test should be free from individual bias. The 1.5-mile run is an objective test since the time used to score the event will likely not change regardless of the test administrator. The number of successfully completed push-ups, however, is likely to differ from one test administrator to another based on their individual enforcement and tolerance of exercise form (e.g., 90° depth criteria at the elbows). Generally speaking, tests that use distance or time as their standard of performance have a higher degree of objectivity than those who employ repetitions.

- *Reliability*: The results of the test should be repeatable. As long as the participant's fitness levels remain constant, the score should remain the same from one test to another. The plank, although arguably safer and more operationally relevant than curl-ups, has poor reliability since the time held to exhaustion can differ greatly from one attempt to the next. This is true for most tests that require an isometric hold for execution (e.g., flexed-arm hang, V-sit, wall squat).

- *Feasibility*: A test should be practical in terms of cost, man power, equipment, and space required. The 1.5-mile run is also considered to be feasible because of its ease of administration and minimal requirement for equipment (i.e., stopwatch). Although performing VO_2max testing may provide slightly more accurate results in terms of aerobic fitness, it is not a feasible option due to its associated cost, required training for test administrators, and equipment (i.e., treadmill, heart rate monitor, metabolic cart).

- *Operationally Relevant*: The physiological requirements of the test should represent sport- or job-specific tasks or skills. Although curl-ups are valid, reliable, and feasible they are not operationally relevant. Rarely do service-members perform repetitive spinal flexion as a specific job task. Instead, they stabilize their core in order to lift, push, pull, or carry. As a result, the plank, although less reliable than curl-ups, is considered more operationally relevant and may be a better testing option over the curl-up.

Additionally, fitness testing should incorporate as many different components of fitness as possible. **TABLE 2.2** provides a comprehensive listing of both health-related and skill-related components of fitness.

In order to prevent excessive fatigue that may affect subsequent performance, field tests should be performed in a specific order. **TABLE 2.3** on the next page indicates the correct order that field tests should be performed as well as examples of each (Baechle & Earle, 2008; Haff & Triplett, 2016).

TABLE 2.2 Components of Physical Fitness

Health Related	Skill Related
Cardiovascular Fitness	Speed
Muscular Endurance	Agility
Muscular Strength	Power
Flexibility	Coordination
Body Composition	Balance
-	Reaction Time

Data from Baechle, T. R., & Earle, R. W. (Eds.). (2008). *Essentials of strength training and conditioning.* (3rd ed.). Champaign, IL: Human Kinetics; Haff, G., & Triplett, N. (Eds.). (2016). *Essentials of strength training and conditioning.* (4th ed). Champaign, IL: Human Kinetics.

TABLE 2.3 Proper Sequence of Field Tests

Field Test Type	Example
Non-Fatiguing	Height/Weight
	Skinfolds
Agility	Pro-Agility
	Illinois Agility
Max Power / Strength	Standing Long Jump
	1RM Bench Press
Sprint	40-yd Dash
Muscular Endurance	Push-Ups
	Curl-Ups
Anaerobic Capacity	300-yd Shuttle
Aerobic Capacity	1.5-Mile Run
	500-yd Swim

Data from Baechle, T. R., & Earle, R. W. (Eds.). (2008). *Essentials of strength training and conditioning.* (3rd ed.). Champaign, IL: Human Kinetics; Haff, G., & Triplett, N. (Eds.). (2016). *Essentials of strength training and conditioning.* (4th ed). Champaign, IL: Human Kinetics.

Criterion performance standards: Use normative data that ranks individuals against an established standard (e.g., pass/fail cut-off score).

Normative performance standards: Use normative data derived from a sample of participants in order to rank individual performance. (e.g., Outstanding = Performance above or equal to the top 10 percentile).

There are two basic means to score field tests: criterion and normative performance standards. **Criterion performance standards** use normative data that ranks individuals against an established standard (e.g., pass/fail cut-off score). **Normative performance standards**, on the other hand, use normative data derived from a sample of participants in order to rank individual performance. (e.g., Outstanding = performance $\geq$ top 10%). Examples of criterion and normative performance standards are provided in the following tables.

Example of Criterion Performance Standards:

U.S. Army Ranger Physical Fitness Test			
Push-Ups	Sit-Ups	Chin-Ups	5-Mile Run
49+	59+	6+	$\leq$ 40 minutes

Example of Normative Performance Standards:

Scoring Categories for U.S. Navy PRT	
Maximum	Performance above or equal or top 2 percentile
Outstanding	Performance above or equal to top 10 percentile, but less than Maximum
Excellent	Performance in top 25 percentile, but less than Outstanding
Good	Performance better than or equal to lowest 25 percentile, but less than Excellent
Satisfactory	Performance in bottom 25 percentile, but above lowest 10 percentile
Failure	Performance in lowest 10 percentile

TABLE 2.4 **Composition of Physical Fitness Tests for the Various Branches of Service**				
	Air Force	**Army**	**Marine Corps**	**Navy**
Aerobic Capacity	1.5-mile Run	2.0-mile Run	3.0-mile Run	1.5-mile Run
Alternate Aerobic	1.0-mile Rockport Walk Test	800-yard Swim 2.5-mile Walk 6.2-mile Bicycle 6.2-mile Cycle Ergometer	5-km Rower	450-meter Swim 500-yard Swim 12-min Stationary Bike
Muscular Endurance (Upper Body)	Push-Ups (1-min)	Push-Ups	Push-Ups Pull-Ups	Push-Ups
Muscular Endurance (Core)	Sit-Ups (1-min)	Sit-Ups	Crunches	Curl-Ups

Fitness Testing in the Military

The Department of Defense Instruction on Physical Fitness and Body Fat Programs Procedures (DoDI 1308.3) mandates that each branch of service (i.e., Air Force, Army, Marine Corps, Navy) develop and implement semi-annual physical fitness tests (PFTs) that evaluate aerobic capacity, muscular strength, and muscular endurance. However, each branch of service is allowed to determine which tests are used to assess each component of fitness (Department of Defense, 2002).

TABLE 2.4 provides a comprehensive overview of the PFT events for each of the different branches of service (Department of Defense, 2002; Navy Physical Readiness Program, 2016b; United States Air Force, 2013; United States Army, 1998; United States Marine Corps, 2016; United States Navy, 2011; United States Navy, 2017).

Over the years, each service branch has made several changes to their respective PFT. For example, with the release of all-Marine bulletin (ALMAR) 022/16 in July 2016, the Marine Corps added push-ups and removed the flexed-arm hang from their PFT. This was the first major change, other than the addition of the Combat Fitness Test (CFT) in 2009, the Marine Corps has made to its physical fitness program since 1972. Similarly, the Navy has made several changes to its Physical Readiness Test (PRT) over the years. However, other than the addition of the 12-minute elliptical test and 12-minute stationary bike tests in 2006 and 2007, respectively, and the subsequent removal of the 12-minute elliptical test in 2018, the PRT has remained relatively unchanged since 1986. TABLE 2.5 on the next page illustrates the different versions of the PRT since its inception in 1980 (Peterson, 2015b; United States Navy, 2017).

Body Composition

Body composition refers to the percentages of fat, muscle, bone, and water within the body. Some of the more common methods (types) of body composition testing are discussed in the next section. TABLE 2.6 on the next page provides body fat percentage ratings for adult males and females (Bryant & Green, 2010).

Body composition: Any method of measure used to describe the percentages of fat, bone, water, and muscle.

TABLE 2.5 Various Versions of the U.S. Navy PRT

	1980	1982	1984	1986	2000	2006	2007	2011	2018
Sit-Reach	-	X	X	X	X	X	X	-	-
Sit-Ups / Curl-Ups	X	X	X	X	X	X	X	X	X
Push-Ups	X	-	-	X	X	X	X	X	X
Flexed Arm Hang	X	-	-	-	-	-	-	-	-
Pull-Ups	X	-	-	-	-	-	-	-	-
1.5-mi. Run	X	X	X	X	X	X	X	X	X
3-min. Run-in-Place	X	X	-	-	-	-	-	-	-
500-yd Swim	-	-	X	X	X	X	X	X	X
450-m Swim	-	-	-	-	X	X	X	X	X
12-min Elliptical Trainer	-	-	-	-	-	X	X	X	-
12-min Stationary Bike	-	-	-	-	-	-	X	X	-

X represents the modalities that were included in the PRT.

Data from Peterson, D. (2015). History of the U.S. Navy Body Composition Program. *Military Medicine*, 180(1), 91-96; United States Army. (01 October 1998). Physical Fitness Training (Field Manual 21-20). Retrieved from http://www1 .udel.edu/armyrotc/current_cadets/cadet_resources/manuals_regulations_files/FM%2021-20%20-%20Physical%20 Fitness%20Training.pdf.

TABLE 2.6 Body Fat Percentage Ratings for Adults

Body Fat Rating	Male	Female
Risky	> 30%	> 40%
Excess Fat	21–30%	31–40%
Moderately Lean	13–20%	23–30%
Lean	9–12%	19–22%
Ultra Lean	5–8%	15–18%
Risky	< 5%	< 15%

Data from Bryant, C. X., & Green, D. J. (Eds.). (2010). *ACE Personal Trainer Manual: The Ultimate Resource for Fitness Professionals*. (4th ed.). San Diego, CA: American Council on Exercise.

Subcutaneous fat: Fat stored below the dermis layer of the skin and is not necessarily hazardous to your health.

Visceral fat: Unseen fat stored around your organs and is linked to several metabolic disorders and diseases.

There are two basic types of fat: subcutaneous and visceral. **Subcutaneous fat** is fat that is stored immediately below the dermis layer of the skin. This type of fat is not necessarily hazardous to your health. **Visceral fat** is the unseen fat stored around your organs (e.g., liver, pancreas, and intestines). This type of fat is considered hazardous to your health and is linked to several metabolic disorders and diseases such as insulin resistance, impaired glucose tolerance, type 2 diabetes, dyslipidemia, and cancer. **FIGURE 2.1** indicates the different types and location of abdominal fat.

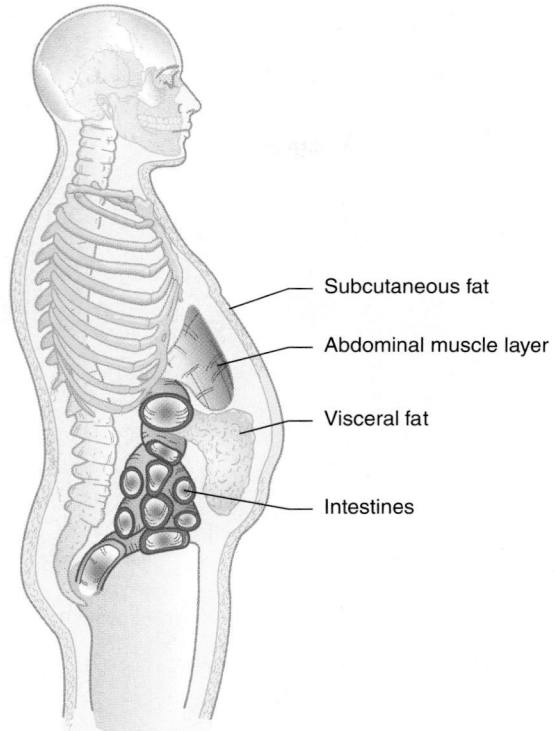

Subcutaneous fat

Abdominal muscle layer

Visceral fat

Intestines

FIGURE 2.1 Subcutaneous vs. Visceral Fat.

FAQ

What is the best way to lose body fat?

Generally speaking, diet is more effective in improving body composition than aerobic training and aerobic training is more effective than strength training. Some success rate statistics for individuals who have lost weight and were able to keep it off for a period of at least one year are provided below.

- **1% success rate:** Exercise alone
- **10% success rate:** Diet alone
- **89% success rate:** Combining diet and exercise

Although it is possible to lose weight with either diet or exercise alone, neither is the preferred approach. The best approach for losing weight, and keeping it off, is with a combination of regular aerobic activity, strength training, and proper dietary strategies.

Body Fat Distribution

Additionally, the location of body fat also plays a critical role in health and disease risk. Specifically, individuals who carry more fat around their waist are more likely to develop the aforementioned metabolic disorders. Generally speaking, females accumulate more fat around their hips and buttocks, thus giving them a pear-shaped (aka **gynoid**) appearance. Conversely, males accumulate more fat around their waist, thus giving them an apple-shaped (aka **android**) appearance. **FIGURE 2.2** on the next page illustrates the difference between the two primary body fat distribution patterns.

Gynoid: Pear-shaped fat distribution pattern mainly around the lower upper body, such as the hips, thighs, and butt.

Android: Apple-shaped fat distribution mainly around the trunk and upper body, such as the abdomen, chest, shoulder, and neck.

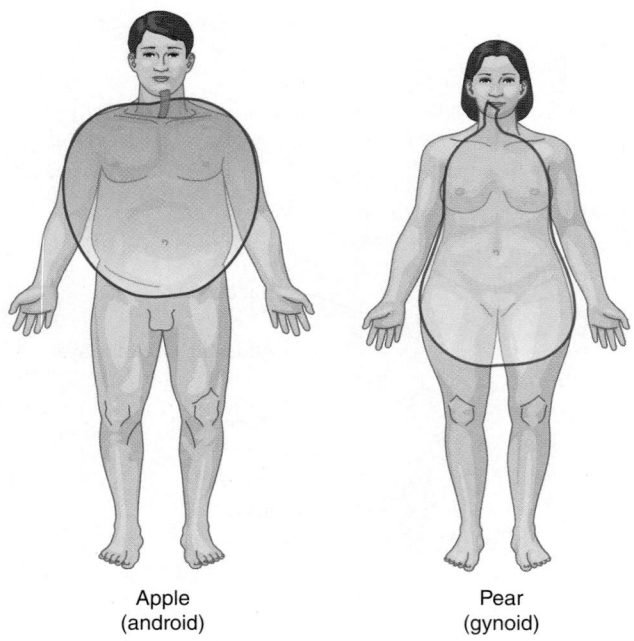

Apple
(android)

Pear
(gynoid)

FIGURE 2.2 Gynoid and Android Fat Distribution Patterns.

FAQ

Why do people who exercise regularly often stop seeing results?

There are a number of reasons why people who exercise on a regular basis stop seeing results. One reason is poor exercise programming. Examples of poor exercise programming include inadequate or infrequent implementation of basic exercise variables such as frequency, duration, and intensity. In other words, you can't keep doing the same thing and expect different results.

Another reason for performance stagnation or plateaus is the lack of essential exercise variation and/or periodization. Periodization means to periodically and systematically change the load (aka the amount of weight used) as well as the number of sets and repetitions (aka volume and intensity).

One of the main reasons why people stop seeing results in terms of their weight loss is because they fail to create a calorie deficit (i.e., burn more calories in a given day than they consume). Even with regular exercise, it is possible to consume too many calories thereby preventing or minimizing weight loss. While running, the average person burns between 90-155 kcal per mile. However, it's easy to consume the same number of calories burned during exercise with poor dietary choices. For example, one 12 ounce beer and one slice of pepperoni pizza have 154 kcal and 320 kcal, respectively. So an individual would have to run between 3 and 5 miles in order to burn off the same number of calories associated with consuming one beer and a slice of pizza. In other words, exercise can't overcome a bad diet. Unfortunately, high-calorie, low-nutritional value foods are easily accessible and affordable. Saying no can be hard, especially when you are too busy to go to the store and the less healthy alternatives can be delivered.

Types of Body Composition Testing

Underwater Weighing (aka Hydrostatic Weighing)

Based on the principle of water displacement, this is an accurate method of determining body composition **FIGURE 2.3**. The participant is required to exhale as much air from their lungs as possible before being submerged because the residual volume (volume of air remaining in the lungs after maximal expiration) can influence results. The difference between the participant's mass (weight) "on land" and underwater is then used to determine volume. Once mass and volume are known, body density can be calculated. Body density is then used in a prediction equation to calculate percent body fat.

Air Displacement Plethysmography (aka BodPod)

Similar to hydrostatic weighing, this method uses air displacement to determine body volume **FIGURE 2.4**. The participant sits inside a small egg-shaped chamber in an effort to measure body mass and volume. This information is then used to calculate body density, which can be entered into various prediction equations to calculate percent body fat.

Dual Energy X-ray Absorptiometry (DEXA)

This method involves scanning the entire body using x-ray beams with two different energy levels; fat and muscle tissue absorb these energies differently **FIGURE 2.5**. Specialized computer software is then used to build an image of underlying tissue and predict body

> **Residual volume:**
> Volume of air remaining in the lungs after maximal expiration.

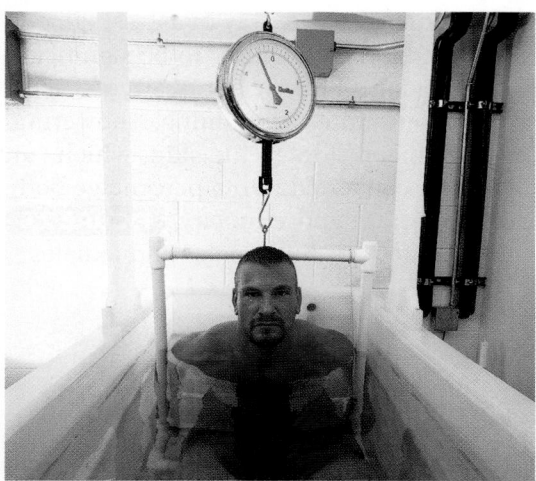

FIGURE 2.3 Hydrostatic Weighing

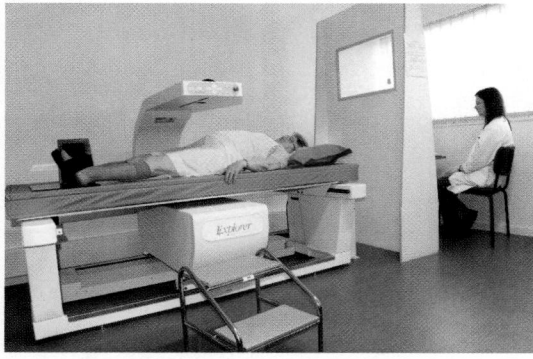

FIGURE 2.5 Duel Energy X-Ray Absorptiometry

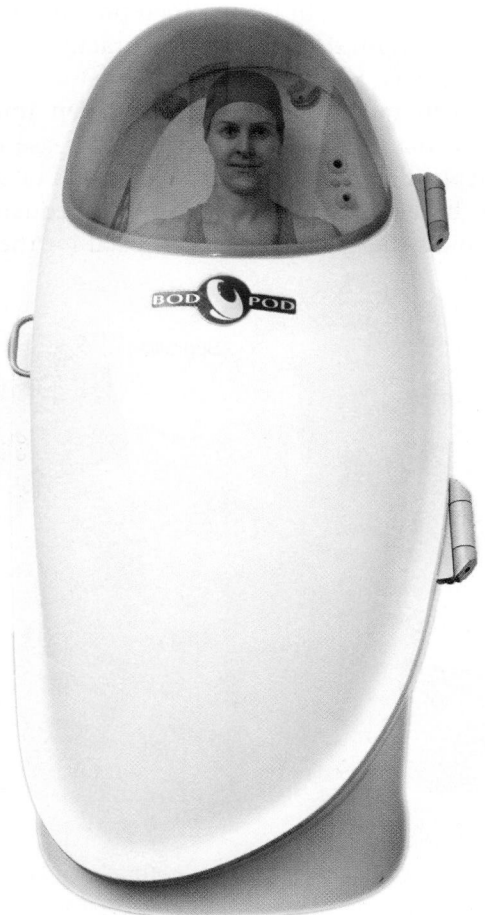

FIGURE 2.4 Air Displacement Plethysmography

composition. Although mostly used for measuring bone density, DEXA also provides an accurate assessment of total fat mass, lean mass, and muscle mass. This method is often considered to be the gold standard for clinical body composition analysis.

Bioelectrical Impedance Analysis (BIA)

This method uses electrodes positioned on the hands and feet and sends a painless electrical current between them. The electrical current moves more easily and quickly through fat-free mass than fat mass (as fat-free mass has a higher proportion of water and conducting electrolytes). The resistance (impedance) to the flow of the signal is related to the amount of fat in the tissue. This information is then used to calculate body density, which can then be used to calculate percent body fat. The participant's hydration level and skin temperature can influence the results.

Near-Infrared Interactance (NIR)

This method uses a fiber optic probe that sends out a beam of near infrared light to a specific area of the body (e.g., biceps). As a result, some of the light is absorbed, some transmitted, and some reflected. A detector within the probe measures the amount of light that penetrates the tissues, which is then entered into a prediction equation, along with age and activity level, to calculate percent body fat.

Skinfolds

This method uses calipers to measure the thickness of the skin at several sites around the body (e.g., triceps, subscapular, biceps, subscapular, abdominal, thigh, calf, iliac crest). When carried out by a trained practitioner, skinfolds are an accurate way of assessing body composition. However, if the practitioner is inexperienced, there is likely to be significant variations in the degree of accuracy (Heaney, Hodgdon, Beckett, & Carter, 1998). Measurements should not be taken immediately after training, swimming, showering, or sauna use as these activities increase the amount of blood flow to the skin, which can increase skinfold thickness. The sum of skinfolds can be converted into a percentage body fat by using a specified prediction equation based on gender and ethnicity. **FIGURE 2.6** depicts the specific locations used for the 3-site skinfold test for both males and females.

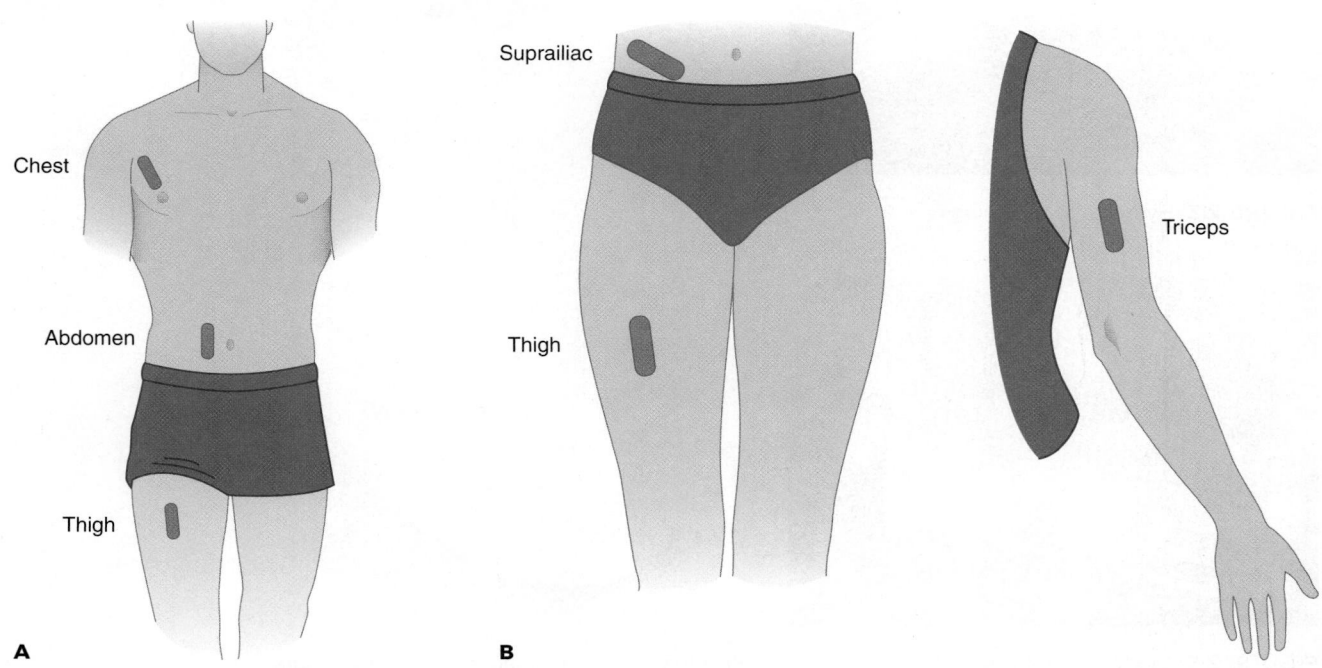

FIGURE 2.6 Locations for 3-Site Skinfold in **(A)** Males and **(B)** Females.

Testing procedures for 7-site and 3-site skinfolds are provided in **TABLE 2.7** (Berardi, 2006). **TABLE 2.8** on pages 37–38 provides percent body fat estimates for both males and females from 3-site skinfolds (Pollock, Schmidt, & Jackson, 1980). To use the table, add the sum of chest, abdominal, and thigh skinfolds for males or triceps, iliac crest, and thigh skinfolds for females. Locate the column that corresponds to the member's height and row that corresponds to the member's sum of skinfolds. Follow the applicable column down and row across until they intersect; this number represents the individual's estimated percent body fat.

TABLE 2.7 Testing Procedures for 7-Site / 3-Site Skinfold Tests

Skinfolds

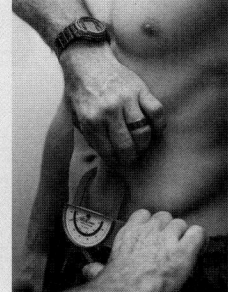

Abdomen. Measurement is taken directly one inch to the left of, and in line with, the umbilicus (belly button) using a vertical pinch (fold) of the skin.

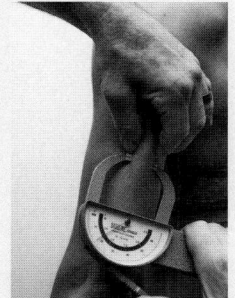

Triceps. Measurement is taken at the back midline of the upper arm halfway between the elbow and acromion process (bony point on top of the shoulder) using a vertical pinch (fold) of the skin. In some cases, it may be necessary to have the subject flex his or her triceps (by extending the arm) in order to separate the muscle from the fat thereby making it easier to take the measurement.

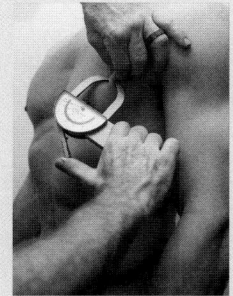

Chest. In men, the measurement is taken on the diagonal line halfway between the armpit and the nipple using a diagonal pinch (fold). In women, in order to account for the wear of upper body undergarments, the measurement is taken one third of the way up between where the male measurement is taken and the armpit.

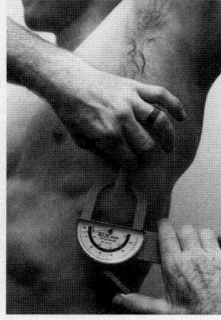

Midaxillary. Measurement is taken on the vertical line between the armpit and the hip and horizontal plane of the xyphoid process (bony spot in the center of the chest) using a vertical pinch (fold) of the skin. It is helpful to have the subject place his or her lower arm on top his or her head while performing the measurement.

(continues)

TABLE 2.7 Testing Procedures for 7-Site / 3-Site Skinfold Tests (continued)

Skinfolds

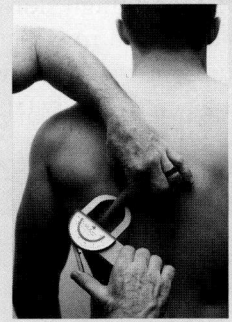

Subscapular. Measurement is taken one inch below and parallel to the bottom of the scapula (shoulder blade) using a diagonal pinch (fold) of the skin.

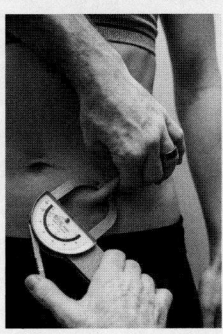

Suprailiac. Measurement is taken one half to one inch above the natural frontal angle of the iliac crest (hip) using a diagonal pinch (fold) of the skin.

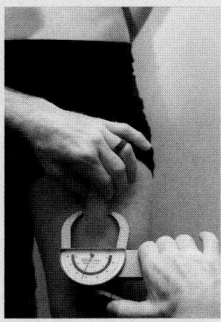

Thigh. Measurement is taken on the front midline of the thigh, halfway between the patella (kneecap) and inguinal crease (the line where leg inserts into hip) using a vertical pinch (fold) of the skin. It is helpful to have the subject bend his or her knee and lift their heel off the ground in order to relax the thigh musculature thereby making it easier to take the measurement.

For the 7-site skinfold test (male/female), perform measurements on all seven sites.

1. Male 7-Site Equations:
- Body Density (Db) = $1.112 - (0.00043499 \times SUM7) + (0.00000055 \times SUM7^2) - (0.00028826 \times Age)$
- % BF = $[(4.57/Db) - 4.142] \times 100$

2. Female 7-Site Equations:.
- Body Density (Db) = $1.097 - (0.00046971 \times SUM7) + (0.00000056 \times SUM7^2) - (0.00012828 \times Age)$
- % BF = $[(4.57/Db) - 4.142] \times 100$

For male 3-site skinfold test, perform chest, abdomen, and thigh measurements. For female 3-site skinfold test, perform triceps, suprailiac, and thigh measurements.

1. Male 3-Site Equations:
- Body Density (Db) = $1.10938 - (0.0008267 \times SUM3) + (0.0000016 \times SUM3^2) - (0.0002574 \times Age)$
- % BF = $[(4.95/Db) - 4.50] \times 100$

2. Female 3-Site Equations:
- Body Density (Db) = $1.0994921 - (0.0009929 \times SUM3) + (0.0000023 \times SUM3^2) - (0.0001392 \times Age)$
- % BF = $[(4.95/Db) - 4.50] \times 100$

Data from Berardi, J. M. (2006). *The precision nutrition: body composition guide*. Science Link, Inc.: Oakland, CA.

TABLE 2.8 Percent Fat Estimates for 3-Site Skinfolds

Males (Age)

Sum of Skinfolds (mm)	<22	23-27	28-32	33-37	38-42	43-47	48-52	53-57	>58
8-10	1.3	1.8	2.3	2.9	3.4	3.9	4.5	5	5.5
11-13	2.2	2.8	3.3	3.9	4.4	4.9	5.5	6	6.5
14-16	3.2	3.8	4.3	4.8	5.4	5.9	6.4	7	7.5
17-19	4.2	4.7	5.3	5.8	6.3	6.9	7.4	8	8.5
20-22	5.1	5.7	6.2	6.8	7.3	7.9	8.4	8.9	9.5
23-25	6.1	6.6	7.2	7.7	8.3	8.8	9.4	9.9	10.5
26-28	7	7.6	8.1	8.7	9.2	9.8	10.3	10.9	11.4
29-31	8	8.5	9.1	9.6	10.2	10.7	11.3	11.8	12.4
32-34	8.9	9.4	10	10.5	11.1	11.6	12.2	12.8	13.3
35-37	9.8	10.4	10.9	11.5	12	12.6	13.1	13.7	14.3
38-40	10.7	11.3	11.8	12.4	12.9	13.5	14.1	14.6	15.2
41-43	11.6	12.2	12.7	13.3	13.8	14.4	15	15.5	16.1
44-46	12.5	13.1	13.6	14.2	14.7	15.3	15.9	16.4	17
47-49	13.4	13.9	14.5	15.1	15.6	16.2	16.8	17.3	17.9
50-52	14.3	14.8	15.4	15.9	16.5	17.1	17.6	18.2	18.8
53-55	15.1	15.7	16.2	16.8	17.4	17.9	18.5	18.7	19.7
56-58	16	16.5	17.1	17.7	18.2	18.8	19.4	20	20.5
59-61	16.9	17.4	17.9	18.5	19.1	19.7	20.2	20.8	21.4
62-64	17.6	18.2	18.8	19.4	19.9	20.5	21.1	21.7	22.2
65-67	18.5	19	19.6	20.2	20.8	21.3	21.9	22.5	23.1
68-70	19.3	19.9	20.4	21	21.6	22.2	22.7	23.3	23.9
71-73	20.1	20.7	21.2	21.8	22.4	23	23.6	24.1	24.7

Females (Age)

Sum of Skinfolds (mm)	<22	23-27	28-32	33-37	38-42	43-47	48-52	53-57	>58
23-25	9.7	9.9	10.2	10.4	10.7	10.9	11.2	11.4	11.7
26-28	11	11.2	11.5	11.7	12	12.3	12.5	12.7	13
29-31	12.3	12.5	12.8	13	13.3	13.5	13.8	14	14.3
32-34	13.6	13.8	14	14.3	14.5	14.8	15	15.3	15.5
35-37	14.8	15	15.3	15.5	15.8	16	16.3	16.5	16.8
38-40	16	16.3	16.5	16.7	17	17.2	17.5	17.7	18
41-43	17.2	17.4	17.7	17.9	18.2	18.4	18.7	18.9	19.2
44-46	18.3	18.6	18.8	19.1	19.3	19.6	19.8	20.1	20.3
47-49	19.5	19.7	20	20.2	20.5	20.7	21	21.2	21.5
50-52	20.6	20.8	21.1	21.3	21.6	21.8	22.1	22.3	22.6
53-55	21.7	21.9	22.1	22.4	22.6	22.9	23.1	23.4	23.6
56-58	22.7	23	23.2	23.4	23.7	23.9	24.2	24.4	24.7
59-61	23.7	24	24.2	24.5	24.7	25	25.2	25.5	25.7
62-64	24.7	25	25.2	25.5	25.7	26	26.2	26.4	26.7
65-67	25.7	25.9	26.2	26.4	26.7	26.9	27.2	27.4	27.7
68-70	26.6	26.9	27.1	27.4	27.6	27.9	28.1	28.4	28.6
71-73	27.5	27.8	28	28.3	28.5	28.8	29	29.3	29.5
74-76	28.4	28.7	28.9	29.2	29.4	29.7	29.9	30.2	30.4
77-79	29.3	29.5	29.8	30	30.3	30.5	30.8	31	31.3
80-82	30.1	30.4	30.6	30.9	31.1	31.4	31.6	31.9	32.1
83-85	30.9	31.2	31.4	31.7	31.9	32.2	32.4	32.7	32.9
86-88	31.7	32	32.2	32.5	32.7	32.9	33.2	33.4	33.7

(continues)

TABLE 2.8 Percent Fat Estimates for 3-Site Skinfolds (continued)

Males (Age)

Sum of Skinfolds (mm)	<22	23-27	28-32	33-37	38-42	43-47	48-52	53-57	>58
74-76	20.9	21.5	22	22.6	23.2	23.8	24.4	25	25.5
77-79	21.7	22.2	22.8	23.4	24	24.6	25.2	25.8	26.3
80-82	22.4	23	23.6	24.2	24.8	25.4	25.9	26.5	27.1
83-85	23.2	23.8	24.4	25	25.5	26.1	26.7	27.3	27.9
86-88	24	24.5	25.1	25.7	26.3	26.9	27.5	28.1	28.7
89-91	24.7	25.3	25.9	26.9	27.1	27.6	28.2	28.8	29.4
92-94	25.4	26	26.6	27.2	27.8	28.4	29	29.6	30.2
95-97	26.1	26.7	27.3	27.9	28.5	29.1	29.7	30.3	30.9
98-100	26.9	27.4	28	28.6	29.2	29.8	30.4	31	31.6
101-103	27.5	28.1	28.7	29.3	29.9	30.5	31.1	31.7	32.3
104-106	28.2	28.8	29.4	30	30.6	31.2	31.8	32.4	33
107-109	28.9	29.5	30.1	30.7	31.3	31.9	32.5	33.1	33.7
110-112	29.6	30.2	30.8	31.4	32	32.6	33.2	33.8	34.4
113-115	30.2	30.8	31.4	32	32.6	33.2	33.8	34.5	35.1
116-118	30.9	31.5	32.1	32.7	33.3	33.9	34.5	35.1	35.7
119-121	31.5	32.1	32.7	33.3	33.9	34.5	35.1	35.7	36.4
122-124	32.1	32.7	33.3	33.9	34.5	35.1	35.8	36.4	37
125-127	32.7	33.3	33.9	34.5	35.1	35.8	36.4	37	37.6

Sum of Chest, Abdominal, and Thigh Skinfolds

Females (Age)

Sum of Skinfolds (mm)	<22	23-27	28-32	33-37	38-42	43-47	48-52	53-57	>58
89-91	32.5	32.7	33	33.2	33.5	33.7	33.9	34.2	34.4
92-94	33.2	33.4	33.7	33.9	34.2	34.4	34.7	34.9	35.2
95-97	33.9	34.1	34.4	34.6	34.9	35.1	35.4	35.6	35.9
98-100	34.6	34.8	35.1	35.3	35.5	35.8	36	36.3	36.5
101-103	35.3	35.4	35.7	35.9	36.2	36.4	36.7	36.9	37.2
104-106	35.8	36.1	36.3	36.6	36.8	37.1	37.3	37.5	37.8
107-109	36.4	36.7	36.9	37.1	37.4	37.6	37.9	38.1	38.4
110-112	37	37.2	37.5	37.7	38	38.2	38.5	38.7	38.9
113-115	37.5	37.8	38	38.2	38.5	38.7	39	39.2	39.5
116-118	38	38.3	38.5	38.8	39	39.3	39.5	39.7	40
119-121	38.5	38.7	39	39.2	39.5	39.7	40	40.2	40.5
122-124	39	39.2	39.4	39.7	39.9	40.2	40.4	40.7	40.9
125-127	39.4	39.6	39.9	40.1	40.4	40.6	40.9	41.1	41.4
128-130	39.8	40	40.3	40.5	40.8	41	41.3	41.5	41.8

Sum of Triceps, Suprailiac, and Thigh Skinfolds

Modified from Pollock M. L., Schmidt D. H., and Jackson A. S., Measurement of cardiorespiratory fitness and body composition in the clinical setting. *Comprehensive Therapy* 1980; 6(9):12-27.

Circumference Measurements

Circumference Measurements (aka Girth Measurements)

Although circumference measurements are a quick and easy method they, by themselves, tell us very little about actual body composition. However, circumference measurements can be an effective means of assessing progress. For example, increases in upper arm girth can be a testament of muscle hypertrophy (increase in size) due to regular strength training. Similarly, a decrease in waist size can be testament of fat loss as a result of regular exercise and healthy dietary practices. The Department of Defense (DoD) uses circumference measurements to estimate percent body fat of its service members through the development and implementation of gender-specific predication equations.

FIGURE 2.7 and **FIGURE 2.8** indicate the location of the various circumference measurement sites for both male and female, as well as the single-site abdominal circumference measurement (taken at the superior border of the iliac crest) (MyHealthyWaist. org, n.d.; Peterson, 2015a; United States Air Force, 2013; United States Navy, 2015, 2016).

Testing procedures for the 3-site / 2-site circumference measurements are provided in **TABLE 2.9** on the next page (Navy Physical Readiness Program, 2016a). The charts used by the DoD to calculate estimated percent body fat from circumference measurements for males and females are provided in **TABLE 2.10** (on pages 41–43) and **TABLE 2.11** (on pages 44–46), respectively (National Heart, Lung and Blood Institute, 1998). The shaded areas in these two tables represent the DoD maximum allowed percent body fat of 26% for males and 36% for females.

When assessing body composition over time, it is recommended to regularly perform skinfolds and/or circumference measurements in addition to weekly / biweekly weight measurements. Individuals employing a well-designed strength and conditioning program may see a slight reduction, no change, or even a slight increase in body weight. Although the individuals are likely losing body fat, changes in actual body weight are hampered by subsequent gains in lean muscle mass. Even so, there will likely be notable changes in the individual's skinfolds and circumference measurements. **FIGURE 2.9** on the next page indicates some of the notable changes in body composition as a result of regular exercise.

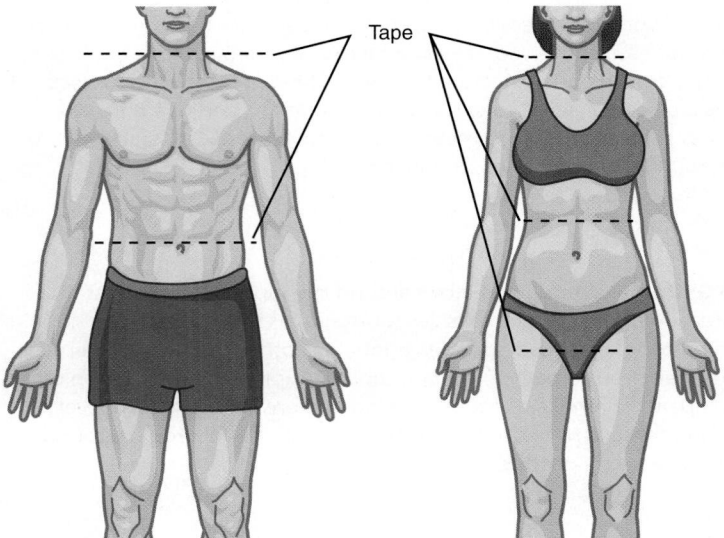

FIGURE 2.7 Location for U.S. Army, Marine Corps, and Navy Circumference Measurements

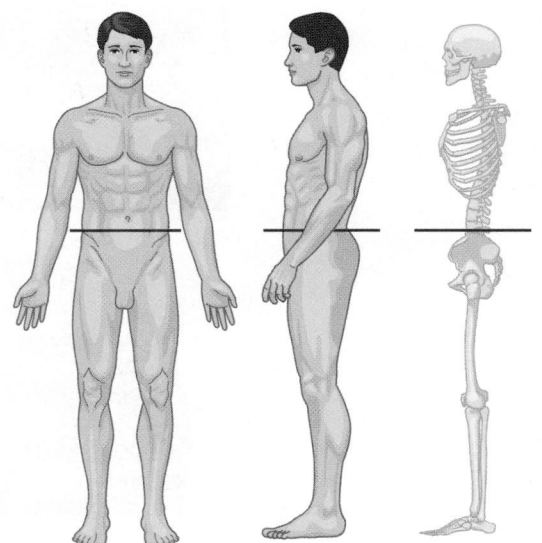

FIGURE 2.8 Location for U.S. Air Force and National Institutes of Health Single-Site Abdominal Circumference Measurement

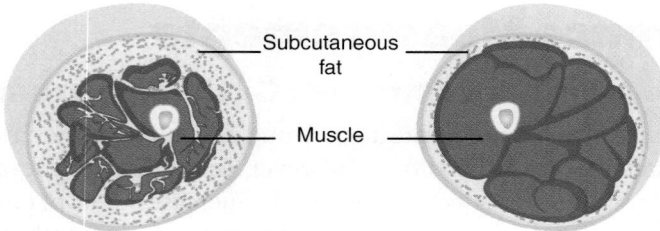

FIGURE 2.9 Changes in Body Composition with Regular Exercise

TABLE 2.9 Testing Procedures for 3-Site / 2-Site Circumference Measurements

Circumference Measurements

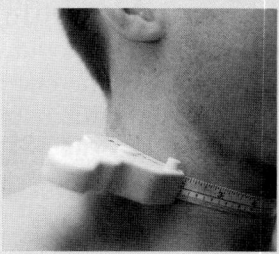

Neck. Measurement is taken on bare skin, just below the larynx (Adam's apple), and perpendicular to the long axis of the neck. Subject should look straight ahead during measurement with shoulders down and relaxed (not hunched). The tape will be as close to horizontal as possible (tape line in the front is at the same height as the tape line in the back). Measurement should not include the shoulder/neck musculature (trapezius). Round measurement up to the nearest ½ inch and record (e.g., round 16 ¾ inches to 17 inches).

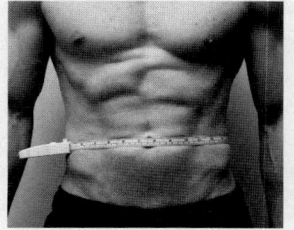

Abdomen. Measurement is taken on bare skin, across the naval (belly button), and with the arms down at the sides. Take measurement at the end of a normal, relaxed exhalation. Discourage subjects from holding their breath during the measurement. Round measurement down to nearest ½ inch and record (e.g., round 34 ¾ inches to 34 ½ inches).

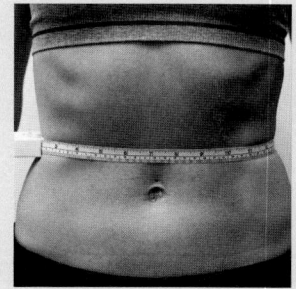

Natural Waist. Measurement is taken on bare skin at the point of minimal abdominal circumference (usually halfway between the navel and the xyphoid process (bony spot in the center of the chest)). When site is not easily observed, take several measurements at probable sites and use smallest value. Ensure the tape is level and that the subject's arms are at their sides. Take measurement at the end of a normal, relaxed exhalation. Round measurement to nearest ½ inch and record (e.g., round 28 ¾ inches to 28 ½ inches).

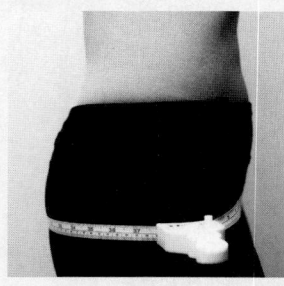

Hip Girth: Measurement is taken around the hips at the greatest protrusion of the gluteus muscles (buttocks) as viewed from the side. Control-top panty hose, spandex tights, and other shaping garments are not allowed to be worn during taping. Apply sufficient tension on the tape to minimize effect of clothing and ensure the tape is level. Round measurement down to nearest ½ inch and record (e.g., round 44 ¾ inches to 44 inches).

For male 2-site circumference measurements, perform neck and abdomen. For female 3-site circumference measurements, perform neck, natural waist, and hip.

Data from Berardi, J. M. (2006). *The precision nutrition: body composition guide.* Science Link, Inc.: Oakland, CA; National Heart, Lung, and Blood Institute. (1998). *Clinical guidelines on the identification, evaluation, and treatment of overweight and obesity in adults: The evidence report.* Bethesda, MD: National Institutes of Health.

TABLE 2.10 Percent Body Fat Estimation for Males

Circumfer-ence Value	Height in Inches																			
	60	60.5	61	61.5	62	62.5	63	63.5	64	64.5	65	65.5	66	66.5	67	67.5	68	68.5	69	69.5
13	<9	<9	<9	<9	<9	<9	<9	<9	<9	<9	<9	<9	<9	<9	<9	<9	<9	<9	<9	<9
13.5	9	<9	<9	<9	<9	<9	<9	<9	<9	<9	<9	<9	<9	<9	<9	<9	<9	<9	<9	<9
14	11	11	11	10	10	10	9	9	9	<9	<9	<9	<9	<9	<9	<9	<9	<9	<9	<9
14.5	12	12	12	11	11	11	11	10	10	10	10	9	9	<9	<9	<9	10	<9	9	<9
15	13	13	13	13	12	12	13	12	11	11	11	11	10	10	10	10	11	9	9	<9
15.5	15	14	14	14	14	13	13	13	13	12	12	12	12	11	11	11	12	11	10	10
16	16	16	15	15	15	15	14	14	14	14	13	13	13	13	12	12	12	12	12	11
16.5	17	17	16	16	16	16	15	15	15	15	14	14	14	14	14	13	13	13	13	12
17	18	18	18	17	17	17	17	16	16	16	16	15	15	15	15	14	14	14	14	14
17.5	19	19	19	18	18	18	18	17	17	17	17	16	16	16	16	16	15	15	15	15
18	20	20	20	19	19	19	19	18	18	18	18	18	17	17	17	17	16	16	16	16
18.5	21	21	21	20	20	20	20	19	19	19	19	19	18	18	18	18	17	17	17	17
19	22	22	22	21	21	21	20	20	20	19	19	19	19	19	19	19	18	18	18	18
19.5	23	23	23	22	22	22	21	21	21	20	20	20	20	20	20	20	19	19	19	19
20	24	24	24	23	23	23	23	22	22	21	21	21	21	20	20	20	20	20	20	20
20.5	25	25	25	24	24	24	24	23	23	22	22	21	22	21	21	21	21	21	21	21
21	26	26	25	25	25	25	24	24	24	23	23	22	23	22	22	22	22	22	22	21
21.5	27	27	26	26	26	26	25	25	25	24	24	23	24	23	23	23	23	23	23	22
22	28	28	27	27	26	26	26	26	26	25	24	24	24	24	24	24	23	24	23	23
22.5	29	29	28	28	27	27	27	26	27	25	25	25	25	25	25	25	24	25	24	24
23	29	29	29	29	28	28	28	27	27	26	26	26	26	26	26	26	25	26	25	25
23.5	30	30	30	29	29	29	28	28	28	27	27	27	27	27	27	27	26	26	26	26
24	31	31	30	30	30	30	29	29	29	28	28	28	28	28	28	27	27	27	27	26
24.5	32	31	31	31	31	30	30	30	30	29	29	29	29	29	28	28	28	28	27	27

(continues)

TABLE 2.10 Percent Body Fat Estimation for Males (continued)

Circumference Value	Height in Inches																			
	70	70.5	71	71.5	72	72.5	73	73.5	74	74.5	75	75.5	76	76.5	77	77.5	78	78.5	79	79.5
15	9	<9	<9	<9	<9	<9	<9	<9	<9	<9	<9	<9	<9	<9	<9	<9	<9	<9	<9	<9
15.5	10	10	9	9	9	<9	<9	<9	<9	<9	<9	<9	<9	<9	<9	<9	<9	<9	<9	<9
16	11	11	11	10	10	10	10	10	9	9	<9	<9	<9	<9	<9	9	<9	<9	<9	<9
16.5	12	12	12	12	11	11	10	10	11	10	10	10	10	10	9	9	<9	<9	<9	<9
17	13	13	13	13	13	12	12	11	12	11	11	11	11	11	10	10	10	10	10	<9
17.5	14	14	14	14	14	13	13	12	13	13	12	12	12	12	12	11	11	10	10	9
18	15	15	15	15	15	14	14	14	14	14	13	13	13	13	13	12	12	11	11	11
18.5	17	16	16	16	16	15	15	15	15	15	14	14	14	14	14	13	13	12	12	12
19	18	17	17	17	17	16	16	16	16	16	15	15	15	15	15	14	14	13	13	13
19.5	18	18	18	18	18	17	17	17	17	17	16	16	16	16	16	15	15	14	14	14
20	19	19	19	19	19	18	18	18	18	18	17	17	17	17	17	16	16	15	15	15
20.5	20	20	20	20	19	19	19	19	19	18	18	18	18	18	17	17	17	16	16	16
21	21	21	21	21	20	20	20	20	20	19	19	19	19	19	18	18	18	17	17	16
21.5	22	22	22	21	21	21	21	21	20	20	20	20	20	19	19	18	18	18	18	17
22	23	23	23	22	22	22	22	22	21	21	21	21	20	20	20	19	20	19	19	18
22.5	24	24	23	23	23	23	23	22	22	22	22	22	21	21	21	20	21	20	20	20

(continues)

TABLE 2.10 Percent Body Fat Estimation for Males (concluded)

Circumference Value	Height in Inches																			
	70	70.5	71	71.5	72	72.5	73	73.5	74	74.5	75	75.5	76	76.5	77	77.5	78	78.5	79	79.5
23	25	24	24	24	24	24	23	23	23	23	23	22	22	22	22	22	21	21	21	21
23.5	25	25	25	25	25	24	24	24	24	24	23	23	23	23	23	22	22	22	22	22
24	26	26	26	26	25	25	25	25	25	24	24	24	24	24	23	23	23	23	23	22
24.5	27	27	27	26	26	26	26	26	25	25	25	25	25	24	24	24	24	24	23	23
25	28	28	27	27	27	27	26	26	26	26	26	25	25	25	25	25	24	24	24	24
25.5	29	28	28	28	28	27	27	27	27	27	26	26	26	26	26	25	25	25	25	25
26	29	29	29	29	28	28	28	28	27	27	27	27	27	27	26	26	26	26	26	26
26.5	30	30	30	29	29	29	29	28	28	28	28	28	27	27	27	27	27	26	26	26
27	31	30	30	30	30	30	29	29	29	29	29	28	28	28	28	28	27	27	27	27
27.5	31	31	31	31	30	30	30	30	30	29	29	29	29	29	28	28	28	28	28	27
28	32	32	32	31	31	31	31	31	30	30	30	30	29	29	29	29	29	29	28	28

To calculate estimated percent body fat for males:
1. Subtract neck circumference from abdominal circumference to obtain circumference value (CV).
2. Locate column that matches member height (rounded up to the nearest half inch) and row that matches member's CV (rounded down to nearest half inch).
3. Follow applicable column down and row across until they intersect; this number represents the member's estimated percent body fat.
4. CVs less than the value in the table represent body fat percentages less than or equal to the smallest body fat percentage in the column.
5. CVs greater than the value in the table represent body fat percentages greater than or equal to the largest body fat percentage in the column.

Data from National Heart, Lung, and Blood Institute. (1998). *Clinical guidelines on the identification, evaluation, and treatment of overweight and obesity in adults: The evidence report.* Bethesda, MD: National Institutes of Health.

TABLE 2.11 Percent Body Fat Estimation for Females

Circumfer-ence Value	Height in Inches																			
	58	58.5	59	59.5	60	60.5	61	61.5	62	62.5	63	63.5	64	64.5	65	65.5	66	66.5	67	67.5
50.5	27	27	27	26	26	26	25	25	25	24	24	23	23	23	23	22	22	22	21	21
51	28	28	28	27	27	27	26	26	26	25	25	24	24	24	24	23	23	23	22	22
51.5	29	29	28	28	28	27	27	27	26	26	26	25	25	25	24	24	24	23	23	23
52	29	29	29	28	28	28	27	27	27	26	26	25	25	25	25	24	24	24	23	23
52.5	30	30	29	29	28	28	28	27	27	26	26	26	26	25	25	25	24	24	24	23
53	31	30	30	29	29	29	28	28	28	27	27	26	26	26	26	25	25	25	24	24
53.5	31	31	31	30	30	30	29	29	28	28	28	27	27	27	26	26	26	25	25	25
54	32	32	31	31	31	30	30	29	29	29	28	28	28	27	27	27	26	26	26	26
54.5	33	32	32	32	31	31	31	30	30	29	29	29	28	28	28	27	27	27	27	26
55	33	33	33	32	32	32	31	31	31	30	30	29	29	29	29	28	28	28	27	27
55.5	34	34	33	33	33	32	32	32	31	31	30	30	30	30	29	29	29	28	28	28
56	35	34	34	34	33	33	33	32	32	31	31	31	30	30	30	29	29	29	29	28
56.5	35	35	35	34	34	34	33	33	33	32	32	31	31	31	31	30	30	30	29	29
57	36	36	35	35	35	34	34	34	33	33	33	32	32	32	31	31	31	30	30	30
57.5	37	37	36	36	36	35	35	35	34	34	34	33	33	33	32	32	32	31	31	31
58	37	37	37	36	36	36	35	35	35	34	34	33	33	33	33	32	32	32	31	31
58.5	38	38	37	37	37	36	36	36	35	35	35	34	34	34	33	33	33	32	32	32
59	38	38	38	37	37	37	36	36	36	35	35	34	34	34	34	33	33	33	32	32
59.5	39	39	38	38	38	37	37	37	36	36	36	35	35	35	34	34	34	33	33	33
60	40	39	39	39	38	38	38	37	37	36	36	36	35	35	35	34	34	34	34	33
60.5	40	40	40	39	39	39	38	38	38	37	37	36	36	36	36	35	35	35	34	34
61	41	41	40	40	40	39	39	39	38	38	38	37	37	37	36	36	36	35	35	35
61.5	41	41	41	40	40	40	39	39	39	38	38	37	37	37	37	36	36	36	35	35
62	42	42	41	41	41	40	40	40	39	39	39	38	38	38	37	37	37	36	36	36
62.5	42	42	42	41	41	41	40	40	40	39	39	38	38	38	38	37	37	37	36	36
63	43	43	42	42	42	41	41	41	40	40	40	39	39	39	38	38	38	37	37	37
63.5	44	43	43	43	42	42	42	41	41	40	40	40	39	39	39	38	38	38	37	37
64	44	44	43	43	43	42	42	42	41	41	41	40	40	40	39	39	39	38	38	38

(continues)

TABLE 2.11 Percent Body Fat Estimation for Females (concluded)

Circumference Value	Height in Inches																			
	68	68.5	69	69.5	70	70.5	71	71.5	72	72.5	73	73.5	74	74.5	75	75.5	76	76.5	77	77.5
56	28	28	27	27	27	26	26	26	25	25	25	25	24	24	24	23	23	23	23	22
56.5	29	28	28	28	27	27	27	26	26	26	26	25	25	25	24	24	24	24	23	23
57	29	29	29	28	28	28	27	27	27	26	26	26	26	25	25	25	24	24	24	24
57.5	30	29	29	29	28	28	28	28	27	27	27	26	26	26	26	25	25	25	25	24
58	30	30	30	29	29	29	28	28	28	28	27	27	27	26	26	26	26	25	25	25
58.5	31	31	30	30	30	29	29	29	28	28	28	28	27	27	27	26	26	26	26	25
59	32	31	31	31	30	30	29	29	29	28	28	28	28	27	27	27	26	26	26	26
59.5	32	32	32	31	31	31	30	30	29	29	29	29	28	28	28	27	27	27	27	26
60	33	32	32	32	31	31	31	30	30	30	30	29	29	29	28	28	28	28	27	27
60.5	33	33	33	32	32	32	31	31	31	30	30	30	30	29	29	29	28	28	28	28
61	34	34	33	33	33	32	32	32	31	31	31	31	30	30	29	29	29	29	28	28
61.5	35	34	34	34	33	33	33	32	32	32	32	31	31	31	30	30	30	29	29	29
62	35	35	34	34	34	33	33	33	32	32	32	32	31	31	31	30	30	30	30	29
62.5	36	35	35	35	34	34	34	33	33	33	33	32	32	32	31	31	31	30	30	
63	36	36	36	35	35	35	34	34	33	33	33	33	33	32	32	32	31	31		
63.5	37	37	36	36	36	35	35	35	34	34	34	34	34	33	33	33	33			
64	37	37	37	36	36	36	35	35	35	34	34	34	34	34	33	33				
64.5	38	38	37	37	37	36	36	36	36	35	35	35	34	34	34					
65	38	38	38	38	37	37	37	36	36	36	35	35	35	35						

(continues)

TABLE 2.11 Percent Body Fat Estimation for Females (concluded)

Circumfer-ence Value	Height in Inches																			
	68	68.5	69	69.5	70	70.5	71	71.5	72	72.5	73	73.5	74	74.5	75	75.5	76	76.5	77	77.5
65.5	39	39	38	38	38	37	37	37	37	36	36	36	35	35	35	35	34	34	34	33
66	40	39	39	39	38	38	38	37	37	37	37	36	36	36	35	35	35	35	34	34
66.5	40	40	39	39	39	39	38	38	38	37	37	37	37	36	36	36	35	35	35	35
67	41	40	40	40	39	39	39	39	38	38	38	37	37	37	36	36	36	36	35	35
67.5	41	41	41	40	40	40	39	39	39	38	38	38	37	37	37	37	36	36	36	36
68	42	41	41	41	40	40	40	40	39	39	39	38	38	38	38	37	37	37	37	36
68.5	42	42	42	41	41	41	41	40	40	39	39	39	39	38	38	38	37	37	37	37
69	43	42	42	42	41	41	41	41	40	40	40	39	39	39	39	38	38	38	38	37
69.5	43	43	43	42	42	42	41	41	41	40	40	40	40	39	39	39	39	38	38	38

To calculate estimated percent body fat for females:
1. Add waist and hip circumferences, then subtract neck circumference to obtain circumference value (CV).
2. Locate column that matches member height (rounded up to the nearest half inch) and row that matches member's CV (rounded down to nearest half inch).
3. Follow applicable column down and row across until they intersect; this number represents the member's estimated percent body fat.
4. CV's less than the value in the table represent body fat percentages less than or equal to the smallest body fat percentage in the column.
5. CV's greater than the value in the table represent body fat percentages greater than or equal to the largest body fat percentage in the column.

Data from National Heart, Lung, and Blood Institute. (1998). Clinical guidelines on the identification, evaluation, and treatment of overweight and obesity in adults: The evidence report. Bethesda, MD: National Institutes of Health.

TABLE 2.12 Relative Risk Ratings for Waist-to-Hip Ratio				
Gender	**Excellent**	**Good**	**Average**	**At Risk**
Males	< 0.85	0.85 - 0.89	0.90 - 0.95	≥ 0.95
Females	< 0.75	0.75 - 0.79	0.80 - 0.86	≥ 0.86

Data from Bryant, C. X., & Green, D. J. (Eds.). (2010). *ACE personal trainer manual: The ultimate resource for fitness professionals.* (4th ed.). San Diego, CA: American Council on Exercise.

Anthropometric Measures Used for Health Risk

Although not typically used to estimate percent body fat, certain anthropometric measurements (e.g., height, weight, abdominal circumference) are often used to assess health risk or establish target weight limits. Some of the more popular anthropometric measurements used include waist-to-hip ratio, waist circumference, and body mass index.

Waist-to-hip ratio (WHR)

Body mass index (BMI), is another method of anthropometric measurement. WHR is considered by some to be an even better predictor of health risk than percent body fat because it takes into consideration the location of fat deposits. Specifically, individuals who carry excess fat around their abdominal area (apple-shaped or android fat distribution pattern) are considered to be at greater risk for certain metabolic disorders and diseases (e.g., insulin resistance, type 2 diabetes, hypertension, hypercholesterolemia) than individuals who carry excess fat around their lower body (pear-shaped or gynoid fat distribution pattern).

WHR is calculated by dividing the waist measurement by the hip measurement (waist [in.] / hips [in.]). However, there is some debate as to which abdominal site to use for the waist measurement. For example, the American Council on Exercise (ACE) proposes using measurements taken at the natural waist (narrowest part of the torso between the xiphoid process and umbilicus). However, the World Health Organization (WHO) recommends using measurements taken at the mid-point (halfway between the lowest rib and the top of the iliac crest) and the National Institutes of Health (NIH) has developed protocols using measurements taken at both the top of the iliac crest and level with the umbilicus. The relative risk ratings for WHR provided in **TABLE 2.12** use measurements taken at the natural waist (Bryant & Green, 2010).

Body mass index (BMI): A weight-to-height ratio, calculated by dividing weight in kilograms by the square of height in meters, which is used as an indicator of obesity and underweight.

Waist Circumference

Unlike WHR, which takes into account the fat distribution around the hips, this method of health risk assessment is based solely on the distribution of fat around the abdomen. Measurements for waist circumference are taken at the level of the umbilicus. As discussed previously, there is a known and strong correlation between excessive abdominal fat and a number of health risks. In fact, research has shown a number of health risks associated with every one inch increase in waist circumference. Specifically:

- 8% increase in blood cholesterol levels
- 10% increase in blood pressure
- 18% increase in triglycerides
- 18% increase in metabolic syndrome risk
- 15% decrease in high-density lipoprotein (HDL)

TABLE 2.13 on the next page depicts the risk categories associated with various waist circumferences for both males and females (Bryant & Green, 2010).

TABLE 2.13 Relative Risk Categories for Various Waist Circumferences

Risk Category	Males (in.)	Females (in.)
Underweight	< 31.5	< 27.5
Normal Weight	31.5–39.0	27.5–35.0
Overweight	39.5–47.0	35.5–43.0
Grade I Obesity	> 47	> 43.5

Data from Bryant, C. X., & Green, D. J. (Eds.). (2010). *ACE personal trainer manual: The ultimate resource for fitness professionals.* (4th ed.). San Diego, CA: American Council on Exercise.

Body mass index (BMI)

This method of measurement provides a descriptive ratio between body weight and height and is calculated by dividing one's weight in kilograms (kg) by the square of one's height in meters (m) [BMI = wt (kg) / ht^2 (m)]. **TABLE 2.14** uses height in inches (in.) and weight in pounds (lbs.) can also be used to determine BMI (National Heart, Lung and Blood Institute, 1998). To use the table, locate the row that corresponds to the individual's height and follow it across until the weight value that is equal to or greater than the individual's weight is located. Once a weight value is selected, follow the applicable column up to determine the BMI. For example, an individual who is 67 in. tall and 180 lbs. would use a weight value of 185 lbs., which correlates to a BMI of 29 (overweight).

Although BMI may be a relatively accurate predictor of health risk for most individuals, it has been shown to over predict individuals who are extremely muscular or have large frames. Additionally, BMI has been shown to under predict older individuals with decreased lean tissue (muscle mass) and excess body fat. **TABLE 2.15** on page 50 is used to categorize BMI (Bryant & Green, 2010).

Body Composition Testing in the Military

Similar to the PFT, the DoD allowed each branch of service to determine the method used in assessing the body composition of its service members. The only stipulation was that the method selected must be easily obtained from the field with minimal amount of training/skill required to perform.

DoD directive 1308.1, titled *Physical Fitness and Body Fat Program*, was published in 1995 and provided the different service branches with three potential means for establishing their respective body composition standards. Specifically, correlating body composition to:

- Physical fitness
- Professional military appearance
- General health

Starting in 1987, all three means were evaluated by the Naval Health Research Center (NHRC) in order to determine which consideration to use as the basis of the Navy's body composition program. Ironically, neither physical fitness nor professional military appearance showed a strong correlation to body composition; only general health.

As a result, all four services eventually ended up using circumference measurements as the basis for their body composition programs. In November 2002, DoDI 1308.3 was released and required each service to use circumference measurements in order to predict the percent body fat of their service members.

However, some of the services begin to question the accuracy and reliability of circumference measurements, stating that they do not take into consideration athletic

TABLE 2.14 Body Mass Index

Ht. (in.)	Normal						Overweight					Obese										Extremely Obese														
BMI	19	20	21	22	23	24	25	26	27	28	29	30	31	32	33	34	35	36	37	38	39	40	41	42	43	44	45	46	47	48	49	50	51	52	53	54
58	91	96	100	105	110	115	119	124	129	134	138	143	148	153	158	162	167	172	177	181	186	191	196	201	205	210	215	220	224	229	234	239	244	248	253	258
59	94	99	104	109	114	119	124	128	133	138	143	148	153	158	163	168	173	178	183	188	193	198	203	208	212	217	222	227	232	237	242	247	252	257	262	267
60	97	102	107	112	118	123	128	133	138	143	148	153	158	163	168	174	179	184	189	194	199	204	209	215	220	225	230	235	240	245	250	255	261	266	271	276
61	100	106	111	116	122	127	132	137	143	148	153	158	164	169	174	180	185	190	195	201	206	211	217	222	227	232	238	243	248	254	259	264	269	275	280	285
62	104	109	115	120	126	131	136	142	147	153	158	164	169	175	180	186	191	196	202	207	213	218	224	229	235	240	246	251	256	262	267	273	278	284	289	295
63	107	113	118	124	130	135	141	146	152	158	163	169	175	180	186	191	197	203	208	214	220	225	231	237	242	248	254	259	265	270	278	282	287	293	299	304
64	110	116	122	128	134	140	145	151	157	163	169	174	180	186	192	197	204	209	215	221	227	232	238	244	250	256	262	267	273	279	285	291	296	302	308	314
65	114	120	126	132	138	144	150	156	162	168	174	180	186	192	198	204	210	216	222	228	234	240	246	252	258	264	270	276	282	288	294	300	306	312	318	324
66	118	124	130	136	142	148	155	161	167	173	179	186	192	198	204	210	216	223	229	235	241	247	253	260	266	272	278	284	291	297	303	309	315	322	328	334
67	121	127	134	140	146	153	159	166	172	178	185	191	198	204	211	217	223	230	236	242	249	255	261	268	274	280	287	293	299	306	312	319	325	331	338	344
68	125	131	138	144	151	158	164	171	177	184	190	197	203	210	216	223	230	236	243	249	256	262	269	276	282	289	295	302	308	315	322	328	335	341	348	354
69	128	135	142	149	155	162	169	176	182	189	196	203	209	216	223	230	236	243	250	257	263	270	277	284	291	297	304	311	318	324	331	338	345	351	358	365
70	132	139	146	153	160	167	174	181	188	195	202	209	216	222	229	236	243	250	257	264	271	278	285	292	299	306	313	320	327	334	341	348	355	362	369	376
71	136	143	150	157	165	172	179	186	193	200	208	215	222	229	236	243	250	257	265	272	279	286	293	301	308	315	322	329	338	343	351	358	365	372	379	386
72	140	147	154	162	169	177	184	191	199	206	213	221	228	235	242	250	258	265	272	279	287	294	302	309	316	324	331	338	346	353	361	368	375	383	390	397
73	144	151	159	166	174	182	189	197	204	212	219	227	235	242	250	257	265	272	280	288	295	302	310	318	325	333	340	348	355	363	371	378	386	393	401	408
74	148	155	163	171	179	186	194	202	210	218	225	233	241	249	256	264	272	280	287	295	303	311	319	326	334	342	350	358	365	373	381	389	396	404	412	420
75	152	160	168	176	184	192	200	208	216	224	232	240	248	256	264	272	279	287	295	303	311	319	327	335	343	351	359	367	375	383	391	399	407	415	423	431
76	156	164	172	180	189	197	205	213	221	230	238	246	254	263	271	279	287	295	304	312	320	328	336	344	353	361	369	377	385	394	402	410	418	426	435	443

Weight (lbs.)

Data from Bryant, C. X., & Green, D. J. (Eds.). (2010). ACE personal trainer manual: The ultimate resource for fitness professionals. (4th ed.). San Diego, CA: American Council on Exercise.

TABLE 2.15 Weight Range Categories for Body Mass Index

Weight Range	BMI Category
Underweight	< 18.5
Normal Weight	18.5–24.9
Overweight	25.0–29.9
Grade I Obesity	30.0–34.9
Grade II Obesity	35.0–39.9
Grade III Obesity	> 40

Body composition assessment (BCA): Method (e.g., circumference measurements, skinfolds) used to estimate a person's percent body fat.

Technical error of measurement (TEM): Variability in the measured scores taken on the same subjects at multiple sessions.

(muscular) builds and, therefore, subsequently overpredict body fat percentages. So, are circumference measurements really the best method for the DoD to use for assessing the body composition of its service members? Or are there other methods currently available that could be used instead that are also easily obtained from the field and require minimal training/skill to perform? **TABLE 2.16** indicates the accuracy of various **body composition assessment (BCA)** techniques (Command Fitness Leader Certification Course, n.d.).

In 1998, NHRC conducted two separate studies to determine the reliability and feasibility of using skinfolds instead of circumference measurements. In both cases, the accuracy of the results and amount of time required to become proficient was far better with circumference measurements than with skinfolds. For example, the **technical error of measurement (TEM)**, variability between scores on the same subjects measured at multiple sessions, went from 85% to 7.43% after 120 trials with skinfolds compared to 1.15% to 0.7% after 75 trials with circumference measurements (Heaney, Hodgdon, Beckett, & Carter, 1998).

As a result, the Navy, along with the Army and Marine Corps, opted to continue using circumference measurements as the basis of their body composition programs. However, in 2009, the Air Force requested and received a waiver to use a single-site abdominal circumference measurement, taken at the superior border of the iliac crest, in lieu of circumference measurements. Beginning in 2016, the Navy has opted to implement the abdominal circumference measurement in addition to circumference measurements in an effort to, according to Naval administrative message (NAVADMIN) 178/15, "account for the body types of today's Sailor."

TABLE 2.16 Prediction Accuracy of Various Body Composition Assessment Techniques

Method	Std. Error (%)
Autopsy	0.01
Hydrostatic Weighing	1.5–3.0
Circumference (Navy)	3.5
Skinfolds	3.0–5.0
Height / Weight	5.0
Bio-Impedance	4.0–5.0
Near Infrared	7.0

Data from Command Fitness Leader Certification Course. *Body composition assessment* (S5620612A) [PowerPoint Presentation]. Navy Physical Readiness Program, Millington, TN.

TABLE 2.17 Maximal Allowable Body Fat Percentages for the Various Branches of Service

Service	Age	%BF Male	%BF Female	AC Male	AC Female
Air Force	-	-	-	> 39*	> 35.5*
	-	-	-	35**	31.5**
Army	17-20	20%	30%	-	-
	21-27	22%	32%	-	-
	28-39	24%	34%	-	-
	40+	26%	36%	-	-
Marine Corps	17–25	18%	26%	-	-
	26–35	19%	27%	-	-
	36–45	20%	28%	-	-
	46+	21%	29%	-	-
Navy	18–21	22%	33%	≤ 39	≤ 35.5
	22–29	23%	34%	≤ 39	≤ 35.5
	30–39	24%	35%	≤ 39	≤ 35.5
	40+	26%	36%	≤ 39	≤ 35.5

* High Risk

** Moderate Risk

Body Composition Standards by Service

TABLE 2.17 provides the maximal allowable body fat percentages (%BF) and abdominal circumference (AC) values by service (Peterson, 2015a; United States Air Force, 2013; United States Army, 1998; United States Marine Corps, 2016; United States Navy, 2011, 2015, 2016).

Reader Challenger: Physical Fitness Test

Listed below are a battery of tests that are easy to administer, either on yourself or on someone else, and provide good insight as to your overall level of physical fitness. To pass, you must meet or exceed the posted standards for each event. Are you up for the challenge?

Event 1. Waist Circumference Measurement

Waist Circumference	
Male	≤ 38 in.
Female	≤ 35 in.

Testing Criteria for Waist Circumference Measurement

Measurement should be taken on the right side of the body with the tape parallel to the floor. Apply the tape to bare skin and across the umbilicus (belly button) with arms down at the sides. **FIGURE 2.10** on the next page depicts the proper positioning of the tape for the waist circumference measurement. Enough tension should be applied so that the tape makes contact with the skin but does not compress the underlying soft tissues. Take the

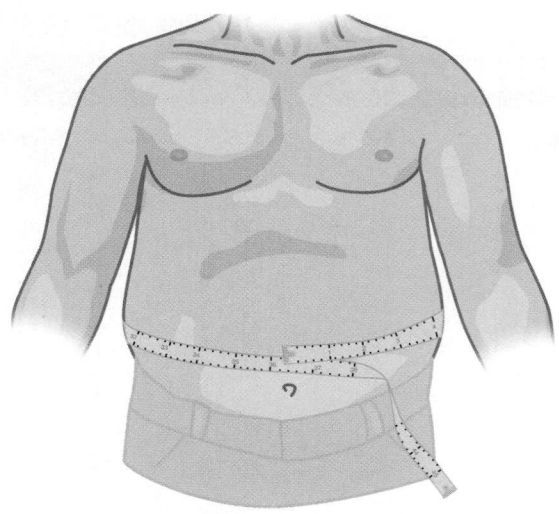

FIGURE 2.10 Waist Circumference Measurement

measurement at the end of normal, relaxed exhalation (do not hold your breath). Round waist circumference measurement down to the nearest ½ inch and record (e.g., round 34 ¾ inches to 34 ½ inches).

Event 2. Physical Fitness Test

Complete the five events below in 30 minutes or fewer.

	Plank	Wall Sit	Chest-to-Deck Push-Ups	Dead Hang Pull-Ups	1-Mile Run
Male	5:00	2:30	50	15	7:00
Female	5:00	2:30	35	6	8:15

Testing Criteria for Plank

Place your elbows on the floor at shoulder width directly below your shoulders. Make a fist with both hands and point them forward. Lift your torso so that your body forms a straight line through your shoulders, hips, knees, and ankles. **FIGURE 2.11** illustrates the proper body position for the plank. Hold this position for as long as possible. The test is ended when you can no longer maintain proper form or any body part other than the forearms and balls of the feet comes in contact with the floor.

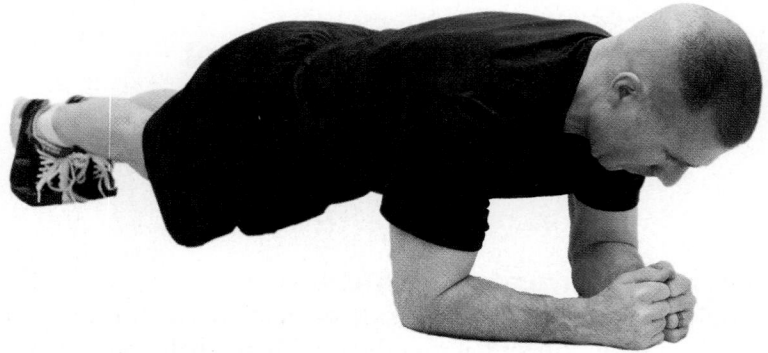

FIGURE 2.11 Proper Body Position for the Plank

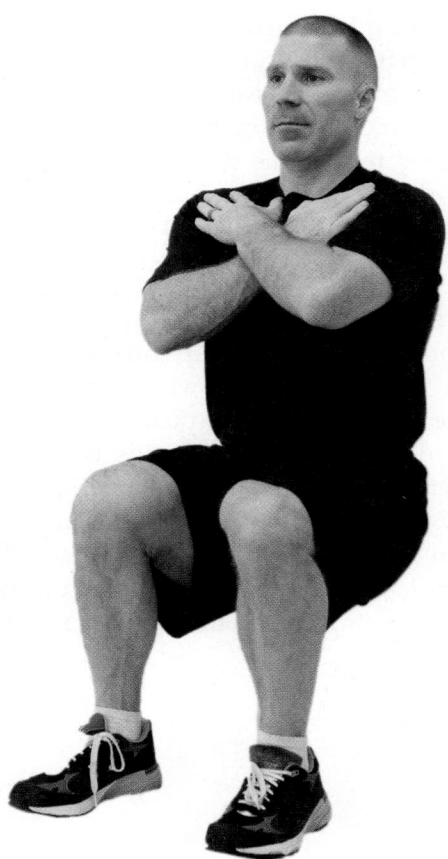

FIGURE 2.12 Proper Body Position for the Wall Sit

Testing Criteria for Wall Sit

Stand comfortably with feet approximately shoulder width apart with your back against a smooth, vertical wall. Arms should be crossed with the right thumb touching the left clavicle (collar bone) and the left thumb touching the right clavicle. Slowly slide your back down the wall until both your knees and hips are at a 90° angle. **FIGURE 2.12** illustrates the proper body position for the wall sit. Hold this position as long as possible. The test is ended when you can no longer maintain proper form (e.g., the hips go below the knees).

Testing Criteria for Chest-to-Deck Push-Ups

The test begins in the front leaning rest position (i.e., the body forms a straight line through the shoulders, hips, knees, and ankles). Weight is supported only by the palms of the hands and the balls of the feet. Hands should be directly under the shoulders or slightly wider than shoulder width (no more than thumb's length). Lower the entire body while keeping the shoulders, hips, knees, and ankles aligned and parallel to the floor until the upper chest (across the nipple line) touches the floor. Upon contact, push the entire body upward and return to the starting position until the arms are fully extended. You may rest only in the up position and while maintaining a straight line through the shoulders, hips, knees, and ankles. Only properly performed repetitions shall be counted. The test is ended if any body part touches the floor other than the hands and feet while in the up position, either hand or foot comes off the floor, or you fail to maintain proper body alignment throughout the test.

Testing Criteria for Dead Hang Pull-Ups

The test begins in the "dead hang" position with arms locked out and the body hanging motionless. Each repetition is to be performed without excessive motion (e.g., kipping), until the chin goes over the bar, and the body is lowered back to the "dead hang" position. Only properly performed repetitions shall be counted. Changes in grip during the test are allowed as long as the feet don't touch the ground and only the hands come in contact with the bar. Both overhand (pronated) and underhand (supinated) grips are allowed.

Testing Criteria for 1-Mile Run

The event consists of running or walking 1.0-mile as quickly as possible, with any combination of running or walking being allowed during the test. The event should be performed on a flat surface (e.g., a standard track or designated route on a road). The time starts as soon as you cross the start line and ends as soon as you cross the finish line. Time is recorded to the nearest second. The 1.0-mile run event can also be performed on a treadmill as long as the incline is set and remains at 1% grade throughout the test (Jones & Doust, 1996). You are allowed to adjust the treadmill speed at any time during the test. The treadmill event is ended if you stop or step off the belt for any reason, grab or hold onto the bar for any reason other than to briefly regain balance, or adjust (either up or down) the incline.

Assessment and Application

Summary

- The implementation of periodic fitness testing is recommended for anyone participating in a sport or exercise program since it offers both the individual and the test administrator a wide variety of useful information (e.g., identify physiological strengths and weaknesses, evaluate the effectiveness of a conditioning program, predict future performance).

- There are several key factors (e.g., validity, reliability, feasibility) that should be considered when choosing a fitness test.

- When administering a battery of tests, special attention should be paid to the sequence of test events since participating in some tests can negatively influence the performance in subsequent tests.

- Although it is possible to lose weight and keep it off by exercise or diet alone, the best approach by far is to use both approaches simultaneously.

- There are numerous ways to assess body composition, with some methods having a higher degree of accuracy than others. Less accurate methods are often used over more accurate methods due to the significant differences in device cost and amount of training required for test administrators to become proficient.

Knowledge Check

1. List some of the purposes of regular fitness testing.
2. List and discuss the five characteristics of a viable fitness test.
3. List the different health-related and skill-related components of fitness.
4. List the order that the National Strength and Conditioning Association (NSCA) recommends field tests be performed in and provide an example of each.
5. Define and differentiate criterion standards and normative standards.
6. Define and differentiate subcutaneous fat and visceral fat.
7. Discuss the best approach for losing body fat.
8. List and discuss the two primary fat distribution patterns.
9. Discuss some of the reasons why individuals who exercise on a regular basis stop seeing results.
10. Define body composition and provide the body fat percentage ratings for both adult males and females.
11. List and discuss the different types of body composition testing provided in the text.
12. In addition to periodic weight measurements, discuss why performing periodic skinfold and/or circumference measurements is also recommended when assessing body composition changes.
13. List and discuss the different types of anthropometric measures provided in the text.
14. Which type of body composition testing is considered to be the gold standard for clinical body composition analysis?
15. List and discuss the reported accuracy of the various body composition assessment techniques.

16. List the components of fitness that the Department of Defense Instruction (DoDI) 1308.3 mandates each branch of service evaluate in their semi-annual physical fitness tests (PFT).
17. Discuss why the Department of Defense (DoD) uses circumference measurements instead of skinfolds to assess body composition.

Activities

Fitness Testing and Assessment

A. Claire and Ethan are looking to assess their body composition as well as improve their physical fitness. First, determine their percent body fat using the skinfold measurements provided in the tables below. Next, determine their percent body fat according to their circumference measurements using Tables 2.10 and 2.11.

B. Using Table 2.13, assess Claire's and Ethan's Risk Category according to their respective waist circumferences.

C. Determine each person's Waist-to-Hip Ratio (WHR) and see which category Claire and Ethan fall into using Table 2.12.

D. Using Table 2.14 and Table 2.15, determine the Body Mass Index (BMI) category for Claire and Ethan. Round to the nearest tenth for the BMI.

E. Using Table 2.1, rate both Claire's and Ethan's fitness (i.e., below average, average, or above average) for their 1.5-mile run, push-ups, sit-ups, and waist circumferences.

Name	Claire		Name	Ethan
Gender	Female		Gender	Male
Weight (lb)	167		Weight (lb)	189
Height (in)	62		Height (in)	73
Age (years)	43		Age (years)	22
3-Site Skinfolds (mm)	Triceps – 29 Suprailiac – 24 Thigh – 46		3-Site Skinfolds (mm)	Chest – 13 Abdomen – 28 Thigh – 18
Circumference Measurements (in)	Waist (Umbilical) – 36 Waist (Natural) – 33 Hip – 40 Neck – 12.5		Circumference Measurements (in)	Waist – 34 Hip – 39 Neck – 14.5
1.5 mile run (min:sec)	14:10		1.5 mile run (min:sec)	13:30
Push-Ups	9		Push-Ups	45
Sit-Ups	23		Sit-Ups	52

References

American College of Sports Medicine. *ACSM, AHA support federal physical activity guidelines.* Retrieved from http://www.acsm.org/about-acsm/media-room/acsm-in-the-news/2011/08/01/acsm-aha-support-federal-physical-activity-guidelines

Baechle, T. R., & Earle, R. W. (Eds.). (2008). *Essentials of strength training and conditioning.* (3rd ed.). Champaign, IL: Human Kinetics.

Berardi, J. M. (2006). *The precision nutrition: Body composition guide.* Oakland, CA: Science Link, Inc.

Bryant, C. X., & Green, D. J. (Eds.). (2010). *ACE personal trainer manual: The ultimate resource for fitness professionals* (4th ed.). San Diego, CA: American Council on Exercise.

Command Fitness Leader Certification Course. *Body composition assessment* (S5620612A) [PowerPoint Presentation]. Navy Physical Readiness Program, Millington, TN.

Department of Defense. (2002, November 5). *Physical fitness and body fat programs procedures* (DoDI 1308.3). Retrieved from http://www.dtic.mil/whs/directives/corres/pdf/130803p.pdf

Haff, G., & Triplett, N. (Eds.). (2016). *Essentials of strength training and conditioning.* (4th ed). Champaign, IL: Human Kinetics.

Heaney, J., Hodgdon, J., Beckett, M., & Carter, J. (1998). The technical error of measurement for selected skinfold and circumference measurements. *Medicine & Science in Sports & Exercise, 30*(5), 276–291.

Jones, A. M., & Doust, J. H. (1996). A 1% treadmill grade most accurately reflects the energetic cost of outdoor running. *Journal of Sports Sciences,* 14, 321–327.

MyHealthyWaist.org. *Waist circumference measurement guidelines.* Retrieved from http://www.myhealthywaist.org/evaluating-cmr/clinical-tools/waist-circumference-measurement-guidelines/index.html.

National Heart, Lung and Blood Institute. (1998). *Clinical guidelines on the identification, evaluation, and treatment of overweight and obesity in adults: The evidence report.* Bethesda, MD: National Institutes of Health.

Navy Physical Readiness Program. (2016a). *Guide 4: The body composition assessment (BCA).* Retrieved from http://www.public.navy.mil/bupers-npc/support/21st_Century_Sailor/physical/Documents/Guide%204-%20Body%20Composition%20Assessment%20(BCA)%202016.pdf.

Navy Physical Readiness Program. (2016b). *Guide 5: Physical readiness test (PRT).* Retrieved from http://www.public.navy.mil/bupers-npc/support/21st_Century_Sailor/physical/Documents/Guide%205-%20Physical%20Readiness%20Test%20%202016.pdf.

Peterson, D. (2015a). History of the U.S. navy body composition program. *Military Medicine, 180*(1), 91–96.

Peterson, D. (2015b). The navy physical fitness test: A proposed revision to the navy physical readiness test. *Strength and Conditioning Journal, 37*(4), 60–68.

Pollock, M. L., Schmidt, D. H., & Jackson, A. S. (1980). Measurement of cardiorespiratory fitness and body composition in the clinical setting. *Comprehensive Therapy, 6*(9), 12–27.

United States Air Force. (2013, October 21). *Fitness program* (Air force instruction 36-2905). Retrieved from http://www.afpc.af.mil/shared/media/document/AFD-131018-072.pdf.

United States Army. (1998, October 1). *Physical fitness training* (Field manual 21-20). Retrieved from http://www1.udel.edu/armyrotc/current_cadets/cadet_resources/manuals_regulations_files/FM%2021-20%20-%20Physical%20Fitness%20Training.pdf.

United States Marine Corps. (2016, July 1). *Changes to the physical fitness test (PFT), combat fitness test (CFT), and body composition program* (ALMAR 022/16). Retrieved from https://fitness.usmc.mil/SitePages/almar.aspx.

United States Navy. (2011, July 11). *Physical readiness program* (OPNAVINST 6110.1J). Retrieved from http://www.usnavy.vt.edu/documents/6110.1H.pdf.

United States Navy. (2015, August 3). *Physical readiness program policy changes* (NAVADMIN 178/15). Retrieved from http://www.public.navy.mil/bupers-npc/reference/messages/Documents/NAVADMINS/NAV2015/NAV15178.txt.

United States Navy. (2016, March 9). *Physical readiness program policy changes* (NAVADMIN 061/16). Retrieved from http://www.public.navy.mil/bupers-npc/reference/messages/Documents/NAVADMINS/NAV2016/NAV16061.txt.

United States Navy. (2017, June 20). *Physical readiness program policy changes* (NAVADMIN 141/17). http://www.public.navy.mil/bupers-npc/reference/messages/Documents/NAVADMINS/NAV2017/NAV17141.txt.

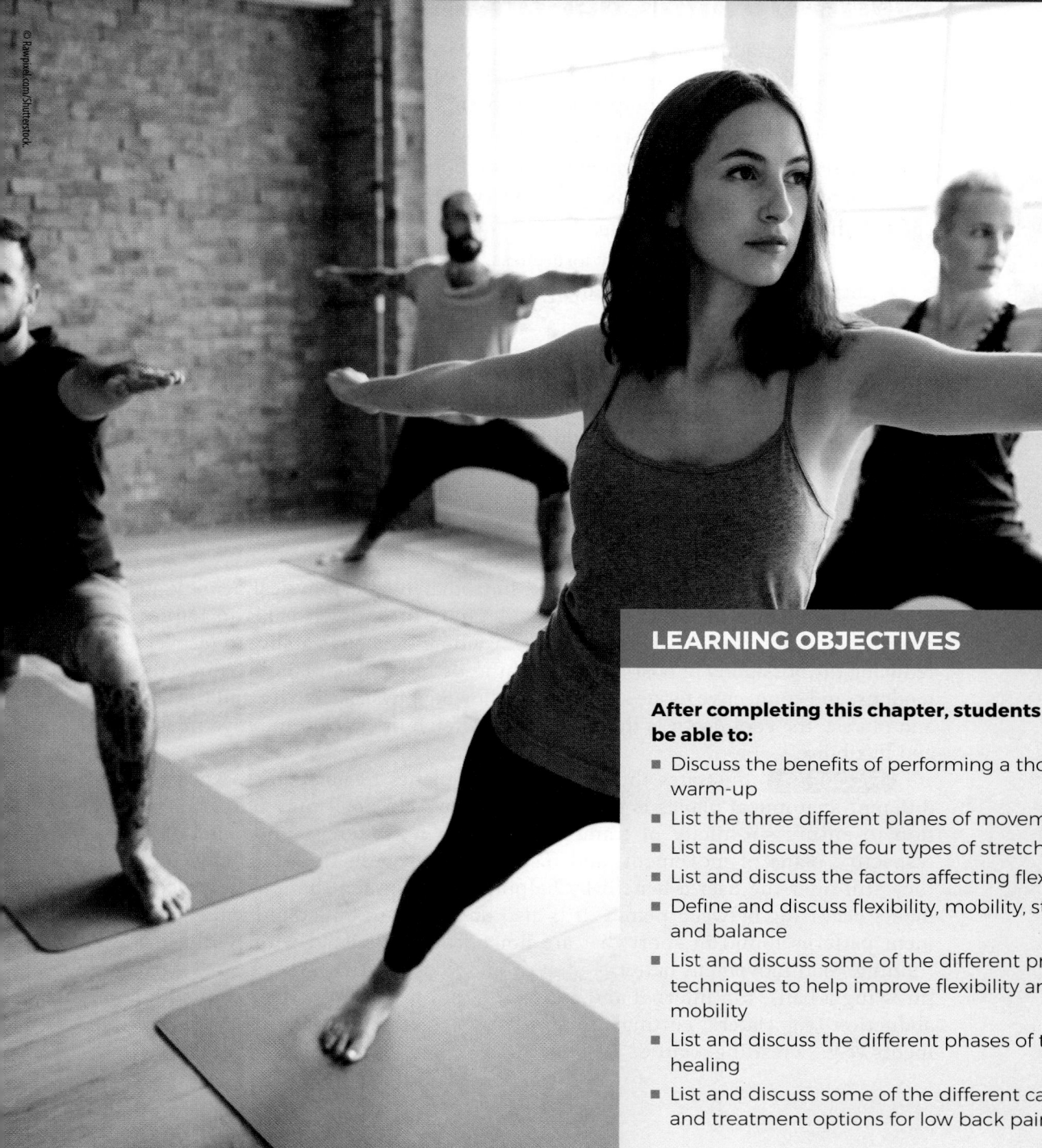

Mobility Training and Low Back Pain

© Rawpixel.com/Shutterstock.

LEARNING OBJECTIVES

After completing this chapter, students should be able to:

- Discuss the benefits of performing a thorough warm-up
- List the three different planes of movement
- List and discuss the four types of stretching
- List and discuss the factors affecting flexibility
- Define and discuss flexibility, mobility, stability, and balance
- List and discuss some of the different prehab techniques to help improve flexibility and mobility
- List and discuss the different phases of tissue healing
- List and discuss some of the different causes of and treatment options for low back pain

Introduction

All athletes, regardless of age or ability, should perform a thorough warm-up prior to physical activity and complete a cool-down afterwards. The purpose of the warm-up is to increase heart rate and blood flow, which subsequently increases muscle temperature, thereby improving muscle elasticity and plasticity. Collectively, this increases the range of motion and decreases the risk of injury. Generally speaking, static stretches are not recommended as part of a warm-up (since this relaxes the muscles) unless the sport or exercise requires an extensive amount of flexibility to be successful (e.g., gymnastics, cheerleading).

Warm-Up and Cool-Down

Warm-up: Gradual increase in exercise intensity intended to prepare the body for the more intense and demanding activity to follow.

Cool-down: Easy exercise completed immediately after more intense activity to allow the body to gradually transition to a resting or near-resting state.

Venous return: Rate of blood flow back to the heart.

A **warm-up** is a gradual increase in exercise intensity intended to prepare the body for the more intense and demanding activity to follow. Performing a thorough warm-up prior to participation in training or competition has been shown to:

- Increase joint flexibility and mobility
- Increase force development and reaction time
- Increase blood flow and oxygen delivery to muscles and connective tissue
- Enhance metabolic reactions
- Increase coordination, body awareness, and reaction time
- Increase muscular strength and power
- Reduce the risk of injury
- Reduce post-exercise muscle soreness

A proper warm-up should begin with gentle range-of-motion exercises and then gradually progress to more dynamic movements. Jumping, bounding, or plyometric movements should be performed last. Additionally, exercises that include movements for all three movement planes should be incorporated. This specifically includes the following:

- Sagittal (forward and back; e.g., back squat)
- Frontal / Coronal (side to side; e.g., lateral shoulder raise)
- Transverse (rotational; e.g., golf swing)

The **cool-down** should be performed immediately after physical activity and involve a gradual reduction in exercise intensity. A proper cool-down helps to improve **venous return** (blood flow back to the heart) thereby aiding the body's ability to recover as well as reducing the possibility of post-exercise lightheadedness and/or fainting. Since the muscles, tendons, and connective tissue are warmer following physical activity, and thus more elastic and pliable, the cool-down is the best time to stretch in order to improve range of motion and flexibility.

FIGURE 3.1 illustrates the three different planes of movement. Knowledge of the different anatomical planes is useful since it can help determine proper exercise selection to ensure specificity of training. Although few exercises operate solely in their respective plane of movement, and instead overlap with the other movement planes, they still offer the user a benefit by helping to strengthen the muscles used for movements occurring between planes. It is also important to target and train specific movement patterns found in sport that are not normally targeted with traditional strength training. Said movement patterns include shoulder internal and external rotation (e.g., throwing a ball), hip internal and external rotation (e.g., pivoting), hip adduction and abduction (e.g., lateral cutting), torso rotation (e.g., batting), and various neck movements (e.g., wrestling; Haff & Triplett, 2016).

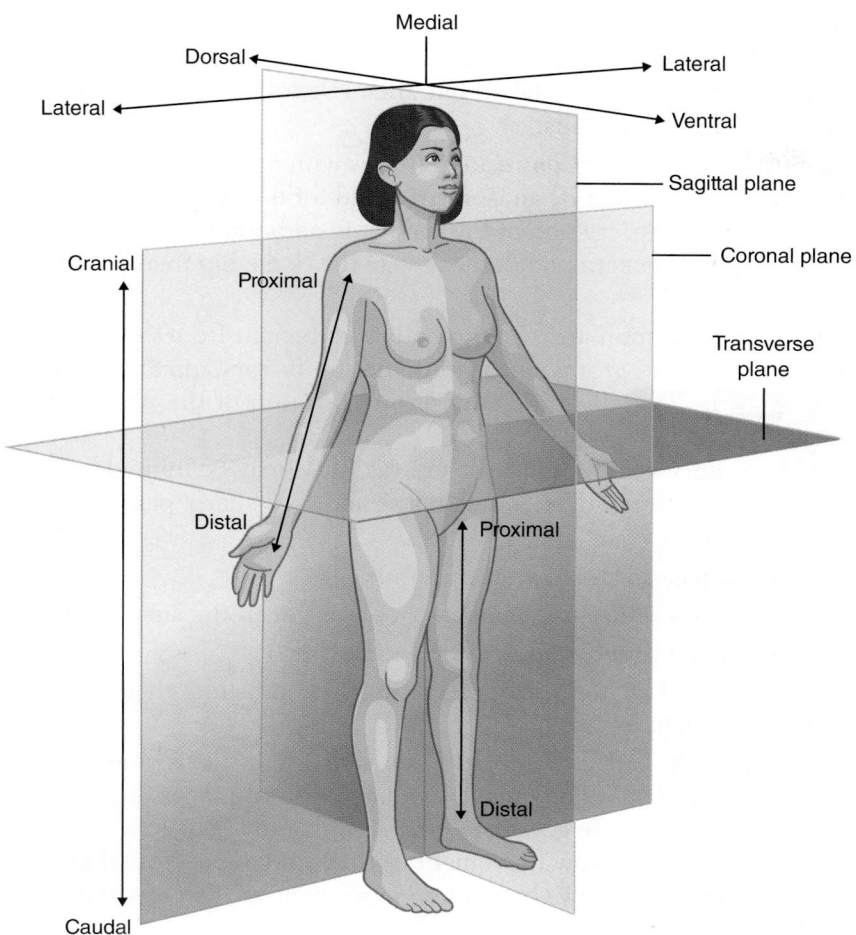

FIGURE 3.1 Planes of Movement

Stretching Types and Guidelines

There are four basic types of stretches: static, ballistic, dynamic (aka mobility drills), and proprioceptive neuromuscular facilitation (PNF). A brief description of each type of stretch is provided in this section.

- *Static:* Stretching that uses a slow and constant stretch with the end position being held for at least 30 seconds.
- *Ballistic:* Stretching that incorporates a bouncing type movement to an unheld end position. Because the muscle is stretched quickly, ballistic stretching causes the muscle to tighten (aka **stretch reflex**) instead of relax, which is counterproductive to the purpose of stretching. This type of stretching greatly increases the risk of injury and is not recommended.
- *Dynamic (aka Mobility Drills):* Stretching that uses sport-specific movements to prepare the muscles and connective tissue for physical activity.
- *Proprioceptive Neuromuscular Facilitation (PNF):* Stretching that uses a partner and involves both passive movement and active muscle actions (both concentric and isometric). There are three basic types of PNF stretching techniques:
  - *Hold-relax:* Begins with a passive pre-stretch that is held for 10 seconds followed by an isometric hold for 6 seconds. Athlete then relaxes and this is followed by a passive stretch for 30 seconds.

Stretch reflex: A muscle contraction in response to stretching, which provides automatic regulation of skeletal muscle length.

Pre-stretch: To extend a limb or body part to its full length or range of motion.

Concentric contraction: A type of muscle activation that increases tension on a muscle as it shortens.

- *Contract-relax:* Begins with a passive **pre-stretch** that is held for 10 seconds followed by **concentric contraction** against partner resistance through the full range of motion (ROM). The athlete then relaxes and this is followed by a passive stretch for 30 seconds.

- *Hold-relax with Agonist Contraction:* Begins with a passive pre-stretch that is held for 10 seconds followed by an isometric hold for 6 seconds. The individual then performs a concentric action of the agonist in addition to a passive stretch. In other words, after the isometric hold, the athlete flexes the hip thereby facilitating a new/ farther ROM.

Some of the more common areas of the body that benefit from PNF stretching include the calves and ankles, chest, groin, hamstrings and hip flexors, quadriceps and hip flexors, and shoulders. **FIGURE 3.2** illustrates the proper position of the partner and athlete for the PNF hamstring stretch.

Be sure not to bounce or force a movement (as ROM may be limited by joint structure) when stretching. Stop stretching if you experience any sharp pains. Stretching is not recommended when:

- The individual has sustained a recent injury
- The individual has acute inflammation in a joint or in the surrounding tissue
- The individual is within 8–12 weeks post fracture

There are a number of anatomical and training-related factors that can affect flexibility. Some of these factors include:

Elasticity: Ability of connective tissue to return to its original length after a passive stretch.

Plasticity: Ability of connective tissue to assume a new or greater length after a passive stretch.

- *Joint Structure:* The type of joint determines its ROM. For example, ball-and-socket joints (e.g., hip and shoulder) move in all anatomical planes and have the greatest ROM. Ellipsoidal joints (e.g., wrist) have significantly less ROM than ball-and-socket joints and only allow movement in the sagittal and frontal planes. Hinge joints (e.g., knee and elbow) only allow movement in the sagittal plane and have the least amount of ROM.

- *Connective Tissue:* The **elasticity** (ability to return to resting length) and **plasticity** (ability to assume a new or greater length) of tendons, ligaments, fascial sheaths,

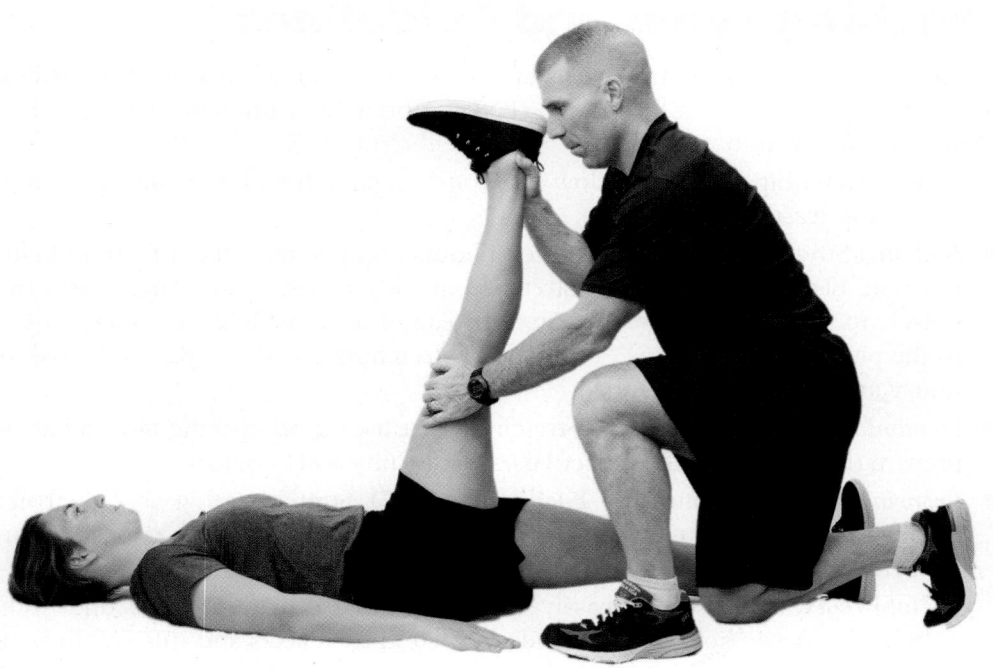

FIGURE 3.2 Proper Positioning for PNF Hamstring Stretch

joint capsules, and skin can affect available ROM. The amount of elasticity and plasticity of the connective tissue can vary greatly between individuals thereby making some more or less flexible than others. Regularly performing stretching exercises can positively influence connective tissue by taking advantage of its plastic potential.

- *Neural Control:* An individual's range of motion is controlled to a large degree by his or her central nervous system (CNS), both via afferent (carrying impulses towards the CNS) and efferent (carrying impulses away from the CNS) mechanisms. These pathways influence the ultimate ROM that the individual is able to attain. Stretching regularly can positively affect the CNS thereby allowing for elicitation of a greater ROM.

- *Gender:* Females tend to be more flexible than males. Differences are most likely due to the structural and anatomical differences between females and males.

- *Age:* Young individuals tend to be more flexible than older individuals. This is likely due to inactivity, reduced ROM in daily activities, as well as **fibrosis** (a process in which fibrous connective tissue replaces degenerating muscle fibers). **FIGURE 3.3** depicts the development of fibrosis (as well as sarcopenia) associated with the aging process (Al-Masri & Bartlett, 2011; Health-Innovations.org, 2015).

> **Fibrosis:** Process in which fibrous connective tissue starts to replace degenerating muscle fibers.

- *Activity Level:* Active individuals tend to be more flexible than sedentary individuals. However, activity alone does not improve flexibility; rather it only improves if the activity involves regular participation in stretching exercises and movements requiring full ROM.

- *Resistance Training with Limited ROM:* Although performing strength training exercises through the full ROM has been shown to actually increase flexibility, heavy resistance training with limited ROM can decrease ROM.

- *Excessive Muscular Bulk:* Large increases in muscle bulk may adversely affect ROM by impeding joint movement. However, the need for large muscles may supersede the need for flexibility in some sports (e.g., bodybuilding).

The American College of Sports Medicine (ACSM) provides the following guidelines for stretching:

- *Frequency:* ≥ 3 days per week
- *Intensity:* Held to a position of mild discomfort

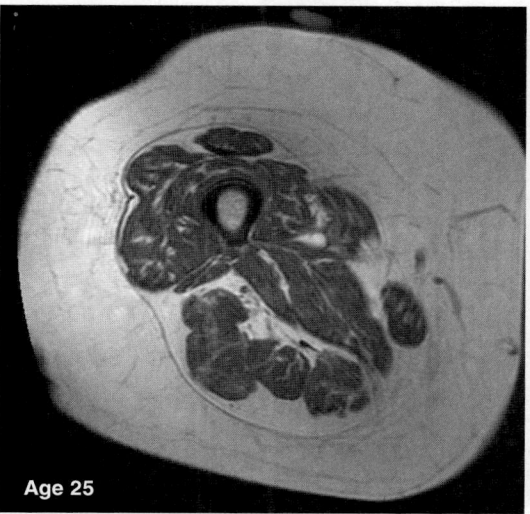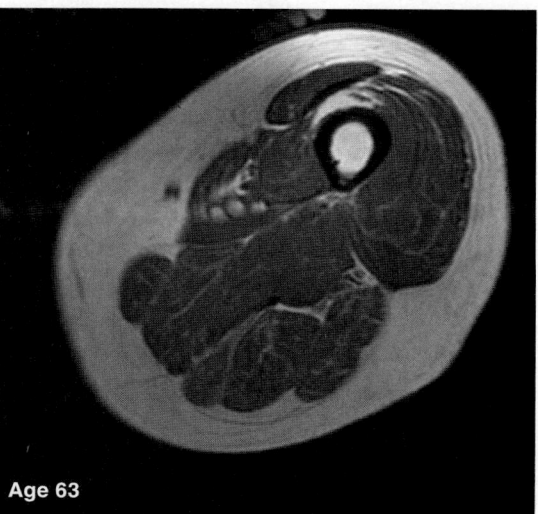

Age 25   Age 63

FIGURE 3.3 Age-Related Loss of Skeletal Muscle Mass

Courtesy of Maria A. Flatarone Singh.

- *Duration:* 10-30 seconds per stretch
- *Repetitions:* 3-5 per stretch
- *Type:* Static

Although holding a stretch for 10–30 seconds is a great start, it is recommended that individuals gradually increase the hold duration over time (e.g., 60 seconds or longer). Current research supports the idea that holding a stretch for 60 seconds is more effective in improving flexibility than either 15- or 30-second holds. Additionally, stretching must be continued over time in order to maintain the benefits.

Dr. Kelly Starrett, a physical therapist, renowned strength and conditioning coach, and author of *Becoming a Supple Leopard*, recommends spending no less than two minutes in each position or until there's noticeable improvement or the realization that there's no additional improvement to be made. In some cases, this may mean spending two minutes or up to 10 minutes in each position.

A sufficient hold duration is necessary in order to stimulate the Golgi tendon organ and allow the muscle to relax. As previously discussed, some fitness experts believe poor flexibility is more of a factor of CNS inhibition than muscle fiber length. Regardless, living an active lifestyle, exercising regularly, and including warm-up exercises before and stretching after each workout is the best way to improve one's flexibility and mobility. **TABLE 3.1** provides 14 popular stretches that can be used to help improve total body flexibility and mobility.

TABLE 3.1 Sample of Recommended Stretches

Sample Stretches

Neck		
Chest	Upper Back	
Triceps	Shoulder	
Quadriceps	Groin	

(continues)

TABLE 3.1 Sample of Recommended Stretches *(continued)*

Sample Stretches

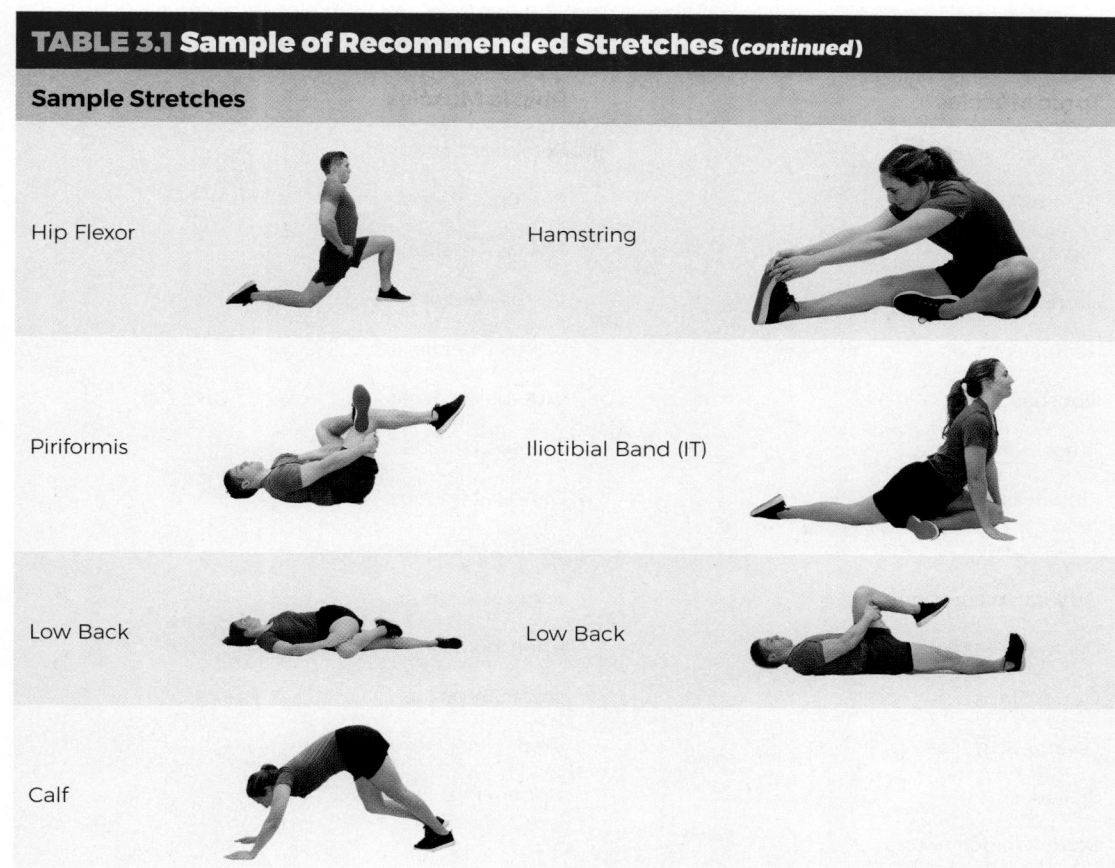

Hip Flexor	Hamstring
Piriformis	Iliotibial Band (IT)
Low Back	Low Back
Calf	

Tonic and Phasic Muscles

Dr. Vladimir Janda, world-renowned physical therapist and researcher, has identified common muscle imbalance syndromes as the leading cause of most back, neck, shoulder, hip, and knee pain. These syndromes lead to specific patterns of tightness and weakness that tend to compromise joint function. Dr. Janda classifies muscles into two basic types (i.e., tonic and phasic) based on function. **Tonic muscles** are primarily flexors and tend to get tighter with age. **Phasic muscles** are primarily extensors and tend to get weaker with age. To correct these syndromes, Dr. Janda recommends regular flexibility training to lengthen the tonic muscles and regular resistance training to strengthen the phasic muscles. **TABLE 3.2** on the next page lists the various tonic and phasic muscles (Prevost, 2015).

Flexibility, Mobility, Stability, and Balance

Flexibility is defined as the ability of a joint to move freely through its entire ROM. **Mobility** is defined as the freedom of a limb to move unhindered through a desired ROM. Individuals with good mobility are able to perform functional movement patterns throughout their entire ROM without restriction. However, individuals with good flexibility may or may not have the core strength, balance, or coordination necessary to perform functional movements properly. **Stability** is defined as the ability to return to a desired position following a disturbance. **Balance** is defined as the ability to maintain static and dynamic equilibrium; in other words, the ability to maintain the body's center of gravity over its base of support. Individuals with poor stability and balance are at a greater risk of falls and lower body injuries. Some of the benefits associated with regular flexibility, mobility, stability, and

Tonic muscles: Flexor muscles that tend to get tighter with age.

Phasic muscles: Extensor muscles that tend to get weaker with age.

Flexibility: Range of motion of the joints or the ability of the joints to move freely through their entire range of motion.

Mobility: Degree to which a joint is allowed to move before being restricted by surrounding tissue.

Stability: Ability to maintain or control joint movement or position.

Balance: The ability to stay upright or stay in control of body movement; coordination is the ability to move two or more body parts under control, smoothly and efficiently. There are two types of balance: static and dynamic.

TABLE 3.2 List of Tonic and Phasic Muscles

Tonic Muscles	Phasic Muscles
Gastroc-Soleus	Peroneus Longus
Tibialis Posterior	Peroneus Brevis
Hip Adductors	Tibialis Anterior
Hamstrings	Vastus Medialis
Rectus Femoris	Vastus Lateralis
Iliopsoas	Gluteus Maximus
Tensor Fascia Lata	Gluteus Medius
Piriformis	Gluteus Minimus
Thoraco-Lumbar Extensors	Rectus Abdominus
Quadratus Lumborum	Serratus Anterior
Pectoralis Major	Rhomboids
Upper Trapezius	Lower Trapezius
Levator Scapulae	Deep Neck Flexors
Scalenes	Upper Limb Extensors
Sternocleidomastoid	-
Upper Limb Flexors	-

balance training include a reduced risk of injuries and low back pain, increased ROM and posture, as well as improved balance.

In addition to stretching there are several other exercises and activities that can be performed to help improve flexibility and mobility. For example 10 to 15 minutes of **prehab** prior to activity can significantly improve range of motion, athletic performance, and reduce the risk of injury. The three basic principles of prehab include the following:

- *Soft-tissue Work:* Using a foam roller or lacrosse ball will help to break up scar tissue and adhesions (aka knots) within the muscle tissue.
- *Dynamic Stretching:* Using a variety of dynamic stretches before beginning an activity will help effectively warm-up the muscles and improve an individual's mobility and range of motion.
- *Movement-specific Activation:* Using a variety of strength training exercises to turn on and activate the specific muscles that will be used in the upcoming activity.

It is sometimes difficult to identify the exact source/cause of restricted ROM and/or pain. For example, low back pain while running long distances may be caused by tight hamstrings. Often, pain felt in one part of the body is the result of an underlying problem located somewhere else; this phenomenon is known as **referred pain**. Referred pain can occur above or below the affected area or on the opposite side of the body. Therefore, regular prehab work should be performed on all muscle groups above and below the affected area as well as on both sides of the body.

One of the common mistakes made with prehab and rehab conditioning is to stop altogether once significant ROM improvements are made and/or the pain starts to subside. Unfortunately, this approach almost guarantees similar issues in the future. Significant losses in flexibility can occur within as little as 7 ± 2 days. Therefore, it is imperative

Prehab: Series of exercises and activities that, if performed regularly, will help to improve athletic performance and reduce the risk of injury.

Referred pain: Pain that is felt in a part of the body other than its actual source.

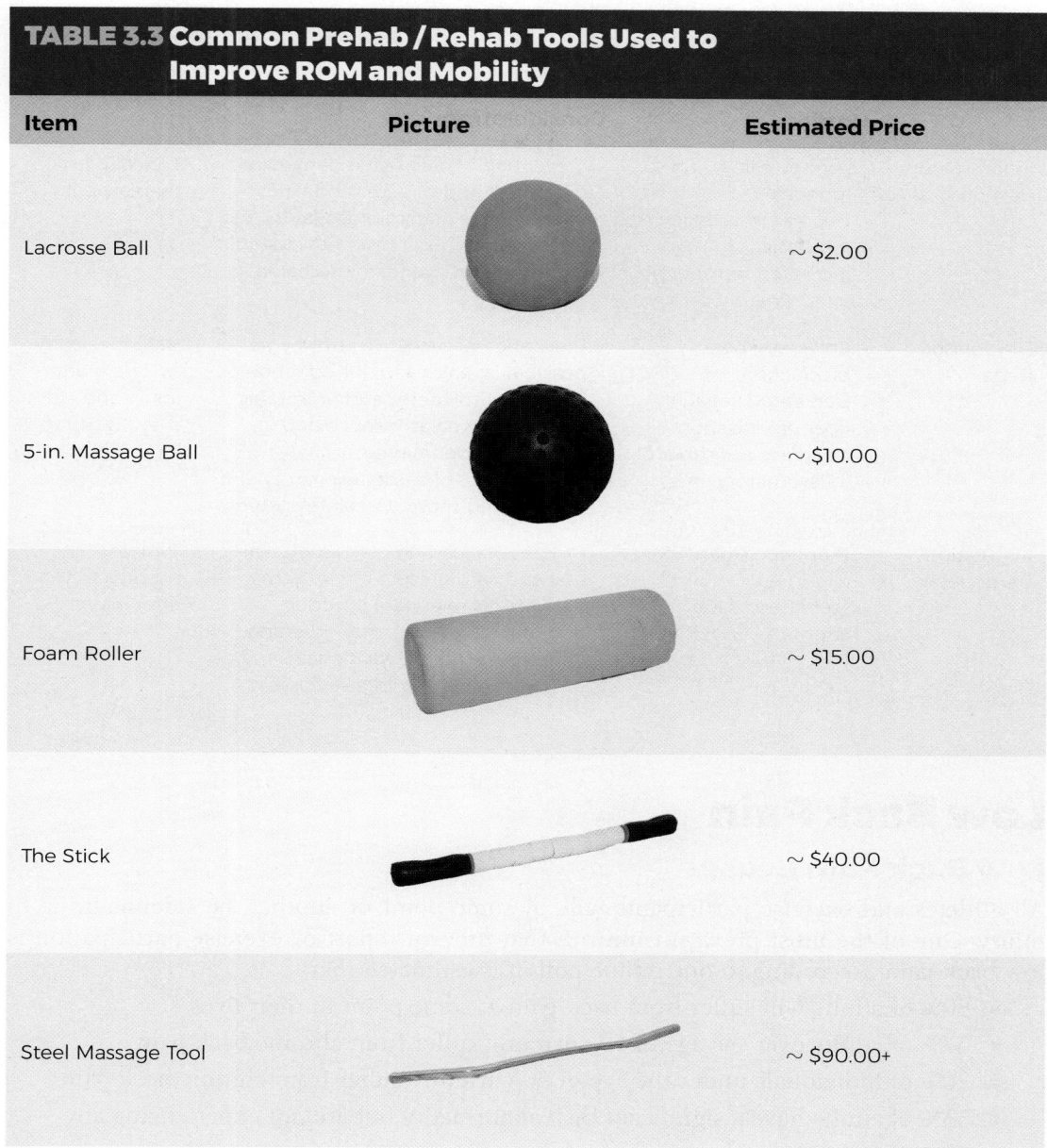

Item	Picture	Estimated Price
Lacrosse Ball		~ $2.00
5-in. Massage Ball		~ $10.00
Foam Roller		~ $15.00
The Stick		~ $40.00
Steel Massage Tool		~ $90.00+

TABLE 3.3 Common Prehab / Rehab Tools Used to Improve ROM and Mobility

to continue regular stretching and prehab work in order to maintain any gains made in function and ROM and prevent detraining.

TABLE 3.3 lists several prehab/rehab tools commonly used to help improve ROM and reduce the risk of injury. In some cases, and depending on location, frequent massage work may help to prevent the onset and/or reduce the extent of **crepitus**, the grinding, cracking, or popping sound that occurs when moving a joint.

Tissue Healing

TABLE 3.4 on the next page describes the process of healing following an injury as well as the training recommendations and considerations that should be followed during the rehabilitation and reconditioning process (Baechle & Earle, 2008; Haff & Triplett, 2016). The timing of these events differs for each type of tissue (e.g., muscle, tendon, ligament, cartilage) and is influenced by a variety of factors including age, previous physical activity, and extent of injury. It is important not to overstress healing tissue; specific criteria must be met in order to safely progress from one healing phase to the next.

Crepitus: Any grinding, creaking, cracking, grating, crunching, or popping sound that occurs when moving a joint.

TABLE 3.4 Different Phases of Tissue Healing

Phase	Characteristics of Healing	Training Recommendations / Considerations	Timeframe
Inflammatory Response	· Pain, swelling, and redness · Decreased collagen synthesis · Increased number of inflammatory cells	· Prevention of new tissue damage via use of rest and passive modalities · Maintenance of cardiorespiratory and surrounding musculoskeletal systems · No active exercise for injured area	Typically less than a week
Fibroblastic Repair	· Collagen fiber production · Decreased collagen fiber organization · Decreased number of inflammatory cells	· Prevention of excessive atrophy via possible (as tolerated) introduction of isometric, isokinetic, and/or isotonic exercise as well as balance and proprioceptive training · Maintenance of cardiorespiratory and surrounding musculoskeletal systems	Begins as early as 2 days after injury and may last up to 2 months
Maturation-Remodeling	· Proper collagen fiber alignment · Increased tissue strength	· Progressive loading of musculoskeletal and cardiorespiratory systems · Possible (as tolerated) introduction of joint-specific strengthening, closed and open kinetic chain, and/or proprioceptive training exercises	Can last months to years after injury

Low Back Pain

Low Back Pain Causes

All athletes and exercise participants will, at some point or another, be sidelined due to injury. One of the most prevalent injuries that prevents sport or exercise participation is low back pain. According to one online poll, it is estimated that:

- 80% of adults will suffer from back pain at some point in their lives
- 57% of adults over the age of 60 currently suffer from chronic back pain
- 20% of individuals under the age of 60 currently suffer from chronic back pain
- 33% of adults have a significant disk abnormality but are not experiencing any pain or symptoms

So how are we to interpret those statistics? In essence, the question is not if we will experience low back pain but when. Low back pain can be a result of or caused by many factors. Ironically, low back pain can be a result of too much activity or not enough. Some of the prominent causes of low back pain include the following:

- Herniated disks
- Spinal stenosis
- Piriformis syndrome
- Arthritis

What we do or don't do can either help prevent low back pain or make it more prevalent. For example, some of the common agitators of low back pain include:

- Prolonged sitting / standing
- Certain sleeping positions (e.g., on your stomach)
- Poor posture
- Certain strength training exercises (e.g., back squat)

As previously mentioned, certain strength training exercises can, in some cases, increase the risk of low back pain or injury. These include exercises that directly place a load on the spine like the back squat, deadlift, and power clean. Additionally, exercises that place a significant amount of compression and shear force on the intervertebral disks can also increase the prevalence of low back pain and/or the risk of injury – especially with the use of heavy weight and/or if the exercise is performed improperly.

Although it would be unfair to simply classify these exercises as dangerous and discourage their use entirely, it is important to recognize that they do pose a slightly greater risk of injury and/or prevalence for low back pain. For individuals who suffer from chronic low back pain, it may be worth considering either using an alternate strength training exercise or modifying certain exercises in order to reduce the risk of injury and low back aggravation.

For example, instead of the back squat, individuals suffering from chronic low back pain could employ front squats, Bulgarian split squats, lying leg press, and/or dumbbell lunges instead. Additionally, individuals with chronic low back pain could deadlift using a trap bar with the weight elevated instead of deadlifting from the floor with a conventional straight bar. Similarly, individuals with chronic low back pain could perform exercises that provide better low back support and avoid high risk phases of movement such as hang cleans instead of power cleans.

Posture

Another predominant agitator of low back pain is poor posture. It makes sense that keeping the spine in a flexed or overextended position (whether sitting, standing, texting) for a prolonged period of time will eventually lead to or exacerbate low back pain. **FIGURE 3.4** below illustrates the differences between a neutral, flexed, and overextended spine.

So how can we identify and correct for poor posture? Dr. Kelly Starrett recommends the two-hand rule and belly-whack test (Starrett & Cordoza, 2015).

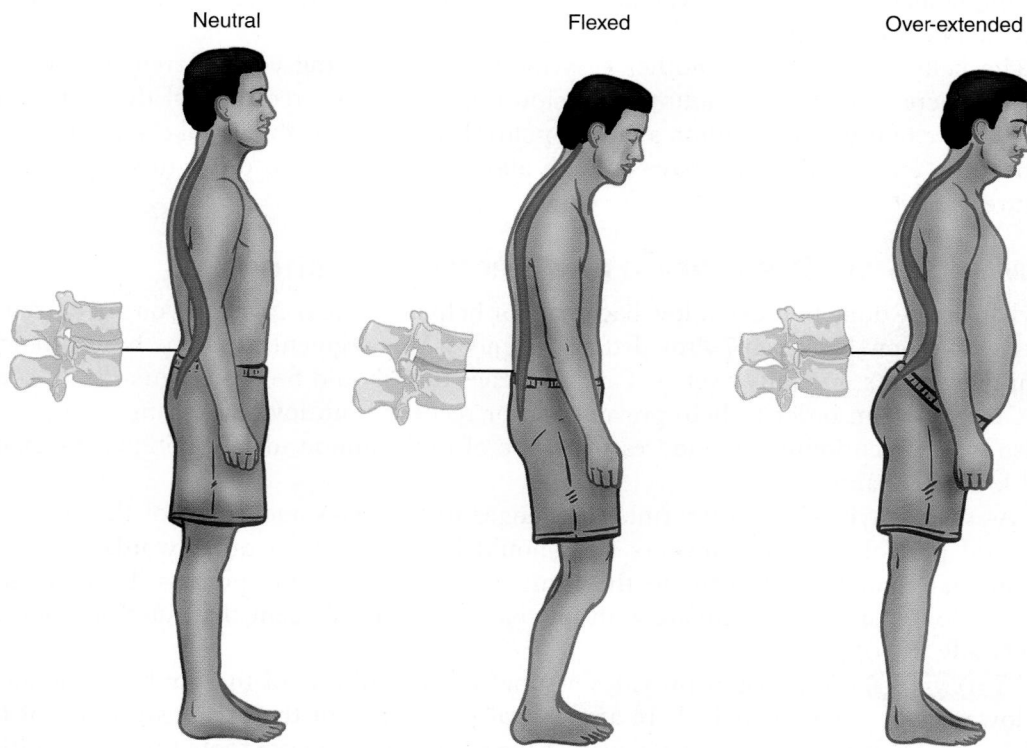

Neutral   Flexed   Over-extended

FIGURE 3.4 Neutral Spinal Position and Common Spinal Faults

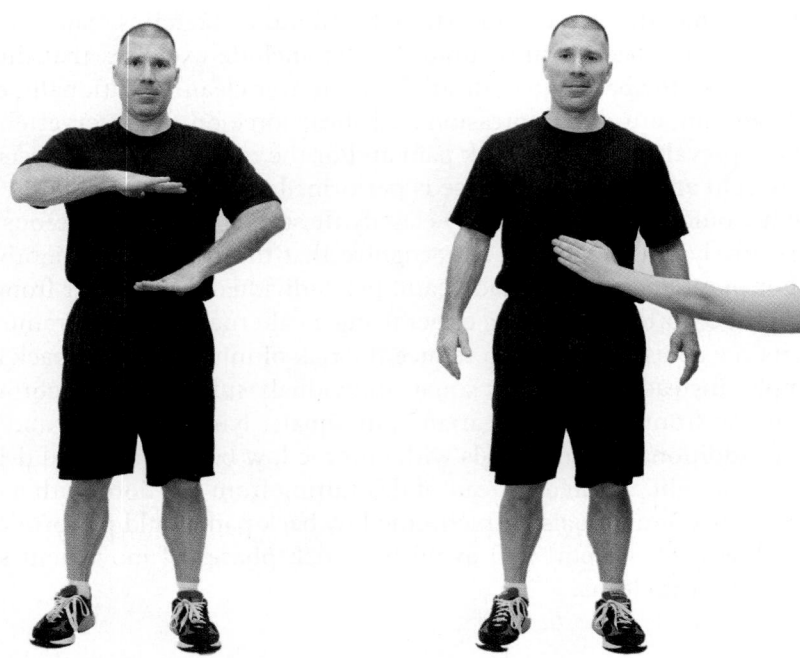

FIGURE 3.5 Two-Hand Rule and Belly-Whack Test

To perform the two-hand rule, place one thumb on the xiphoid process (sternum) and the other thumb on the iliac crest (top of the pelvis) with the fingers splayed and palms facing down and parallel with the floor. When the spine is in a neutral position, both hands are parallel, as shown in **FIGURE 3.5**. When the spine is flexed, the hands move closer together. When the spine is overextended, the hands move farther apart. The two-hand rule is a simple method of raising awareness to the current position of your spine and making adjustments as necessary.

The belly-whack test is another easy method of assessing your current posture. In essence, there is a certain amount of tension (albeit modest) required of the abdominal musculature in order to maintain a braced neutral spine. Being able to take a quick whack to the belly ensures that you have enough abdominal tension in order to support good posture.

Low Back Pain Prevention and Recovery Techniques

So what can be done to prevent low back pain or help facilitate recovery if you are currently experiencing low back pain? Provided at the end of this segment are some basic strength training exercises, mobility exercises and stretches that should be done regularly (in some cases everyday) in order to help prevent and/or recover from low back pain. However, it is also worth mentioning and addressing some of the common misperceptions associated with low back pain.

As with graying hair and wrinkles, changes to the disks and bones of the spine are a natural part of the aging process and should be expected. In other words, there are incremental changes that occur to the spine as part of the aging process. Even so, said changes do not necessarily equate with low back pain or represent the cause of low back pain (Cady, 2016).

FIGURE 3.6 on the right provides a superior view of one of the lumbar vertebra of the lower spine. As depicted, there are several places within the boney structure of the vertebra that could be compressing against the spine and/or nerve roots thereby resulting in pain (e.g., thickening of the pedicle, lamina, and/or hypertrophy of the facet joints).

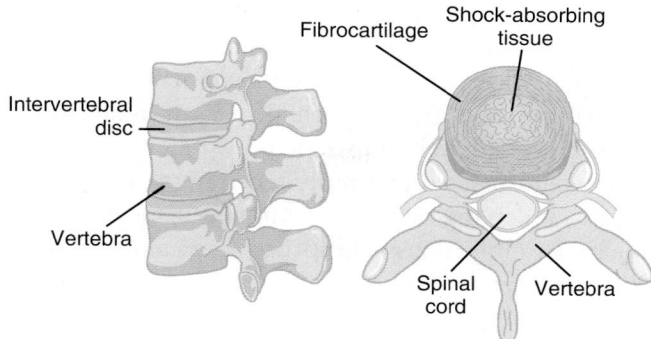

FIGURE 3.6 Anatomy of a Vertebra

All of these adaptations can possibly be the result of regular participation in strength training. In other words, said adaptations in and of themselves are not necessarily bad, but when combined with age-related disk abnormalities may result in acute and/or chronic low back pain.

According to current research, almost all adults have some form of "spinal abnormality" (Cady, 2016). That said, just because you have a spinal abnormality does not guarantee that you will have low back pain. Similarly, it is also possible to have low back pain without a documented spinal abnormality (as seen on a **magnetic resonance imaging (MRI)**).

So what does that mean? In essence, we cannot rely solely on MRI results to determine whether or not we should have low back pain. In fact, MRI findings can sometimes persuade both the patient and physician into believing that these so-called "abnormalities" are responsible for low back pain when in fact they are not. **FIGURE 3.7** shows the relationship between age and the percentage of individuals *with no back pain* but who have a documented disk abnormality as depicted on an MRI.

It is also important to remember that although MRI results provide an extremely detailed picture of the disks and bones of the spine, they are not without their limitations. For example, MRI pictures are taken while the patient is lying down; however, the patient's pain may only occur when he or she is sitting or performing certain movements. In other words, the underlying cause of the pain may not be detected by the MRI while the patient is lying down. Additionally, and in most cases, back pain will resolve on its own within a couple of weeks. So seeking invasive treatment options (e.g., **corticosteroid injections**, surgery) immediately upon the onset of low back pain may not be necessary.

Magnetic resonance imaging (MRI): A procedure that uses magnetism, radio waves, and a computer to create pictures from inside the body.

Corticosteriod injection: A shot used to provide short-term pain relief and reduce swelling and inflammation in a joint, tendon, or bursa.

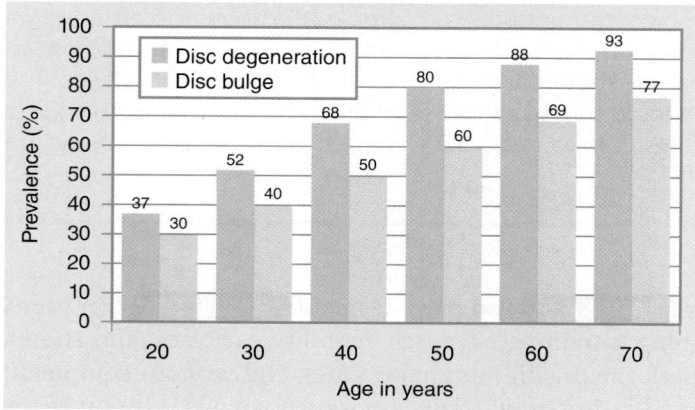

FIGURE 3.7 Percentage of Patients with Documented Disc Abnormalities but no Symptoms

Data from Cady, M. (2016). Paindemic: A practical and holistic look at chronic pain, the medical system, and the anti-pain lifestyle. New York, NY: Morgan James Publishing.

Individuals may want to consider more invasive options when they have associated pain, numbness, or weakness in the same nerve-related pathway as indicated by the disk abnormality on the MRI. If there is only back pain but no associated weakness, pain, numbness, or reflex changes, the disk abnormality is unlikely to be causing a serious problem (Cady, 2016). Unfortunately, most people prefer to have something done to formally treat their back pain instead of simply receiving reassurance that it will get better on its own. Ironically, receiving verbal reassurance instead of unnecessary MRIs and treatments could save them a lot in terms of future medical costs and pain. Instead, most of what patients should and can be doing to address or prevent lowback pain is independent of their actual MRI results.

Low Back Strength Training, Mobility Exercises, and Stretches

Although most physicians may recommend waiting a few weeks before scheduling an MRI or treatment options to see if the patient's back pain will resolve on its own, very few, if any, recommend remaining completely sedentary in the interim.

For example, Dr. Kelly Starrett recommends that individuals get up and stand every 10-15 minutes in order to avoid the negative health effects of prolonged sitting. Additionally, he recommends four minutes of mobility work for every 30 minutes of continuous sitting. When frequent mobility work is not an option (e.g., long car rides), Dr. Starrett recommends using some kind of lumbar support that will help give support and keep the low back in a better position (Starrett & Cordoza, 2015).

In terms of back pain recovery and prevention, getting up and performing regular movement is paramount. Movement helps to loosen the muscles, prevent unnecessary loss of ROM, as well as bring blood and nutrients to the area to help facilitate healing. Although the exact recommendations for exercise type, frequency, volume, and intensity will likely differ for individuals suffering from acute vice chronic back pain, in both instances individuals are encouraged to regularly perform a variety of strength training exercises, mobility exercises, and stretches.

FAQ

Should physical activity recommendations change based on profession?

Research suggests that remaining sedentary for long periods every day can be detrimental to your health. So how much physical activity is required to offset the harmful effects of sitting? A recent study found that using a ratio to determine physical activity recommendations may be better than implementing a fixed number of minutes per week (Ekelund et al., 2016). For example, individuals who sit for 8 hours a day should exercise at least 1 hour per day. Individuals who sit for 6 hours a day should exercise for at least 30 minutes per day. The study also found that exercise doesn't have to be performed all at once, or rigorously, in order to be effective.

TABLE 3.5, **TABLE 3.6** (on page 74), and **TABLE 3.7** (on page 75) provide some basic low back strength training exercises, mobility exercises, and stretches. These simple exercises can be performed with minimal training and without equipment. These exercises should be performed at least once daily (more if tolerated). If you frequently suffer from low back pain and/or are suffering from low back pain currently, it is important not to be overly aggressive when performing these exercises as doing so may lead to the worsening of

TABLE 3.5 Sample Low Back Strength Training Exercises

Low Back Strength Training Exercises

	Beginner	Intermediate / Advanced
Plank		
Plank Runners		
Side Planks		
Glute Bridges		
Bird Dogs		

pain and/or symptoms. Instead, perform a low-intensity warm-up (e.g., slow walk, stationary bike, elliptical trainer) for 10–15 minutes, followed by 3–5 strength training exercises, followed by 3–5 mobility exercises for 2–5 minutes each, followed by 3–5 stretches for 30–90 seconds (or longer as tolerated). Eventually (e.g., few days to weeks), the pain should begin to lessen or subside completely.

Ironically, individuals often reduce the frequency of performing these exercises and stretches, or stop them altogether, as they begin to feel better. Obviously, this is not recommended. The unfortunate reality with low back pain relief is that it is transient and reversible. If regular strength training and mobility work are not performed, the benefits of and results from this training will slowly start to diminish and eventually dissipate altogether over time.

TABLE 3.6 Sample Low Back and Hip Mobility Exercises

Low Back and Hip Mobility Exercises

Cow to Cat Pose	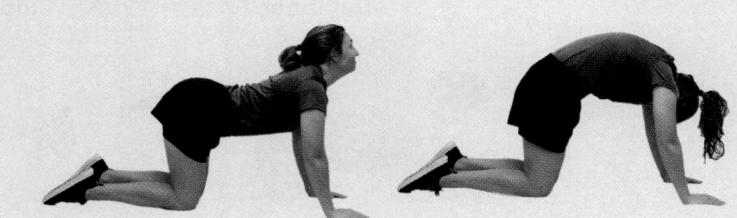
Child's to Cobra Pose	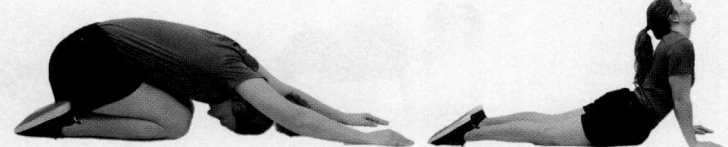
Rocking (Forward & Back) Frog Pose	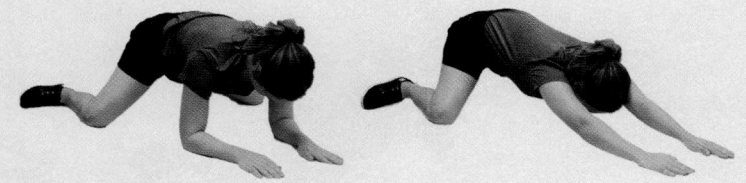
Squat to Hip Hinge	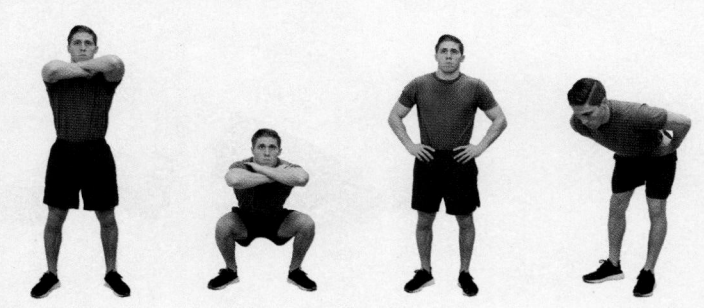
Alternating Side Lunges	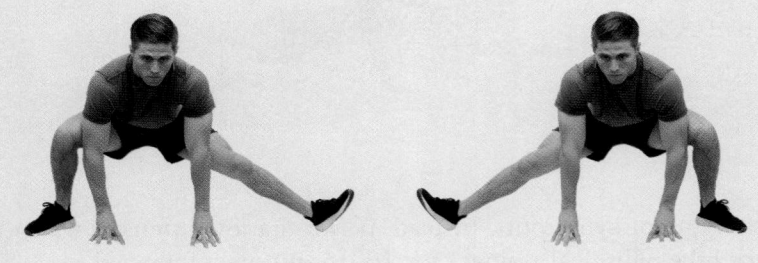
Rocking (Forward & Back) Single Leg Flexion with External Rotation	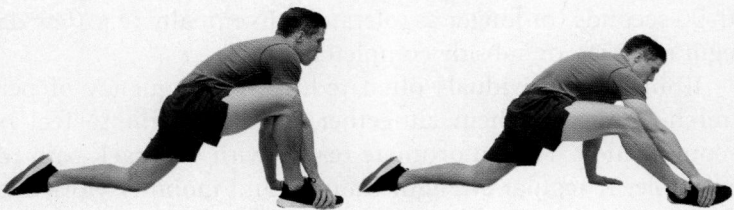

TABLE 3.7 Sample Low Back and Hip Stretches

Low Back and Hip Stretches

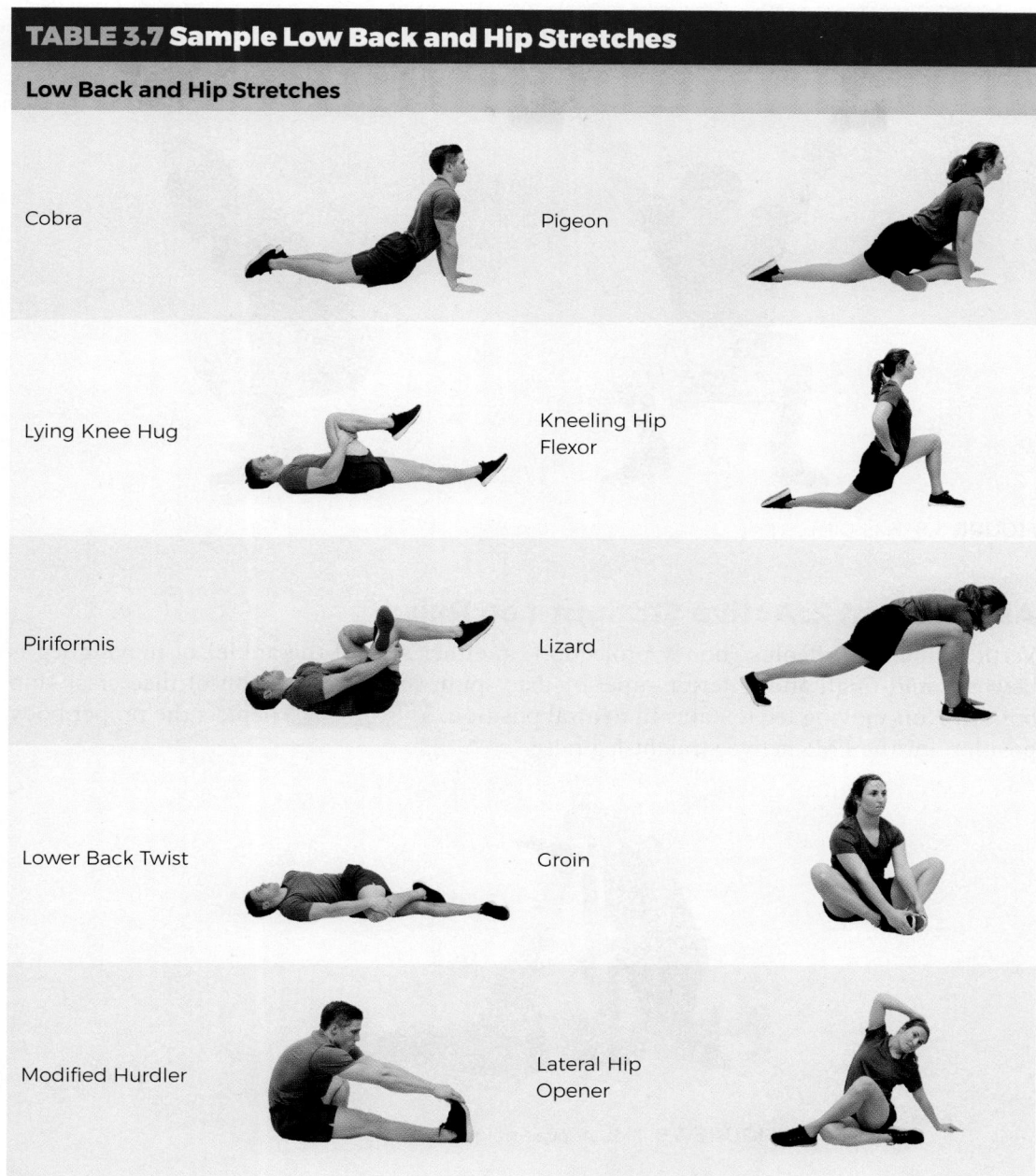

Cobra		Pigeon	
Lying Knee Hug		Kneeling Hip Flexor	
Piriformis		Lizard	
Lower Back Twist		Groin	
Modified Hurdler		Lateral Hip Opener	

Reader Challenge: Mobility

Provided below are three simple assessments from the Functional Movement Screen (FMS). To pass, you must be able to perform each assessment using the specified testing criteria provided. How did you do?

Assessment 1. Deep Squat

Upper torso is parellel with the tibia (lower leg bone). Femur (upper leg bone) is below horizontal. Knees are aligned over feet. Bar is aligned over feet. FIGURE 3.8 on the next page depicts the proper body position for the FMS deep squat.

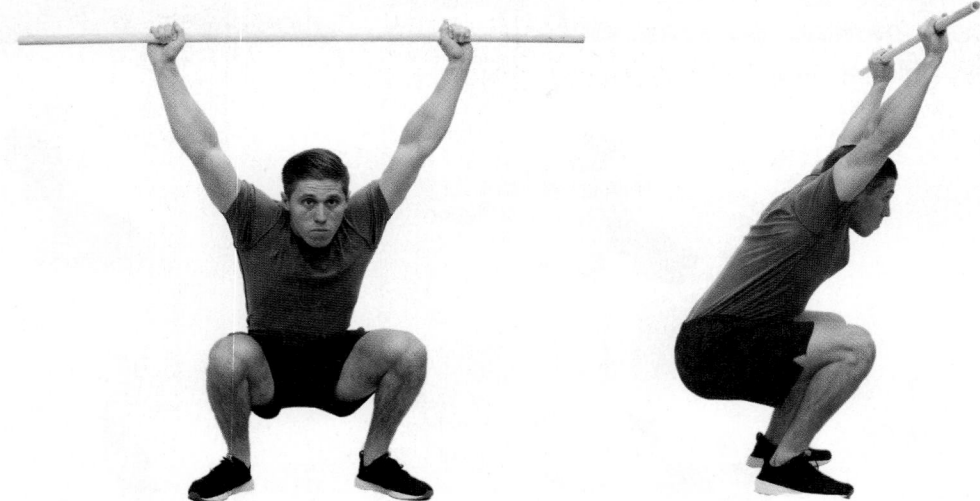

FIGURE 3.8 FMS Deep Squat

Assessment 2. Active Straight-Leg Raise

Vertical line of malleolus (boney projection on either side of the ankle) of moving leg is between mid-thigh and anterior superior iliac spine (boney projection of iliac crest [hip bone]). Non-moving leg remains in neutral position. **FIGURE 3.9** depicts the proper body position for the FMS active straight-leg raise.

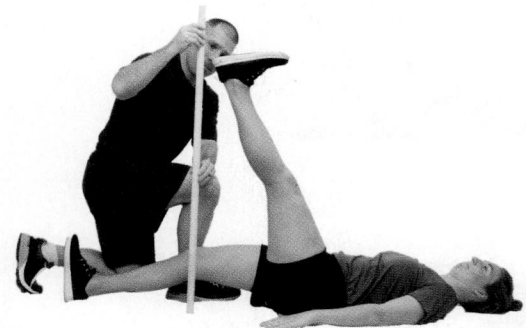

FIGURE 3.9 FMS Active Straight-Leg Raise

Assessment 3. Trunk Stability Push-Up

Males align thumbs with top of head. Females align thumbs with chin. Lift body as a single unit with no lag in the spine. **FIGURE 3.10** depicts the proper body position for males for the FMS trunk stability push-up. **FIGURE 3.11** depicts the proper body position for females for the FMS trunk stability push-up.

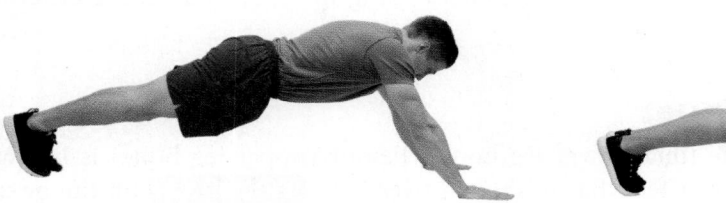

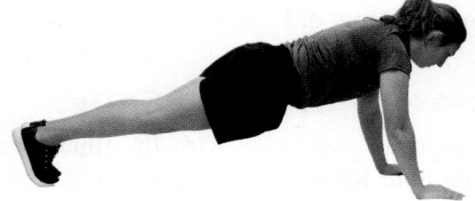

FIGURE 3.10 FMS Trunk Stability Push-Up (Male)   **FIGURE 3.11** FMS Trunk Stability Push-Up (Female)

Assessment and Application

Summary

- Although often overlooked or left out, a proper and thorough warm-up and cool-down are essential for performance, recovery, and injury prevention.

- Since exercise and sport are rarely one dimensional, it is important to perform regular mobility work in all three planes of movement.

- Although all four types of stretches can improve flexibility and range of motion, ballistic stretching is not recommended due to its higher risk of injury. Proprioceptive neuromuscular facilitation (PNF) stretching has been shown to be the most effective but requires the use of a trained partner.

- The American College of Sports Medicine (ACSM) recommends that stretching be performed at least three days per week. However, several strength and conditioning professionals are now recommending that at least 12–15 minutes be dedicated daily to mobility work.

- Tonic muscles (flexor muscles) tend to tighten with age, whereas phasic muscles (extensor muscles) tend to weaken with age. To combat this, it is recommend to regularly stretch tonic muscles and to perform strength training exercises for the phasic muscles.

- Ten to 15 minutes of prehab work prior to performing physical activity can significantly improve performance, range of motion, and reduce the risk for injury.

- Understanding and applying the recommendations for the three basic phases of tissue healing can help facilitate a faster recovery and prevent further injury.

- Even though there are a number of different causes of low back pain, the recommended treatment for recovery and prevention is generally the same. Performing low back specific stretches and mobility exercises daily will significantly help to prevent and recover from chronic low back pain.

- Researchers now believe that prolonged sitting is detrimental to one's health. To combat the harmful effects of sitting, individuals should get up and stand every 10–15 minutes or perform at least four minutes of physical activity for every 30 minutes of continuous sitting.

Knowledge Check

1. Define warm-up and cool-down and discuss some of the associated benefits of each.
2. List the three planes of movement.
3. Define and discuss the four basic types of stretches.
4. Which type of stretch is not recommended and why?
5. Discuss the circumstances when stretching is not recommended.
6. List and discuss the anatomical and training-related factors that affect flexibility.
7. What are the American College of Sports Medicine (ACSM) and American Heart Association (AHA) recommended guidelines for stretching?
8. Define elasticity, plasticity, and fibrosis and discuss their impact on flexibility and range of motion.

9. List 10 popular stretches aimed at improving total body flexibility as well as the specific muscle group which they target.
10. Define tonic and phasic muscles and provide training recommendations for each.
11. Define and discuss flexibility, mobility, and stability.
12. Define prehab and discuss some of its associated benefits.
13. List and discuss the different phases of tissue healing.
14. Discuss the detrimental effects of prolonged sitting as well as the exercise recommendations to counteract them.
15. List and discuss some of the different causes of and treatment options for low back pain.

Activities

Warm-Up, Cool-Down, and Stretching

A. Ethan suffers with chronic low back pain and is looking for advice on treatment. What training advice would you recommend?

References

Al-Masri, L., & Bartlett, S. (2011). *100 Questions & answers about sports nutrition and exercise.* Burlington, MA: Jones & Bartlett.

Baechle, T. R., & Earle, R. W. (Eds.). (2008). *Essentials of strength training and conditioning.* (3rd ed.). Champaign, IL: Human Kinetics.

Cady, M. (2016). *Paindemic: a practical and holistic look at chronic pain, the medical system, and the anti-pain lifestyle.* New York, NY: Morgan James Publishing.

Ekelund, U., Steene-Johannessen, J., Brown, W., Fagerland, M., Owen, N., Powell, K., Bauman, A., & Lee, I. (28 July 2016). *Does physical activity attenuate, or even eliminate, the detrimental association of sitting time with mortality? A harmonized meta-analysis of data from more than 1 million men and women. The Lancet.* Retrieved from http://www.thelancet.com/journals/lancet/article/PIIS0140-6736(16)30370-1/fulltext.

Haff, G., & Triplett, N. (Eds.). (2016). *Essentials of strength training and conditioning.* (4th ed). Champaign, IL: Human Kinetics.

Health-innovations.org. (2015). *Researchers identify precise cause of muscle weakness and loss due to aging.* Retrieved from https://health-innovations.org/2015/09/09/researchers-identify-precise-cause-of-muscle-weakness-and-loss-due-to-aging/

Prevost, M. (2015). *Built to endure* [eBook]. Retrieved from http://built-to-endure.blogspot.com/

Starrett, K., & Cordoza, G. (2015). *Becoming a supple leopard.* (2nd ed.). Las Vegas, NV: Victory Belt Publishing, Inc.

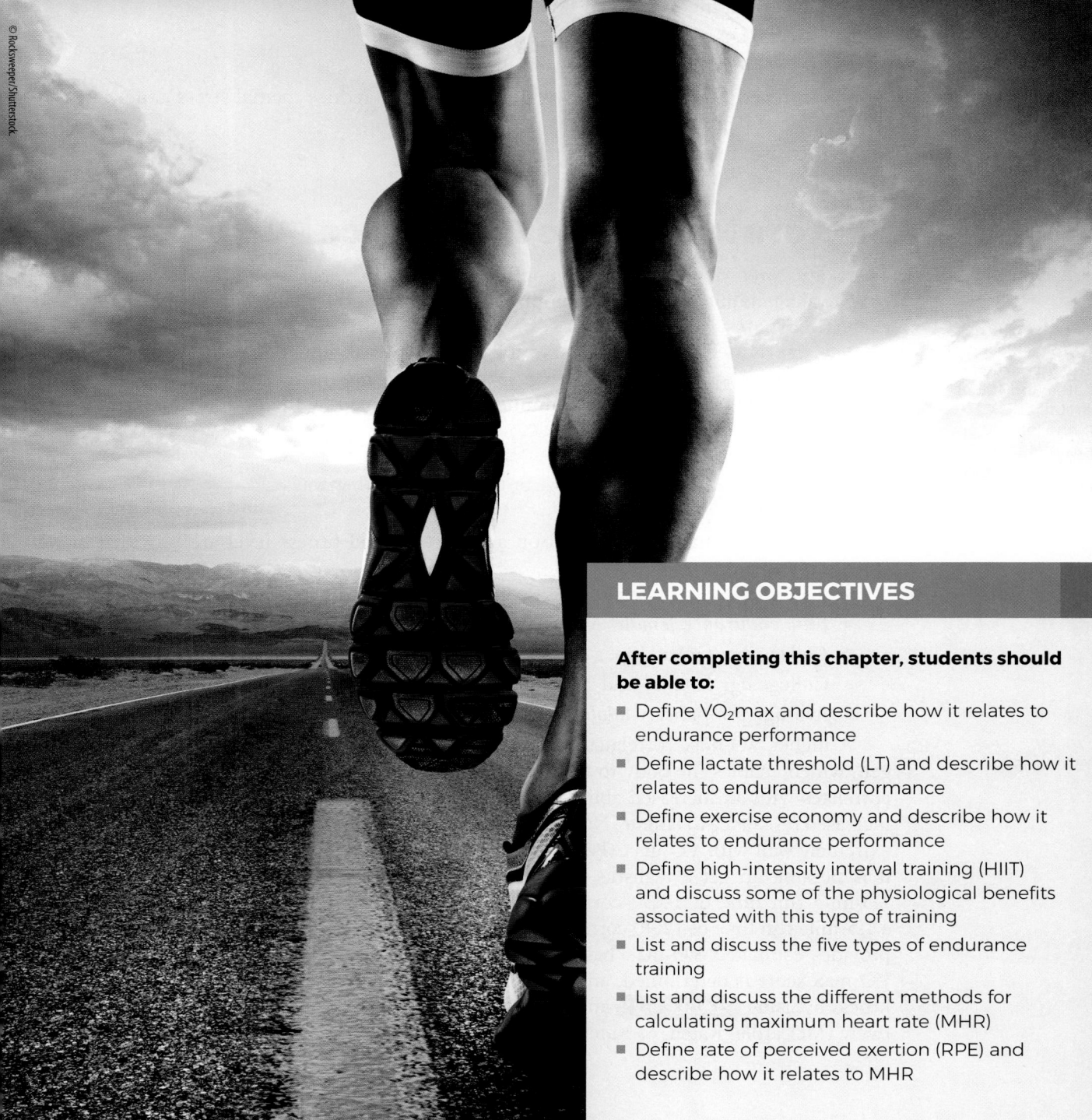

Endurance Training

LEARNING OBJECTIVES

After completing this chapter, students should be able to:

- Define VO$_2$max and describe how it relates to endurance performance
- Define lactate threshold (LT) and describe how it relates to endurance performance
- Define exercise economy and describe how it relates to endurance performance
- Define high-intensity interval training (HIIT) and discuss some of the physiological benefits associated with this type of training
- List and discuss the five types of endurance training
- List and discuss the different methods for calculating maximum heart rate (MHR)
- Define rate of perceived exertion (RPE) and describe how it relates to MHR

Introduction

Cardiovascular fitness: Ability of the heart and lungs to supply oxygen to the working muscle tissues as well as the ability of the muscles to use that oxygen to produce energy for movement.

Endurance training (aka aerobic capacity) is a method of training designed to improve cardiovascular fitness. **Cardiovascular fitness** is defined as the ability of the heart, lungs, and other organs to consume, transport, and utilize oxygen. Some of the benefits associated with regular endurance training include the following:

- Higher VO$_2$max
- Increased O$_2$ carrying capacity
- Decreased resting heart rate
- Increased cardiac muscle strength
- Increase in size and number of mitochondria
- Increase in the number of functional capillaries
- Faster recovery time
- Lower blood pressure and blood lipids
- Improved hormonal profile (which may help to reduce mental stress and symptoms of depression)
- Increase in fat-burning enzymes

Factors Related to Endurance Performance

There are three major factors that influence endurance performance: maximal aerobic power (aka maximal oxygen consumption, maximal oxygen uptake), lactate threshold, and exercise economy.

VO$_2$max: Maximum amount of oxygen that an individual can utilize during intense or maximal exercise. It is measured as milliliters of oxygen used in one minute per kilogram of body weight (ml/kg/min).

VO$_2$max is defined as the maximum amount of oxygen the body can take in and utilize during a specified period (e.g., 1 minute) of high intensity exercise. VO$_2$max is expressed mathematically as the amount of O$_2$ consumed by the body in a minute / body weight in lbs.

$$\frac{\text{ml of O}_2 \text{ consumed}}{\text{Body Weight (kg)}} \text{ or to say it in another way, } \frac{\text{Fitness}}{\text{Fatness}}$$

Projected VO$_2$max scores based on age, gender, and fitness level are provided below (McCormick, n.d.) :

- *Elite endurance male*: Upper 70s into 80s ml/kg/min
- *Elite endurance female*: Mid 60s to 70 ml/kg/min
- *College age male*: Upper 30s to 40 ml/kg/min
- *College age female*: Mid 30s ml/kg/min
- *Average pre-puberty adolescent*: 40s to 50 ml/kg/min

A higher VO$_2$max correlates with a body's increased ability to extract and utilize oxygen, which enables the body to train harder and longer. Additionally, a higher VO$_2$max also correlates with an increased ability of the body to buffer lactate production, which leads to increased resistance to fatigue. Numerous studies have shown that 1.5-mile run time correlates extremely well with VO$_2$max (Baechle & Earle, 2008; Haff & Triplett, 2016) In other words, it is possible to get a realistic estimation of one if you know the other. For example, a 1.5-mile run time of 10:30 correlates with a VO$_2$max score of 48.6 ml/kg/min. Similarly, a 1.5-mile run time of 12:40 correlates with a VO$_2$max score of 39.8 ml/kg/min. **TABLE 4.1** provides estimated VO$_2$max based on actual 1.5-mile run times (Cooper, 1968). Once a VO$_2$max score is determined, an individual can classify their current level of cardiovascular fitness by using **TABLE 4.2** and **TABLE 4.3** (on page 82) for males and females, respectively (McCardle, Katch, & Katch, 2015).

TABLE 4.1 Estimated VO$_2$max Score Based on 1.5-Mile Run Time

Run Time	Estimated VO$_2$max	Run Time	Estimated VO^{2}max	Run Time	Estimated VO$_2$max	Run Time	Estimated VO$_2$max
6:10	80.0	9:30	54.7	12:50	39.2	16:10	30.5
6:20	79.0	9:40	53.5	13:00	38.6	16:20	30.2
6:30	77.9	9:50	52.3	13:10	38.1	16:30	29.8
6:40	76.7	10:00	51.1	13:20	37.8	16:40	29.5
6:50	75.5	10:10	50.4	13:30	37.2	16:50	29.1
7:00	74.0	10:20	49.5	13:40	36.8	17:00	28.9
7:10	72.6	10:30	48.6	13:50	36.3	17:10	28.5
7:20	71.3	10:40	48.0	14:00	35.9	17:20	28.3
7:30	69.9	10:50	47.4	14:10	35.5	17:30	28.0
7:40	68.3	11:00	46.6	14:20	35.1	17:40	27.7
7:50	66.8	11:10	45.8	14:30	34.7	17:50	27.4
8:00	65.2	11:20	45.1	14:40	34.3	18:00	27.1
8:10	63.9	11:30	44.4	14:50	34.0	18:10	26.8
8:20	62.5	11:40	43.7	15:00	33.6	18:20	26.6
8:30	61.2	11:50	43.2	15:10	33.1	18:30	26.3
8:40	60.2	12:00	42.3	15:20	32.7	18:40	26.0
8:50	59.1	12:10	41.7	15:30	32.2	18:50	25.7
9:00	58.1	12:20	41.0	15:40	31.8	19:00	25.4
9:10	56.9	12:30	40.4	15:50	31.4		
9:20	55.9	12:40	39.8	16:00	30.9		

Data from Cooper, K. H. (1968). A means of assessing maximal oxygen intake. *Journal of the American Medical Association*, 203, 201–204.

TABLE 4.2 VO$_2$max Score Classification for Males

| Classification | Male (Age) | | | | |
	≤ 29	30–39	40–49	50–59	60–69
Poor	≤ 24.9	≤ 22.9	≤ 19.9	≤ 17.9	≤ 15.9
Fair	25–33.9	23–30.9	20–26.9	18–24.9	16–22.9
Average	34–43.9	31–41.9	27–38.9	25–37.9	23–35.9
Good	44–52.9	42–49.9	39–44.9	38–42.9	36–40.9
Excellent	≥ 53	≥ 50	≥ 45	≥ 43	≥ 41

TABLE 4.3 VO$_2$max Score Classification for Females					
	Female (Age)				
Classification	**≤ 29**	**30–39**	**40–49**	**50–59**	**60–69**
Poor	≤ 23.9	≤ 19.9	≤ 16.9	≤ 14.9	≤ 12.9
Fair	24–30.9	20–27.9	17–24.9	15–21.9	13–20.9
Average	31–38.9	28–36.9	25–34.9	22–33.9	21–32.9
Good	39–48.9	37–44.9	35–41.9	34–39.9	33–36.9
Excellent	≥ 49	≥ 45	≥ 42	≥ 40	≥ 37

Data from McArdle, W. D., Katch, F. I., & Katch, V. L. (2015). *Exercise physiology: nutrition, energy, and human performance.* (8th ed.). Baltimore, MD: Wolters Kluwer Health.

On average, every pound gained equates to roughly a 3–4 second slower 1.5-mile run time. Conversely, every pound lost equates to roughly a 3–4 second faster 1.5-mile time (Prevost, 2015). Understanding the relationship between VO$_2$max and 1.5-mile run time, it is possible to manipulate the VO$_2$max formula in an effort to determine how much fitness someone would need to gain or weight they would need to lose in order to attain a specific VO$_2$max score.

For example, say a 165 lb. (75 kg) female has been running consistently for several months and wants to achieve a 1.5-mile run time of 12:40. Her current VO$_2$max score, as determined by testing in a human performance lab, was 37.2 ml/kg/min (which equates to a 13:30 1.5-mile run time).

$$\frac{2790 \text{ ml/min}}{75 \text{ kg}} = 37.2 \text{ ml/kg/min}$$

Even if her current fitness level remains the same, we can still manipulate the VO$_2$max formula in order to determine what her body weight (i.e., denominator) would need to be in order to achieve a VO$_2$max score of 39.8 (which equates to a 12:40 1.5-mile run time). She would need to lose roughly 11 lbs. (75 − 70.1 = 4.9 kg; 4.9 × 2.2 = 10.78 lbs.) in order to improve her VO$_2$max score from 37.2 to 39.8 ml/kg/min.

$$\text{Required body weight (kg)} = \frac{2790 \text{ ml/min}}{39.8 \text{ ml/kg/min}} = 70.1 \text{ kg}$$

With that said, losing weight is not always the recommended approach to improving VO$_2$max. For example, it would be contraindicated for individuals who already have a low percentage of body fat to lose weight as the majority of weight loss would come from water and/or muscle mass. Instead, it would be better for those individuals to perform regular speed and pace/tempo training in an effort to improve their overall level of fitness (i.e., numerator).

After the age of 40, VO$_2$max decreases by roughly 10% per decade until it falls to 20 ml/kg/min. Participation in regular endurance training increases the VO$_2$max of untrained individuals (up to 25–30%); however, similar improvements in well trained endurance athletes are less likely.

Recommendations for maximizing an individual's VO$_2$max include adequate training volume and intensity. Specifically, low to moderate intensity endurance work (70–80% of max heart rate) should be performed for at least 20 minutes per endurance training session, 3–6 times per week, and total between 6–7 hours per week (Baechle & Earle, 2008; Haff & Triplett, 2016). Although performing more than this can lead to improvements in exercise economy and a higher sustainable running pace, it is not believed to result in further increases in VO₂max. Additionally, high-intensity interval training (between 90–100% VO₂max) should be performed one to two times per week at a 1:3 to 1:5 work to rest ratio (Baechle & Earle, 2008; Haff & Triplett, 2016).

Some of the physiological adaptations associated with high-intensity endurance training aimed at improving VO₂max include increases in (Al-Masri & Bartlett, 2011; Baechle & Earle, 2008; Haff & Triplett, 2016):

- Maximal cardiac output
- Resting and maximal stroke volume
- Left ventricular chamber size
- Blood volume, red blood cell mass, and hemoglobin
- Capillary density

The byproduct of **glycolysis** (breakdown of carbohydrates (glycose) into adenosine triphosphate (ATP)) is **lactate** (byproduct of anaerobic metabolism caused by insufficient supply of oxygen to the tissues). During exercise, lactate production increases, which subsequently leads to an increase in muscle acidity (due to an increased number of available hydrogen ions). Increased muscle acidity is one the primary factors responsible for muscle fatigue. So although increased lactate production is not the culprit of muscle fatigue, it is a good indicator.

Lactate threshold (LT) is defined as the point in exercise at which lactate starts to accumulate in the blood at a faster rate than it can be removed. Research suggests that one's lactate threshold is a better predictor of cardiovascular fitness than VO₂max (Baechle & Earle, 2008; Haff & Triplett, 2016). In essence, LT defines your upper limit in terms of a sustainable pace during training and competition. After blood lactate starts to accumulate above resting levels, it becomes impossible for the muscles to sustain that pace thereby resulting in fatigue. Identifying and correctly using one's LT can help determine the correct exercise intensity in which to train or compete at in order to maximize performance and avoid muscle fatigue.

At some run intensities, the body reaches a steady state, called **maximal lactate steady state (MLSS)**, in which the level of lactate no longer increases and remains relatively stable. **FIGURE 4.1** shows how, at certain run intensities (i.e., miles per hour), the body is able to reach and maintain a lactate steady state (Prevost, 2015). However, at 9 mph the individual

Glycolysis: Process in cell metabolism by which carbohydrates and sugars, especially glucose, are broken down to produce ATP and pyruvic acid.

Lactate: Byproduct of glucose utilization by muscle cells during anaerobic glycolysis.

Lactate threshold: The intensity of exercise at which lactate begins to accumulate in the blood at a faster rate than it can be removed.

Maximal lactate steady state (MLSS): Highest blood lactate concentration and work load that can be maintained over time without a continual blood lactate accumulation.

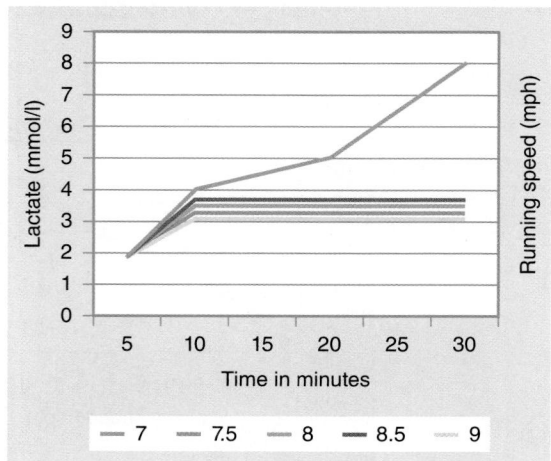

FIGURE 4.1 Lactate Steady States at Various Run Paces

Data from Liang, H., & Ward, W. F. (2006). PGC-1α: A key regulator of energy metabolism. *Advances in physiology education, 30*(4), 145-151.

can no longer maintain a steady state and the level of lactate continues to climb. In this example, the individual's MLSS is at 8 mph. Running any faster would eventually result in fatigue.

Ironically, two athletes with the same VO₂max can have significantly different running paces due to differences in their LT. As shown in **FIGURE 4.2**, athlete 1 and athlete 2 have the same VO₂max but athlete 1's lactate threshold occurs at 60% of his or her VO₂max, whereas athlete 2's lactate threshold occurs at 70% of his or her VO₂max. In other words, while both athletes have the same VO₂max, athlete 1 is only able to sustain a max running speed of 6.8 miles per hour (mph) whereas athlete 2 is able to sustain a max running speed of 7.8 miles per hour. As a result, athlete 2 would cover the required distance faster and, therefore, finish the race first.

LT determines how much of the aerobic upper limit can be used or sustained for long periods of time. For example, in untrained individuals, LT is 60–70% of VO₂max. In well trained endurance athletes, LT is 75–80% of VO₂max. In elite endurance athletes, LT is 90% or more of VO₂max (McCormick, n.d.).

Some of the physiological adaptations associated with high-intensity endurance training aimed at improving LT include (Baechle & Earle, 2008; Haff & Triplett, 2016):

- Increase in mitochondrial density
- Increase in pyruvate dehydrogenase (PDH) activity
- Increase in β-oxidative enzymes
- Muscle fiber shift from Type IIb (fast twitch) to Type IIa (slow twitch)

Collectively, these adaptations help to improve the aerobic capacity of the muscle, thereby improving endurance training tolerance and performance.

Recommendations for increasing LT include high-intensity interval training (90–110% VO₂max). Additionally, sufficient time should be afforded for rest between intervals in order to allow for maximal lactate clearance (1:3 to 1:5 work-to-rest ratio) (Baechle & Earle, 2008; Haff & Triplett, 2016).

Exercise economy, usually measured in terms of oxygen consumption (ml/kg/min), is defined as the amount of energy required to maintain a constant speed of movement or generate a specific amount of power. Exercise economy has been shown to be another important predictor of endurance performance, although not to the same extent as VO₂max and LT, and it can explain some of the endurance performance differences between individuals. Some of the factors that influence exercise economy include neuromuscular coordination, percentage of type I muscle fibers, elastic energy storage, joint stability, and flexibility (Training 4 Endurance, 2017). **FIGURE 4.3** shows how exercise

Exercise economy: Relates to the quantity of oxygen (ml/kg/min) required to move at a given speed or generate a specific amount of power and influenced by a number of factors including: neuromuscular coordination, percentage of type I muscle fibers, elastic energy storage, and joint stability and flexibility.

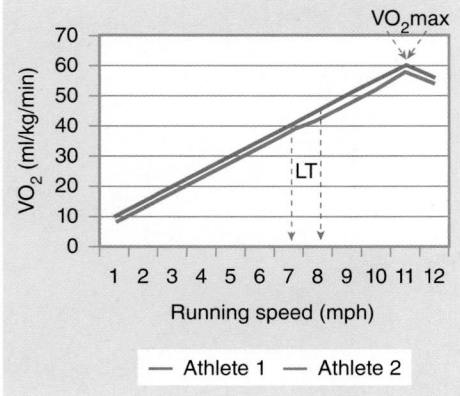

FIGURE 4.2 Lactate Threshold Comparison between Athletes

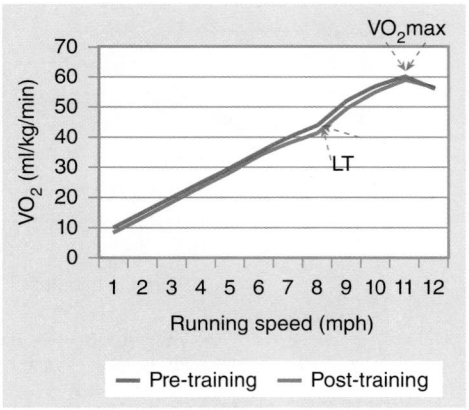

FIGURE 4.3 Influence of Exercise Economy on Lactate Threshold and VO₂max

Modified from Hoeger, W. K., Hoeger, S. A., Hoeger, C. I., & Fawson, A. L. (2017). *Lifetime Physical Fitness and Wellness.* (14th ed). Boston, MA: Cengage Learning.

FAQ

Hypoxia training: Hype or hoax?

Hypoxia training is a relatively new training concept that uses a specially designed mask or device (e.g., vascular occlusion training) to reduce the amount of oxygen being taken in by the lungs and/or being delivered to the working muscles. The idea behind hypoxia training is that if you regularly train in a hypoxic state, the body will eventually adapt and become more efficient at consuming, delivering, and utilizing oxygen. Unfortunately, such claims are not supported by current research. Although a few studies have shown some improvements in time to exhaustion, reduced blood lactate accumulation, and cardiovascular performance with hypoxia training, said improvements were modest at best (Laurentino, et al., 2008; McConnell & Romer, 2004; Prevost, 2015). Additionally, most strength and conditioning professionals believe that hypoxia training may be counterproductive. This is because the physiological adaptations associated with chronic exercise are dependent upon the training stimulus. In other words, since the body cannot exercise at the same intensity or duration in a hypoxic state, the training stimulus has to be reduced to compensate. So even though you feel like you are training harder, in reality, you are not. As training intensity and/or duration are reduced, so are the subsequent training adaptations. Bottom line: if you wish to include hypoxia training into your overall strength and conditioning program, it should be performed in addition to and not in lieu of conventional endurance training.

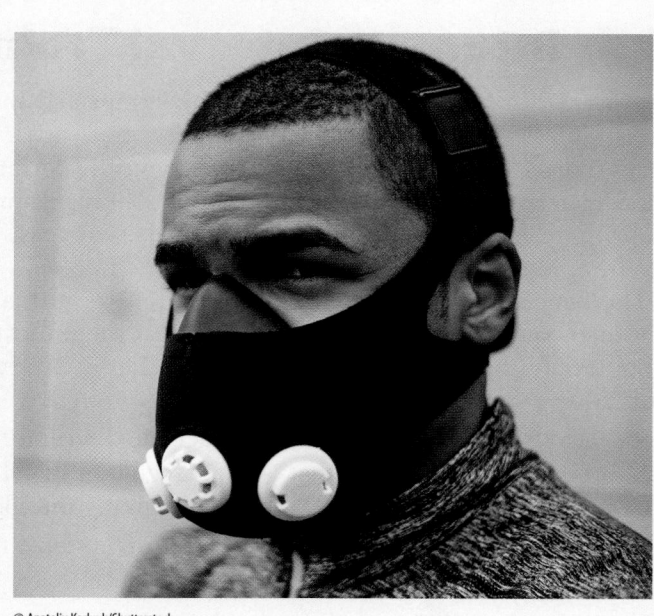
© Anatoliy Karlyuk/Shutterstock.

> **Hypoxia training:** A type of training that uses a specially designed mask or device to reduce the amount of oxygen being taken in by the lungs and/or being delivered to the working muscles. In theory, doing so allows the body to become more efficient at consuming, delivering, and utilizing oxygen.

economy can improve endurance performance even when VO$_2$max and LT remain unchanged (Ivy, 2016).

Although not considered a major component another factor that can influence endurance performance is muscle fiber type. Although a small percentage (i.e., 3–4%) of type IIb fibers can be converted to type IIa fibers with chronic endurance training (and vice versa), the vast majority of fast-twitch to slow-twitch fibers appears to be genetically determined. The genetic distribution of slow- and fast-twitch fibers is often used as one of the primary factors that determines which sport or activity an athlete ultimately competes in. For example, athletes with a higher percentage of slow-twitch fibers tend to compete in long distance events (e.g., 10-km, half marathon, marathon); whereas athletes with a higher percentage of fast-twitch fibers tend to compete in speed events (e.g., 100-meter, 200-meter, 400-meter sprints).

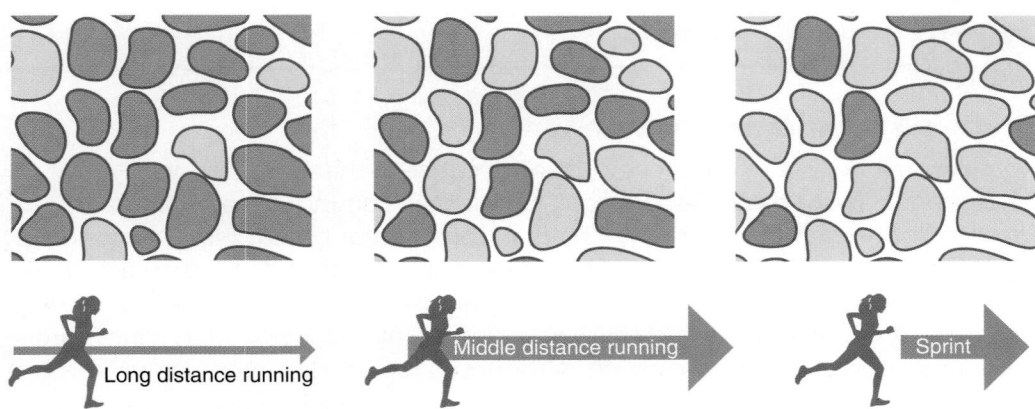

FIGURE 4.4 Fiber Type Differences between Endurance Athletes

FIGURE 4.4 illustrates the difference in fiber type percentages for long, middle, and short distance endurance athletes. Red circles represent slow-twitch (type I) fibers whereas white circles represent fast-twitch (type II) muscle fibers.

High-Intensity Interval Training

High-intensity interval training: A form of interval training that alternates short periods of intense anaerobic exercise with less-intense recovery periods.

High-Intensity Interval Training (HIIT) involves repeated short to long bouts of high-intensity exercise interspersed with recovery periods. Short intervals can be performed well above 100% VO_2max; whereas, long intervals are typically performed closer to VO_2max. The sport should dictate the type of interval used (i.e., short or long). For example, sprinters would benefit more from performing short intervals; whereas, marathon runners would benefit more from long intervals.

The benefits associated with regular HIIT are virtually identical to those found with traditional endurance training regimens but at a significantly lower training volume. Some of the specific benefits include (Baechle & Earle, 2008; Haff & Triplett, 2016; Liang & Ward, 2006):

- Activates peroxisome-proliferator activated receptor γ coactivator (PGC-1α) in human skeletal muscle that is a key regulator in cellular energy metabolism, which stimulates mitochondrial biogenesis, making muscle tissue more oxidative in nature
- Stresses oxygen transport and utilization systems fully, thereby providing an extremely effective endurance training stimulus
- Improves insulin and glucose sensitivity in obese and diabetic patients

Additionally, HIIT may be a safer method of endurance training for individuals with heart disease. For example, short bursts of high-intensity endurance activity has been shown to induce large magnitude increases in cellular and peripheral vascular stress, while, at the same time, effectively protecting the heart from those stresses due to its brief duration. This relative central insulation allows individuals to train at much higher intensity than they would be able to otherwise.

Types of Endurance Training

Long slow distance (LSD) training: A form of continuous training performed at a constant pace of low to moderate intensity over an extended distance or duration.

There are several different types of endurance training programs, each with their own specific guidelines in terms of exercise frequency, intensity, duration, and progression. **TABLE 4.4** shows the different types of endurance training as well as their respective guidelines for exercise prescription (Baechle & Earle, 2008; Haff & Triplett, 2016).

Long slow distance (LSD) training, aka low intensity steady state, is a form of continuous endurance training that is performed at a constant pace at low to moderate

TABLE 4.4 Types of Aerobic Endurance Training

Endurance Type	Intensity	Duration	Frequency	Work:Rest Ratio
Long Slow Distance	70–80% MHR	30–120 min	1+	–
Pace/Tempo	80–90% MHR	20–30 min	1–2	–
Interval	>90% MHR	3–5 min	1–2	1:1
Repetition	≤100% MHR	30–90 sec	1	1:5
Fartlek	70–90% MHR	20–60 min	1	–

Data from Baechle, T. R., & Earle, R. W. (Eds.). (2008). *Essentials of strength training and conditioning.* (3rd ed.). Champaign, IL: Human Kinetics; Haff, G., & Triplett, N. (Eds.). (2016). *Essentials of strength training and conditioning.* (4th ed). Champaign, IL; Haff, G., & Triplett, N. (Eds.). (2016). Essentials of Strength Training and Conditioning. (4th ed). Champaign, IL: Human Kinetics.

intensity over an extended distance or period of time. Physiological adaptations associated with LSD training include improved cardiovascular and thermoregulatory function, improved mitochondrial energy production and oxidative capacity, and increased fat utilization. Due to its moderate training intensity, LSD effectively improves endurance and maximum oxygen uptake in undertrained or moderately trained individuals but is less effective in well-trained athletes, who require higher training intensities in order for additional physiological adaptations to occur.

For endurance athletes, more mileage per week is almost always better. However, there does seem to be a point of diminishing return. For most athletes, this appears to be around 60 miles per week. **FIGURE 4.5** below shows the nominal improvements made with extremely high weekly running mileage (Prevost, 2015).

With novice runners, there appears to be a minimum effective dose of LSD training. Exceeding this threshold significantly increases the participant's risk of injury. The following table provides run mileage and injury incidence on US Army recruits over a 12-week period (United States Army, 2008). The group that ran less mileage actually had faster 2-mile run times and a significantly lower injury rate.

Run Mileage	Injury Incidence	2-Mile Run Time
130 miles	54%	13:45
56 miles	41%	13:28

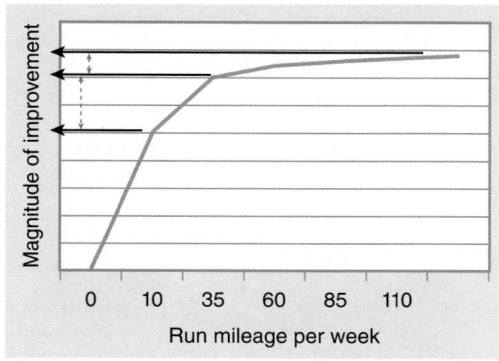

FIGURE 4.5 Nominal Improvement with Weekly Run Mileage

Modified from Liang, H., & Ward, W. F. (2006). PGC-1α: A key regulator of energy metabolism. *Advances in Physiology Education*, 30(4), 145-151.

Pace/tempo training: A form of endurance training that uses intensities at or slightly higher than race pace intensity.

Interval training: A form of endurance training that involves high-intensity intervals (typically 3-5 minutes in duration) close to VO_2max.

Repetition training: A form of endurance training that uses high-intensity intervals (typically 30-90 seconds in duration) at intensities greater than VO_2max.

Fartlek: Swedish for "speed play," is a form of endurance training that combines long slow distance (LSD) with interval training.

Pace/tempo training, aka lactate threshold (LT) or threshold run, is another form of endurance training that uses intensities at or slightly higher than race pace intensity. There are two ways to conduct pace/tempo training: steady or intermittent. Steady pace/tempo training uses a training intensity equal to LT for 20–30 minutes. Intermittent pace/tempo training also uses a training intensity equal to LT but employs a series of intervals with brief recovery periods in between. When employing pace/tempo training it is important not to train above LT. In fact, it is better to increase training distance than intensity. The primary purpose of pace/tempo training is to develop a sense of race pace and improve the body's ability to sustain that pace. The physiological adaptations associated with pace/tempo training include improved running economy and increased LT (Baechle & Earle, 2008; Haff & Triplett, 2016).

Interval training involves high-intensity endurance training close to VO_2max. The work intervals should last between 3–5 minutes with a similar amount of time afforded for rest (periods of low-intensity endurance exercise) in between (i.e., work:rest ratio of 1:1). Interval training is very stressful and should not be performed more than twice per week until a firm base of aerobic conditioning (by way of LSD) has been attained. The physiological adaptations associated with interval training include increased VO_2max and enhanced anaerobic metabolism (Baechle & Earle, 2008; Haff & Triplett, 2016).

Another form of endurance training used to develop speed and endurance is **repetition training (REPS)**. Repetition training involves short bursts of high-intensity endurance training at intensities above VO_2max. The work intervals should last between 30 and 90 seconds with 4–6 times the amount of time afforded for rest in between (i.e., work:rest ratio of 1:5). The physiological adaptations associated with REPS include improved running speed and economy and increased anaerobic metabolism (Baechle & Earle, 2008; Haff & Triplett, 2016). This type of training is also beneficial for providing athletes with the necessary push at the end of an all-out endurance event.

Fartlek, which is Swedish for "speed play," is yet another endurance training method that combines LSD with interval training. Fartlek training blends easy running (at LSD pace) with short bursts of high-intensity interval training. The physiological adaptations associated with Fartlek training include enhanced VO_2max, increased LT, and improved running economy and fuel utilization (Baechle & Earle, 2008; Haff & Triplett, 2016). Due to its versatility and variability, Fartlek training may also help to reduce the monotony and boredom often associated with long-term endurance training.

TABLE 4.5 provides some specific examples for each of the different endurance training methods.

TABLE 4.5 Sample Exercises for the Various Types of Endurance Training

LSD	Pace / Tempo	Interval	Repetition	Fartlek
Run 3–5 miles	5-min Easy / 10-min Hard Repeats	4–6 × 400m Sprints	8–10 × 100m Sprints	Indian Runs
Run 30+ minutes	Treadmill Tempo Run	2–3 × 800m Sprints	6–8 × 200m Sprints	Sprint straightaways / walk curves
		1-mile Repeats	6–8 × 300-yd Shuttle	

Data from Baechle, T. R., & Earle, R. W. (Eds.). (2008). *Essentials of strength training and conditioning.* (3rd ed.). Champaign, IL: Human Kinetics; Haff, G., & Triplett, N. (Eds.). (2016). *Essentials of Strength Training and Conditioning.* (4th ed). Champaign, IL; Haff, G., & Triplett, N. (Eds.). (2016). *Essentials of Strength Training and Conditioning.* (4th ed). Champaign, IL: Human Kinetics.

Most of the examples listed above are either widely known or easily researched. However, the **treadmill tempo run** is a new approach to pace / tempo training aimed at targeting a specific run time. The example provided is tailored for the 1.5 mile run:

- *Step 1*: Subtract 30 seconds from last 1.5 mile run time = Desired Run Time
- *Step 2*: 90 ÷ Desired Run Time = Required Miles per Hour (MPH)
- *Step 3*: Run 1.5-miles at Required MPH. Walk as required; however, only the distance run counts toward 1.5 mile distance
- *Step 4*: When able to run 1.5 mile without stopping, increase incline to 0.5%
- *Step 5*: When able to run 1.5 mile at 0.5% incline without stopping, increase incline to 1.0%
- *Step 6*: When able to run 1.5 mile at 1.0% incline without stopping, subtract 30 seconds from Desired Run Time and repeat

Desired Run Time	Required MPH
15:00	6.0
14:30	6.2
14:00	6.4
13:30	6.7
13:00	6.9
12:30	7.2
12:00	7.5
11:30	7.8
11:00	8.2
10:30	8.5
10:00	9.0
09:30	9.5
09:00	10.0
08:30	10.6
08:00	11.3

Treadmill tempo run: New type of pace/tempo training aimed at targeting a desired run time for a specific race distance (e.g., 1.5-miles).

The treadmill tempo run approach is extremely versatile and can be used to train for specific race paces for a variety of different distances (e.g., 1.0 mile, 1.5 mile, 2.0 mile, 3.0 mile, 5 km, 10 km). However, this method is not as effective in preparing for race distances greater than 10 km since the required pace is too slow to produce the physiological adaptations associated with LT training. As previously shown, the number 90 is used to determine the desired run time for a race distance of 1.5 mile. The following table provides similar values for other common race distances.

Race Distance (mi.)	Required Dividend	Seconds to Subtract
1.0	60	10–20
1.5	90	15–30
2.0	120	20–45
3.0	180	30–60
3.1 (5 km)	180.6	30–60
6.2 (10 km)	361.2	60–90

Faster runners should be more conservative with the number of seconds to subtract whereas novice or slower runners should be more liberal. For example, someone who is already running a 1.5-mile run time of 8:30 should only subtract 15 seconds whereas someone running a 1.5-mile run time of 12:40 would benefit more from subtracting 30 seconds. A good way to gauge whether you need to subtract additional, or fewer, seconds is by counting how many times you had to stop and walk. If you had to stop more than three times in a session, you likely subtracted too many seconds. Conversely, if you did not have to stop or stopped only once, it is likely that you did not subtract enough seconds. If performed consistently once a week, the entire process generally takes 4–6 weeks to complete.

Let's perform a sample calculation. Let's say your last 10-km run time was 36:00 and the goal for your next 10-km race is 34:50. This equates to a 70-second difference, which is in line with the "seconds to subtract" recommendation.

These are the necessary steps required to calculate the required miles per hour in order to complete a desired 10-km run time of 34:50:

- Divide 361.2 (required dividend) by 34.83 (numeric representation of a 34:50 run time) in order to determine required MPH
- $361.2 \div 34.83 = 10.37$
- The required MPH to complete a desired 10-km run time of 34:50 = 10.4 mph

Training should be tailored to develop and maximize VO_2max and LT as these are two of the primary factors influencing endurance performance. **FIGURE 4.6** plots the different types of endurance training and their association with VO_2max and LT. Notice that endurance training programs that consist of only LSD training do little to improve LT and VO_2max.

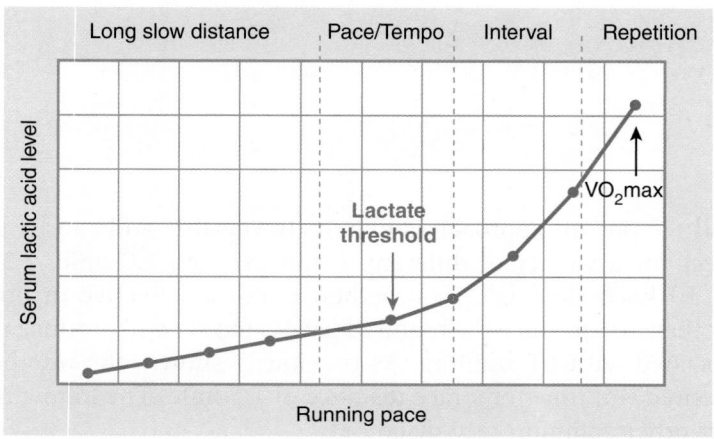

FIGURE 4.6 Relationship between Endurance Training Type, VO₂max, and Lactate Threshold

The type and amount of recommended endurance training will differ depending on the race distance and duration. For example, individuals training for endurance events lasting roughly 30 minutes or fewer (e.g., 1.5-mile, 2.0-mile, 3.0-mile, 5-km runs) would benefit more from a conditioning program that frequently employs pace/tempo, speed, and some LSD work. Conversely, individuals training for endurance events lasting longer than 30 minutes (e.g., half marathon, marathon, 50-miler) would benefit more from a conditioning program consisting predominantly of LSD and possibly some pace/tempo work. Pace/tempo training may still be beneficial for ultra-endurance athletes as it has been shown to increase running economy and LT; both of which may help to improve run times for longer distance runs. The following table provides the necessary information (i.e., required dividend and time to subtract) in order to tailor pace/tempo training to ultra-endurance races.

Race Distance (mi.)	Required Dividend	Minutes to Subtract
Half Marathon (13.1 mi.)	786	3–5
Marathon (26.2 mi.)	1572	10–20
50-Miler	3000	45–60
100-Miler	6000	90–120

Although there are five distinct types of endurance training, categorization can be reduced to three basic types of endurance training as shown in the following table. Specifically, LSD, pace/tempo, and speed. Since Fartlek training is a combination of LSD and pace/tempo, including said training into one's endurance training program is not necessary as long as LSD and pace/tempo are already being performed. Additionally, since both interval and repetition training utilize the same energy pathways (i.e., phosphagen and/or glycolysis) and result in similar physiological adaptations (e.g., increased VO_2max and anaerobic metabolism), the two types of training could be combined and used interchangeably. For example, if your endurance training program calls for two days per week of speed training, one session could employ interval training and the other repetition.

LSD	Pace / Tempo	Interval	Repetition	Fartlek
Run 3–5 miles	5-min Easy / 10-min Hard Repeats	4–6 × 400-m Sprints	8–10 × 100-m Sprints	Indian Runs
Run 30+ minutes	Treadmill Tempo Run	2–3 × 800-m Sprints 1-mile Repeats	6–8 × 200-m Sprints 6–8 × 300-yd Shuttle	Sprint straightaways / walk curves

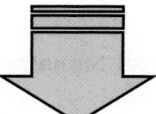

LSD	Pace / Tempo	Speed	
Run 3–5 miles	5-min Easy / 10-min Hard Repeats	4–6 × 400-m Sprints	8–10 × 100-m Sprints
Run 30+ minutes	Treadmill Tempo Run	2–3 × 800-m Sprints 1-mile Repeats	6–8 × 200-m Sprints 6–8 × 300-yd Shuttle

> **FAQ**
>
> ## What type of cardio is recommended for strength athletes?
>
> If the goal is to facilitate fat loss but retain muscle mass, low-intensity endurance training (e.g., walking, elliptical trainer, biking, swimming) is recommended. However, if the goal is to maximize fat loss in minimal time, high-intensity interval training (HIIT) is recommended. In either case, excessive LSD running (run volume > 15 miles per week) is not recommended for athletes primarily training for size, strength, or power.

Maximum Heart Rate Prediction Equations

As described earlier, endurance training type recommendations are often based on an individual's maximum heart rate (MHR). Here are some of the more popular equations used to estimate MHR.

Age Predicted Max Heart Rate (APMHR)	Tanaka, Monahan, and Seals	Karvonen	Female Specific
220 − Age	208 − (0.7 × Age)	· APMHR − Resting Heart Rate (RHR) = Heart Rate Reserve (HRR) · HRR × Desired Exercise Intensity + RHR	206 − (.88 × Age)

Using the above formulas and information provided below, let's perform some sample calculations:

- 22-year-old Female
- Resting Heart Rate of 72 beats per minute (bpm)
- Desired Training Zone of 65–80% Max Heart Rate

	APMHR	Tanaka, Monahan, and Seals	Karvonen	Female Specific
Formula	220 − Age = MHR	208 − (0.7 × Age) = MHR	APMHR − RHR = HRR	206 − (0.88 × Age) = MHR
Calculation	220 − 22	208 − 15.4	198 − 72	206 − (0.88 × 22)
Estimated MHR / HRR	198 bpm	193 bpm	126 bpm	187 bpm

	APMHR	Tanaka, Monahan, and Seals	Karvonen	Female Specific
Formula	MHR × 0.65 ÷ MHR × 0.80	MHR × 0.65 ÷ MHR × 0.80	(HRR × 0.65) + RHR ÷ (HRR × 0.80) + RHR	MHR × 0.65 ÷ MHR × 0.80
Calculation	198 × 0.65 ÷ 198 × 0.80	193 × 0.65 ÷ 193 × 0.80	(126 × 0.65) + 72 ÷ (126 × 0.80) + 72	187 × 0.65 ÷ 187 × 0.80
Target Heart Rate Range	129–158 bpm	125–154 bpm	154–173 bpm	121–145 bpm

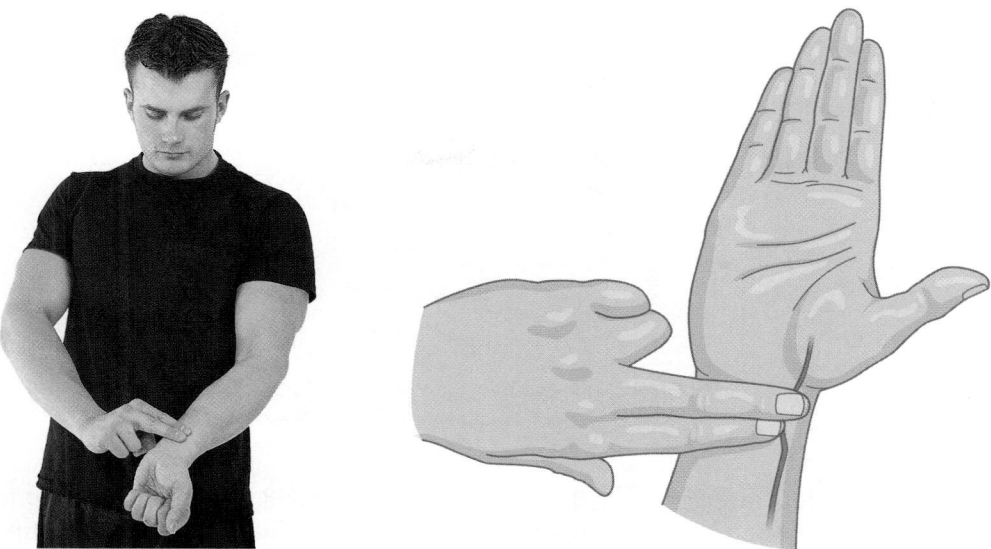

FIGURE 4.7 How to Calculate Your Resting Heart Rate

Use the following steps to calculate your resting heart rate (RHR):

- Resting heart rate is best taken first thing in the morning prior to getting out of bed. If that is not an option, it should be taken after sitting quietly for about half an hour.
- As demonstrated in **FIGURE 4.7**, take your pulse on the wrist (thumb side) over the radial artery.
- Using the tips of your first two fingers (not your thumb), press lightly over the radial artery.
- Count your pulse for 10 seconds and then multiply that number by 6 to determine your heart rate in beats per minute (bpm).

TABLE 4.6 can be used to assess resting heart rate (Hoeger, Hoeger, Hoeger, & Fawson, 2017) Generally speaking, a lower resting heart equates to greater level of aerobic fitness.

These various formulas produce significant differences in the recommended target heart rate ranges for the same individual. Therefore, estimated MHR (compared with measured) is not a reliable predictor of exercise intensity. In fact, research has shown that MHR can vary significantly among individuals regardless of age or fitness level (Prevost, 2015).

TABLE 4.6 Resting Heart Rate Ratings

Heart Rate (bpm)	Rating
≤ 59	Excellent
60–69	Good
70–79	Average
80–89	Fair
≥ 90	Poor

Data from Hoeger, W. K., Hoeger, S. A., Hoeger, C. I., & Fawson, A. L. (2017). *Lifetime Physical Fitness and Wellness*. (14th ed). Boston, MA: Cengage Learning.

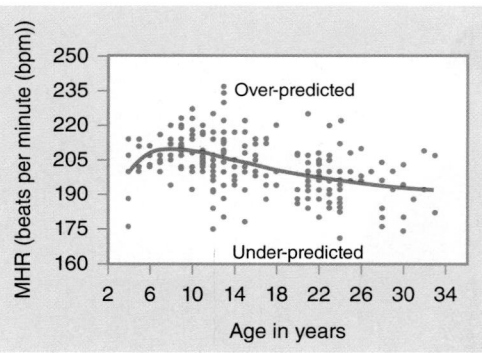

FIGURE 4.8 Accuracy of Max Heart Rate Equations
Modified from McCormick, W. Aerobic Training [PowerPoint Presentation]. Loyola Marymount University, Los Angeles, CA.

The blue dots in (**FIGURE 4.8**) represent measured MHR (not estimated) for individuals of various ages; the red line represents the 220 - Age value for each age group (Robergs, 2002). In some cases the APMHR equation over-predicted measured MHR and in other cases it under-predicted measured MPR. This means that if the 220 - Age equation was used to prescribe exercise intensity; some individuals would be overtraining while others would be undertraining.

Other methods of accessing exercise intensity are the **rate of perceived exertion (RPE)** and **talk test**. (**TABLE 4.7**) illustrates a strong collection correlation between RPE, talk test, and MHR (Command Fitness Leader Certification Course, n.d.). Therefore, if an individual does not have the ability to measure his or her MHR, or have access to a heart rate monitor, using RPE or the talk test may be an easier and just as reliable means of monitoring exercise intensity.

Current research clearly supports that regular strength training improves run performance, whether that be in terms of run economy or time to exhaustion. In order

Rate of perceived exertion (RPE): A method of measuring physical activity intensity level based on how hard you feel like your body is working.

Talk test: A simple way to measure exercise intensity. In general, during moderate-intensity activity you can talk, but not sing. During vigorous-intensity activity, you will not be able to say more than a few words without pausing for a breath.

TABLE 4.7 Correlation between Rate of Perceived Exertion, the Talk Test, and % of Max Heart Rate

RPE Chart		Talk Test	%MHR
1	**Very Light Activity** Watching TV, riding in a car, etc.		
2-3	**Light Activity** Feels like you can maintain for hours	Breathing is easy, can sing	
4-6	**Moderate Activity** Feels like you can exercise for hours	Can carry a conversation	**52-66**
7-8	**Virgorous Activity** On the verge of becoming uncomfortable	Short of breath, can speak a sentence or two	**61-85** **86-91**
9	**Very Hard Activity** Very difficult to maintain exercise intensity	Can only speak one word at a time	**92**
10	**Maximum Effort Activity** Feels almost impossible to keep going	Completely out of breath, unable to talk	

Data from Command Fitness Leader Certification Course. Exercise principles and programming (S5620612A) [PowerPoint Presentation]. Navy Physical Readiness Program, Millington, TN.

Is running counterproductive to strength training?

Depends on frequency, intensity, and duration of endurance training. Although regular strength training has shown to improve endurance performance, excessive endurance training can impact strength, size, and power gains. The exact amount of endurance training required to negatively impact strength training is unclear; however, it is recommended to keep total run mileage to under 15 miles per week.

to prevent some of the common problems associated with run gait (e.g., hip drop, foot crossover), added focus should be placed on training the core. **TABLE 4.8** provides several recommended strength training exercises that are beneficial for runners to perform.

Although the vast majority of recommendations provided are specific to running, the same basic training principles can be applied to other types of endurance training such as cycling, swimming, elliptical trainers, rowing machines, or a combination thereof.

TABLE 4.8 Recommended Strength Training Exercises for Runners

Sample Exercise
Walking Lunges
Bulgarian Split Squats
Loaded Carries
Stiff-Leg Deadlifts
Kettlebell Swings

Assessment and Application

Summary

- Cardiovascular fitness is the ability of the heart, lungs, and organs to consume, transport, and utilize oxygen.

- VO_2max is the maximum amount of oxygen that the body can take in and utilize in one-minute of high-intensity exercise. Knowing what your VO_2max score is and how to effectively train to improve it is important as VO_2max correlates well to certain distance run times (e.g., 1.5-mile).

- Lactate threshold (LT) is the point in exercise where lactate production starts to exceed lactate removal in the blood. Research has shown LT to be a better predictor of one's cardiovascular fitness than VO_2max.

- Exercise economy is the amount of energy required to maintain a particular running speed or generate a specific amount of power. Exercise economy does have a significant impact on endurance performance, although not to the same extent as VO_2max and LT.

- Although the rationale behind hypoxia sounds compelling, it is not supported by current research. Therefore, any hypoxia training should be done in addition to and not in lieu of conventional endurance training.

- High-intensity interval training (HIIT) is a type of endurance training that utilizes repeated short to long bouts of high-intensity exercise combined with short recovery periods. Research has shown that the benefits of HIIT are almost identical to that of traditional endurance training.

- There are five distinct types of endurance training (i.e., long slow distance (LSD), pace/tempo, interval, repetition, Fartlek) each with their own specific training guidelines in terms of exercise intensity, duration, frequency, and rest.

- Although an easy and popular method to use, maximum heart rate prediction equations have been shown to be an unreliable means of assessing and prescribing exercise intensity.

Knowledge Check

1. List and discuss the three major factors that influence endurance performance.
2. How much weight would athlete A need to lose (in lbs.) if his or her current weight was 145 lbs., level of aerobic fitness was 3200 ml O_2, and his or her goal VO_2max score was 50.0 ml O_2?
3. Discuss some of the different training recommendations for increasing lactic threshold.
4. Discuss how muscle fiber type can influence endurance performance.
5. Define hypoxia training and discuss some of the proposed benefits associated with it.
6. Define high-intensity interval training (HIIT) and list some of the benefits associated with this type of endurance training.
7. List and discuss the different endurance training types including the intensity, duration, frequency, and rest assignments for each.
8. Provide specific training examples for each of the different endurance training types.

9. Provide specific endurance training exercises that can be used to improve VO$_2$max.
10. Calculate the required miles per hour (mph) for someone wanting to use the treadmill tempo run method in order to achieve a 12:40 1.5-mile run time.
11. What would the run time (aka desired run time) be for someone running 5K at 7.8 miles per hour (mph) using the treadmill tempo run method?
12. Calculate the estimated maximum heart rate (MHR) and target heart rate range (THRR) of 60–85% for a 22-year-old female with a resting heart rate (RHR) of 68 beats per minute (bpm) using both the Karvonen and female-specific methods.
13. Describe the relationship between MHR, rate of perceived exertion (RPE), and the talk test.
14. Provide specific examples of some strength training exercises that are beneficial for endurance athletes.

Activities

Endurance Training

A. Using Claire's and Ethan's 1.5 mile run time of 14:10 and 13:30, respectively, determine their VO$_2$max scores using **Table 4.1**.
B. Using these VO$_2$max scores for Claire and Ethan, determine the amount of weight each would need to lose if they wanted to achieve their 1.5 mile goal run time. Claire's goal run time is 12:40; Ethan's goal run time is 10:30. Assume their level of aerobic fitness remains the same.
C. Generate a treadmill tempo run workout for both Claire and Ethan using their current run times and their goal run times for the 1.5 mile run.
D. Determine the max heart rates (MHR) for both Claire and Ethan using all applicable equations (all four equations for Claire, and all but the female-specific equation for Ethan). Then, determine the training heart ranges in beats per minute (bpm) if Ethan is looking to train between 80% and 90% of his MHR, and Claire is looking to train between 65% and 80% of her MHR. Assume that Claire's resting heart rate (RHR) is 66 bpm and Ethan's RHR is 72 bpm.

References

Al-Masri L., & Bartlett, S. (2011). *100 Questions & answers about sports nutrition and exercise.* Burlington, MA: Jones & Bartlett.

Baechle, T. R., & Earle, R. W. (Eds.). (2008). *Essentials of strength training and conditioning.* (3rd ed.). Champaign, IL: Human Kinetics.

Command Fitness Leader Certification Course. *Exercise principles and programming* (S5620612A) [PowerPoint Presentation]. Navy Physical Readiness Program, Millington, TN.

Cooper, K. H. (1968). A means of assessing maximal oxygen intake. *Journal of the American Medical Association*, 203, 201–204.

Haff, G., & Triplett, N. (Eds.). (2016). *Essentials of strength training and conditioning.* (4th ed). Champaign, IL: Human Kinetics.

Hoeger, W. K., Hoeger, S. A., Hoeger, C. I., & Fawson, A. L. (2017). *Lifetime physical fitness and wellness.* (14th ed). Boston, MA: Cengage Learning.

Ivy, J. (2016). *Exercise training and conditioning: what works and why.* Nutrition for Sports, Exercise and Weight Management Workshop. Arlington, VA.

Laurentino, G., Ugrinowitsch, C., Aihara, A. Y., Fernandes, A. R., Parcell, A. C., Ricard, M., & Tricoli, V. (2008). Effects of strength training and vascular occlusion. *International Journal of Sports Medicine, 29*(8), 664–667.

Liang, H., & Ward, W. F. (2006). PGC-1α: a key regulator of energy metabolism. *Advances in Physiology Education, 30*(4), 145–151.

McArdle, W. D., Katch, F. I., & Katch, V. L. (2015). *Exercise physiology: nutrition, energy, and human performance.* (8th ed). Baltimore, MD: Wolters Kluwer Health.

McConnell, A. K., & Romer, L. M. (2004). Respiratory muscle training in healthy humans: resolving the controversy. *International Journal of Sports Medicine*, 25(4), 284–93.

McCormick, W (n.d.). *Aerobic training* [PowerPoint Presentation]. Loyola Marymount University, Los Angeles, CA.

Prevost, M. (2015). *Built to endure* [eBook]. Retrieved from http://built-to-endure.blogspot.com/.

Robergs, R. A. (2002). The surprising history of the HRmax = 220 - age equation. *Journal of Exercise Physiology*, 5(2), 1–10.

Training 4 Endurance (2017). *Exercise economy / economy of motion*. Retrieved from http://training4endurance.co.uk/physiology-of-endurance/exercise-economy/

United States Army. (2008, July 23). *Recommendations for Prevention of Physical Training (PT)-Related Injuries: Results of a Systematic Evidence-Based Review by the Joint Services Physical Training Injury Prevention Work Group (JSPTIPWG)*. Retrieved from http://oaaction.unc.edu/files/2014/10/Bullock-08-JSPTIPWG-final-report.pdf

Strength Training

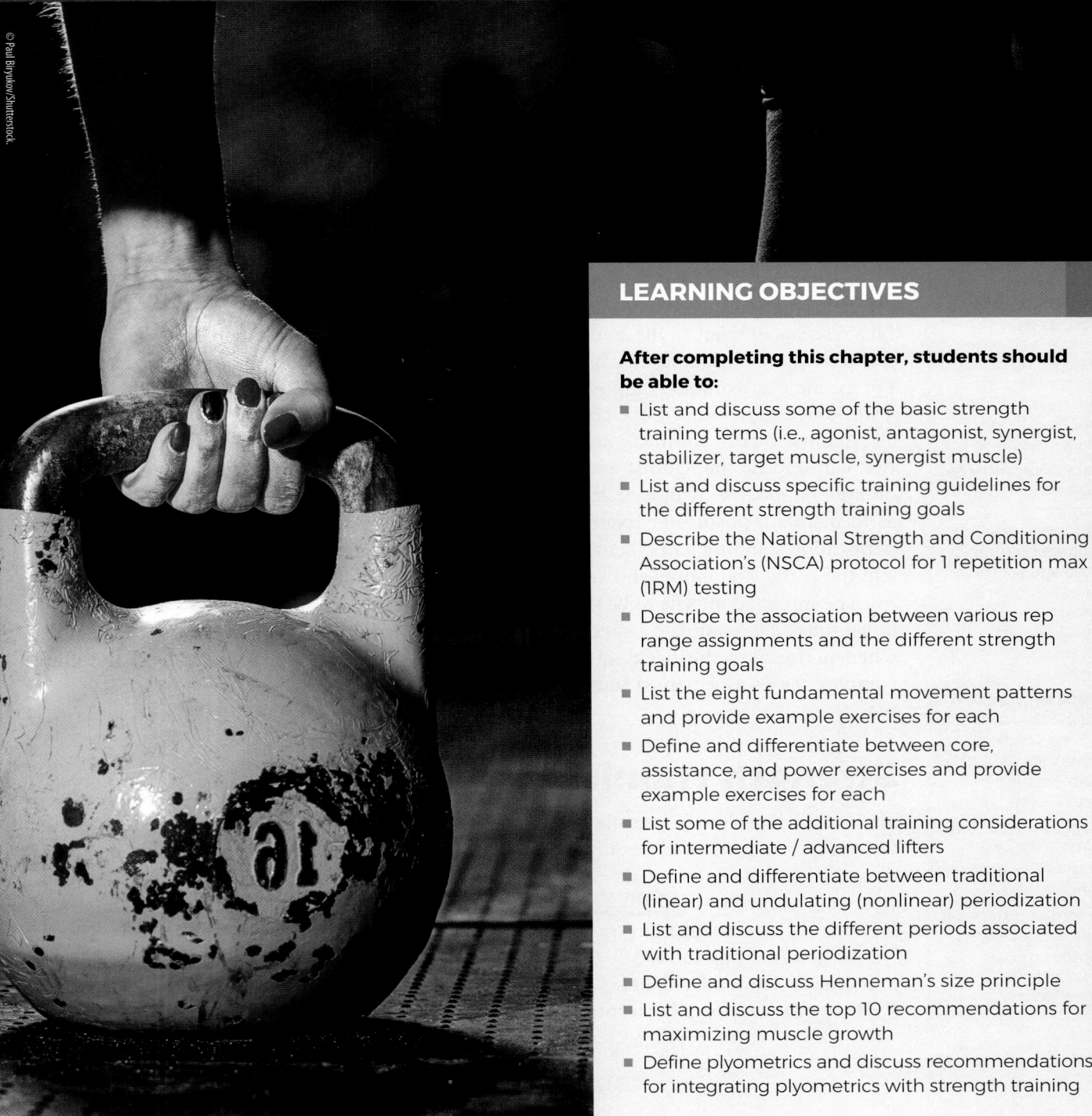

LEARNING OBJECTIVES

After completing this chapter, students should be able to:

- List and discuss some of the basic strength training terms (i.e., agonist, antagonist, synergist, stabilizer, target muscle, synergist muscle)
- List and discuss specific training guidelines for the different strength training goals
- Describe the National Strength and Conditioning Association's (NSCA) protocol for 1 repetition max (1RM) testing
- Describe the association between various rep range assignments and the different strength training goals
- List the eight fundamental movement patterns and provide example exercises for each
- Define and differentiate between core, assistance, and power exercises and provide example exercises for each
- List some of the additional training considerations for intermediate / advanced lifters
- Define and differentiate between traditional (linear) and undulating (nonlinear) periodization
- List and discuss the different periods associated with traditional periodization
- Define and discuss Henneman's size principle
- List and discuss the top 10 recommendations for maximizing muscle growth
- Define plyometrics and discuss recommendations for integrating plyometrics with strength training

Strength training (aka Resistance training): Type of physical exercise specializing in the use of resistance in order to improve the strength, anaerobic endurance, and size of skeletal muscle.

Repetition (rep): A complete motion of a particular exercise or movement pattern.

Set: A group of repetitions sequentially performed before the athlete stops to rest.

Load: Amount of weight assigned to an exercise set.

Volume: The total amount of weight lifted in a training session.

Agonist muscle: Most skeletal muscle is arranged in opposing pairs. The contracting muscle is the agonist muscle during an exercise.

Antagonist muscle: Most skeletal muscle is arranged in opposing pairs. The contracting muscle is the agonist muscle during an exercise. The antagonist muscle is the opposite (opposing) the agonist muscle.

Stabilizer muscle: A muscle that contracts with no significant movement to maintain posture or fixate a joint.

Target muscle: The primary muscle intended to train or exercise.

Synergist muscle: A muscle that assists another muscle to accomplish a movement.

Introduction

Strength training (aka resistance training) is a training method that uses resistance to produce power, size, strength, and anaerobic endurance gains in skeletal muscle. Some of the benefits associated with regular strength training include increased muscle proteins (i.e., actin, myosin), collagen proteins (found in tendons and ligaments), and osteoproteins (found in the bones), which results in a stronger and more injury-resistant musculoskeletal system. Additional benefits include increased myofibrils (slender threads of a muscle fiber), capillaries, and intramuscular energy stores as well as better muscle fiber recruitment. Secondary benefits include improved physical capacity (amount of work that can be performed), higher metabolic function, and reduced risk of injury (Al-Masri & Bartlett, 2011; Baechle & Earle, 2008; Haff & Triplett, 2016; Westcott, 1995).

Basic Strength Training Terms

Before going into specific strength training guidelines and recommendations, it is important to first understand some basic strength training terms.

A **repetition (rep)** refers to the complete motion of a particular exercise or movement pattern. For example, one rep of a pushup is when you begin with the arms extended and the body in the front leaning rest position, lower your body down until the arms are at 90 degrees at the elbows, then push the body back up until the arms are once again extended. A **set** is the specific number of reps performed sequentially before resting. For example, two sets of 10 rep push-ups means you completed 10 reps of push-ups, two separate times. **Load** (aka resistance) refers to the amount of weight being lifted, such as a 50 lb. kettlebell. **Volume** refers to the total number of exercises, sets, and reps you complete in a particular workout. For example, a workout composed of 4 exercises, 6 sets of 10 reps has a higher volume than a workout composed of 3 exercises, 2 sets of 15 reps.

A muscle that contracts and causes motion is called the **agonist muscle**. A muscle that can oppose the agonist and/or move the joint in the opposite direction is called the **antagonist muscle**. A muscle that contracts but performs no significant movement, such as to maintain posture or fixate a joint, is called a **stabilizer muscle**. For example, when performing standing barbell curls, the biceps are the agonist, the triceps are the antagonist, and the rectus abdominis and erector spinea are the stabilizers.

The intended muscle to be trained is called the **target muscle**. A muscle that assists the target muscle to complete a specific movement is called the **synergist muscle**. For example, when performing the back squat, the quadriceps are the target muscles, and the glute complex serves as synergist muscles.

Strength Training Goals

Similar to endurance training, there are several different approaches (or goals) to strength training, each requiring specific rep, set, and rest recommendations. In short, these different training goals can be divided into four basic categories: strength, power, size, and endurance. **TABLE 5.1** depicts the load, rep, set, and rest recommendations for each respective strength training goal (Baechle & Earle, 2008; Haff & Triplett, 2016).

As described in Table 5.1, repetition and set recommendations are often based on an individual's 1RM. Listed here are the National Strength and Conditioning Association's (NSCA) protocol for 1RM testing.

TABLE 5.1 Recommended Load and Volume Assignments Based on Training Goal

Training Goal	Load (% 1RM)	Goal Reps	Goal Sets	Rest
Endurance	≤ 67	≤ 12	2–3	≤ 30 sec.
Hypertrophy	67–85	6–12	3–6	30–90 sec.
Strength	≤ 85	≤ 6	2–6	2–5 min.
Power	75–90	1–5	3–5	2–5 min.

Data from Baechle, T. R., & Earle, R. W. (Eds.). (2008). *Essentials of strength training and conditioning.* (3rd ed.). Champaign, IL: Human Kinetics; Haff, G., & Triplett, N. (Eds.). (2016). *Essentials of strength training and conditioning.* (4th ed). Champaign, IL: Human Kinetics.

- *Step 1*: Warm-up using light resistance that easily allows for 5–10 repetitions
- *Step 2*: Allow for a 1-minute rest period
- *Step 3*: Estimate a warm-up load that can be completed for 3–5 repetitions
- *Step 4*: Allow for a 2-minute rest period
- *Step 5*: Estimate a conservative, near-maximal load that can be completed for 2–3 repetitions
- *Step 6*: Allow for a 2–4 minute rest period
- *Step 7*: Make a load increase and attempt 1RM
- *Step 8*: If successful, allow for a 2–4 minute rest period, make a load increase, and attempt a new (heavier) 1RM
- *Step 9*: If unsuccessful, allow for a 2–4 minute rest period, make a load decrease, and attempt a new (lighter) 1RM
- *Step 10*: Continue increasing or decreasing the load until a 1RM is determined

FIGURE 5.1 shows how **1-repetition maximum (RM)** ranges are associated with the different strength training goals (Baechle & Earle, 2008; Haff & Triplett, 2016). Note that the bold yellow areas indicate the primary training goal for different repetition ranges. The larger fonts indicate a greater correlation between certain repetition ranges and specific training goals; whereas smaller fonts indicate less correlation.

As shown in the chart, certain repetition ranges are associated with specific physiological adaptations (e.g., 2–6 reps = gains in strength; 6–12 reps = gains in size; 12–20+ reps = gains in muscle endurance). This is important since some athletes have multiple strength training goals. For example, athletes interested in gaining both strength and size would benefit from

> **1-Repetition maximum (1RM):** Greatest amount of weight that can be lifted for one repetition.

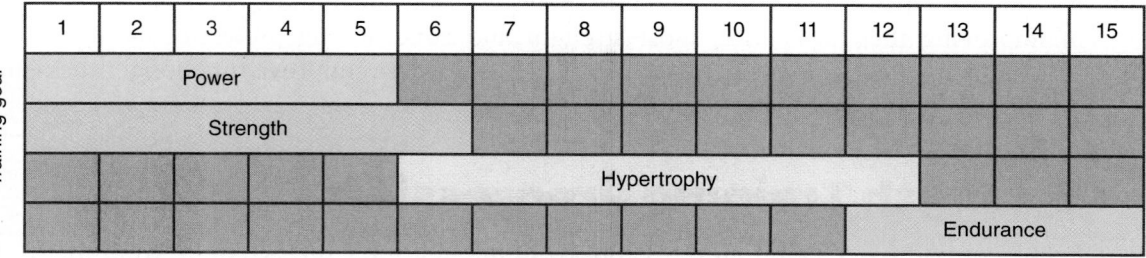

Repetitions

FIGURE 5.1 Association of Rep Ranges with Various Training Goals

Data from Haff, G., & Triplett, N. (Eds.). (2016). *Essentials of Strength Training and Conditioning.* (4th ed). Champaign, IL: Human Kinetics.

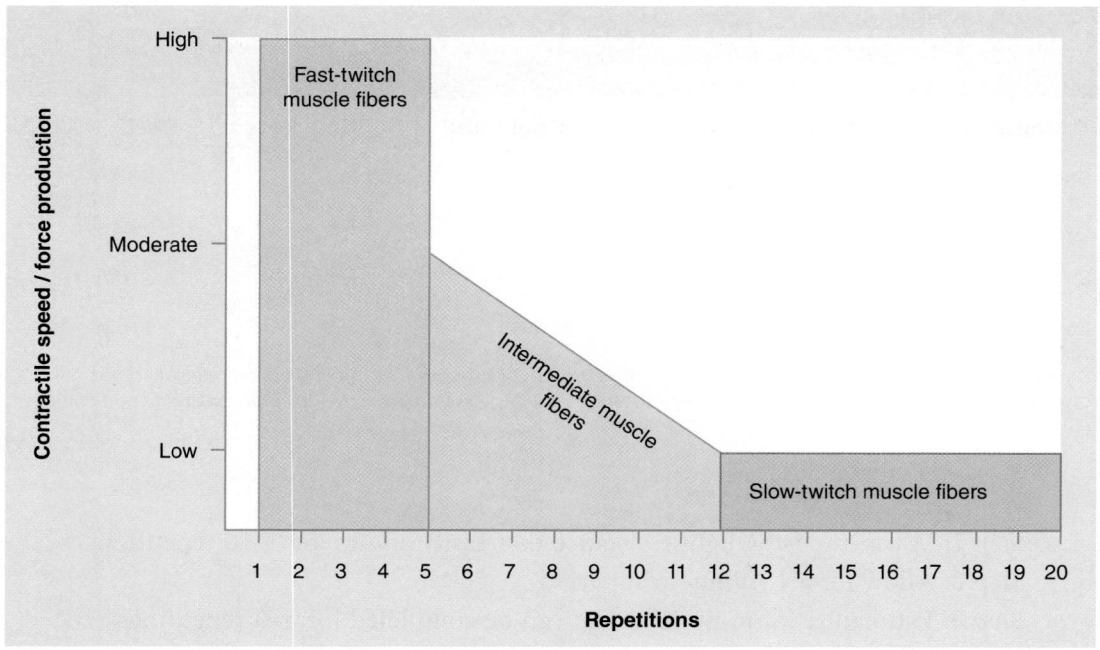

FIGURE 5.2 Associated Repetition Ranges per Fiber Type

using sets of 6 repetitions. Similarly, athletes interested in gaining both size and endurance would benefit from using sets of 12 repetitions.

FIGURE 5.2 shows the importance of training at a variety of repetition ranges since each muscle fiber type (e.g., type I (slow-twitch), type II (fast-twitch)) responds differently to various repetition ranges. For example, type I muscle fibers are more aerobic (endurance) in nature and respond better to lighter weights and higher repetitions; type II muscle fibers are more anaerobic (strength/power) in nature and respond better to heavier weights with fewer repetitions or explosive movements (e.g., Olympic lifts).

Regardless of the training goal (i.e., strength, power, size, or muscular endurance), there are certain exercises, or movement patterns, that should be incorporated in order to promote maximal gains in terms of sport performance, injury prevention, and quality of life.

In all, there are eight fundamental movement patterns that should be used in any strength training regimen. **TABLE 5.2** lists the eight different fundamental movement patterns and provides an example for each.

The recommendation to design resistance training programs around specific movement patterns is a relatively new concept. Previously, most resistance training programs were designed to target specific muscle groups (e.g., chest, back, shoulders, arms, legs). Although the traditional approach has worked well for bodybuilders and those interested in improving their aesthetics, most strength and conditioning professionals now agree that targeting specific movement patterns is a better way to improve functional fitness and prepare their athletes for sport participation.

Strength Training Progression

Before providing specific progression recommendations for strength training, it is worth discussing some fundamental guidance regarding exercise progression as a whole. Specifically, the movement of each exercise should be mastered before adding an external load. For example, prior to performing back squats with a loaded bar, body weight squats should be performed until the proper technique (e.g., no knee

TABLE 5.2 Eight Fundamental Movement Patterns and Sample Exercises for Each

Movement Pattern	Sample Exercise		
Horizontal Push	Bench Press		
Horizontal Pull	Bent Over Row		
Vertical Push	Military Press		
Vertical Pull	Lat Pulldown		
Squat	Back Squat		
Hip Hinge	Good Mornings		
Loaded Carry	Farmers Carry		
Core	Russian Twists		

TABLE 5.3 Training Recommendations Based on Training Status

Training Status	Training Type	Training Frequency (sessions per week)
Beginner	· Core Exercises · Mostly Machines · Linear Progression	2–3
Intermediate	· Mostly Core Exercises · Increase Intensity · Introduce Power Exercises	3–4
Advanced	· Mostly Core · Power Exercises · Some Assistance · Periodized Intensity	4–7

Data from Baechle, T. R., & Earle, R. W. (Eds.). (2008). *Essentials of Strength Training and Conditioning.* (3rd ed.). Champaign, IL: Human Kinetics; Haff, G., & Triplett, N. (Eds.). (2016). *Essentials of Strength Training and Conditioning.* (4th ed). Champaign, IL: Human Kinetics.

Varus: Form deficiency caused by the oblique displacement of a limb towards the midline of the body.

Valgus: Form deficiency caused by the oblique displacement of a limb away from the midline of the body.

Core exercise: Recruit one or more large muscle areas, involve two or more primary joints, and receive priority because of their direct application to the sport.

Assistance exercise: Recruit smaller muscle areas, involve only one primary joint, and are considered less important to improving sport performance.

Power exercise: Structural exercises that are performed very quickly or explosively.

Structural exercise: Exercises that load the spine directly or indirectly.

varus or **valgus**) and range of motion are both mastered. In some cases, this may take several training sessions, weeks, or even months. However, failing to do so may result in diminished training gains, reduced range of motion over time, and/or increased risk of injury.

When determining training frequency, the following factors should also be considered: training status, load (aka amount of weight), types of exercises, and concurrent training or activities. **TABLE 5.3** provides training type and frequency recommendations based on training status (Baechle & Earle, 2008; Haff & Triplett, 2016).

Core exercises are movements that recruit one or more major muscle groups (e.g., chest, back, quadriceps), involve two or more joints, and receive priority due to their direct application to sport. **Assistance exercises** are movements that recruit smaller muscle groups (e.g., biceps, triceps), involve only one joint, and are considered less important in terms of improving sport performance. A movement is classified as a **power exercise** when it is performed very quickly or explosively and it loads the spine either directly or indirectly. Exercises that load the spine are referred to as **structural exercises**.

The order in which strength training exercises are performed is also important in order to ensure proper form, prevent muscular fatigue, and reduce the risk of injury. Specifically, power exercises should be performed first, followed by core exercises. Assistance exercises should be performed last, if at all. The following table provides examples of power, core, and assistance exercises.

Power	Core	Assistance
Power Clean	Squat	Bicep Curls
Push Press	Bench Press	Tricep Extensions
Snatch	Deadlift	Leg Curls
Plyometrics	Overhead Press	Lateral Raises
Kettlebell Swings	Bent Over Row	Calf Raises

In addition to performing the correct number of reps and sets for a specific training goal, applying the correct amount of rest time between sets is another important training consideration. In terms of rest between sets there are two basic approaches: inactive and

TABLE 5.4 Load Increase Recommendations

	Beginner / Early Intermediate	Late Intermediate / Advanced
Upper Body Exercises	2.5–5 lbs.	5–10 lbs.
Lower Body Exercises	5–10 lbs.	10–15 lbs.

Data from Baechle, T. R., & Earle, R. W. (Eds.). (2008). *Essentials of Strength Training and Conditioning*. (3rd ed.). Champaign, IL: Human Kinetics; Haff, G., & Triplett, N. (Eds.). (2016). *Essentials of Strength Training and Conditioning*. (4th ed.). Champaign, IL: Human Kinetics.

active. Inactive rest involves no additional activity or exercises being performed between sets. **Active rest** involves performing low-intensity exercises or movements (e.g., stretching or low-intensity endurance training) between sets. Another approach to active rest is to train opposing (aka antagonist) muscle groups between sets. For example, alternating between upper body (e.g., military press) and lower body exercises (e.g., leg press) or pushing (e.g., bench press) and pulling exercises (e.g., lat pull-down). When exercises are performed in short succession it is referred to as **circuit training**.

Another important consideration is load progression (i.e., when to add weight and by how much). The **2-for-2 Rule** states that when you can perform two or more repetitions over the assigned repetition goal in the last set for two consecutive workouts, weight should be added to that exercise for the next training session. **TABLE 5.4** provides some general recommendations regarding load progression in terms of training status and exercise type (i.e., upper body, lower body) (Baechle & Earle, 2008; Haff & Triplett, 2016).

Training Considerations for Intermediate / Advanced Lifters

Intermediate and advanced lifters should also consider additional training options such as **cluster sets** and the **rest-pause technique**. Cluster sets incorporate short intra-set rest periods (e.g., 5–20 seconds) to allow for an increase in both training intensity and volume. For example, instead of doing four sets of 6 reps, you would perform four sets of 2 reps (not to failure) with a 20 second intra-set rest in between using a heavier load. There are a couple of different ways to perform the rest-pause technique. One of the more popular approaches is to perform three sets to concentric (muscle shortening) failure with a 15 second intra-set rest in between. For example, pick a weight you can perform 8–12 reps with good form. Perform the first set to failure then rest 15 seconds; then perform the second set to failure then rest 15 seconds, followed by the third and final set to failure. You will notice that the amount of repetitions performed will drop significantly between sets. In fact, it is not uncommon to only be able to perform 1–2 reps on the last set.

Another increasingly popular method of introducing progression and variation into a traditional resistance training program is by using chains and resistance bands. Both methods are currently employed by numerous powerlifters, especially for lifts like the bench press and squat, and are growing in popularity for other athletes in a variety of sports. Despite their popularity, the scientific research on these methods is largely unsubstantiated (Haff & Triplett, 2016).

When using chains, researchers recommend that the chain be suspended from the bar without touching the floor until the athlete is in the lowest position of the squat or until the bar touches the chest in the bench press. As the bar is lowered, the chains pile on the floor

Active rest: A means of recovery during or post workout that involves either stretching or exercising at lower intensity.

Circuit training: A form of conditioning or resistance training that incorporates both strength building and muscular endurance. A "circuit" is one completion of all prescribed exercises in the program.

2-for-2 Rule: Progression recommendation in strength training requiring weight to be added when you can perform two or more repetitions over the assigned repetition goal in the last set for two consecutive workouts.

Cluster sets: Sets that incorporate intra-set rest periods that allow for better manipulation of volume and intensity.

Rest-pause technique: A method that involves stopping during the completion of a set, resting for a short period and then continuing on with the set.

Stretch-shortening cycle (SSC): An active stretch (eccentric contraction) of a muscle followed by an immediate shortening (concentric contraction) of that same muscle.

Amortization phase: One of the three plyometric phases of movement that occurs between the concentric and eccentric phases and is considered to be the most crucial phase in the body's ability to produce power.

Eccentric contraction: A type of muscle activation that increases tension on a muscle as it lengthens.

Concentric contraction: A type of muscle activation that increases tension on a muscle as it shortens.

Olympic lifting: Type of strength (power) training in which athletes attempt to lift near maximum loads that are mounted on barbells.

and the mass of the barbell decreases, which may allow for a more rapid stretch-shortening cycle (SSC) (active stretch of a muscle followed by an immediate shortening of that same muscle) thereby resulting in a faster amortization phase (time between the concentric and eccentric phases and considered the most crucial phase in the production of power) as the athlete shifts from the eccentric contraction (muscle lengthening) to concentric contraction (muscle shortening) phase of movement. Most strength and conditioning professionals recommend the use of chains only for athletes with significant strength training experience.

When using resistance bands, researchers recommend using bands to substitute 20–35% of the total load (weight) used (Haff & Triplett, 2016). Similar to chains, the greatest amount of tension and resistance load is provided at the lockout position of the exercise. As the athlete approaches the lockout position of the exercise, the bands impart greater resistance. The theory is that continued use of resistance bands (and chains) will translate into greater strength and power gains over time; however, current research has yet to substantiate this claim. However, band composition varies significantly depending on the type of thermoplastic or elastomer used in manufacturing. Additionally, bands of the same type can sometimes differ as much as 8-19% in mean tension, which can significantly affect the balance and load distribution of the exercise being performed (Haff & Triplett, 2016).

Another consideration for intermediate or advance lifters is Olympic lifting (e.g., snatch, clean and jerk, power cleans). Although this type of strength training can promote gains in muscular size and strength, it is primarily used to develop muscular power. Additionally, Olympic lifts are more technique oriented (requiring a certain amount of skill to perform safely/correctly) than traditional strength training exercises (e.g., bench press, back squat, deadlift) and, therefore, have a higher risk for injury. Because of this, utilization of Olympic lifts may not be suitable for everyone. Although they makes sense for those athletes requiring a great deal of explosive power in order to be successful on the field or court (e.g., football, basketball, volleyball), they may not be the best approach for those individuals using strength training for the sole purpose of general fitness, hypertrophy, and/or strength.

FAQ

Which type of strength training is best: bodybuilding, powerlifting, or Olympic lifting?

When deciding which strength training approach is appropriate, it is important to keep in mind that the body responds to the training stimulus. For example, if exposed to high volume (3–5+ sets) and moderate load (6–12 reps), the muscles will get larger (hypertrophy); if exposed to moderate volume (2–6 sets) and heavier loads (≤ 6 reps), the muscles will get stronger; and, if required to move moderate to heavy loads very quickly, the muscles will become more powerful (explosive).

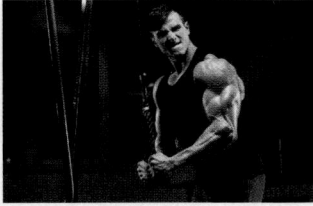
© Nikolas_jkd/Shutterstock.

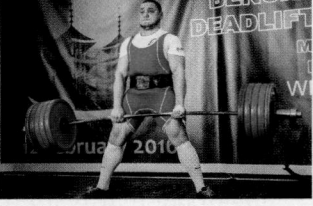
© sportpoint/Shutterstock.

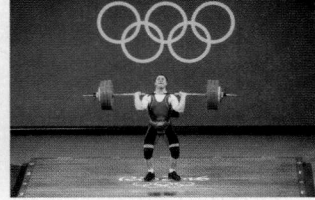
© Stringer/Anadolu Agency/Getty Images.

Although each type of strength training results in muscular size, strength, and power, the extent of the physiological adaptations can differ significantly among approaches. As depicted in the picture, bodybuilding is the best approach to build size (mass); powerlifting is the best approach to build strength, and Olympic lifts are the best approach to build power (explosiveness). So pick the approach that best matches your overall strength training goal (i.e., size, strength, or power). In some cases, a combination of two or all three may be the right answer. For example, an offensive lineman in football would benefit from bigger (bodybuilding), stronger (powerlifting), and more powerful (Olympic lifting) muscles. As a result, most sports employ a periodization model that includes a designated hypertrophy, strength, and power phase into their overall strength and conditioning program.

Although Olympic lifting is likely the best approach for developing power (explosiveness), it may not be suitable for everyone. Olympic lifts (e.g., snatch, clean and jerk, power cleans) are extremely technical and thus require extensive coaching in order to perform correctly. Individuals with limited resistance training experience and/or access to a qualified strength and conditioning coach would likely be better served using machines or less complicated strength training exercises (e.g., bench press, back squat, deadlift, overhead press). Olympic lifts also pose a greater risk for injury and, therefore, may not be recommended for individuals with certain injuries or ailments (e.g., torn rotator cuff, herniated disk). For those individuals training for hypertrophy, Olympic lifting does not produce the same degree of muscular size and strength that bodybuilding and powerlifting do. Because Olympic lifts are performed quickly, they do not produce the same amount of muscle strain or damage on the muscle during the eccentric (muscle lengthening) phase of movement as bodybuilding and powerlifting do.

Periodization

Periodization is a strategy that promotes long-term training and performance improvements with preplanned, systematic variations in training specificity, intensity, and volume that are organized into periods (aka cycles) within an overall program. Additionally, periodization involves shifting training priorities from non-sport-specific activities of high volume and low intensity to sport-specific activities of low volume and high intensity over many weeks to prevent overtraining and optimize performance. **FIGURE 5.3** provides a graphic depiction of the linear periodization model and the relationship between training volume, intensity, and competition in sport.

There are two basic types of periodization: linear (aka traditional) and nonlinear (aka undulating). **Linear periodization** employs gradual changes in exercise programming with a series of training cycles (i.e., macrocycles, mesocycles, microcycles). In other words, linear periodization uses a systematic approach to exercise prescription that transitions from high volume and low intensity to low volume, high intensity in an attempt to maximize gains in strength, power, size, and endurance. On the other hand, **Nonlinear periodization** uses daily

Periodization: A form of strength training that uses a strategic implementation of training phases (e.g., hypertrophy, strength, power). These phases periodically increase and decrease both volume and intensity in order to prevent overtraining and maximize gains.

Linear periodization: Traditional model with gradual progressive increases in intensity over time.

Non-linear periodization: An alternative method that involves large fluctuations in load and volume assignments.

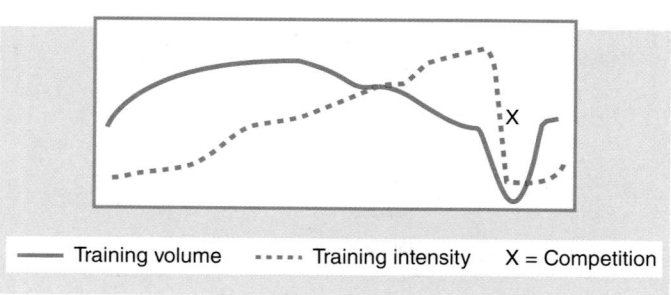

—— Training volume   ····· Training intensity   X = Competition

FIGURE 5.3 Relationship between Training Volume and Intensity in Linear (Traditional) Periodization

Linear vs. non-linear periodization

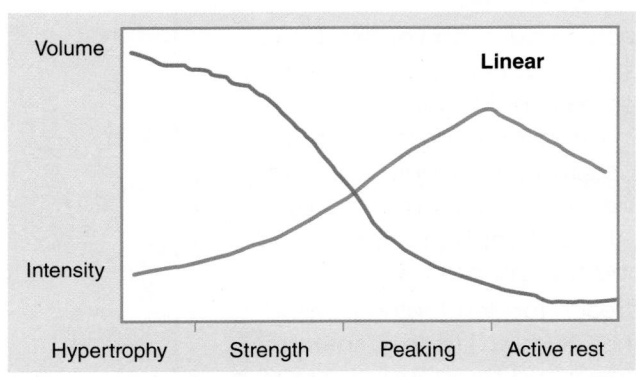 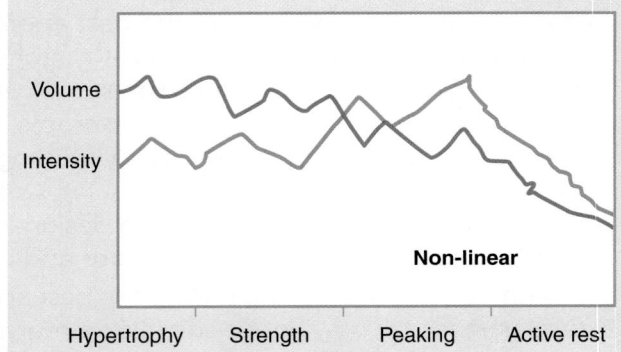

FIGURE 5.4 Differences in Training Volume and Intensity Recommendations between Linear (Traditional) and Nonlinear (Undulating) Periodization

fluctuations, instead of week- or month-long cycles, in volume, intensity and load assignments to accomplish these same goals. **FIGURE 5.4** illustrates some of the differences between linear and nonlinear periodization in terms of training volume and intensity (University of New Mexico, n.d.).

Provided in the following tables are examples of linear and nonlinear (undulating) training programs.

Linear Periodization Example											
Endurance			**Hypertrophy**			**Strength**			**Power**		
Week	**Reps**	**Sets**	**Week**	**Reps**	**Sets**	**Week**	**Reps**	**Sets**	**Week**	**Reps**	**Sets**
1	≥ 12	2	5	6–12	3	10	≤ 6	3	15	1–5	3
2	≥ 12	3	6	6–12	4	11	≤ 6	4	16	1–5	4
3	≥ 12	4	7	6–12	5	12	≤ 6	5	17	1–5	5
4	Deload		8	6–12	6	13	≤ 6	6	18	Deload	
			9	Deload		14	Deload				

Nonlinear (Undulating) Periodization Example					
	Week	**Monday** **Max Effort** **Lower Body**	**Wednesday** **Max Effort** **Upper Body**	**Friday** **Dynamic Effort** **Lower Body**	**Sunday** **Dynamic Effort** **Upper Body**
Core Exercises	1	Work up to 1RM	Work up to 1RM	12 × 2 @ 75% 1RM	9 × 3 @ 60% 1RM
	2			12 × 2 @ 80% 1RM	9 × 3 @ 60% 1RM
	3			10 × 2 @ 85% 1RM	9 × 3 @ 60% 1RM
Assistance Exercises (3–5 sets of 8–12 reps ea.)		Hamstrings Glutes Lower Back Core	Shoulders Triceps Chest Upper Back	Hamstrings Glutes Lower Back Core	Shoulders Triceps Chest Upper Back

*If preferred, the same set, rep, and load assignment for DE LB can be applied to DE UB.

Which type of periodization is best: linear (traditional) or nonlinear (undulating)?

Research has shown that both linear and nonlinear periodization models are effective in developing significant gains in terms of muscle size and strength. For example, the Westside Barbell Program recommends the use of non-linear periodization and argues that it is the best and fastest approach for increasing 1RM scores in the core lifts. However, Renaissance Periodization, another credible strength and conditioning program, advocates for linear periodization (Israetel, n.d.). Therefore, deciding which method to use is up to the individual athlete and his or her respective training goals and objectives. It is possible that the best approach is trying both methods to see which one works better or to systematically transition from one method to the other in order to promote variability and prevent training plateaus. However, it may be counterproductive or contraindicative for some athletes to perform weekly 1RM attempts as muscle damage and soreness can significantly affect sport performance (e.g., gymnasts, tennis players).

As mentioned previously, there are numerous other studies showing just the opposite (i.e., that linear periodization produces greater size and strength gains than nonliner periodization).

Linear Periodization Terms, Periods, and Seasons

In linear (traditional) periodization, there are three basic phases (aka terms): macrocycle, mesocycle, and microcycle. A **macrocycle** usually represents an entire training year, but it can also last for a period of many months up to several years. A **mesocycle** represents two or more cycles within the macrocycle, each one lasting several weeks to several months. A **microcycle** typically represents only one week, but it can last for up to four weeks. The purpose of a periodization training model is to prevent training burnout and/or overtraining.

In traditional (linear) periodization, there are four basic periods: preparatory, first transition, competition, and second transition (aka rest).

- *Preparatory Period*: The initial time of the year when there are no competitions and only a limited number of sport-specific skill practices or scrimmages. This period includes very limited sport-specific training and the primary emphasis is to establish a base level of conditioning in order to increase the athlete's tolerance for more intense training. There are three separate phases within the preparatory period, each with distinct differences in training intensity and volume. As each phase progresses, training intensity will increase with a subsequent decrease in training volume.
  - *Hypertrophy/Endurance Phase*: Low to moderate intensity (e.g., 50–75% of 1 repetition max (RM)) and high to moderate volume (e.g., 3–6 sets of 10–20 reps)
  - *Basic Strength Phase*: High intensity (e.g., 80–90% of 1RM) and moderate volume (e.g., 3–5 sets of 4–8 reps)
  - *Strength/Power Phase*: High intensity (e.g., 75–95% of 1RM) and low volume (e.g., 3–5 sets of 2–5 reps)

Macrocycle: The longest of the three cycles of traditional periodization. It represents the overall training period and generally lasts an entire year or longer.

Mesocycle: One of the three cycles of traditional periodization and represents a specific block of training designed to accomplish a particular training goal. Mesocylces typically last a month but can range anywhere from 2 weeks to several months.

Microcycle: The shortest of the three cycles of traditional periodization and typically lasts about a week.

- *First Transition Period*: Time between the preparatory and competitive periods, which is used as a break between high-volume training and high-intensity training. The cross-over point between training intensity and volume generally occurs during this period.
- *Competition Period*: The goal for the competition period is to peak strength and power through increases in training intensity with subsequent decreases in training volume. This phase also includes a high amount of sport-specific training and drills and is mostly intended for performance maintenance than for trying to improve athletic potential.
  - *Peaking*: Use high intensity (e.g., ≥93% of 1RM) and low volume (e.g., 1–3 sets of 1–3 reps)
  - *Maintenance*: Use moderate intensity (e.g., 80–85% of 1RM) and moderate volume (e.g., 2–3 sets of 6–8 reps)
- *Second Transition Period (Active Rest)*: Period of time between the competitive season and next preparatory period, which consists of recreational activity and generally does not involve resistance training.

TABLE 5.5 shows the four periods associated with linear (traditional) periodization (Baechle & Earle, 2008; Haff & Triplett, 2016).

In traditional (linear) periodization, there are also four basic seasons: off-season, pre-season, in-season, and post-season.

- *Off-season*: Period of time between the postseason and six weeks, although this can vary significantly between sports, before the first contest of the following season. During this time, the primary focus is on resistance training.
- *Pre-season*: Period of time leading up to the first contest that commonly contains the late stages of the preparatory period and the first transition period. During this time, emphasis should be on sport-specific training. Resistance training should be performed 3 times per week with an emphasis on strength and power gains. Plyometric and anaerobic endurance training are also frequently used.

TABLE 5.5 Linear (Traditional) Periodization Model for Resistance Training

Period	Preparatory ——————→		First Transition	Competition		Second Transition
Season	**Off-Season**		**Pre-Season**	**In-Season**		**Post-Season**
Phase	Endurance and Hypertrophy	Basic Strength	Strength / Power	Peaking *OR* Maintance		Active Rest
Intensity	Low to Moderate	High	High	Very High	Moderate	
	50–75% 1RM	80–90% 1RM	75–95% 1RM	≥ 93% 1RM	80–85% 1RM	
Volume	High to Moderate	Moderate	Low	Very Low	Moderate	Recreational Activities
	3–6 sets	3–5 sets	3–5 sets	1–3 sets	2–3 sets	
	10–20 reps	4–8 reps	2–5 reps	1–3 reps	6–8 reps	

Data from Baechle, T. R., & Earle, R. W. (Eds.). (2008). *Essentials of strength training and conditioning.* (3rd ed.). Champaign, IL: Human Kinetics; Haff, G., & Triplett, N. (Eds.). (2016). *Essentials of strength training and conditioning.* (4th ed). Champaign, IL: Human Kinetics.

Season	Post-season				Active rest	Off-season			Active rest	Pre-season			Active rest	In-season		Active rest
Training goal	Endurance					Hypertrophy /strength				Power/peaking				Maintenance		
Month	May	Jun	Jul	Aug		Sep	Oct	Nov		Dec	Jan	Feb		Mar	Apr	

FIGURE 5.5 Relationship between Periodization Periods and Sport Seasons

- *In-season*: Period of time containing all scheduled contests and tournament games. During this time, the primary focus is to maintain and possibly improve strength, power, flexibility, and anaerobic conditioning. Additional time should be devoted to sport-specific skill and strategy development. Resistance training should be limited to 30 minutes, 1-3 times per week, alternated with plyometric training.

- *Post-season*: Period of time after the final contest and before the start of next season's off-season or preparatory period. During this time, emphasis should be placed on active or relative rest with no formal or structured workouts. Recreational activities should be performed at low intensity and volume.

FIGURE 5.5 shows the four distinct seasons associated with the linear (traditional) periodization model (Haff & Triplett, 2016).

Strength Training for Size

The Henneman's size principle states that under load, muscle fibers are recruited from smallest to largest. In other words, slow-twitch (type I) fibers are activated before fast twitch (type II) fibers. If the primary training goal is size, training across a wide spectrum of repetition ranges (e.g., 12+, 6–10, 1–5) is recommended. Lighter loads with high repetitions will target and develop the slow-twitch fibers whereas higher loads with few repetitions will target and develop the fast-twitch fibers. However, if the goal is maximal strength, heavy loads are recommended over lighter loads.

As discussed previously, each muscle fiber type responds differently to various load and repetition assignments. Slow-twitch muscle fibers respond better to lighter weights and higher repetitions (e.g., 12+). Fast-twitch muscle fibers respond better to heavier weights, lower repetitions (e.g., 1–6), and/or explosive movements. Intermediate fibers (type IIa and IIb) have both type I and type II characteristics and likely respond best to load and repetition assignments somewhere in between (e.g., 6–12). Therefore, in order to maximize muscle growth, an individual would benefit from training at a variety of load and repetition assignments in order to target and develop each muscle fiber type individually.

Muscle fiber type percentage is genetically determined and different for each person and from muscle group to muscle group. Even so, individuals who possess predominantly slow-twitch fibers can still significantly increase their muscle size and strength through a well-designed strength training program by using a variety of load and repetition assignments. The majority of size and strength gains achieved are likely due to the fast-twitch type IIa fibers converting into type IIb fibers by a process called **fiber type transition**. Although all types of muscle fibers can become more aerobic or anaerobic in nature depending on the type of training employed, slow-twitch fibers cannot transition to become fast-twitch fibers nor can fast-twitch fibers transition to become slow-twitch fibers. **FIGURE 5.6** on the next page shows the different types of fibers within the muscle as well as the targeted repetition ranges for each (Baechle & Earle, 2008; Haff & Triplett, 2016).

Recommendations about the ideal number of sets per muscle group in order to maximize gains in size is a topic of much debate. Some researchers say more is better, while others argue less is more. Mike Mentzer, Mr. Universe 1978 and founder of Heavy Duty training, was a proponent of a single set to failure while performed slowly (i.e., 4 seconds

Henneman's size principle: Under load, motor units are recruited from smallest to largest.

Fiber type transition: Adaptation of specific muscle fibers (typically the intermediate muscle fibers) to become more aerobic or anaerobic in nature as a result of training.

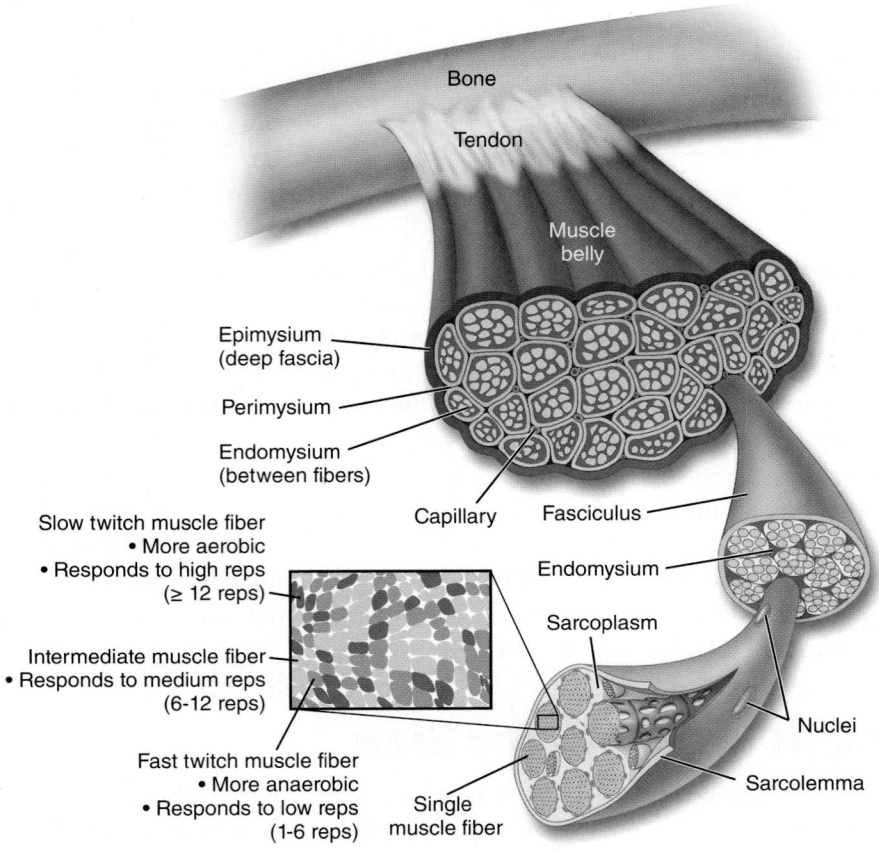

FIGURE 5.6 Recommended Rep Ranges Based on Fiber Type

up and 4 seconds down). A significant amount of research has been done on this topic to try and answer this age-old question. Although significant gains in size have been documented with single set exercise programs, research seems to suggest they are not optimal. Instead, multiple sets per muscle group appear to be better suited to maximize results in terms of both strength and size gains.

TABLE 5.6 illustrates the results of the required number of sets per muscle group from a variety of scientific studies (Krieger, 2014). As you can see, 6 sets per muscle group seems to be the most common recommendation in terms of the ideal number of sets across multiple studies.

TABLE 5.6 Required Number of Sets per Muscle Group to Achieve Specific Training Adaptations

Training Adaptation	Number of Sets per Muscle Group
Maximum Gains in Strength	• 4 (Rhea) • 8 (Rhea; competitive athletes) • 6-7 (Ostrowski) • 8 (Marshall) • 6+ (Krieger)
Maximum Gains in Size	• 4-6 (Wernborn) • 6-7 (Ostrowski) • 6+ (Krieger)
Maximum Increase in Protein Synthesis and Anabolic Signaling	• 6 (Kumar)

Data from Israetel, M. Raw Powerlifting Priorities [PowerPoint Presentation]. University of Central Missouri, Warrensburg, MO.

FAQ

How many sets of strength training exercises should I perform?

The exact number of sets required for maximal size and strength gains is debatable. Most researchers believe that at least six sets per muscle group are needed. Failing to perform enough sets will not maximize the physiological adaptations associated with regular strength training. However, performing too many sets can lead to overtraining and increase the risk of injury. A realistic goal is to perform between 9–20 total sets of all strength training exercises performed (not including warm-up sets) per training session.

Researchers have proposed several additional recommendations for maximizing gains in size and strength. Following are 10 recommendations to help maximize muscle growth:

- Train across a wide variety of repetition ranges (e.g., 1–2, 3–5, 6–12).
- Train using max loads (> 85% of 1RM).
- Train using compound, multi-joint exercises (e.g., squats, bench press, deadlift, power cleans).
- Incorporate eccentric training (muscle lengthening phase of a movement in which 30–40% percent more weight can be used than can be lifted concentrically); e.g., performing negatives (using a weight greater than one's 1RM) on the bench press.
- Incorporate high-tension exercises (i.e., exercises where a specific muscle is tensed then moved against that tension through a specified ROM); e.g., the Maltese and Iron Cross in men's gymnastics.
- Incorporate both progression and variation into exercise programming, e.g., periodically change up the repetitions and exercises used.
- Accelerate sub-max loads (50–85% of 1RM). In other words, expedite the concentric phase of the movement when using lighter loads.
- Perform multiple sets (≥ 6 sets).
- Allow for adequate rest and recovery (e.g., 24 hours for moderate strength training / 72–96 hours for intense strength training).
- Consume a high-calorie and nutrient-dense diet (e.g., 500–1000 extra kcal per day) with the majority of additional calories coming from carbohydrate, not protein, sources. Additional carbohydrates in the diet are needed in order to provide energy and help prevent gluconeogenesis (making of glucose from protein). A lack of adequate carbohydrate in the diet will result in available protein being used for energy rather than for muscle growth (synthesis).

Plyometrics

Plyometrics (aka jump training), which is Greek for "more measure," is a specific type of strength training that employs exercises that require the muscle to exert maximum force in the shortest possible time. Plyometrics are quick, powerful movements that involve **counter-movements** (downward movement immediately followed by an upward movement or vice versa) and the stretch-shortening cycle (SSC) (active stretch followed by an immediate shortening of the same muscle). In other words, a rapid eccentric muscle action stimulates the stretch reflex and storage of the muscle's elastic energy, thereby increasing the force produced during the subsequent concentric action. The aftereffect response associated with counter-movements and the SSC is referred to as **post-activation potentiation**.

Eccentric training: A strength training technique that exaggerates the lengthening phase of a movement and allows for 30-40 percent more weight to be lifted than can be done concentrically (muscle shortening phase). (Also known as negative training).

High-tension exercises: Exercises in which one tenses a specific muscle then moves that muscle against tension as if simulating that a heavy weight were being lifted.

Gluconeogenesis: Formation of glucose from precursors other than carbohydrates (e.g., amino acids, glycerol from fats, or lactate produced by muscle during anaerobic glycolysis).

Plyometrics: A form of conditioning in which muscles exert maximum force in short intervals of time with the goal of increasing muscular power.

Counter-movements: Movement in which the athlete begins from an upright standing position, initiates a downward movement by flexing the knees and hips, then immediately extends the knees and hips again to jump vertically off the ground.

Post-activation potentiation: A theory that purports that the contractile history of a muscle influences the mechanical performance of subsequent muscle contractions.

Complex training: A form of conditioning that combines resistance training with plyometric training.

TABLE 5.7 Recommended Training Volumes for Plyometric Training

Training Status	Volume
Beginner	80–100 reps/contacts
Intermediate	100–120 reps/contacts
Advanced	120–140 reps/contacts

Data from Baechle, T. R., & Earle, R. W. (Eds.). (2008). *Essentials of strength training and conditioning.* (3rd ed.). Champaign, IL: Human Kinetics; Haff, G., & Triplett, N. (Eds.). (2016). *Essentials of strength training and conditioning.* (4th ed). Champaign, IL: Human Kinetics.

Although extremely effective in improving explosiveness and speed, plyometric training is extremely taxing on the body. As a result, one can expect greater stress on muscles, connective tissues, and joints. This is especially true when performing:

- Single-leg exercises
- Exercises at elevated heights
- Exercises at greater speed
- Exercises while at a heavier body weight (220+ lbs.)

Exercise volume is generally expressed in terms of the total number of sets and repetitions performed in a single training session. Although similar assignments can be applied to plyometric training, volume is normally expressed in terms of the number of repetitions, contacts (aka landings), throws performed, or distance covered. **TABLE 5.7** provides plyometric volume recommendations for the number of contacts to be performed in a single training session (Baechle & Earle, 2008; Haff & Triplett, 2016).

When combining plyometric training with strength training, special consideration should be given with regard to exercise programming. For example, in order to allow adequate rest between exercises and ensure proper technique throughout the training session, one recommendation is to combine lower body resistance training with upper body plyometrics and vice versa. **TABLE 5.8** provides recommendations for integrating plyometric and strength training (Baechle & Earle, 2008; Haff & Triplett, 2016).

However, heavy resistance training can be combined with plyometrics for the same muscle group as long as adequate recovery time is afforded. Similarly, plyometric training can be performed immediately following low-intensity strength training (i.e., 30% 1RM) as another technique to try and maximize gains in muscular power. This advanced form of conditioning is referred to as **complex training**.

TABLE 5.8 Sample Schedule for Combing Plyometric and Resistance Training

Day	Strength Training	Plyometrics
Monday	High-Intensity Upper Body	Low-Intensity Lower Body
Tuesday	Low-Intensity Lower Body	High-Intensity Upper Body
Thursday	Low-Intensity Upper Body	High-Intensity Lower Body
Friday	High-Intensity Lower Body	Low-Intensity Upper Body

Data from Baechle, T. R., & Earle, R. W. (Eds.). (2008). *Essentials of strength training and conditioning.* (3rd ed.). Champaign, IL: Human Kinetics; Haff, G., & Triplett, N. (Eds.). (2016). *Essentials of strength training and conditioning.* (4th ed). Champaign, IL: Human Kinetics.

TABLE 5.9 Recommended Upper Body and Lower Body Plyometric Drills

Upper Body Drills	Lower Body Drills
Two-Hand Overhead Throw	Depth Jump w/ Standing Long Jump
Chest Pass	Lateral Box Jumps
Power Drop	Jump to Box
Two-Hand Side-to-Side Throw	Depth Jumps
45° Sit-Up	Depth Jumps w/ Lateral Movement

Plyometric exercises are divided into two primary categories: upper body drills and lower body drills. Upper body drills include various throws (generally with medicine balls) and push-ups. Lower body drills include various jumps in place, standing jumps, multiple jumps and hops, bounds, box drills, and depth jumps. **TABLE 5.9** gives some specific examples of upper body and lower body plyometric drills (Baechle & Earle, 2008; Haff & Triplett, 2016).

Reader Challenge: Strength

So how strong is strong enough? **TABLE 5.10** provides some recommendations from two of the top strength and conditioning coaches in the field (Prevost, 2015). Participate in some or all of the below assessments and compare your performance to the below criteria. How did you do?

TABLE 5.10 How Strong is Strong Enough?

Dan John's List		Rob Shaul's List	
Upper Push	Expected: BW Bench Press	Front Squat	1.5 × BW
	Game Changer: BW Bench Press for 15 reps	Deadlift	2.0 × BW
Upper Pull	Expected: 5 Pull-Ups	Bench Press	1.5 × BW
	Game Changer: 15 Pull-Ups	Push Press	1.1 × BW
Hip Hinge	Expected: 1.5 × BW Deadlift	Squat Clean	1.25 × BW
	Game Changer: 2.0 × BW Deadlift	Squat Clean + Push Press	1.1 × BW
Squat	Expected: BW Squat		
	Game Changer: BW Squat for 15 reps		
Core	Expected: Farmer's Walk with ½ BW per hand		
	Game Changer: Farmer's Walk with BW per hand	BW = Bodyweight	

Data from Krieger, J. Single vs. multi-set training: how many sets for optimum results? [PowerPoint Presentation]. NSCA Personal Trainers Conference, Washington, D.C. 02-04 October, 2014.

Assessment and Application

Summary

- There are four distinct training goals (i.e., endurance, hypertrophy, strength, power) associated with strength training and each has their own specific training guidelines in terms of load assignments, goal sets, goal reps, and rest.

- There is some overlap among the different training goals in terms of their recommended rep ranges. This allows for some physiological adaptations to occur simultaneously.

- Regardless of the training goal, there are eight fundamental movement patterns that should be incorporated into a strength training program in order to promote maximal gains in sport performance and injury prevention.

- Gains in muscular size, strength, and power are possible with all three types of strength training (i.e., bodybuilding, powerlifting, Olympic lifting). However, bodybuilding is tailored more to developing size; powerlifting is tailored more to developing strength; and Olympic lifting is tailored more to developing power.

- Periodization is a strategy that is used to promote long-term training and performance improvements with the implementation of preplanned, systemic variations in training specificity, intensity, and volume.

- There are two basic types of periodization: traditional (linear) and undulation (nonlinear). Traditional periodization employs a systematic approach to exercise progression and occurs gradually over several weeks or months. Undulating periodization, on the other hand, uses daily fluctuations in load, volume, and intensity assignments in order to accomplish these same goals.

- There is much debate about the best approach of periodization (i.e., traditional (linear) or undulating (nonlinear)). It basically comes down to personal preference since both approaches have a demonstrated history of improving size, strength, and power.

- Research suggests that at least six sets per muscle group is required in order to promote maximal gains in terms of muscular size and strength.

- Plyometrics is a specific type of strength training that exerts near maximum force of the muscles in a very short period of time via the employment of quick, powerful movements / exercises. Special consideration should be taken when attempting to safely and effectively combine strength and plyometric training.

Knowledge Check

1. List and discuss some of the benefits associated with regular strength training.
2. Define and differentiate agonist, antagonist, stabilizer, target muscle, and synergist muscle.
3. List and discuss the different strength training goals including the load, repetition, set, and rest assignments for each.
4. Using the repetition continuum chart provided in the text, what is the recommended number of repetitions per set for someone whose strength training goals include improvements in both strength and size (hypertrophy)?

5. List and provide specific examples of the eight fundamental movement patterns.
6. List some of the specific strength training recommendations for beginner, intermediate, and advanced lifters.
7. Define core, assistance, and power exercises and provide specific examples of each.
8. Define and discuss the 2 for 2 rule.
9. List and discuss some of the additional strength training considerations for intermediate and advanced lifters.
10. Discuss the similarities and differences between bodybuilding, powerlifting, and Olympic lifting.
11. Discuss the similarities and differences between traditional (linear) and undulating (nonlinear) periodization.
12. Define and discuss the four basic periods associated with linear (aka traditional) periodization.
13. Define and discuss the four basic seasons associated with linear (aka traditional) periodization.
14. List and discuss the 10 recommendations for maximizing muscle growth.
15. According to research, what is the general consensus regarding the minimal number of sets required to maximize muscular size and strength gains?
16. Define and discuss plyometric training.
17. Discuss some of the recommendations for integrating plyometric and strength training.

Activities

Strength Training

A. Claire knows that she needs to start strength training; however, she has little exposure to and experience with this type of training. Design a basic strength training plan for Claire to include specific exercise, set, rep recommendations. Be sure to include an exercise for each of the 8 fundamental movement patterns.
B. Discuss why you chose the exercises, reps, and set recommendations you did for your plan.

References

Al-Masri L., & Bartlett, S. (2011). *100 Questions & answers about sports nutrition and exercise*. Burlington, MA: Jones & Bartlett

Baechle, T. R., & Earle, R. W. (Eds.). (2008). *Essentials of strength training and conditioning*. (3rd ed.). Champaign, IL: Human Kinetics.

Haff, G., & Triplett, N. (Eds.). (2016). *Essentials of strength training and conditioning*. (4th ed). Champaign, IL: Human Kinetics.

Israetel, M. *Raw powerlifting priorities* [PowerPoint Presentation]. University of Central Missouri, Warrensburg, MO.

Krieger, J. *Single vs. multi-set training: How many sets for optimum results?* [PowerPoint Presentation]. NSCA Personal Trainers Conference, Washington, D.C., October 02-04, 2014.

Prevost, M. (2015). *Built to endure* [eBook]. Retrieved from http://built-to-endure.blogspot.com/.

University of New Mexico. *Periodization planning overview* [PowerPoint Presentation]. Retrieved from https://www.unm.edu/~lkravitz/Teaching%20Aerobics/PeriodSlidesExp2.pdf

Westcott, W. (1995). *Strength fitness: physiological principles and training techniques*. New York, NY: WCB/McGraw-Hill.

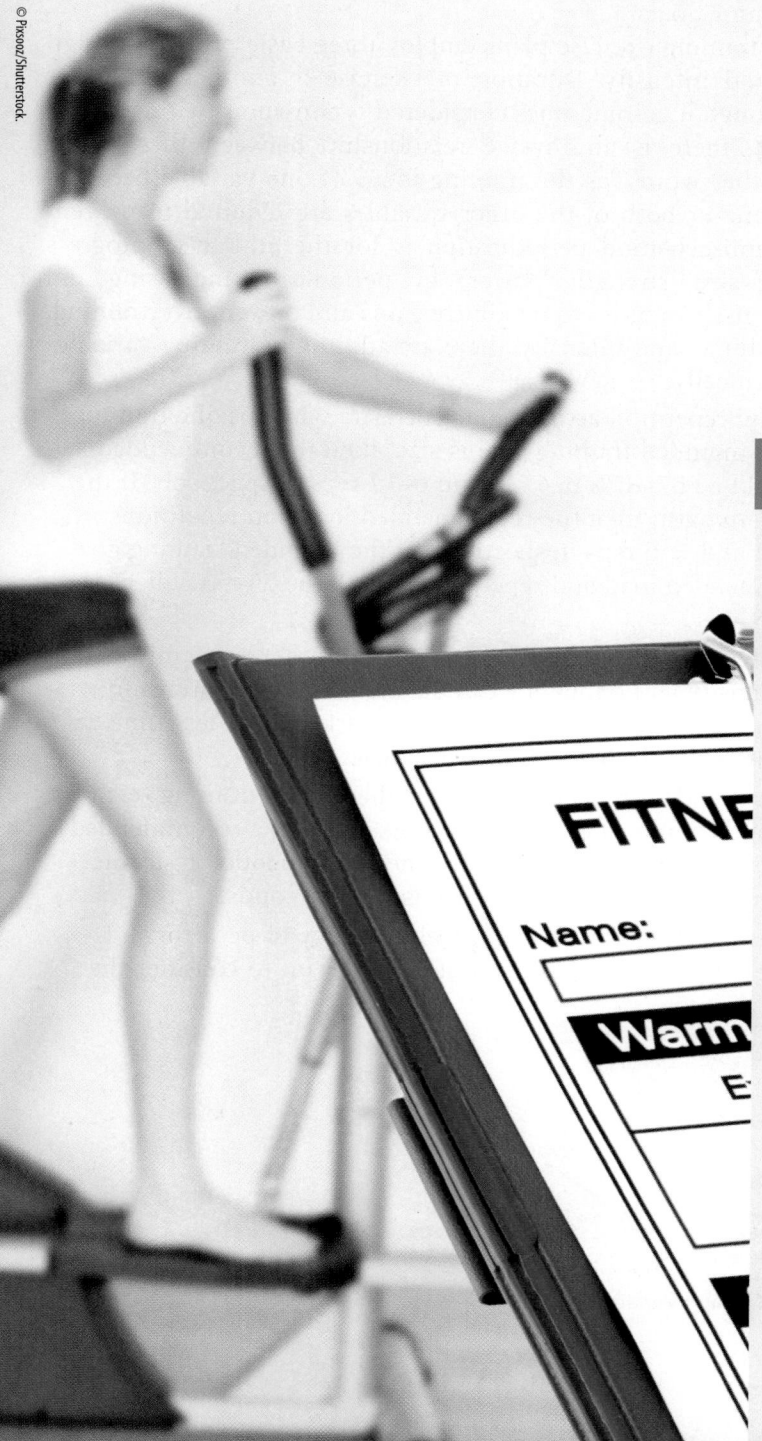

CHAPTER 6

Exercise Programming

LEARNING OBJECTIVES

After completing this chapter, students should be able to:

- Discuss the inverse relationship between exercise frequency, intensity, and volume
- List and discuss the other key exercise program design variables
- Define and discuss the purpose of a needs analysis
- Discuss some of the common mistakes associated with exercise programming
- List and discuss some of the different training priorities to consider when designing an exercise program
- List the American College of Sports Medicine (ACSM) and American Heart Association's (AHA) guidelines for endurance, strength, and mobility training
- Design a personalized exercise plan
- List and discuss some of the specific exercise programming considerations for children
- List and discuss some of the specific exercise programming considerations for pregnant women
- List and discuss some of the specific exercise programming considerations for senior adults

Introduction

Although the below quote was written for endurance athletes, the underlying message is appropriate for all athletes regardless of sport or training goal (Baechle & Earle, 2008).

> *"A common trend with many endurance athletes is to adopt and embrace the training practices of other highly successful or well-known endurance athletes. Although this strategy may be effective for a few, most endurance athletes would be better served by constructing their own training regimen based on a good working knowledge of the sound principles and an understanding of their own physical limitations and needs."*

This chapter will discuss the basics behind developing an effective strength and conditioning program. Although it will provide sample exercise plans, its intent is to equip you with the understanding and resources necessary to develop a plan tailored specifically for you and your respective training goals.

All endurance and strength training exercise plans employ three basic program design variables: frequency, volume, and intensity. Duration of exercise is another important design variable to consider, although it is sometimes considered synonymous with volume. As shown in **FIGURE 6.1**, there is an inverse relationship between these three variables (Antonio, 2015). In other words, as the training focus of one variable becomes more prevalent, reductions in one or both of the other variables are required to prevent overtraining or injury. The premise behind periodization is for the athlete to progress through different phases (i.e., size, strength, power) by periodically increasing and decreasing both volume and intensity in order to maximize gains and prevent overtraining.

In addition to frequency, volume, and intensity, there are additional training variables that need to be considered, specifically:

- *Load/Repetitions*: Load and repetition assignments correlate with specific training goals. For example, if the intended training goal is size, then the recommended load and repetitions should be 67–85% of 1RM and 6–12 reps, respectively. If the intended training goal is strength, then the recommended load and repetitions should be ≥ 85% of 1RM and ≥ 6 reps, respectively. If the intended training goal is power, then the recommended load and repetitions should be 75–90% of 1RM and 1–5 reps, respectively.

- *Exercise Duration*: As previously discussed, the influence of other program variables such as exercise intensity and frequency can dictate recommendations for duration. In other words, the harder or more often you workout, the less time required in order to facilitate the desired training response.

- *Rest/Recovery*: Rest recommendation change based on the type of training (e.g., endurance training, strength training) employed. For example, the recommended work:rest ratio for interval training is 1:1. Similarly, the recommended rest time between sets when training for muscular endurance is ≤ 30 seconds.

- *Exercise Order*: Certain exercises require a great deal of energy to perform and, therefore, can be extremely fatiguing. As a result, it is important to consider the

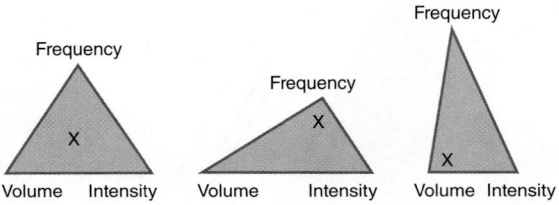

FIGURE 6.1 Relationship between Training Variables

TABLE 6.1 Exercise Recommendations for Sport-Specific Movement Patterns

Movement Pattern	Related Exercise
Ball Dribbling / Passing	Close-Grip Bench Press, Dumbbell Bench Press, Tricep Push-Down, Reverse Curl, Hammer Curl
Ball Kicking	Unilateral Hip Adduction and Abduction, Forward Step Lunge, Leg (Knee) Extension, Leg Raise
Freestyle Swimming	Lat Pull-Down, Lateral Shoulder Raise, Forward Step Lunge, Upright Row, Barbell Pull-Over
Jumping	Power Clean, Push Jerk, Back Squat, Front Squat, Standing Calf Raise
Racket Stroke	Flat Dumbbell Fly, Bent-Over Lateral Raise, Wrist Curl, Wrist Extension
Rowing	Power Clean, Bent-Over Row, Seated Row, Hip Sled, Horizontal Leg Press, Deadlift, Good Morning
Running / Sprinting	Forward Step Lunge, Step-Up, Leg (Knee) Extension, Leg (Knee) Curl, Toe Raise (Dorsiflexion)
Throwing / Pitching	Barbell Pull-Over, Overhead Triceps Extension, Shoulder Internal and External Rotation

Data from Antonio, R. (2015). *Deciphering the ideal training frequency for muscle growth*. Retrieved from http://www.thinkeatlift.com/deciphering-the-ideal-training-frequency-for-muscle-growth/.

order that exercises are performed. In terms of strength training, it is recommended to perform exercises in the following order: power (e.g., power clean), core (e.g., squat), then assistance (e.g., bicep curls).

- *Exercise Selection*: Thought should also be given to what exercises should be performed. For example, both the back squat and leg press are effective exercises for lower body size and strength development. However, the back squat may be a more appropriate exercise choice to perform for a football lineman since it more closely mimics the stance and body position of that sport. **TABLE 6.1** provides some specific exercise recommendations for sport-specific movement patterns (Baechle & Earle, 2008: Haff & Triplett, 2016).

Needs Analysis

Another effective tool used to develop an effective strength and conditioning program is a **needs analysis**; a two-stage process that evaluates the requirements of the sport as well as an assessment of the athlete (Baechle & Earle, 2008; Haff & Triplett, 2016).

The first priority of a needs analysis is evaluating the unique characteristics of the sport. This includes the sport's fundamental movement patterns and the musculature involved (**movement analysis**); muscular endurance, strength, size, and power requirements (**physiological analysis**); as well as the joints/muscles most susceptible to injury and possible causal factors (**injury analysis**). Therefore, it is important to pick and employ exercises that, if used regularly, will help provide dynamic support to susceptible areas of the body in order to prevent and/or reduce injury risk.

The second priority of a needs analysis is evaluating the needs of the respective athlete. This includes the athlete's previous training history, injury status, and their primary

Needs analysis: A two-stage process in developing a strength and conditioning program to include an evaluation of the sport and an assessment of the athlete.

Movement analysis: Part of the needs analysis that evaluates body and limb movement and muscular involvement of the sport.

Physiological analysis: Part of the needs analysis that evaluates the strength, power, size, and muscular endurance priorities of the sport.

Injury analysis: Part of the needs analysis that evaluates common sites for joint and muscle injuries as well as causative factors.

FAQ

How much physical activity is recommended?

The Centers for Disease Control and Prevention (CDC) provide specific physical activity recommendations for adults in order to lose weight and reduce the risk of certain metabolic diseases (e.g., cardiovascular disease, high blood pressure, metabolic syndrome, type 2 diabetes, certain types of cancer).

Provided below are specific recommendations for various training goals (Centers for Disease Control and Prevention, n.d.):

- **Reduce the risk of disease:** 100–115 minutes (~800–900 kcal) of moderate-intensity aerobic activity, or 50–60 minutes of vigorous-intensity aerobic activity, per week. This equates to ~14–20% reduction in disease risk. Provided below are some examples of moderate-intensity and vigorous-intensity exercises (World Health Organization, n.d.).
- **Prevent weight gain / improve fitness:** 150–250 minutes (~1200–2000 kcal) of moderate-intensity aerobic activity, or 75–125 minutes of vigorous-intensity aerobic activity per week.
- **Lose weight:** 250–300 minutes (~2000+ kcal) of moderate-intensity aerobic activity, or 125–150 minutes of vigorous-intensity aerobic activity per week.

The good news is that if you train to lose weight you will also reduce your risk for disease, prevent future weight gain, and improve your current level of fitness at the same time.

The American College of Sports Medicine (ACSM) and the American Heart Association (AHA) also provide physical activity guidelines for adults regarding the type and amount of exercise that should be performed (American College of Sports Medicine [ACSM], 2011). Specifically:

- **Aerobic Activity:** At least 150 minutes of moderate-intensity aerobic activity, or 75 minutes of vigorous-intensity aerobic activity per week.
- **Strength Training:** A minimum of 2 nonconsecutive days per week using 8–10 different exercises involving the major muscle groups (e.g., back, chest, hips, legs, shoulders, abdominals).
- **Flexibility:** Flexibility training should be performed at least 2–3 days per week for at least 10 minutes per day.
- **Balance:** To reduce the risk of injury from falls, adults (especially senior adults) should regularly perform exercises that help maintain or improve balance (e.g., yoga, Pilates, tai chi, qigong, dance).

Moderate-Intensity	Vigorous-Intensity
Brisk Walking	Running
Dancing	Brisk Walking Uphill
Gardening	Fast Cycling
Housework / Domestic Chores	Aerobics
General Building Tasks	Fast Swimming
Traditional Hunting / Gathering	Heavy Shoveling / Digging
Sport Participation for Leisure	Competitive Sport Participation
Carrying / Moving Moderate Loads (< 20 kg)	Carrying / Moving Heavy Loads (> 20 kg)

training goal (e.g., improve, strength, size, speed). The following information should be reviewed when assessing the athlete's training history:

- Type of training program used (e.g., endurance, strength)
- Length of time spent and level of intensity used in previous training program
- Level of experience performing certain exercise techniques (e.g., Olympic lifts)

Although athletes may want to improve in two or more areas, it is generally recommended that they concentrate on only one training goal at a time (e.g., strength focus and then power).

In addition to a needs analysis, Dan John, a renowned strength and conditioning coach and author, also uses the "Point A to Point B" example in providing exercise prescription recommendations to athletes. In short, Point A establishes "where are you now." This includes evaluating current injuries, training history, current strengths and weaknesses, available time and equipment, and exercise preferences and dislikes. Point B establishes "where you want to be" and includes identifying specific training goals in detail (John, 2013).

Point A ⟶ Point B

Effective exercise prescription provides the basic programming
for how to safely transition from Point A to Point B

Some of the common mistakes associated with exercise programming include:

- Doing too much too soon
- Loading bad movement (e.g., putting weight on a bar before mastering proper exercise technique)
- Trusting fad recommendations over scientific research (e.g., the *INSANITY* approach to exercise "flips traditional interval training on its head" by performing long bursts of maximum-intensity exercises followed by short periods of rest. Unfortunately, this approach to exercise violates known minimum recovery times for high-intensity interval training and, as a result, can quickly lead to overtraining and/or injury).
- Spending more time on what you're good at than what you need to work on
- Being too vague or unrealistic with your training goals or expectations
- Being too competitive – either with someone else or a previous version of yourself

Dr. Mike Israetel, a professor of Exercise Science at Temple University and competitive powerlifter, bodybuilder, and Brazilian Jiu-Jitsu grappler, provides the following list of training priorities to consider (Israetel, n.d.). Essentially, some variables are more important than others in terms of their role and influence and, therefore, should be given priority (**FIGURE 6.2** on the next page);

- *Specificity*: The principle of specificity implies that in order to become better at a particular exercise or skill, you must perform that exercise or skill. To become a better runner, you must run; to become a better cyclist, you must cycle; and to become a better swimmer, you must swim.
- *Overload*: The principle of overload means exposing the body to a greater stress or load than it is normally accustomed to in order to facilitate certain physiological adaptations.
- *Fatigue Management*: The principle of fatigue management refers to deliberately implementing designated rest periods; either complete rest or continued exercising but with reduced volume and intensity, after several weeks of hard training in order to allow the body time to fully recover.
- *Stimulus Recovery Adaptation (SRA)*: The principle of SRA implies that physiological adaptations take place during recovery, not training. As a result, frequency recommendations for each of the different types of exercise should be based on the amount of time required to recover.
  - *Moderate endurance training*: 24 hours
  - *Moderate strength / intense endurance training*: 48 hours
  - *Intense strength training*: 72–96 hours

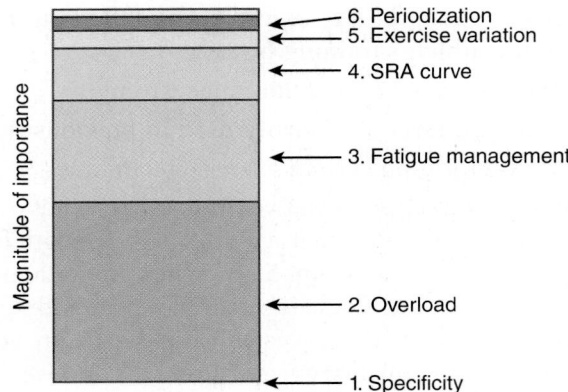

FIGURE 6.2 Important Training Priorities to Consider

Data from Foster, C., Wright, G., Battista, R., and Porcari, J. (2007). Training in the aging athlete. *Current Sports Medicine Reports*, (6), 200-206.

- *Variation*: The principle of variation recommends periodic rotation of exercises in order to prevent training plateaus and/or overtraining.
- *Periodization (aka Phase Potentiation)*: A form of strength training that uses a strategic implementation of training phases (e.g., hypertrophy, strength, power). These phases periodically increase and decrease both volume and intensity in order to prevent overtraining and maximize gains. The order in which these phases are performed is also important. Specifically, the hypertrophy phase should be performed before the strength phase and the strength phase should be performed before the peaking (aka power) phase. In other words, the first step in the process is to build new muscles (hypertrophy phase). The next step is to make the new muscle stronger (strength phase). The final step is to express new gains in strength in terms of a 1RM (peaking phase). Although not required, the endurance phase should be performed prior to the hypertrophy phase.

Exercise Programming Considerations

There are 11 different components of physical fitness. The first five components of physical fitness relate directly to one's health and, therefore, are considered to be the most important. These include cardiovascular endurance, muscular strength, muscular endurance, flexibility, and body composition. The remaining six components of physical fitness are skill related and correlate with sports and daily activities. These include agility, balance, coordination, power, reaction time, and speed. **FIGURE 6.3** depicts the different components of physical fitness.

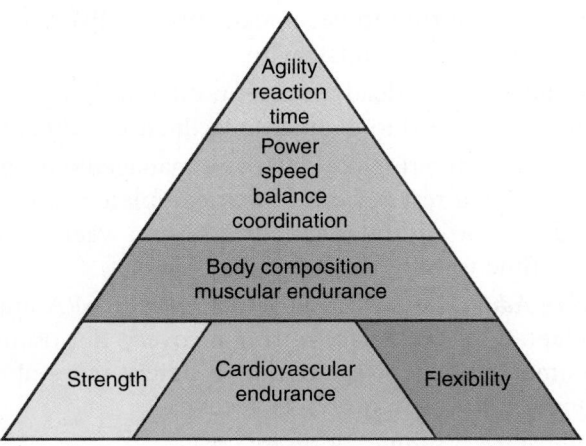

FIGURE 6.3 Various Components of Fitness

Fitness Trident

As seen in Figure 6.3, there is an established hierarchy between the different components of fitness. Although each component plays an integral role in one's overall fitness level, some components are considered more essential than others, and, therefore, should receive training priority. For example, athletes should first focus on developing a foundation of strength and endurance before training for power and/or speed. Similarly, training for balance and coordination will subsequently improve one's agility and reaction time.

The ACSM and AHA recommend the following guidelines regarding exercise type and duration:

- *Strength Training*: Minimum of 2 nonconsecutive days per week
- *Endurance Training*: Minimum of 3 days per week (estimation based on the 150 minutes [moderate-intensity] to 75 minutes [vigorous-intensity] recommendations)
- *Mobility/Flexibility*: Minimum of 2–3 days per week

However, Dr. Kelly Starrett disagrees with current ACSM and AHA guidelines regarding the minimum frequency recommended for mobility training. Instead of a minimum of 2–3 days per week, Dr. Starrett is a proponent of "no days off" when it comes to mobility training. In fact, they recommend that at least 10–15 minutes be dedicated to mobility training every day (Starrett & Cordoza, 2015). A few minutes of mobility work every day will help to improve your range of motion, posture, and function. However, when you take a day off from mobility work, the muscles start to stiffen and begin to lose their vital range of motion. As a result, your movement and posture will reflect that adaptation. Bottom line: Although it is recommended to periodically take time off from strength and endurance training, you should never take a day off from mobility training.

As shown in **FIGURE 6.4**, there are three fundamental components of physical fitness; muscular strength, cardiovascular endurance, and mobility (which includes flexibility). Together, these three components of physical fitness comprise the **fitness trident** and they should constitute the primary foundation of any strength and conditioning program.

To better illustrate this point, imagine your current strength and conditioning plan is a three-legged stool and each leg represents one of the prongs on the fitness trident (i.e., strength, endurance, mobility). Ideally, each leg of the stool would be exactly the same length. Accomplishing this ensures that the training plan is well-balanced and capable of providing a solid foundation for improved athletic potential and reduced risk of injury. Unfortunately, this is not the case for most individuals. Instead, most training plans ensure that one leg of the stool is considerably longer or shorter than the others. This results in

Fitness trident: Depicts the three most important components of fitness and foundation of any strength and conditioning program. Specifically: strength, endurance, and mobility.

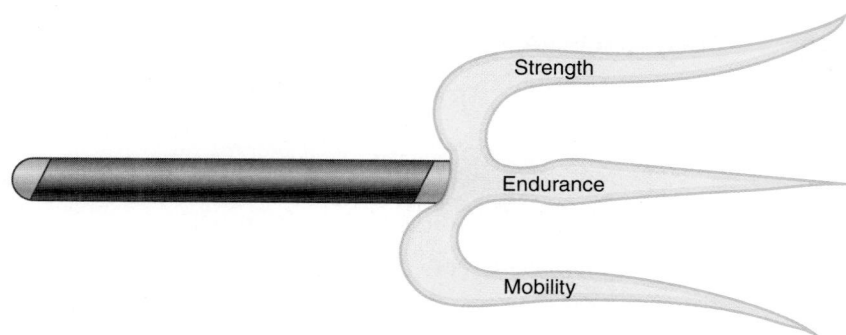

FIGURE 6.4 Fitness Trident

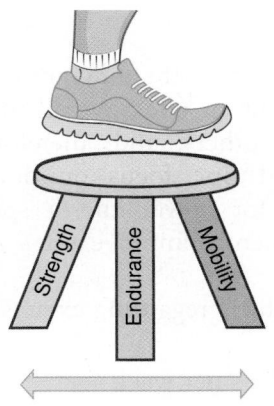

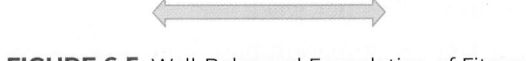

FIGURE 6.5 Well-Balanced Foundation of Fitness

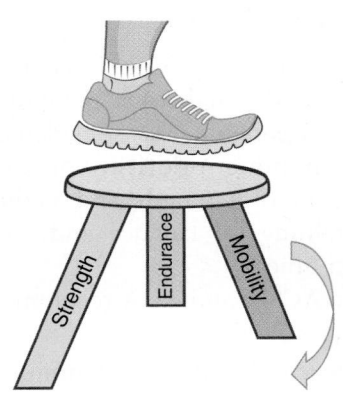

FIGURE 6.6 Unbalanced Foundation of Fitness

decreased athletic potential and an increased risk of injury. For example, **FIGURE 6.5** and **FIGURE 6.6** describe a well-balanced fitness plan and an unbalanced fitness plan, respectively. The foot shown in these figures represents the rigors of training and sport participation. Since all three legs of the stool are the same length in Figure 6.5, it can easily support the rigors of training and sport participation. In Figure 6.6, the three legs of the stool are of different lengths and it cannot support the rigors of training or sport participation and, therefore, topples over.

So how does one transition from an unbalanced training plan to a balanced one? The answer is to aggressively train the shorter leg(s) of the stool while maintaining (not increasing) the length of the longest one. Individuals often continue to train their longest leg because it is what they enjoy most or are good at. Instead, they should train to maintain but not improve (add) fitness to that leg. This can be done by reducing the training volume, intensity, or both of the longer leg. Simultaneously, they should increase the training volume, intensity, or both of the shorter leg(s). Training to improve fitness in the longer leg should not resume until all three legs of the stool are roughly the same length.

Based on these guidelines, the following exercise programming recommendations are provided for endurance, strength, and mobility training. Specifically, the following tables provide training type and frequency recommendations based on number of days per week you are able to train.

	Strength Training	
Option	**Days per Week**	**Split Type**
A	2	2-Day Split / Total Body
B	3	Alternate 2-Day Split / 3-Day Split
C	4	2-Day Split × 2
D	5	3-Day Split (Option 1)
E	6	3-Day Split × 2
F	7	3-Day Split (Option 2)

Endurance Training		
Option	**Days per Week**	**Training Type**
A	3	1 LSD / 1 Pace/Tempo / 1 Speed
B	4	2 LSD / 1 Pace/Tempo / 1 Speed
C	5	2 LSD / 1 Pace/Tempo / 2 Speed
D	6	2 LSD / 2 Pace/Tempo / 2 Speed
E	7	3 LSD / 2 Pace/Tempo / 2 Speed

Mobility Training		
Option	**Days per Week**	**Training Type**
A	2	Static Stretching
B	3	Yoga
C	4	Pilates
D	5	**Tai Chi**
E	6	**Qigong**
F	7	Dance

Tai chi: An ancient Chinese form of exercise that was originally created as a fighting art. The words Tai Chi Chuan loosely translate to mean supreme ultimate exercise or skill.

Qigong: A Chinese system of physical exercises and breathing control similar to tai chi.

The following table better explains some of the different split options associated with strength training (e.g., 2-day split, 3-day split).

Strength Training								
Split Type	**Week**	**Workout 1**	**Workout 2**	**Workout 3**	**Workout 4**	**Workout 5**	**Workout 6**	**Workout 7**
2-Day Split	-	Upper Body *	Lower Body *	-	-	-	-	-
Total Body	-	Total Body	Total Body	-	-	-	-	-
Alternate 2-Day Split	1, 3, 5	Upper Body *	Lower Body *	Upper Body *	-	-	-	-
	2, 4, 6	Lower Body *	Upper Body *	Lower Body *	-	-	-	-
3-Day Split	-	Back/Bi's	Legs/Shoulders	Chest/Tri's	-	-	-	-
2-Day Split × 2	-	Upper Body *	Lower Body *	Upper Body *	Lower Body *	-	-	-
3-Day Split (Option 1)	1, 4	Chest/Tri's	Back/Bi's	Legs/Shoulders	Chest/Tri's	Back/Bi's	-	-
	2, 5	Legs/Shoulders	Chest/Tri's	Back/Bi's	Legs/Shoulders	Chest/Tri's	-	-
	3, 6	Back/Bi's	Legs/Shoulders	Chest/Tri's	Back/Bi's	Legs/Shoulders	-	-

(continues)

		Strength Training (*continued*)						
Split Type	Week	Workout 1	Workout 2	Workout 3	Workout 4	Workout 5	Workout 6	Workout 7
3-Day Split × 2	-	Back/Bi's	Legs/Shoulders	Chest/Tri's	Back/Bi's	Legs/Shoulders	Chest/Tri's	-
3-Day Split (Option 2)	1, 4	Chest/Tri's	Back/Bi's	Legs/Shoulders	Chest/Tri's	Back/Bi's	Legs/Shoulders	Chest/Tri's
	2, 5	Back/Bi's	Legs/Shoulders	Chest/Tri's	Back/Bi's	Legs/Shoulders	Chest/Tri's	Back/Bi's
	3, 6	Legs/Shoulders	Chest/Tri's	Back/Bi's	Legs/Shoulders	Chest/Tri's	Back/Bi's	Legs/Shoulders

* Upper Body / Lower Body Split Routine can be substituted for Push-Pull Split Routine

The next table shows various training plan options for combining endurance, strength, and mobility training into one comprehensive program. The various options are based on the desired number of training days per week. To use this table, you must first reference the endurance, strength, mobility tables on the previous page as well as take into consideration the minimal training frequency guidelines for each training type as provided by ACSM and AHA.

For example, say you wanted to work out 5 days per week. Based on the information provided in the following table, you have the option of performing endurance training either 3 times per week (Endurance Option A), 4 times per week (Endurance Option B), or 5 times per week (Endurance Option C). Similarly, you have the option of performing strength and mobility training 2 times per week (Strength/Mobility Option A), 3 times per week (Strength/Mobility Option B), 4 times per week (Strength/Mobility Option C), or 5 times per week (Strength/Mobility Option D).

	Comprehensive Training Plan Options		
Days per Week	Endurance	Strength	Mobility
3	A	A, B	A, B
4	A, B	A, B, C	A, B, C
5	A, B, C	A, B, C, D	A, B, C, D
6	A, B, C, D	A, B, C, D, E	A, B, C, D, E
7	A, B, C, D, E	A, B, C, D, E, F	A, B, C, D, E, F

Using the 5 days per week training plan example, you could opt to run 3 days a week, strength train 2 days per week, and mobility train 4 days per week. Ultimately, the frequency used for each type of training is left up to the individual but should be based on several factors to include desired training goal, current fitness level, and injury status. The following table provides several examples of comprehensive training programs based on the desired number of training days per week.

	Monday	Tuesday	Wednesday	Thursday	Friday	Saturday	Sunday
3-Day Program (Basic)	Speed Lower Body Mobility	Off	LSD Mobility	Off	Tempo Upper Body Mobility	Off	Off
4-Day Program (Basic)	Speed Lower Body Mobility	Tempo Mobility	Off	Upper Body Mobility	LSD	Off	Off

	Monday	Tuesday	Wednesday	Thursday	Friday	Saturday	Sunday
5-Day Program (Basic)	Lower Body	LSD Mobility	Tempo Mobility	Upper Body	Speed Mobility	Off	Off
6-Day Program (Endurance Focus)	LSD Mobility	Lower Body	Tempo Mobility	Upper Body	LSD Mobility	Speed Mobility	Off
7-Day Program (Strength Focus)	Lower Body Mobility	Upper Body Mobility	Tempo	Lower Body Mobility	Upper Body Mobility	Speed	LSD

Putting it all Together

These recommendations help to determine exactly how many days per week one should be performing endurance, strength, and mobility training. With those recommendations in mind, the next step is to plot out a weekly training template aimed at addressing and working toward a specific goal (e.g., lose weight, run faster, lift more, get bigger).

Step 1: Determine Training Schedule

Determine the exact number of days per week for endurance training (ET), strength training (ST), mobility work, and off days. This determination is made by considering the overall training goal, the available time to exercise, and the current injury status. Additionally, special consideration should be paid to the stimulus recovery adaptation (SRA) recommendations. Specifically:

- *Moderate endurance training*: 24 hours
- *Moderate strength / intense endurance training*: 48 hours
- *Intense strength training*: 72–96 hours

For example, performing lower body strength training on Monday followed by sprint training on Tuesday would not be advised since this violates the 48 hours of recovery recommendation. Instead, a better option would be to either perform both lower body strength training and sprints on Monday, then wait 72 hours before repeating or wait at least 48 hours between conducting lower body strength training and speed work. Similarly, performing 5 sets of bench press on Monday and then a push-up ladder workout on Tuesday would not be recommended.

Additionally, as previously discussed, there should be an inverse relationship between training frequency, volume (and/or duration), and intensity. For example, if you do not want to exercise every day ($\downarrow$ frequency), you will need to exercise longer ($\uparrow$ volume/duration) on the days that you do exercise in order to achieve the same level of training stimulus. Similarly, if your workouts become significantly harder ($\uparrow$ intensity), you will need to reduce training frequency and/or volume in order to prevent overtraining and reduce the risk of injury. Generally speaking, as long as the weekly totals are the same in terms of intensity and total volume, the training effect should be the same whether you work out three days a week or seven.

The following table is a sample weekly exercise plan for someone training predominantly for size and strength gains but who also wants to maintain or possibly improve his or her aerobic fitness levels. This individual opted to train seven days a week in order to prevent doubling up on ET and ST in the same day.

Mon	Tues	Wed	Thurs	Fri	Sat	Sun
Strength	Strength	Endurance Mobility	Strength	Strength	Endurance Mobility	Endurance Mobility

Step 2: Determine Training Type

Determine the type of training you plan on doing each day (i.e., ET, ST, or Mobility). In terms of ET, determine whether you will be performing long slow distance (LSD), pace/tempo (P/T), or speed work. In terms of ST, determine which split option you will be performing. Some different split training options (all depicting the 8 fundamental movement patterns) include:

- Push / Pull
- Upper Body / Lower Body
- Total Body
- Muscle Group (e.g., Back / Biceps; Chest / Triceps; Legs / Shoulders / Abs)

Mon	Tues	Wed	Thurs	Fri	Sat	Sun
ST	ST	ET Mobility	ST	ST	ET Mobility	ET Mobility
UB	LB	LSD	UB	LB	Pace/Tempo	Speed

Step 3: Finalize Workout Plan

Determine the exact workout you will be performing each training day. For example, here are some recommendations for the different ET methods.

LSD	Pace / Tempo	Interval	Repetition	Fartlek
Run 3–5 miles	5-min Easy / 10-min Hard Repeats	4–6 × 400-m Sprints	8–10 × 100-m Sprints	Indian Runs
Run 30+ minutes	Treadmill Tempo Run	2–3 × 800-m Sprints	6–8 × 200-m Sprints	Sprint straightaways / walk curves

Similarly, here are some possible split options for employing the eight different fundamental movement patterns.

Upper Body	Lower Body
Horizontal Push	Squat
Horizontal Pull	Hip Hinge
Vertical Push	Loaded Carry
Vertical Pull	Core

Push	Pull
Horizontal Push	Horizontal Pull
Vertical Push	Vertical Pull
Squat	Hip Hinge
Core	Loaded Carry

Back / Biceps / Traps	Chest / Shoulders / Triceps	Legs / Abs
Horizontal Pull	Horizontal Push	Squat
Vertical Pull	Vertical Push	Hip Hinge
Loaded Carry	-	Core

Some of the different training options for improving mobility and flexibility include yoga, Pilates, tai chi, qigong, dance as well as traditional warm-up and stretching exercises.

After determining the number and type of training days per week, and ensuring this programming does not violate established SRA recommendations, we are finally able to construct a 1-week training template.

Mon	Tues	Wed	Thurs	Fri	Sat	Sun
ST	ST	ET Mobility	ST	ST	ET Mobility	ET Mobility
UB	LB	LSD	UB	LB	P/T	Speed
· 5 × 5 Bench Press · 5 × 5 Bent Over Row · 5 × 5 Military Press · 5 × 5 Lat Pulldown	· 5 × 5 Back Squat · 5 × 5 Stiff Leg Deadlift · 5 × 15-yd Farmer's Carry · 5 × 15 Knee-Ups	3-mi. Run 20-min. Total Body Stretching	Same as Mon	Same as Tues	Treadmill Tempo Run 45-min. Yoga	8 × 200-m Repeats 20-min. Total Body Stretching

In order for fitness gains to continue over time, training programs should incorporate **progressive overload**. In terms of ST, this can be done by periodic and systemic changes (aka periodization) in the amount of weight (load), sets, and/or repetitions. In addition to monthly variations in load, sets, and repetitions, it is also recommended to use a different set of exercises for each of the ST phases (i.e., endurance, hypertrophy, strength, power). For example, employ incline dumbbell press as a chest exercise during the muscular endurance phase and then switch to barbell bench press for the hypertrophy phase, etc.

The chart below lists possible exercises for each of the eight fundamental movement patterns that could be employed during the four different ST phases.

Progressive overload: Gradual increase in volume, intensity, frequency, or time in order to prevent training plateaus and achieve the targeted goal.

	Endurance	Hypertrophy	Strength	Power
Squat	Goblet Squats	Front Squat	Leg Press	Back Squat
Hip/Hinge	Kettlebell Swing	Good Mornings	Stiff Leg Deadlift	Deadlift
Horizontal Pull	1-Arm Row	Seated Row	Bent-Over Row	1-Arm Row
Horizontal Push	Incline	DB Bench	Decline	Bench
Vertical Pull	Lat Pulldowns (Wide)	Pull-Ups	Lat Pulldowns (Narrow)	Weighted Pull-Ups
Vertical Push	Seated DB	Standing DB	Seated BB	Standing BB
Loaded Carry	Suitcase Carry	Waiter's Walk	Weighted Walking Lunges	Farmer's Walk
Core	Plank	Russian Twist	Weighted Rope Crunch	Med Ball Curl-Ups
DB = Dumbbell			BB = Barbell	

Week	Reps	Sets	Training Goal
1	≥ 12	2	
2	≥ 12	3	Muscular Endurance
3	≥ 12	4	
4			Deload
5	6–12	3	
6	6–12	4	Hypertrophy (Size)
7	6–12	5	
8	6–12	6	
9			Deload
10	≤ 6	3	
11	≤ 6	4	Strength
12	≤ 6	5	
13	≤ 6	6	
14			Deload
15	1–5	3	
16	1–5	4	Power
17	1–5	5	
18			Deload

The previous chart details a comprehensive 18-week ST program using traditional linear periodization. Notice the deliberate change in the number of repetitions and sets that are used throughout the program.

Additionally, notice the strategic implementation of deload weeks at the end of each training phase. Deload weeks are necessary in order to prevent overtraining. There are several options for deload weeks. One option is to continue using the same ST exercises but decreasing training intensity and volume by 25% and 50%, respectively. Another option is to use bodyweight and/or plyometric exercises instead, while keeping training frequency and volume the same. In either case, long periods of inactive rest should be avoided in order to prevent unnecessary detraining.

Although the proposed ST program is likely sufficient for the novice or recreational athlete, individuals wanting to maximize size and strength gains may require a more robust ST regime. Remember that in order for any ST program to be effective and prevent training plateaus over time, it must continue to introduce overload, progression, and variation.

Introducing these concepts can be done in a number of ways. For example, one could either increase the recommended set assignments per week or use the proposed assignments and train each muscle group 2–3 times per week. Another option would be to keep the set assignments the same but add 1–2 additional exercises per muscle group (e.g., back squats and leg press; bench press and incline bench; etc.).

The following table provides several ST linear (traditional) and nonlinear (undulating) periodization options. These options can be used with the basic 18-week ST program previously provided.

For example, individuals interested in ST 4 days per week could begin with the basic format provided in Linear Periodization Option A for the first 18 weeks, transition to the format provided in Linear Periodization Option B for the next 18 weeks, and repeat. Similarly, individuals could also begin with the format provided in Non-Linear Periodization Option A for the first 18 weeks, transition to Non- Linear Periodization Option B for the next 18 weeks, and then repeat. A third option could be for individuals to start with Linear Periodization Option A for 18 weeks, Linear Periodization Option B for the next 18 weeks, Non-Linear Periodization Option A for the next 18 weeks, and then transition to Non- Linear Periodization Option B for the final 18 weeks, and then repeat.

As you can see, ST design and programming does not need to be overly cumbersome or complicated in order to be effective. By using a deliberate and systemic approach to ST, individuals can continue incorporating overload, progression, and variation over time. In doing so, individuals are more likely to maximize ST gains, prevent training plateaus, reduce the risk of injury, and avoid exercise monotony.

	Linear Periodization (Option A)	Linear Periodization (Option B)	Non-Linear Periodization (Option A)	Non-Linear Periodization (Option B)
Mon	Phase Specific Load & Volume Assignments	Phase Specific Load & Volume Assignments	Musc. End. or Hypertrophy Load & Volume Assignments	Musc. End. or Hypertrophy Load & Volume Assignments
Tues	Phase-Specific Load & Volume Assignments	Phase-Specific Load & Volume Assignments	Musc. End. or Hypertrophy Load & Volume Assignments	Musc. End. or Hypertrophy Load & Volume Assignments
Wed	Off	Off	Off	Off
Thurs	Same Load, Volume, & Exercises as Mon	Same Load & Volume as Mon but Different Exercises	Same exercises as Mon but Strength or Power Load & Volume Assignments	Strength or Power Load & Volume Assignments + Different Exercises
Fri	Same Load, Volume, & Exercises as Tues	Same Load & Volume as Tues but Different Exercises	Same exercises as Tues but Strength or Power Load & Volume Assignments	Strength or Power Load & Volume Assignments + Different Exercises
Sat	Off	Off	Off	Off
Sun	Off	Off	Off	Off

In terms of ET, this can be done by weekly increases in run distance and/or time, or by reducing the amount of recovery time between intervals (e.g., from a 1:5 to 1:4 work:rest ratio). Additionally, on speed days one can rotate between interval (e.g., 400-meter, 800-meter sprints) and repetition (e.g., 100-meter, 200-meter sprints) training methods each week. Provided in the next table is a sample 6-week ET program depicting a reasonable approach to exercise variation and progression specific to ET.

Week	ET Type	Frequency	Duration	Sets	Rest Interval
1	LSD	3	20	N/A	N/A
	Pace/Tempo	N/A	N/A	N/A	N/A
	Speed	N/A	N/A	N/A	N/A
2	LSD	3	25	N/A	N/A
	Pace/Tempo	N/A	N/A	N/A	N/A
	Speed	N/A	N/A	N/A	N/A
3	LSD	3	30	N/A	N/A
	Pace/Tempo	1	15	N/A	1:1
	Speed	N/A	N/A	N/A	N/A
4	LSD	2	30	N/A	N/A
	Pace/Tempo	1	15	N/A	1:1
	Speed	1	N/A	3–4	1:5
5	LSD	2	35	N/A	N/A
	Pace/Tempo	1	20	N/A	< 1:1
	Speed	1	N/A	4–5	1:5
6	LSD	1	35	N/A	N/A
	Pace/Tempo	1–2	20	N/A	< 1:1
	Speed	1–2	N/A	5–6	1:4

FAQ

Which should be performed first: endurance or strength training?

If the overall training goal is weight loss or general fitness, then it doesn't matter. However, if the overall training goal is endurance, then endurance training should be performed first. If the overall training goal is for size, strength, or power, strength training should be performed first.

Exercise Programming Considerations for Children

There are considerable variations in the growth rates and development among children. For example, two different 14-year-old children can differ in height by as much as 9 inches and in weight by over 40 pounds (Haff & Triplett, 2016). The degree of maturation has been shown to be directly linked to physical fitness and athletic performance. There are several different methods for assessing the maturation process in children. **Chronological age** is defined by a child's age in months or years. **Biological age** is defined in terms of a child's skeletal age, somatic (term relating to the body) maturity, or sexual maturation. Ironically, two children can have the same chronological age but differ by several years in terms of their biological age. **Training age** is defined by the length of time a child has participated in a formalized conditioning program. It is important to understand that even though two children may have the same training age, there can be significant differences in terms of their physical fitness (e.g., cardiovascular endurance, speed, muscular strength) and technical competency.

Peak muscle mass generally occurs between the ages of 16 and 20 for girls and between 18 and 25 in boys. Boys generally achieve peak gains in muscular strength about 1.2 years after **peak height velocity** and 0.8 years after **peak weight velocity**. Although girls also typically achieve peak gains in muscular strength after peak height velocity, there is greater variation in the relationship between strength, height, and weight for girls than for boys. Children can be at an increased risk of injury during periods of peak height velocity, which generally occurs around age 12 and 14 in girls and boys, respectively. As a result, it may be a good idea to modify conditioning programs by decreasing training volume, intensity, or both during periods of rapid growth. Instead, conditioning programs should focus on proper movement patterns, target flexibility restrictions, and correct muscle imbalances (Haff & Triplett, 2016).

On average, peak strength gains are attained in untrained girls by the age of 20 and between the ages of 20 and 30 for untrained boys. Although most bones have fused by the early 20s for both genders, girls typically achieve full bone maturity about two to three years before boys. Children who mature earlier tend to have a more **mesomorphic** (muscular and broader shoulders) or **endomorphic** (rounder and broader hips) build, whereas those who mature later tend to have a more **ectomorphic** (slender and tall) build.

Due to numerous hormonal and physiological differences (e.g., lack of myelination of numerous motor neurons until sexual maturity), children should not be expected to respond to training in the same way or reach the same skill level as adults. However, there is no scientific evidence to suggest that participation in a well-designed strength and conditioning program will delay or accelerate the growth or maturation process in children. In fact, the osteogenic benefits of physical activity, especially weight-bearing activities (e.g., resistance training), have been shown to be critical for proper skeletal remodeling and growth (Haff & Triplett, 2016).

Although epiphyseal plate fractures have been reported in adolescents, these cases involved training programs that employed the use of heavy overhead lifts in unsupervised settings (Haff & Triplett, 2016). There have not been any reported cases of epiphyseal plate fracture in training studies employing resistance training programs that adhered to established training guidelines. Therefore, as long as children and adolescents are properly trained and follow established training guidelines, the risk of an epiphyseal plate fracture is minimal. In fact, it is likely that the forces placed on the joints during normal play far exceed those generated from sound resistance training programs.

Regular participation in a well-designed strength and conditioning program has been shown to promote the following health- and fitness-related improvements (Haff & Triplett, 2016):

- Increased muscular strength, muscular endurance, power, and agility
- Improved motor skills and athletic performance
- Improved body composition and self-esteem/confidence
- Improved bone density
- Decreased risk for injury and certain diseases (e.g., diabetes, heart disease)

Chronological age: Number of years that an individual has lived.

Biological age: Subjective age based on an individual's development.

Training age: Number of years that an individual has spent training and participating in various sports.

Peak height velocity: Period of adolescent maturation where the maximum rate of growth occurs.

Peak weight velocity: Period of adolescent maturation associated with a rapid increase in body weight due to significant increases in the amount of muscle and bone mass.

Mesomorph: Body type that is compact and muscular.

Endomorph: Body type that is round and with a high proportion of body fat.

Ectomorph: Body type that is lean and delicate.

TABLE 6.2 Resistance Training Guidelines for Children	
Frequency	2–3 nonconsecutive days per week
Intensity	Can incorporate loads up to 1RM as long as training sessions are supervised and proper technique is enforced
Volume	1–3 sets of 6–15 reps using a variety of single and multi-joint exercises
Progression	Increase resistance gradually (5–10%) as strength and technique improves

Data from Centers for Disease Control and Prevention. *The Benefits of physical activity.* Retrieved from http://www.cdc.gov/physicalactivity/basics/pa-health/index.htm#PreventFalls.

Although there is no minimal age requirement for participation in strength and conditioning program, children should have the emotional maturity to receive and follow directions for this type of training. Research has shown that children as young as five years of age have benefited from resistance training (Haff & Triplett, 2016). Strength gains of upwards of 30–40% have been reported in untrained preadolescent children employing short-term (8–20 weeks) resistance training programs. However, special consideration should be given to each child's technical competency, training age, training goal, and maturity level when designing a strength and conditioning program.

In addition to gains in physical fitness and athletic performance, the goal of any strength and conditioning program for children should include educating them about their bodies, promoting a life-long commitment to physical activity, and having fun. Advanced multi-joint exercises (e.g., snatch, clean and jerk) can be incorporated into the training program but the primary focus should be on developing the proper form and technique instead of on the amount of weight being lifted. It is recommended that children begin with an unloaded barbell, long wooden stick, or PVC pipe when learning new exercises.

TABLE 6.2 provides several additional recommendations and guidelines for strength training programs for children (Haff & Triplett, 2016).

Exercise Programming Recommendations for Pregnancy

Recently, exercise programming recommendations for pregnant females has changed significantly. For a long time, medical professionals proposed that pregnant females refrain from participating in a regular exercise program for fear that doing so might negatively affect the development of the fetus (Bryant & Green, 2010). Specifically, the concern was that exercise would redirect blood flow to the working muscles thereby reducing the amount of oxygen and glucose being delivered to the fetus. However, it was later determined that women who exercise regularly before and during pregnancy actually increase the amount of blood, oxygen, and nutrients being delivered to the uterus, thereby negating the risk of fetal ischemia (inadequate blood supply to an organ or part of the body) during exercise (ACSM. 2014). However, it is recommended that pregnant women avoid exercising in the supine position after the first trimester in order to prevent a restriction of blood flow to the fetus (ACSM, 2014; Bryant & Green, 2010).

Since the mid-1990s, medical professionals have encouraged pregnant females to exercise regularly throughout their pregnancy since doing so provides numerous benefits for both the mother and fetus. For example, exercising regularly during pregnancy may have a positive impact on fetal birth weight. Specifically, women who exercise regularly during pregnancy are less likely to deliver babies who are overweight or underweight.

Ischemia:
Inadequate blood supply to an organ (especially the heart) or part of the body.

Some additional benefits (for the mother) of exercising regularly during pregnancy include a reduced risk of (ACSM, 2014; Bryant & Green, 2010):

- Excessive weight gain
- Gestational diabetes
- Pregnancy-induced hypertension
- Pregnancy-induced incontinence
- Preeclampsia
- Cesarean delivery
- Low back pain (due to center of gravity changes as the fetus grows)

Although the exercise prescription for pregnant women is generally consistent with recommendations for non-pregnant women, it may be necessary to adjust it based on the pregnant woman's symptoms, discomforts, and abilities (ACSM, 2014). These adjustments are necessary due to the numerous anatomical and physiological changes that can make physical activity more difficult than normal. Some of these changes include (ACSM, 2014):

- Increased oxygen uptake (VO_2) during weight-dependent exercises (although VO_2 remains unchanged for weight-independent exercises)
- Increased heart rate
- Increase of up to 50% in blood volume (ironically, without a subsequent increase in systolic and diastolic blood pressure (likely due to a decrease in total peripheral resistance))
- Increased minute ventilation (abbreviated VE; volume of gas inhaled or exhaled from the lungs per minute) due to increased ventilatory sensitivity

Since pregnancy raises the resting heart rate and lowers the maximum heart rate, using heart rate to gauge exercise intensity is not recommended. Instead, pregnant women should use the rate of perceived exertion (3–4 on a 1–10 scale) or the "talk test" (able to carry on a conversation while exercising) to monitor exercise intensity (ACSM, 2014; Bryant & Green, 2010). Pregnant women should avoid contact sports or any sport/activity that requires extensive jumping or presents an increase in the the risk of falling. Some examples include soccer, football, basketball, softball, volleyball, and horseback riding. Women who were sedentary before pregnancy, are morbidly obese, or have a pregnancy-induced medical condition (e.g., gestational diabetes mellitus, pregnancy-induced hypertension) should seek medical clearance from their physician before beginning an exercise program. Additionally, these women should begin slowly and gradually increase their levels of physical activity. Due to increased metabolic demands during pregnancy, pregnant women should also increase their daily caloric intake (~300 additional calories) and drink plenty of water. **TABLE 6.3** provides specific physical activity recommendations that should be followed during pregnancy.

Incontinence: Lack of voluntary control over urination or defecation.

Minute ventilation: Amount of air (in liters) that a person breathes per minute. Minute ventilation is calculated by multiplying respiratory rate and tidal volume (normal volume of air displaced between normal inhalation and exhalation).

TABLE 6.3 Physical Activity Recommendations for Pregnant Women

Frequency	At least 3 days per week, preferably daily
Intensity	Moderate / 3-4 RPE (on 1-10 scale)
Duration	15 – 30 min
Mode	Aerobic activity (e.g., walking, cycling, elliptical training, swimming) Strength Training (40–60% of 1RM / 3 sets of 12–15 reps)

Data from American College of Sports Medicine. ACSM, AHA *support federal physical activity guidelines.* Retrieved from http://www.acsm.org/about-acsm/media-room/acsm-in-the-news/2011/08/01/acsm-aha-support-federal-physical-activity-guidelines; Baechle, T. R., & Earle, R. W. (Eds.). (2008). *Essentials of strength training and conditioning.* (3rd ed.). Champaign, IL: Human Kinetics.

Pregnant women should stop exercising immediately if they experience any of the following symptoms (ACSM, 2014; Bryant & Green, 2010):

Dyspnea: Difficult or labored breathing.

- Vaginal bleeding / amniotic fluid leakage
- Dyspnea (difficult or labored breathing) / chest pain
- Headache / dizziness
- Muscle weakness
- Calf pain or swelling
- Preterm labor / uterine contractions
- Decreased fetal movement

In most cases, postpartum exercise may begin as early as 4–6 weeks after delivery. However, women who deliver via cesarean will likely require a recovery period of longer than 6 weeks (ACSM, 2014). Additionally, a significant amount of detraining is likely to occur during the initial postpartum period, so women should begin exercising again slowly and gradually increase their levels of physical activity.

Exercise Programming Considerations for Senior Adults

The physiological mechanisms associated with the aging process are not well understood. For most individuals, biological function and physical performance tend to peak somewhere between 20–35 years of age. However, there appears to be significant differences in function and performance between individuals at any given age. In fact, it is possible for a well-trained 65-year old to outperform a sedentary 25-year old. As a result, exercise prescription recommendations should be based on biological age rather than chronological age.

Even with continued training, decrements in function and performance are inevitable. For example, the slow onset of atherosclerosis and arteriosclerosis begin to decrease oxygen supply, thereby negating aerobic capacity. Additionally, cross-links develop between adjacent collagen fibers within the tendons and ligaments, thereby reducing their flexibly, range of motion, and muscle contractile performance. Finally, metabolism also slows by about 10% from 25 to 65 years of age thereby increasing an individual's percent body fat.

It is uncertain how much of these decrements are inevitable and how much are due to a progressive decrease in the amount and intensity of physical activity over the years. It does appear, however, that regular participation in physical activity will slow down or at least reduce the extent that these physiological decrements occur.

The peak age of athletic performance varies widely among sports. For example, the peak age for sports requiring significant flexibility (e.g., gymnastics) is mid to late adolescents (up to 18 years of age). For most aerobic sports (e.g., triathlons, marathons), the peak age is somewhere in the mid-20s. For anaerobic events (e.g., powerlifting), the peak age can extend out as far as the late 30s or early 40s.

FIGURE 6.7 illustrates the sharp decline in world record performances with age for endurance, skill, and power events (Foster, Wright, Battista, & Porcari, 2007). Note the sharp decline after the age of 30.

Here are some specific physiological changes associated with aging (Al-Masri & Bartlett, 2001; Baechle & Earle, 2008; Haff & Triplett, 2016; Shepard, 1998):

Catecholamines: Class of aromatic amines (organic compound derived from ammonia) that includes neurotransmitters such as epinephrine and dopamine.

- *Decreased VO$_2$max:* Decreases by 0.5–1.0 ml/kg/min per decade from 25 to 65 years of age with possible acceleration thereafter. Reduction in VO$_2$max is likely due to decreases in maximal heart rate, stroke volume, and arterio-venous oxygen difference.
- *Decreased Maximal Heart Rate:* Decreases due to a decreased responsiveness of cardiac muscle to circulating catecholamines (i.e., neurotransmitters, such as epinephrine and dopamine, which affect the sympathetic nervous system).

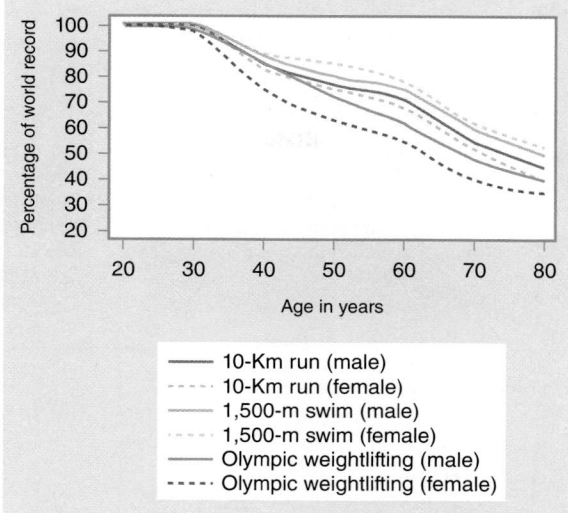

FIGURE 6.7 Age-Related Decline in Athletic Performance

Data from Bryant, C. X., & Green, D. J. (Eds.). (2010). *ACE personal trainer manual: The ultimate resource for fitness professionals.* (4th ed.). San Diego, CA: American Council on Exercise.

- *Decreased Stroke Volume*: Decreases as a result of impaired venous filling due to poor peripheral venous tone (likely due to the onset of atherosclerosis/arteriosclerosis) and a slower relaxation and contractility of the left ventricular wall.

- *Decreased Arterio-Venous Oxygen Difference*: Decreases from 140–150 ml/dl in a young adult to 120–130 ml/dl in seniors.

- *Decreased Peak Strength*: Strength tends to peak around 25 years of age then plateaus through 35–40 years of age, with a 25% loss in peak force production by age 65. Although the exact reason is unknown, most researchers suspect reduced innervation and degeneration of type II (fast twitch) muscle fibers. Interestingly, changes are greater in the legs than in the arms and in females more than in males.

- *Decreased Flexibility*: The buildup of cross-links between adjacent **collagen** fibers significantly reduce the elasticity of tendons, ligaments, and joint capsules.

- *Decreased Bone Mass*: There is a progressive decrease in calcium content and deterioration of the organic matrix of the bones. As with peak strength, decrements are more pronounced in females than in males (likely due to hormone profile differences between the genders). Calcium loss can begin as early as age 30.

> **Collagen:** Main structural protein found in connective tissue.

As previously discussed, senior adults are encouraged to participate in the same type of physical activities as younger adults. However, training and injury status should be considered before designing and participating in any exercise program. For example, strength training with free weights may not be recommended for some seniors, especially if they have no previous experience or have not participated in regular strength training for some time. Additionally, certain movements or exercises (e.g., deadlift, power cleans) may be contraindicative for some seniors based on previous injuries and certain medical conditions (e.g., herniated disks, degenerative joints, arthritis). Here are some training recommendations for seniors (Haff & Triplett, 2016):

- Get a medical screening before participation and get advice concerning the most appropriate type of activity

- Warm-up for 5–10 minutes before each training session

- Perform static stretching exercises after each training session

- Avoid holding one's breath during exercise to avoid an abnormal increase in blood pressure

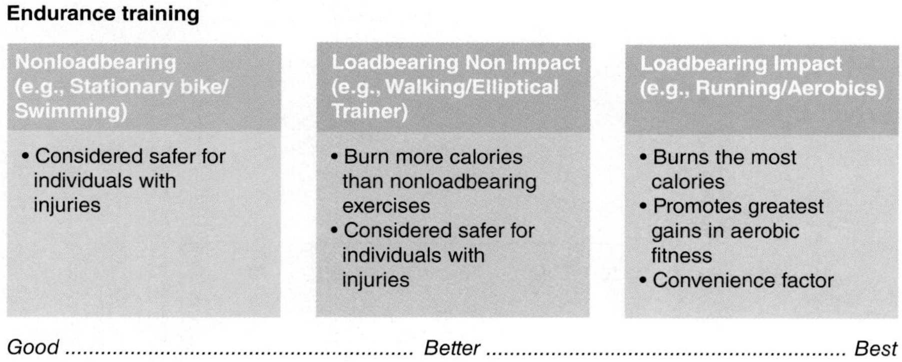

Endurance training

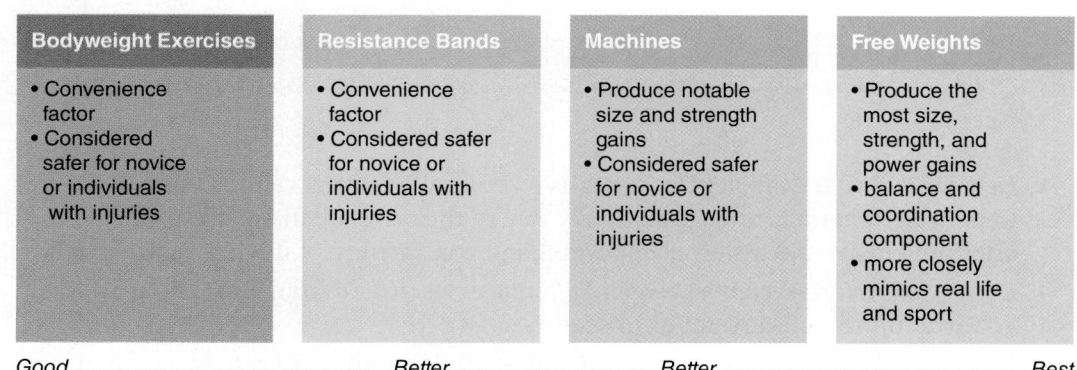

Nonloadbearing (e.g., Stationary bike/ Swimming)	Loadbearing Non Impact (e.g., Walking/Elliptical Trainer)	Loadbearing Impact (e.g., Running/Aerobics)
• Considered safer for individuals with injuries	• Burn more calories than nonloadbearing exercises • Considered safer for individuals with injuries	• Burns the most calories • Promotes greatest gains in aerobic fitness • Convenience factor

Good .... Better .... Best

FIGURE 6.8 Endurance Training Considerations for Seniors

Strength training

Bodyweight Exercises	Resistance Bands	Machines	Free Weights
• Convenience factor • Considered safer for novice or individuals with injuries	• Convenience factor • Considered safer for novice or individuals with injuries	• Produce notable size and strength gains • Considered safer for novice or individuals with injuries	• Produce the most size, strength, and power gains • balance and coordination component • more closely mimics real life and sport

Good .... Better .... Better .... Best

FIGURE 6.9 Strength Training Considerations for Seniors

- Allow 48 to 72 hours of recovery between exercise sessions
- Perform all exercises within a ROM that is pain free

FIGURE 6.8 and **FIGURE 6.9** provide some considerations and benefits associated with different types of endurance and strength training for senior adults.

Assessment and Application

Summary

- There is an inverse relationship between exercise intensity, volume, and frequency. As one of these parameters increases, reductions will need to be made in the other two in order to prevent overtraining and/or injury.

- The CDC recommends that 100–115 minutes of moderate-intensity aerobic activity be performed each week to reduce the risk of disease; 150–200 minutes of moderate-intensity aerobic activity per week to prevent weight gain and/or improve fitness; and 250–300 minutes per week to lose weight. However, these time requirements can be cut in half if vigorous-intensity aerobic activity is performed instead.

- A needs analysis is an effective means of exercise prescription that bases exercises selection and programming on detailed evaluations of both the individual and their sport.

- Although there are 11 different components of fitness, some are more important than others and have training priority. The three fundamental components of fitness include muscular strength, cardiovascular endurance, and mobility and are collectively known as the Fitness Trident.

- Recommendations from ACSM state that endurance training should be performed at least 3 days per week; strength training should be performed at least 2 days per week; and mobility training should be performed at least 2 to 3 days per week. However, it is important to understand that these are the recommended minimums. If you are lacking in a particular area, you should do more than the recommended minimums.

- The order in which exercises are performed does appear to matter when combining strength and endurance training into a single training session. Therefore, whichever component of fitness (i.e., strength or endurance) needs the most work should be performed first. However, if strength training and endurance training are performed on the same day but at different times (e.g., morning and evening workouts), then the order has no consequence.

- Research has shown that regular strength and endurance training have been shown to be both safe and effective for children. However, research has also shown that children don't respond to training the same way as adults. Therefore, training sessions for children should focus more on learning technique and having fun than the amount of weight lifted.

- Research has shown that exercising during pregnancy has numerous benefits for both the mother and fetus. Although the exercise prescription for a pregnant woman are generally consistent with the recommendations for a non-pregnant woman, it may be necessary to adjust them based on the pregnant woman's symptoms, discomforts, and abilities. Postpartum exercise may begin as early as 4–6 weeks after delivery. However, women who deliver via cesarean will likely require a recovery period of more than 6 weeks.

- Research has shown that senior adults respond favorably to regular strength and endurance work. In fact, seniors can perform the same type of strength and endurance exercises as younger adults as long as they are free from injury and properly conditioned. However, as with the case of children, seniors require a slightly different exercise progression and recovery program than their younger peers.

Knowledge Check

1. List the three basic program design variables used for all endurance and strength training exercise plans.
2. In addition to the three basic program design variables, list the other training variables that need to be considered for endurance and strength training programming.
3. List and differentiate between the physical activity recommendations provided from the CDC, ACSM, and AHA.
4. Provide some sport-specific exercises that a soccer player should include in their lower body strength training program.
5. Define and discuss a needs analysis.
6. List some of the common mistakes associated with exercise programming.
7. List the six different training priorities discussed by Dr. Mike Israetel.
8. List the 11 different components of fitness.
9. Define SRA and list the frequency recommendations for moderate endurance training, intense endurance training, moderate strength training, and intense strength training.
10. Discuss the Fitness Trident and list the three components of physical fitness that comprises it.
11. List and discuss some of the recommendations for combining endurance and strength training.
12. Define and differentiate biological and chronological age.
13. List some of the health- and fitness-related improvements associated with regular strength training in children.
14. List and discuss some of the specific strength training recommendations and guidelines for children.
15. List and discuss some of the physiological changes associated with aging.
16. List and discuss some of the specific training recommendations and guidelines for senior adults.

Activities

Exercise Programming

A. Keeping SRA considerations and the ACSM/AHA minimal frequency recommendations in mind, and using the individual information provided below, fill in appropriate workout recommendations for each training day in the provided weekly training plan.

Name	Claire
Gender	Female
Weight (lb)	167
Height (in)	62
% Body Fat	37
Age (years)	43

	Training Goals	1) Lose Weight 2) Train for a 10K race
	Current Training Plan	1) Runs 2–3 miles a couple times per week 2) Currently does no strength training work at all 3) Will stretch for 3–5 minutes after some but not every run workout
	Injury Assessment	Currently seeing a PT for Peteollofemoral Pain Syndrome *[Note: Patellofemoral pain is a common knee problem in which pain is felt under and around the kneecap. The pain can get worse when performing physical activity or sitting for a long period of time.]*

	Monday	Tuesday	Wednesday	Thursday	Friday	Saturday	Sunday
Type of Training							
Type of Workout							
Exact Workout							

Name	Ethan
Gender	Male
Weight (lb)	189
Height (in)	73
% Body Fat	17
Age (years)	22
Training Goals	1) Gain muscle 2) Increase weight on his bench, back squat, and deadlift
Current Training Plan	1) Lifts weights 5 days a week. Performs bench / squat / deadlift on M / W / F; shoulders / arms / back on T / Th. Employs the same exercises, number of sets & reps, as well as exercises every workout. Current plan incorporates no variation or progression. Has reached a plateau in terms of body weight and strength gains. 2) Currently does no cardio or mobility work.
Injury Assessment	Periodically suffers with low back pain

	Monday	Tuesday	Wednesday	Thursday	Friday	Saturday	Sunday
Type of Training							
Type of Workout							
Exact Workout							

References

Al-Masri L., & Bartlett, S. (2011). *100 Questions & answers about sports nutrition and exercise.* Burlington, MA: Jones & Bartlett.

American College of Sports Medicine. (2011). *ACSM, AHA support federal physical activity guidelines.* Retrieved from http://www.acsm.org/about-acsm/media-room /acsm-in-the-news/2011/08/01/acsm-aha-support-federal-physical-activity-guidelines

American College of Sports Medicine. (2014). *Resource manual for guidelines for exercise testing and prescription.* (7th ed.). Philadelphia, PA: Lippincott, Williams & Wilkins.

Antonio, R. (2015). *Deciphering the ideal training frequency for muscle growth.* Retrieved from http:// www.thinkeatlift.com/deciphering-the-ideal-training-frequency-for-muscle-growth/

Baechle, T. R., & Earle, R. W. (Eds.). (2008). *Essentials of strength training and conditioning.* (3rd ed.). Champaign, IL: Human Kinetics.

Bryant, C. X., & Green, D. J. (Eds.). (2010). *ACE personal trainer manual: the ultimate resource for fitness professionals.* (4th ed.). San Diego, CA: American Council on Exercise.

Centers for Disease Control and Prevention. *The Benefits of physical activity.* Retrieved from http://www.cdc.gov/physicalactivity/basics/pa-health/index.htm#PreventFalls

Foster, C., Wright, G., Battista, R., & Porcari, J. (2007). Training in the aging athlete. *Current Sports Medicine Reports*, (6), 200–206

Haff, G., & Triplett, N. (Eds.). (2016). *Essentials of strength training and conditioning.* (4th ed.). Champaign, IL: Human Kinetics.

Israetel, M. *Raw powerlifting priorities* [PowerPoint Presentation]. University of Central Missouri, Warrensburg, MO.

John, D. (2013). *Intervention: course corrections for the athlete and trainer.* Aptos, CA: On Target Publications.

Shepard, R. (1998). *Aging and exercise.* Encyclopedia of Sports Medicine and Science. Retrieved from http://www.sportsci.org/encyc/agingex/agingex.html#THE PHENOMENON OF

Starrett, K., & Cordoza, G. (2015). *Becoming a supple leopard: the ultimate guide to resolving pain, preventing injury, and optimizing athletic performance.* Las Vegas, NV: Victory Belt Publishing Inc.

World Health Organization. *What is moderate-intensity and vigorous-intensity physical activity?* Retrieved from http://www.who.int/dietphysicalactivity/physical_activity_intensity/en/

General Nutrition

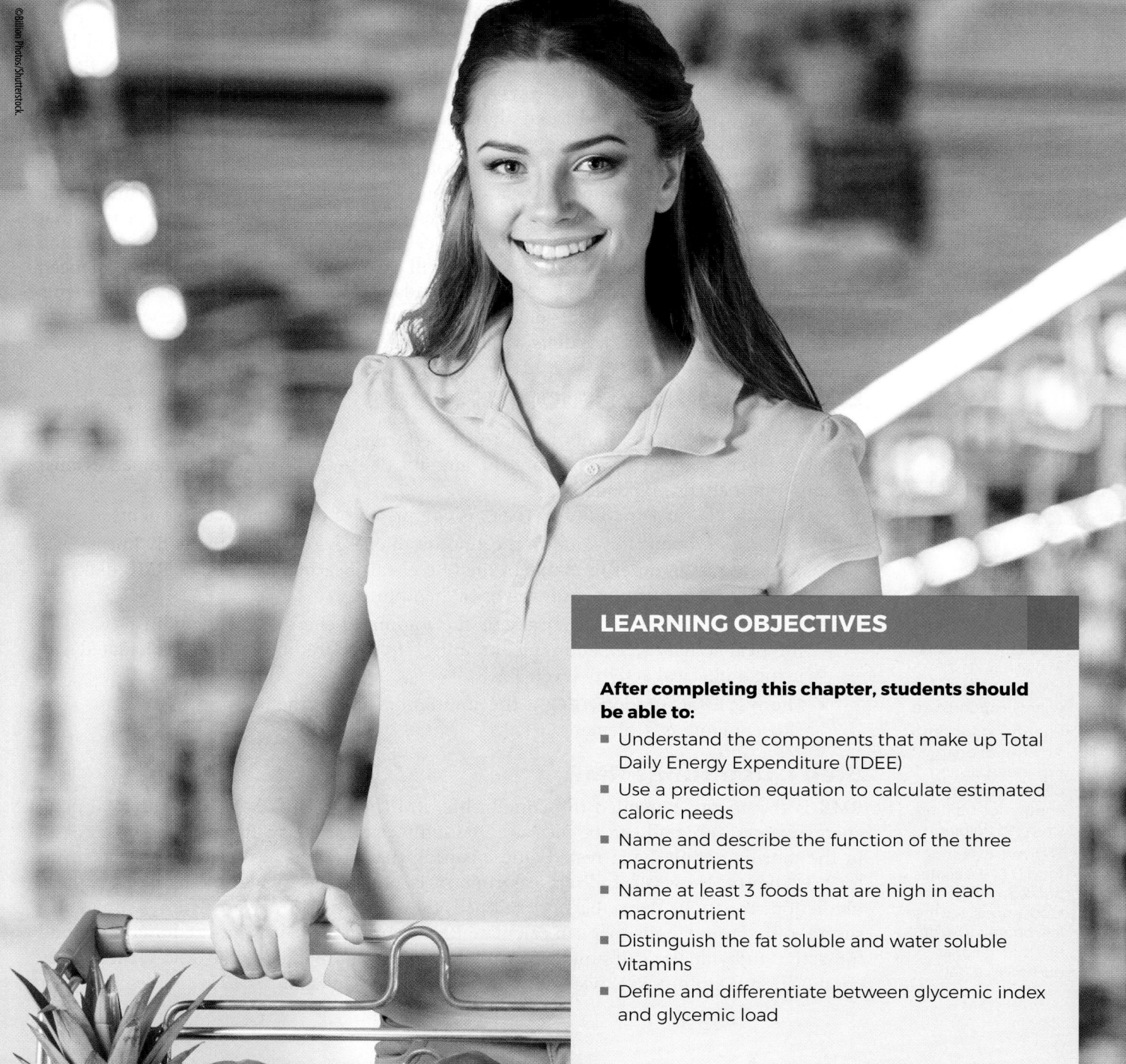

LEARNING OBJECTIVES

After completing this chapter, students should be able to:

- Understand the components that make up Total Daily Energy Expenditure (TDEE)
- Use a prediction equation to calculate estimated caloric needs
- Name and describe the function of the three macronutrients
- Name at least 3 foods that are high in each macronutrient
- Distinguish the fat soluble and water soluble vitamins
- Define and differentiate between glycemic index and glycemic load

Introduction

Although a complex science, nutrition is the study of how the food you and I consume helps our bodies grow, develop and remain healthy. Food is composed of many nutrients and other elements that the body uses to function. A food's nutritional value should always be considered when choosing what to eat. You should think about what a food is offering to help you become a stronger, healthier individual. It is also important to consider a variety of food. Instead of always choosing food with the highest amount of protein, you should also try finding foods that are high in other nutrients such as vitamin C, iron, or other vitamins and minerals. Nutritional balance is very important.

Since so many people lead busy lives, they often eat just to eat, frequently unaware of what or how much they are consuming. Society does not value the benefits of food. Instead, many people look for a quick fix to lose weight or gain muscle. The more practical approach is to focus on what food can provide instead of using supplements to make up for a poor diet. People should apply smart dietary strategies that can be supported long term instead of simply avoiding specific macronutrients (e.g., fats, carbohydrates). Eating a healthy well-balanced diet will always be beneficial. Mass marketing helps manufactures sell their product; this has led to an abundance of supplements, pre-packed, and highly processed foods that are consumed without regard to their nutritional quality.

Consumers often try fad diets because of the influence of marketing. They believe that this is the new "healthy" way to eat or that they will just try the diet for a little while to quickly lose some unwanted weight. Athletes and active individuals' don't realize that their performance can dramatically decrease if calories or entire food groups are restricted beyond needed levels. Therefore, this chapter will focus on key points of healthy, balanced eating for life. Topics will include how to calculate caloric needs, what macronutrients are, how to determine macronutrient needs, and an overview of some key vitamins and minerals. Supplements and fad diets will be covered in Chapter 9.

Determining Caloric Needs

One of several key components for optimal performance is energy balance. To evaluate energy balance, you need to compare the amount of energy (calories) consumed against the amount of energy expended.

Total Daily Energy Expenditure (TDEE) is comprised of three main components:

- **Resting Metabolic Rate (RMR):** the amount of energy (calories) the body burns while at rest in order to maintain life (e.g., heart beating, breathing). RMR makes up 70–75% of our total daily energy expenditure.
- **Energy Expenditure (EE):** represents the amount of energy expended during physical activity (e.g., endurance training, strength training). This is calculated using a physical activity level (PAL).
- **Thermic Effect of food (TEF):** is the amount of calories the body burns at rest. (Rosenbloom & Coleman, 2012).

Step 1: Determine RMR

RMR is the energy expended to maintain life. RMR makes up 70–75% of our total daily energy expenditure and can be measured by indirect calorimetry. It should be taken early in the morning while lying rested, and ensuring that no food has been consumed for at least 12 hours. However, indirect calorimetry is not always available; therefore, several prediction equations have been developed to estimate RMR. **TABLE 7.1** illustrates several different methods that can calculate RMR. Mifflin-St. Jeor is most common method for active individuals. Cunningham can be used for individuals who know their body composition (Dunford & Doyle, 2015; Rosenbloom & Coleman, 2012).

Total daily Energy Expenditure (TDEE): The total amount of calories an individual burns in a day.

Resting metabolic rate (RMR): Energy expended to maintain life. RMR makes up 70-75% of our total daily energy expenditure.

Energy expenditure: Amount of energy expended during physical activity (e.g., endurance training, strength training).

Thermic Effect of food (TEF): Calories burned to digest food, and accounts for roughly 10% of the total calories burned in a day.

TABLE 7.1 Resting Metabolic Rate Prediction Equations

	Harris-Benedict	Cunningham	Mifflin-St. Jeor
Male	66.4730 + 13.7516W + 5.0033H − 6.7750A	500 + 22FFM	10W + 6.25H − 5A + 5
Female	665.0955 + 9.5634W + 1.8496H − 4.6756A	500 + 22FFM	10W + 6.25H − 5A − 161

W = weight (kg); H = height (cm); A = age (years); FFM = fat free mass (kg)

To convert lb to kg, divide weight in lbs. by 2.2; To convert in. to cm, multiple height in inch by 2.54

FAQ

Sample RMR calculation using Mifflin-St. Jeor Equation:

Female / 25 years / 5'5" / 150 lb

Step 1: 150 lb ÷ 2.2 = 68.03 kg

68.03 × 10 = 680.3

Step 2: 5'5" = 65 in × 2.54 = 165.1 cm

165.1 × 6.25 = 1,031.875

Step 3: 680.3 + 1031.875 = 1712.175

Step 4: 25 y × 5 = 125

Step 5: 1,712.175 − 125 = 1587.175

Step 6: 1587.175 − 161 = 1426.175 (round to nearest whole number)

       RMR = 1426 kcal

Step 2: Determine EE

To determine caloric expenditure from physical activity, multiply RMR, by the appropriate PAL. **TABLE 7.2** indicates the PAL ranges for various amounts of activity (Institute of Medicine, 2005; Rosenbloom & Coleman, 2012; Williams, 2007).

For example, using a 150-lb. (68 kg) active female, take the RMR of 1,426 and multiply it by the activity factor of 1.75 to determine how many calories she would need to consume to account for her activity level. She would need 2495 kcal (1426 × 1.75 = 2495 kcal).

Step 3: Determine TEF

TEF can account for up to 10% of the total calories burned in a day. However, this percentage can vary greatly depending on the type of food consumed (e.g., nutrient dense foods yield a higher TEF than processed foods). To calculate TEF for our active female, take her 2495 kcal needs × 10% to determine that she could expend up to an additional 250 extra kcal.

TABLE 7.2 Physical Activity Level (PAL)

Physical Activity Category	Mean Value PAL (Range)	Kcal	Example
Sedentary	1.25 (1.1–1.39)	2,165 kcal/day	Spends most of day sitting
Low Activity	1.5 (1.40–1.59)	2,593.8 kcal/day	Participates in sports 1–3 days/week
Active	1.75 (1.6–1.89)	3,026.2 kcal/day	Exercises 1 hr/day
Very Active	2.20 (1.90–2.5)	3,804.4 kcal/day	>1 hr/day or exercises multiple times/day

Finalize TDEE

Total calorie estimates should be rounded to the nearest 100. For our example, TDEE = 2500–2750 kcal per day. This was determined by rounding 2495–2500 kcal and adding the 250 kcal from TEF.

Macronutrient Distribution

After calculating daily caloric need, the next step is to determine the macronutrient breakdown. Macronutrients are carbohydrates, protein, and fat, that provide the body with energy (or calories). The Institute of Medicine (IOM) provides the following distribution recommendations for the different macronutrients:

Nutrition facts label: Lists nutrients supplied and is based on a daily diet of 2000 kilocalories (kcal). The label was mandated by the 1990 Nutrition Labeling and Education Act (NEA).

- Carbohydrate (CHO): 45–65%
- Protein (PRO): 10–35%
- Fat (FAT): 20–35%

Once the total daily caloric intake and macronutrient distribution ranges have been determined, the last step is to identify possible food options that collectively meet the macronutrient and calorie requirements for each day. To do this use the nutrition facts label provided on food labels in order to determine the type and amount of food to eat. **FIGURE 7.1** illustrates a sample food label and shows how to calculate the calories for each macronutrient.

The New and Improved Nutrition Facts Label – Key Changes

The U.S. Food and Drug Administration has finalized a new Nutrition Facts label for packaged foods that will make it easier for you to make informed food choices that support a healthy diet. The updated label has a fresh new design and reflects current scientific information, including the link between diet and chronic diseases.

1. Servings

The number of "servings per container" and the "Serving Size" declaration have increased and are now in larger and/or bolder type. Serving sizes have been updated to reflect what people actually eat and drink today. For example, the serving size for ice cream was previously ½ cup and now is ¾ cup.

There are also new requirements for certain size packages, such as those that are between one and two servings or are larger than a single serving but could be consumed in one or multiple sittings.

2. Calories

"Calories" is now larger and bolder.

3. Fats

"Calories from Fat" has been removed because research shows the type of fat consumed is more important than the amount.

4. Added Sugars

"Added Sugars" in grams and as a percent Daily Value (%DV) is now required on the label. "Added Sugars" include sugars that have been added during the processing or packaging of a food. Scientific

Current Label

Nutrition Facts
Serving Size 2/3 cup (55g)
Servings Per Container About 8

Amount Per Serving

Calories 230   Calories from Fat 72

	% Daily Value*
Total Fat 8g	**12%**
Saturated Fat 1g	**5%**
Trans Fat 0g	
Cholesterol 0mg	**0%**
Sodium 160mg	**7%**
Total Carbohydrate 37g	**12%**
Dietary Fiber 4g	**16%**
Sugars 1g	
Protein 3g	

Vitamin A	10%
Vitamin C	8%
Calcium	20%
Iron	45%

* Percent Daily Values are based on a 2,000 calorie diet. Your daily value may be higher or lower depending on your calorie needs.

		Calories:	2,000	2,500
Total Fat	Less than		65g	80g
Sat Fat	Less than		20g	25g
Cholesterol	Less than		300mg	300mg
Sodium	Less than		2,400mg	2,400mg
Total Carbohydrate			300g	375g
Dietary Fiber			25g	30g

New Label

Nutrition Facts

1 8 servings per container
Serving size   2/3 cup (55g)

2 **Amount per serving**
Calories   230

	% Daily Value*
3 **Total Fat** 8g	**10%**
Saturated Fat 1g	**5%**
Trans Fat 0g	
Cholesterol 0mg	**0%**
Sodium 160mg	**7%**
Total Carbohydrate 37g	**13%**
Dietary Fiber 4g	**14%**
Total Sugars 12g	
4 Includes 10g Added Sugars	**20%**
Protein 3g	

5 Vitamin D 2mcg	10%
Calcium 260mg	20%
Iron 8mg	45%
Potassium 235mg	6%

6 * The % Daily Value (DV) tells you how much a nutrient in a serving of food contributes to a daily diet. 2,000 calories a day is used for general nutrition advice.

data shows that it is difficult to meet nutrient needs while staying within calorie limits if you consume more than 10 percent of your total daily calories from added sugar.

5. Nutrients

The lists of nutrients that are required or permitted on the label have been updated. Vitamin D and potassium are now required on the label because Americans do not always get the recommended amounts. Vitamins A and C are no longer required since deficiencies of these vitamins are rare today. The actual amount in grams in addition to the %DV must be listed for vitamin D, calcium, iron, and potassium.

The daily values for nutrients have also been updated based on newer scientific evidence. The daily values are reference amounts of nutrients to consume or not to exceed and are used to calculate the %DV.

6. Footnote

The footnote at the bottom of the label has changed to better explain the meaning of %DV. The %DV helps you understand the nutrition information in the context of a total daily diet.

Manufacturers will need to use the new label by July 26, 2018, and small businesses will have an additional year to comply. During this transition time, you will see the current Nutrition Facts label or the new label on products.

July 2016

FDA

For more information about the new Nutrition Facts label, visit:
www.fda.gov/Food/GuidanceRegulation/GuidanceDocumentsRegulatoryInformation/LabelingNutrition/ucm385663.htm

FIGURE 7.1 Nutrition Facts Label

The bottom area of the food label indicates that carbohydrates and proteins have four calories per gram (kcal/g) whereas fat has nine calories per gram. This allows us to calculate the exact number of carbohydrates, protein, and fat calories per serving. In the illustrated example, the product provided 124 kcal (31 g × 4 kcal/g) from carbohydrate (CHO), 20 kcal (5 g × 4 kcal/g) from protein (PRO), and 117 kcal (13 g × 9 kcal/g) from fat (FAT).

When reading food labels, pay close attention to serving sizes. In the above example, there are two servings per container. So, if someone ate the entire container (i.e., both servings), they would consume a total of 522 kcal (261 × 2).

Carbohydrates

Carbohydrates come in simple forms such as sugars and complex forms such as starches and fiber. The body breaks down most sugars and starches into glucose, which the body uses to fuel its cells. **Fiber** is a type of carbohydrate found in plants that does not break down. Fiber helps you feel full faster and stay full longer, which can help in terms of weight control. Fiber also helps the process of digestion and helps prevent constipation. **FIGURE 7.2** illustrates how to find high fiber foods, which are foods that have a **percent daily value (DV)** of at least 20%.

Types of Carbohydrates

Carbohydrates are separated into three different categories: **monosaccharides** (simple, one sugar molecules), **disaccharides** (composed of two monosaccharides), and **polysaccharides** (composed of long chains of monosaccharides). Simple carbohydrates include the monosaccharides and disaccharides. Complex carbohydrates are polysaccharides; examples include starches and fiber. Monosaccharides digest the quickest, while polysaccharides take the longest. However, polysaccharides also help you feel full and prevent blood sugar spikes. Added sugars (e.g., syrup, honey, table sugar and brown sugar) should be kept to a minimum since they have no nutritional value and add extra calories. On the next page, **TABLE 7.3** indicates different types of simple and complex carbohydrates. These are further divided into three different classifications: monosaccharides, disaccharides and polysaccharides. Examples of the different categories of sugar are listed in **TABLE 7.4**.

Fiber: Fiber is a carbohydrate substance found in plants. Fiber helps you feel full faster and stay full longer – which can help in terms of weight control. Fiber also aids in digestion and helps prevent constipation.

percent daily value (DV): An area on the nutrition facts label that helps consumers determine the level of various nutrients in a standard serving of food. DV are based on an intake of 2000 calories.

Monosaccharide: Single sugar unit, such as glucose.

Disaccharide: Two monosaccharides linked together.

Polysaccharide: Several monosaccharides linked together.

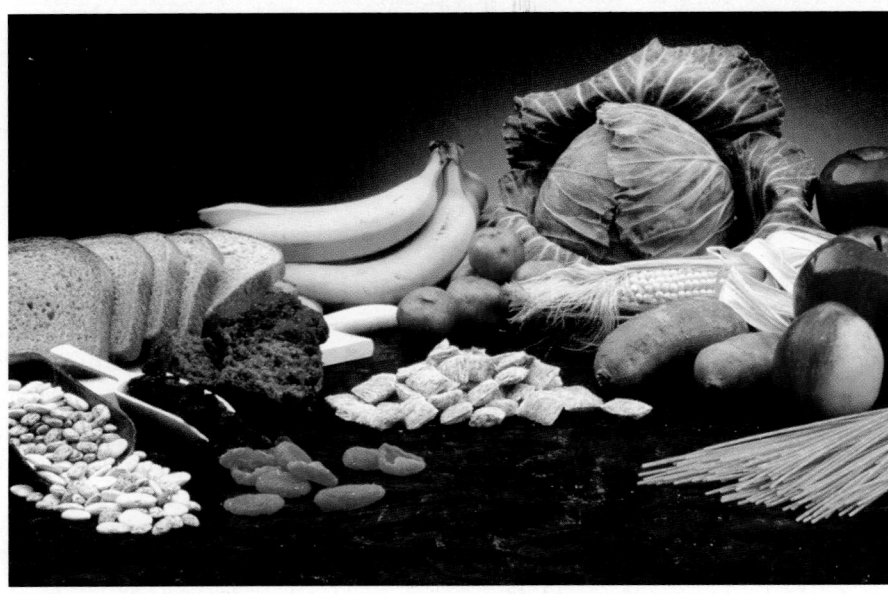

FIGURE 7.2 Carbohydrate Foods

TABLE 7.3 Simple and Complex Carbohydrates

Simple (Monosaccharides)	Complex (Disaccharides and Polysaccharides)	
Galactose	Lactose	Glycogen
Glucose	Maltose	Starch
Fructose	Sucrose	Fiber

TABLE 7.4 Classification of Carbohydrates

Monosaccharides		Disaccharides		Polysaccharides	
Galactose	form of sugar found in milk	Lactose	galactose + glucose; found in milk, ice-cream and dairy products	Glycogen	contains many branched chains of glucose and is the stored form of carbohydrate in the muscles and liver
Glucose	simplest form of carbohydrate and is type of sugar that circulates in the blood after foods are broken down	Maltose	glucose + glucose; found in bread and cereals	Starch	straight or branched chains of glucose; found in grains, legumes, and starchy vegetables
Fructose	form of sugar found in fruits	Sucrose	glucose + fructose (aka table sugar)	Fiber	straight or branched chains of monosaccharides; bond that links the sugar units cannot be separated by the body, therefore we absorb less carbohydrate from these foods

TABLE 7.5 Carbohydrate Food Sources

Grains	Bread, rice, pasta, cold cereal, oatmeal, grits, quinoa
Fruit	All fruits
Starchy Vegetables	Potatoes, corn, beans, peas
Dairy	Milk, yogurt

Glycemic index: Instead of counting the total amount of carbohydrates in foods in their unconsumed state, Glycemic Index (GI) measures the actual impact of these foods on blood sugar. Foods are ranked as being very low, low, medium, or high in their GI value. Low-GI diets have been associated with decreased risk of cardiovascular disease, type 2 diabetes, metabolic syndrome, stroke, depression, chronic kidney disease, formation of gall stones, neural tube defects, formation of uterine fibroids, and cancers of the breast, colon, prostate, and pancreas.

Carbohydrate Food Choices

Many foods contain carbohydrates. Grains including breads, rice, pasta, cereals, all fruits and starchy vegetables, such as potatoes, corn, beans, and peas all contain carbohydrates. Non-starchy vegetables do not contain enough carbohydrates to be considered a good source. Dairy products are also a good source of carbohydrates. **TABLE 7.5** identifies many different carbohydrate sources. It is best to eat a variety of carbohydrate sources in order to consume a variety of nutrients found in each of the food categories.

Glycemic Index

Glycemic index (GI) classifies a food by how high and for how long it raises blood glucose. Blood glucose levels rise after ingestion of carbohydrate. The rate at which blood glucose levels rise is based off how quickly the carbohydrate is digested and absorbed. The faster the carbohydrate is digested and absorbed, the higher the GI ranking. White bread is typically used as the example for a high glycemic index food. Carbohydrate-containing foods can be classified as high, moderate, or low glycemic index relative to pure glucose (GI = 100). The below table provides a list of some common carbohydrate sources and their GI rankings.

High GI (≥ 70)	Glucose, dextrose, high fructose corn syrup, white bread, white rice, corn flakes, breakfast cereals, maltose, maltodextrins, sweet potato, white potato, pretzels, bagels
Moderate GI (56-69)	white sugar or sucrose, not intact whole wheat or enriched wheat, pita bread, basmati rice, unpeeled boiled potato, grape juice, raisins, prunes, pumpernickel bread, cranberry juice, regular ice cream, banana
Low GI (≤ 55)	fructose; beans (black, pinto, kidney, lentil, peanut, chickpea); small seeds (sunflower, flax, pumpkin, poppy, sesame, hemp); walnuts, cashews, most whole intact grains (durum/spelt/kamut wheat, millet, oat, rye, rice, barley); most vegetables, most sweet fruits (peaches, strawberries, mangos); mushrooms; chili

Low-GI diets have been associated with decreased risk of cardiovascular disease, type 2 diabetes, metabolic syndrome, stroke, depression, chronic kidney disease, gall stones, uterine fibroids, and various types of cancer (i.e., breast, colon, prostate, pancreas). Additionally, a low GI meal has been shown to elicit a greater rate of fat oxidation during exercise as compared to a high GI meal. Although GI can be a valuable nutritional tool, it can be influenced by one or more of the following:

- Carbohydrates of similar type or sources can vary in their GI rankings
- Soil used to grow carbohydrates can influence their GI rankings
- GI rankings vary significantly when fiber, protein, and/or fat are consumed with carbohydrates
- Undigested food from a previous meal or snack can influence the rate of digestion and absorption of subsequent meals or snacks
- Carbohydrate consumed in liquid form are generally digested and absorbed faster than when consumed in solid form
- Time of day (due to fluctuations in gut motility and digestive enzyme production) can influence the rate at which carbohydrates are digested and absorbed

Glycemic Load

Glycemic Load (GL) was developed to evaluate the quality of carbohydrate in addition to the total grams of carbohydrate provided by the food. Glycemic load can be calculated by multiplying the glycemic index of the food by the grams of carbohydrate in a serving, divided by 100. For a typical serving of a food, glycemic load would be considered high with GL ≥ 20, intermediate with GL of 11–19, and low with GL ≤ 10.

The GL allows consumers to make a more accurate assessment of their dietary choices. For example, carrots have a higher glycemic index than ice cream; however, ice cream is not necessarily healthier for us than carrots. Carrots may raise blood glucose more quickly, but with the GL we can tell we would need to eat a lot of carrots to do that. Keep in mind these methods only apply to the food you are referencing and if you have a meal with a variety of foods, which most people do, that would impact the digestion rate and effect how quickly blood glucose rises. For example, fiber, fat and protein all slow or delay the spike in blood glucose you would normally see from eating a high glycemic index food.

What does the GL mean for the consumer? Often people tolerate moderate to higher glycemic foods if eating within an hour prior to exercise. However, throughout the day,

Glycemic Load: Takes into account the number of grams of carbohydrate in a food to determine how quickly the food raises blood glucose levels. It can be calculated by multiplying the glycemic index of the food by the grams of carbohydrate in a serving of that food, divided by 100.

after exercise, off days or if you are someone that gets hungry midway through exercise, it is recommended you eat moderate to lower glycemic index carbohydrate choices. These types of carbohydrates are generally more satiating (feeling of being full), provide more nutrients and help stabilize blood sugar levels better. Examples include choosing whole wheat bread instead of white bread and oatmeal instead of Special K.

Protein

Amino acids: Amino acids are the building blocks of proteins. The body absorbs amino acids through the small intestine into the blood.

Indispensable amino acids: Amino acids that must be consumed in the diet because they can not be manufactured in the human body.

Proteins are made up of essential and nonessential **amino acids** (organic compounds that are the building blocks from which all proteins are constructed). The body manufactures 13 essential amino acids, also known as **indispensable amino acids**. We must consume essential amino acids in our diet because our bodies cannot make them. Animal sources of protein contain all 13 essential amino acids. Plant proteins are often considered an incomplete protein because they are often missing at least one indispensable amino acid. The key, however, is to eat a variety of vegetables, whole grains and beans so that there will be no issue consuming all 13 essential amino acids.

Protein plays a crucial role in muscle repair, recovery, and growth. Protein can be used as a fuel source if someone does not consume enough calories or carbohydrates. However, if an individual uses protein as a fuel source, it means they are breaking down their muscles to obtain fuel to keep functioning. Performance will begin to decrease soon after this point. **TABLE 7.6** shows the various essential and nonessential amino acids (Rosenbloom & Coleman, 2012).

Recommended Protein Intake

How much protein does an individual need? The Recommended Daily Allowance (RDA) for protein is 0.8 g/kg/day. For a 150-lb. person that is 54 grams (0.8 × 70 = 54). Most people consume at least the RDA for protein; even vegetarians are able to meet the RDA for protein. Active individuals need slightly more. Even those with the highest requirements can meet their needs through food and subsequently do not require supplementation. For example, if the 150-lb person were an athlete performing a strenuous workout, they would need 1.6–2.0g/kg or (108–136 grams of protein per day. That could easily be met with 6 servings of protein containing 20 grams each. And while some people will consume a protein shake instead of a food source, mostly for convenience, there is no benefit to drinking a shake instead of eating a food source. **TABLE 7.7** lists the recommended protein intake for different activity levels (Thomas, Erdman & Burke, 2016).

TABLE 7.6 Essential and Nonessential Amino Acids

Essential Amino Acids		Nonessential Amino Acids	
Histidine	Threonine	Alanine	Glutamine*
Isoleucine	Tryptophan	Arginine*	Glycine*
Leucine	Valine	Asparagine	Proline*
Lysine		Aspartic Acid	Serine
Methionine		Cysteine*	Tyrosine*
Phenylalanine		Glutamic Acid	

* Considered conditionally essential by the Institute of Medicine (IOM)

TABLE 7.7 Recommended Protein Intake

Sedentary	0.8 g/kg/day
Low intensity or Short Duration Activity	1.0–1.2 g/kg/day
Moderate Intensity or Medium Duration Activity	1.2–1.6 g/kg/day
Long Duration or Strenuous Activity	1.6–2.0 g/kg/day

Data from Thomas, D. T., Erdman, K. A., & Burke, L. M. (2016). American College of Sports Medicine joint position statement. Nutrition and athletic performance. *Medicine & Science in Sports & Exercise, 48*(3), 543–568.

Protein Food Sources

Protein is found in a variety of foods. Protein content is highest in meat and poultry products, however dairy, whole grains, nuts, seeds and beans are also good sources. **TABLE 7.8** lists examples of high protein foods. **FIGURE 7.3** describes animal sources of protein while **FIGURE 7.4** on the next page lists non-animal sources of protein.

TABLE 7.8 Protein Sources

Meat	Kidney beans
Fish/Tuna	Black beans
Poultry	Soy beans
Eggs	Nuts
Greek Yogurt	Seeds
Milk	Peanut butter

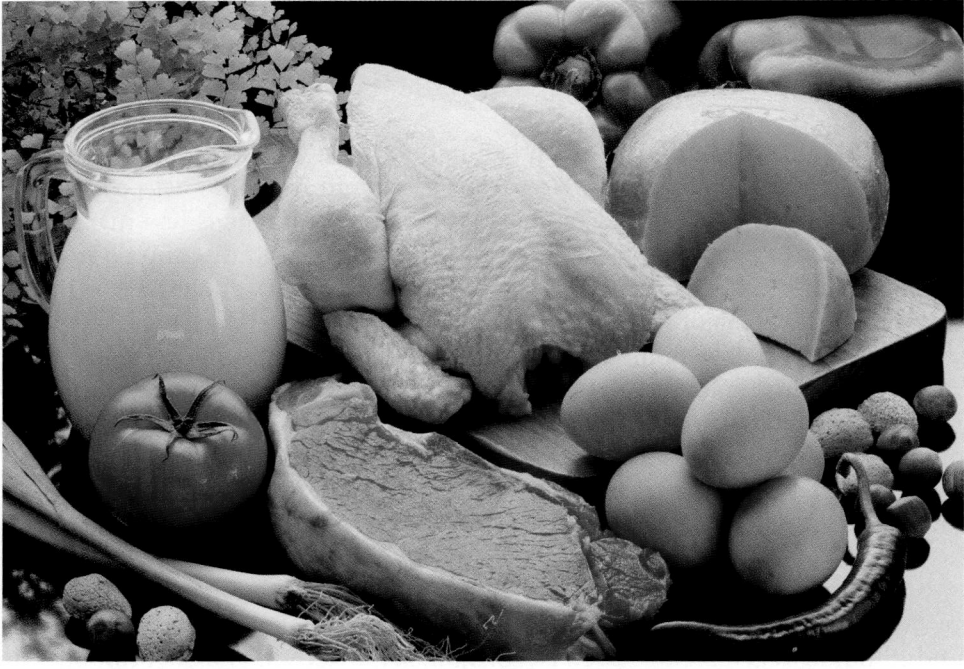

FIGURE 7.3 Animal Protein Sources
© age fotostock/Alamy Stock Photo.

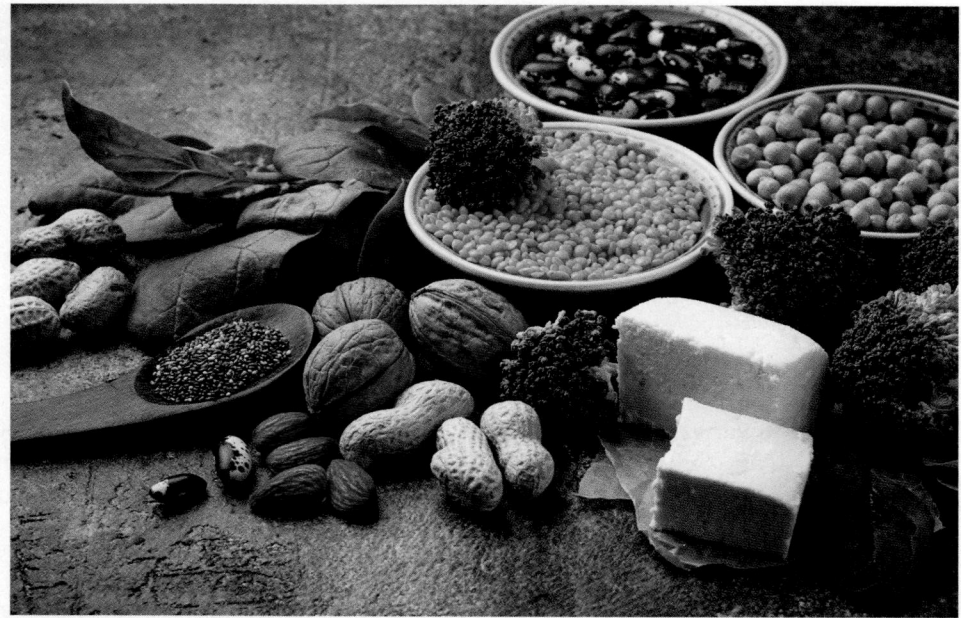

FIGURE 7.4 Non-Animal Protein Sources
© Yulia Furman/Shutterstock.

Cholesterol: Cholesterol is a waxy, fat-like substance found in all cells of the body. The body needs some cholesterol to make hormones, vitamin D, and substances that help in digestion. The body can manufacture all the cholesterol it needs; however, cholesterol can also be found in food (animal products). High levels of cholesterol in the blood can increase the risk of heart disease.

Fatty acids: Fatty acids are a major component of fats and are used by the body for energy and tissue development.

Monounsaturated fat: Type of fat found in avocados, canola oil, nuts, olives and olive oil, and seeds. Monounsaturated fats (aka "healthy fats") are thought to help lower cholesterol and reduce heart disease risk. However, monounsaturated fat has the same number of calories as other types of fat and may contribute to weight gain if eaten in excess.

Polyunsaturated fat: Type of fat that is liquid at room temperature. There are two types of polyunsaturated fatty acids (PUFAs).

Fat

Fat is needed in the diet for proper physiological growth, development, and function as well as the absorption of fat soluble vitamins. Due to its high caloric content, a high intake of fat increases an individual's risk for obesity and chronic disease. Too little fat could also be harmful to one's health. Fat provides texture, aroma and flavor to foods. Fat is found in animal products including meat, cheese, and dairy. Fat is also in plant sources such as avocado, nuts, and oils and it is hidden in baked goods, salad dressing, pizza, and donuts.

Types of Fat

Cholesterol is an animal sterol. It is manufactured in the liver and. Since it is made by the body we do not need to consume it. However, it is found in all animal products so most Americans consume it. The daily recommended cholesterol intake is less than 300 mg per day. Those who consume a lot of meat and dairy products in their diet should monitor their cholesterol consumption. Generally, the leaner the meat the less cholesterol is present.

Fatty Acids are a major component of fats and are used by the body for energy production and tissue development. These are important dietary sources of fuel because they can produce large amounts of ATP (energy).

Monounsaturated Fat is a type of fat found in avocados, canola oil, nuts, olives and olive oil, and seeds. Monounsaturated fats (aka "healthy fats") are thought to help lower cholesterol and reduce heart disease risk. However, monounsaturated fat has the same number of calories as other types of fat and may contribute to weight gain if eaten in excess.

Polyunsaturated Fat is a type of fat that is liquid at room temperature. There are two types of polyunsaturated fatty acids (PUFAs): omega-6 and omega-3. Omega-6 fatty acids are found in liquid vegetable oils such as corn oil, safflower oil, and soybean oil. Omega-3 fatty acids come from plant sources such as canola oil, flaxseed, soybean oil, walnuts, as well as from fish and shellfish.

Saturated Fat is a type of fat that is solid at room temperature. Among other foods, saturated fat is found in full-fat dairy products (e.g., butter, cheese, cream, ice cream, and whole milk), coconut oil, lard, palm oil, ready-to-eat meats, and the skin and fat of chicken and turkey. Saturated fats have the same number of calories as other types of fat, and may contribute to weight gain if eaten in excess. The daily recommendation for saturated fat is less than 7% of total calories.

Trans Fat is a type of fat that is created when liquid oils are changed into solid fats in order to increase the shelf life of certain foods such as shortening and some margarines. Trans fats are found in crackers, cookies, and snack foods. Trans fats are believed to raise LDL (bad) cholesterol and lower HDL (good) cholesterol. Products are now required to list trans-fats as part of the Nutrition Facts label.

Healthy Fat Sources

The daily recommended intake of calories from fat is 20–35%, with the highest percentage allocated for infants and children. There are no current recommendations for fat intake related to exercise, however, fat acts as a calorie buffer for those having a hard time reaching caloric needs. Fat does take longer to digest so it shouldn't be consumed shortly before exercising. Fats such as peanut butter, avocado, and nuts or seeds should be eaten throughout the day to better meet an individual's caloric needs. **TABLE 7.9** lists some common healthy fat sources and **FIGURE 7.5** shows healthy fat options.

TABLE 7.9 Healthy Fat Sources

Almonds, Walnuts	Salmon
Avocado	Peanut butter
Cooking oils	Sunflower seeds

Saturated fat: Type of fat that is solid at room temperature. Saturated fat is found in full-fat dairy products (e.g., butter, cheese, cream, ice cream, and whole milk), coconut oil, lard, palm oil, ready-to-eat meats, and the skin and fat of chicken and turkey, among other foods. Saturated fats have the same number of calories as other types of fat, and may contribute to weight gain if eaten in excess.

Trans fat: Type of fat that is created when liquid oils are changed into solid fats, like shortening and some margarines. This is done to make food last longer without going bad. Trans fats are found in crackers, cookies, and snack foods. Trans fats are believed to raise LDL (bad) cholesterol and lower HDL (good) cholesterol.

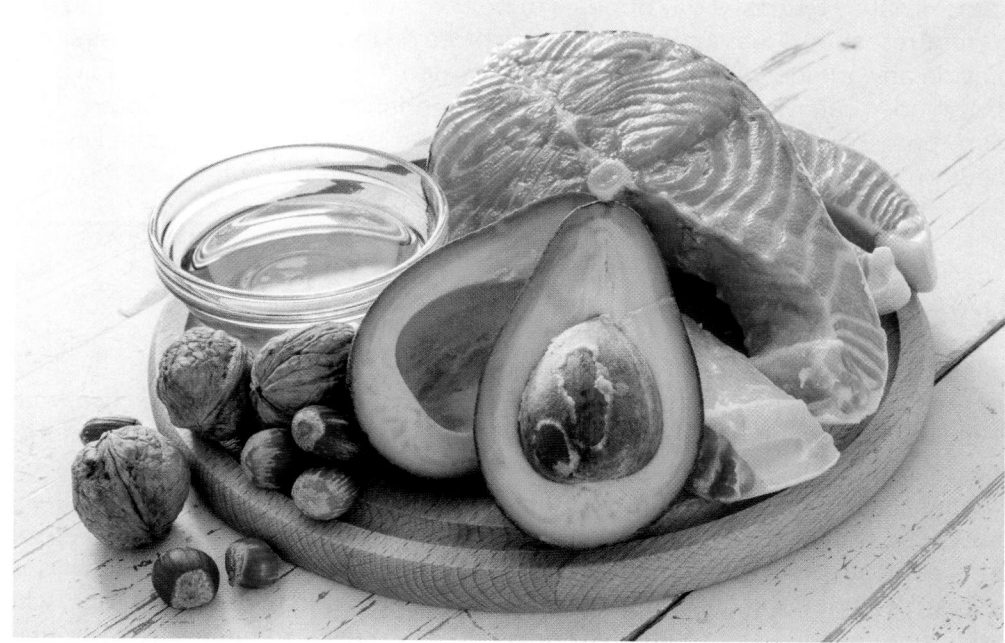

FIGURE 7.5 Healthy Fats
© Oleksandra Naumenko/Shutterstock.

Nutritional Modifications for Weight Gain or Weight Loss

Tips for Weight/Muscle Gain

- Increase caloric intake 500–1000 kcal per day
- Add 14 grams of protein per day, as long as it's not more than 2.0 g/kg/day
- Have a carbohydrate and protein source at each meal and snack
- Aim for 3 meals and 3 snacks or 6 meals per day
- Gain no more than 1–2 lbs. per week

Tips for Weight/Fat Loss

- Determine the kcal needs using current weight and prediction equations, then create a caloric deficit of no more than 500–750 kcal per day
- Maintain a regular eating schedule; do not skip meals
- Continue to eat vegetables; they help keep you full
- Eat balanced meals and snacks
- Eat at least 1.0 g/kg of protein or more if exercising, especially if in a caloric deficit
- Lose no more than 1–2 lbs. per week

FAQ

How can you gain 5 lbs. of muscle without gaining excess body fat?

The best way nutritionally to gain 5 lbs. of lean body mass is to increase your caloric intake; eat a well-balanced diet, high in fruits, vegetables, and whole grains; and consume protein at regular intervals throughout the day (20–30 g approximately 5 times a day appears to be the most beneficial according to current research). Please note that excess protein (above daily needs) does not provide any additional benefit for muscle growth. This is assuming the individual has an adequate workout routine that is also enhancing muscle anabolism. Many times, athletes only focus on protein or one component, while the key is to focus on the consistency and quality of their diet over time for the best results.

Vitamins: Various organic substances, either found in food or produced by the body, that are essential in minute quantities and act as coenzymes/precursors of coenzymes in the regulation of certain metabolic processes. Vitamins do not provide energy or serve as building units.

Micronutrients

Vitamins are various organic substances that are found in food or produced by the body. They are essential in small quantities and act as coenzymes or precursors of coenzymes for the regulation of certain metabolic processes. Vitamins do not provide energy (calories) or serve as building units (Williams, 2007).

Vitamins are separated into two different groups: water-soluble and fat-soluble vitamins. The water-soluble vitamins include vitamin C and the B vitamins. Fat-soluble vitamins are vitamins A, D, E, and K. The biggest difference between the two classes are that excessive amounts of fat-soluble vitamins will be stored in the adipose tissue, whereas excessive amounts of water-soluble vitamins will be excreted in the urine. Also, the over consumption of water-soluble vitamins are less likely to produce toxic effects. **TABLE 7.10** indicates the water-soluble and fat-soluble vitamins (Grosvenor & Smolin, 2012).

TABLE 7.10 Water-Soluble and Fat-Soluble Vitamins

Water-Soluble		Fat-Soluble
Thiamin	Vitamin C	Vitamin A
Riboflavin	Pantothenic Acid	Vitamin D
Niacin	Vitamins B$_6$ & B$_{12}$	Vitamin E
Biotin	Folate	Vitamin K

Data from Grosvenor, M., & Smolin, L. (2012). *Visualizing Nutrition: Everyday Choices.* (2nd Ed). New York, NY: John Wiley & Sons, Inc.

Minerals consist of inorganic elements found in foods that are essential for maintaining certain metabolic functions. Minerals are needed by the body in small amounts. Their main functions include maintaining structures (including bone) and regulating chemical reactions and body processes. The major minerals are needed by the body in amounts greater than 100 mg per day, while less than 100 mg per day are needed for the trace minerals. **TABLE 7.11** shows the major and trace minerals (Grosvenor & Smolin, 2012).

Electrolytes are minerals found in body fluids. They are ions with an electrical charge that must remain in balance for the body to function properly. The major electrolytes are sodium, chloride, potassium, magnesium, calcium, and phosphate. When someone is dehydrated, their body does not have enough fluid or electrolytes, which can lead to cramping, and sometimes to other complications (like irregular heartbeat, weakness, twitching, seizures, and/or numbness). It is important to keep the body's electrolytes in balance. **TABLE 7.12** lists the various electrolytes along with their recommended daily intake, sources, major functions, and the upper limit that can be taken without potential toxic effects.

Minerals: Consist of inorganic elements found in foods that are essential to certain metabolic functions. Examples include sodium, potassium, chloride, calcium, phosphate, sulfate, magnesium, iron, copper, zinc, manganese, iodine, selenium, and molybdenum.

Electrolytes: Electrolytes are minerals found in body fluids. They include sodium, potassium, magnesium, and chloride. When you are dehydrated, your body does not have enough fluids and electrolytes.

TABLE 7.11 Minerals

Major Minerals		Trace Minerals	
Sodium	Calcium	Iron	Chromium
Potassium	Phosphorus	Copper	Fluoride
Chloride	Magnesium	Zinc	Manganese
	Sulfur	Selenium	Molybdenum

Data from Grosvenor, M., & Smolin, L. (2012). *Visualizing Nutrition: Everyday Choices.* (2nd Ed). New York, NY: John Wiley & Sons, Inc.

TABLE 7.12 Electrolytes of Interest

Nutrient	Source	Recommended Intake	Major Functions	Upper Limit
Water	Water, beverages, soup, fruit, and other foods	2.7+ L/day (females) 3.7+ L/day (males)	Regulate temperature and pH, transporter of nutrients	N/A
Sodium	Table salt, processed foods	<2300 mg/day	Nerve transmission, muscle contraction, fluid balance	2300 mg/day
Potassium	Fresh fruits and vegetables, whole grains, milk, meat	≥ 4700 mg/day	Nerve transmission, muscle contraction, fluid balance	N/A
Chloride	Table salt, processed foods	<3600 mg/day, 2300mg is ideal	Fluid balance	3600 mg/day

Modified from Grosvenor MB and Smolin LA. *Visualizing Nutrition: Everyday Choices.* (2012). (2nd Ed). New York, NY: John Wiley & Sons.

	TABLE 7.13 Sources, Function, Intake, and Upper Limit of Select Minerals				
Nutrient	**Source**	**Recommended Intake**	**Major Functions**	**Upper Limit**	
Calcium	Dairy, fish, leafy greens, fortified foods	1000–1200 mg/day	Bone formation, enzyme activation, nerve impulse, muscle contraction	N/A	
Phosphorus	Meat, poultry, fish, eggs, dairy, cereals, soft drinks	700 mg/day	Bone formation, acid-base balance	2300 mg/day	
Magnesium	Milk, yogurt, greens, whole grains, beans, nuts, seeds	310–420 mg/day	Protein synthesis, nerve transmission, muscle contraction, fluid balance	N/A	
Sulfur	Protein-based foods, preservatives	Unknown	Part of amino acid and vitamins, assists acid-base balance	N/A	

Modified from Grosvenor MB and Smolin LA. *Visualizing Nutrition: Everyday Choices.* (2012). (2nd Ed). New York, NY: John Wiley & Sons, Inc.

Major Minerals for Bone Health

Calcium is important for the body because it helps support bone health and plays a role in muscle contractions. Ninety-nine percent of the calcium in the body is found in the bones. Many of the studies done on calcium intake indicate that 70% or more of athletes, both male and female, are not consuming enough calcium. Diets high in fruits, vegetables, whole grains, and low-fat dairy have been found to decrease urinary calcium excretion and, therefore, are thought to help conserve calcium and preserve bone. The adverse effects of low calcium intake on bone mineralization may be enhanced by high phosphorus intakes.

Phosphorus is the second most abundant mineral in bone; however, excess can be detrimental. When excess phosphorous is consumed, it turns on a hormone that intensifies calcium resorption (aka loss) from bones. Phosphorous comes from processed foods (crackers, deli meats, cheeses, beverages, etc.); phosphates and polyphosphates are added to these products to help preserve shelf life.

Magnesium is found in abundant supply in many foods. Green leafy vegetables such as spinach, legumes, nuts, seeds, and whole grains are all good sources. Most foods containing dietary fiber provide magnesium (Grosvenor & Smolin, 2012). **TABLE 7.13** provides a brief overview of the major minerals.

Trace Minerals

Trace minerals are only needed in small amounts and most can be found in many foods. Iodine is not found in many foods, but table salt in the United States is fortified with iodine. Iron deficiency is the most common deficiency in the world and one of the only deficiencies still seen in developed countries. Iron's major function is to help transport and utilize oxygen. The majority of it is in the form of hemoglobin, a protein-iron compound of the red blood cell (RBC). Iron deficiency is often associated with lower bone density and stress fracture risk in athletes.

Heme: Non-protein part of hemoglobin found in animal products.

There are two forms of iron **heme** (non-protein part of hemoglobin and some other biological molecules) found in animal products, and non-heme found in vegetable products. While there appears to be more iron in non-heme sources, it has less bioavailability than

TABLE 7.14 Source, Intake, Function and Upper Limit for Minerals

Nutrient	Source	Recommended Intake	Major Functions	Upper Limit
Iron	Red meats, leafy greens, dried fruit, legumes, grains, fortified cereal	8 mg/day (males) 18 mg/day (females) +20% for athletes	Part hemoglobin, holds oxygen in muscles, proteins needed for ATP production and immune function	45 mg/day
Zinc	Meat, seafood, whole grains, dairy, beans, nuts	8–11 mg/day	Protein synthesis, growth and development, wound healing, antioxidant enzyme	40 mg/day
Selenium	Meat, seafood, eggs, whole grains, nuts, seeds	55 µg/day	Antioxidant, spares vitamin E, synthesis thyroid hormones	400 µg/day
Iodine	Iodized salt, seafood, dairy, seaweed	150 µg/day	Needed synthesis of thyroid hormones	1110 µg/day
Manganese	Nuts, legumes, whole grains, leafy vegetables, tea	1.8-2.3 mg/day	Carbohydrate and cholesterol metabolism	11 mg/day

Modified from Grosvenor MB and Smolin LA. *Visualizing Nutrition: Everyday Choices.* (2012). (2nd Ed). New York, NY: John Wiley & Sons, Inc.

heme sources and; therefore, higher amounts need to be consumed. Iron is best absorbed when consumed with vitamin C sources.

Zinc is another common mineral found in animal products and is important for many enzymatic reactions needed for energy metabolism. Zinc is also associated with immune functions. **TABLE 7.14** provides an overview of the trace minerals.

Putting it all Together

Now that you have learned about the benefits of and required amounts for the different macronutrients and micronutrients, the next step is to put it all together into an effective, long-term nutrition plan. This will help ensure you are eating a well-balanced diet within the required calorie range for your specific performance goal (e.g., improve athletic performance, lose, gain weight). If you have sport-specific nutrition goals, please see Chapter 8 for additional guidance. **FIGURE 7.6** on the next page provides examples for typical meal plans. **TABLE 7.15**, **TABLE 7.16**, and **TABLE 7.17** (on pages 161–162) can help create meal plans that are broken down by food category and can help those interested in either maintaining their current weight, losing weight, or gaining weight.

Maintaining Weight

Calculate your daily calorie needs using the prediction equations provided earlier in the chapter. Then, locate the calorie requirements in Table 7.16 to determine how many servings of each food group you need per day.

The good news is there are numerous resources readily available that can make tracking daily caloric intake relatively quick and easy. For example, websites like www.supertracker .usda.gov or www.choosemyplate.gov provide nutrition facts for millions of different foods and can help users construct individual diet plans. Additionally, Appendix A at the end of

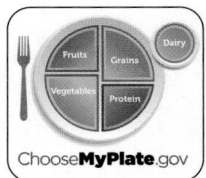

MyPlate Daily Checklist

Find your Healthy Eating Style

Everything you eat and drink matters. Find your healthy eating style that reflects your preferences, culture, traditions, and budget—and maintain it for a lifetime! The right mix can help you be healthier now and into the future. The key is choosing a variety of foods and beverages from each food group— *and making sure that each choice is limited in saturated fat, sodium, and added sugars.* Start with small changes —**"MyWins"**—to make healthier choices you can enjoy.

Food Group Amounts for 2200 Calories a Day

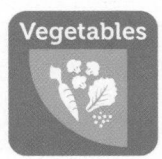 Vegetables	 Fruits	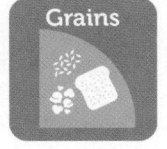 Grains	 Dairy	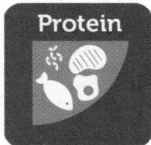 Protein
3 cups	**2 cups**	**7 ounces**	**3 cups**	**6 ounces**
Vary your veggies Choose a variety of colorful fresh, frozen, and canned vegetables—make sure to include dark green, red, and orange choices.	**Focus on whole fruits** Focus on whole fruits that are fresh, frozen, canned, or dried.	**Make half your grains whole grains** Find whole-grain foods by reading the Nutrition Facts label and ingredients list.	**Move to low-fat or fat-free milk or yogurt** Choose fat-free milk, yogurt, and soy beverages (soy milk) to cut back on your saturated fat.	**Vary your protein routine** Mix up your protein foods to include seafood, beans and peas, unsalted nuts and seeds, soy products, eggs, and lean meats and poultry.

 **Drink and eat less sodium, saturated fat, and added sugars. Limit:**
- Sodium to **2300 milligrams** a day.
- Saturated fat to **24 grams** a day.
- Added sugars to **55 grams** a day.

Be active your way: Children 6 to 17 years old should move **60 minutes** every day. Adults should be physically active at least **2 1/2 hours** per week. **Use SuperTracker to create a personal plan based on your age, sex, height, weight, and physical activity level.** SuperTracker.usda.gov

FIGURE 7.6 MyPlate Eating Plan

Courtesy of U.S. Department of Agriculture.

the text also provides nutrition facts for a large variety of foods without requiring Internet access (U. S. Department of Agriculture, 2015).

Losing Weight

Calculate your daily calorie needs with the prediction equations provided earlier in the chapter or using Table 7.15. Then, subtract 250-500 kcal from your total daily calories to determine the calorie level you should use to plan your meals from Table 7.16. NOTE: males should not consume less than 1800 kcal/day and females should not consume less than 1500 kcal/day without being supervised by a physician. If your calculation displays a lower number, please use 1500 kcal/day if you are female and 1800 kcal/day if you are a male.

TABLE 7.15 MyPlate Food Intake Pattern Calorie Levels

Age	Activity Level (Males)			Activity Level (Females)		
	Sedentary*	Mod. Active*	Active*	Sedentary*	Mod. Active*	Active*
2	1000	1000	1000	1000	1000	1000
3	1000	1400	1400	1000	1200	1400
4	1200	1400	1600	1200	1400	1400
5	1200	1400	1600	1200	1400	1600
6	1400	1600	1800	1200	1400	1600
7	1400	1600	1800	1200	1600	1800
8	1400	1600	2000	1400	1600	1800
9	1600	1800	2000	1400	1600	1800
10	1600	1800	2200	1400	1800	2000
11	1800	2000	2200	1600	1800	2000
12	1800	2200	2400	1600	2000	2200
13	2000	2200	2600	1600	2000	2200
14	2000	2400	2800	1800	2000	2400
15	2200	2600	3000	1800	2000	2400
16	2400	2800	3200	1800	2000	2400
17	2400	2800	3200	1800	2000	2400
18	2400	2800	3200	1800	2000	2400
19–20	2600	2800	3000	2000	2200	2400
21–25	2400	2800	3000	2000	2200	2400
26–30	2400	2600	3000	1800	2000	2400
31–35	2400	2600	3000	1800	2000	2200
36–40	2400	2600	2800	1800	2000	2200
41–45	2200	2600	2800	1800	2000	2200
46–50	2200	2400	2800	1800	2000	2200
51–55	2200	2400	2800	1600	1800	2200
56–60	2200	2400	2600	1600	1800	2200
61–65	2000	2400	2600	1600	1800	2000
66–70	2000	2200	2600	1600	1800	2000
71–75	2000	2200	2600	1600	1800	2000
76+	2000	2200	2400	1600	1800	2000

*Calorie levels are based on the Estimated Energy Requirements (EER) and activity levels from the Institute of Medicine Dietary Reference Intakes Macronutrients Report, 2002.

Sedentary: Less than 30 minutes a day of moderate physical activity in addition to daily activities.

Mod. active: At least 30 minutes up to 60 minutes a day of moderate physical activity in addition to daily activities.

Active: Sixty or more minutes a day of moderate physical activity in addition to daily activities.

Reproduced from U.S. Department of Agriculture, Center for Nutrition Policy and Promotion. (2012). MyPlate food intake pattern calorie levels. Online: http://www.MyPlate.gov

TABLE 7.16 Number of Servings per Food Group for Various Calorie Levels

Caloric Needs	1500	1800	2000	2200	2400	2600	2800	3000	3200	3400	3600	3800	4000
Grain (serving)	5	5	6	7	8	9	10	10	11	11	12	12	12
Fruit (serving)	3	3	3-4	4	4	4	4-5	4-5	4-5	4-5	4-5	4-5	4-5
Vegetable (cups)	2	2.5	2.5	3	3	3.5	3.5	4	4.5	4.5	4.5	5	5
Protein (oz.)	6	6	6	6	6.5	6.5	7	7.5	8	8	9	10	11
Dairy (serving)	2	2.5	2.5	3	3	3	3	3	3.5	4	4	4	4

Reproduced from U.S. Department of Agriculture, Center for Nutrition Policy and Promotion. (2016).

TABLE 7.17 Number of Servings of Food Groups per Meal for Various Calorie Levels

Caloric Needs	1500	1800	2000	2200	2400	2600	2800	3000	3200	3400	3600	3800	4000
Grain (serving)	1-2	1-2	2	2-3	2-3	3-4	3-4	3-4	3-4	4-5	4-5	5-6	5-6
Fruit (serving)	1	1	1	1	1	1	1-2	1-2	1-2	1-2	1-2	1-2	1-2
Vegetable (cups)	1	1	1	1.5	1.5	1.5-2	1.5-2	2	2-2.5	2-2.5	2.5	2.5-3	2.5-3
Protein (oz.)	3	3	3	3	3.5	3.5	4	4.5	4.5	4.5	5	5.5	6
Dairy (serving)	1	1	1.5	1.5	1.5	1.5	1.5	1.5	2	2	2	2	2

Data from MyPlate.gov

Gaining Weight

Calculate your calories with the prediction equations provided earlier in the chapter. Next, add 250-500 kcal to your total daily calories to determine the calorie level you should use to plan your meals from Table 7.16.

Table 7.16 illustrates how many servings of each food group to consume per day to meet your caloric requirements. It can also be used to determine how to spread out your calories during the day and you can use the second table to help guide your food selections. Table 7.17 provided examples of how many servings of each food group to have per meal. This will vary depending on how many snacks you have throughout the day. Experts recommend eating every 3-4 hours; therefore, you may need to eat at least 1-2 snacks per day. Serving sizes for each of the food groups are displayed in **TABLE 7.18** .

TABLE 7.18 Portion Sizes

Grains (½ cup)	Fruits (½ cup)	Vegetables (1 cup raw; ½ cup cooked)	Proteins (3–4 oz.)	Dairy Products (1 cup)	Fats (1 tablespoon)
• 1 slice bread • 1 small tortilla • ½ cup cooked oatmeal • 1 cup cold cereal • ⅓ cup cooked rice • ½ cup cooked pasta • ½ cup corn/peas	• 17 small grapes • ½ cup cut-up fruit • ¼ cup dried fruit • 1 small apple/orange • ½ large banana • ¼ cup 100% juice	• 1 cup raw veggies • 2 cups raw lettuce/spinach • ½ cup cooked veggies • ¼ cup 100% vegetable juice	• 3 oz. meat/fish/poultry • 1 egg or 2 egg whites • 1 tbsp. peanut butter • ¼ cup beans • 2 tbsp. nuts	• 1 cup milk • 1 cup soy/almond milk • 1 cup yogurt • 1.0 oz. cheese • ½ cup cottage cheese	• 1 tbsp. butter/margarine • 1 tbsp. low-fat mayonnaise • 1 tbsp. salad dressing • 1 tsbp. vegetable oil • ⅛ avocado

Serving sizes:
- ½ cup = size of a cupped hand
- 1 cup = size of a fist
- 3–4 oz. = size of the palm of the hand
- 1 tablespoon = size of the thumb

Case Scenario

Sam is a 21-year-old male who is 5'10" (178 cm) and 185 lbs. (84 kg) and exercises for one hour thrice a week. Using the Mifflin equation with an activity factor of 1.5, his daily caloric needs are:

- **Weight Maintenance:** 3200–3300 kcal/day
- **Weight loss:** 2600–2700 kcal/day
- **Weight gain:** 3700–3800 kcal/day

Time	Meal	Food Selection
0600	Breakfast	1 C oatmeal (2 grains), 3 scrambled eggs (3 oz. protein), banana (fruit), 2 pc whole wheat toast (2 grain) with 2T peanut butter (1 oz. protein)
0930	Snack	Yogurt with berries (dairy and fruit)
1215	Lunch	6" turkey sub (3 grain, 3 oz. meat), 1 C salad (1 veg), 1 C milk (1 dairy), 1 C carrots (1 veg), 1 apple (1 fruit), 1 serving pretzels (1 grain)
1500	Snack	-
1830	Dinner	1.5 C Pasta (3 grains), 1 pc garlic bread (1 grain), 3 meatballs (3 oz. protein), side salad (1 veg), 1 C broccoli (1 veg), 1C milk
2030	Snack	1 oz. almonds + ½ C fruit salad

Daily Total Provided (3200 kcal): 11 Grains, 10 oz. Protein, 4C vegetables, 4 Fruits, 3 Dairy.

Assessment and Application

Summary

- Total daily calorie expenditure can be calculated by evaluating resting metabolic rate, exercise expenditure, and the thermic effect of food.
- The three macronutrients are carbohydrate, fat, and protein.
- Micronutrients are vitamins and minerals.
- Vitamins are classified into either water soluble or fat soluble.
- When trying to lose weight, active men should not consume less than 1800 kcal/day and active females should not consume less than 1500 kcal/day.

Knowledge Check

1. List and discuss the three components of total daily energy expenditure (TDEE).
2. Using the Harris-Benedict equation, calculate the RMR for a 22-year-old male who is 5'10" and weighs 185 lbs.
3. Assuming the individual is "active," calculate the caloric expenditure from physical activity using the RMR calculated from question 2.
4. Assuming an individual consumes a total of 2200 kcal per day and desires a macronutrient breakdown of 60% carbohydrate (CHO), 20% protein (20%), and 20% fat (FAT), calculate the required number of calories that should be consumed for CHO, PRO, and FAT.
5. List and discuss the three categories of carbohydrates.
6. What are two main differences between simple and complex carbohydrates?
7. Glycemic Index (GI) is a method of classifying food by how high and for how long it raises blood glucose levels. Glycemic Load (GL) is a method of evaluating the quality of food (i.e., carbohydrates) to help consumers make smarter dietary choices.
8. Name three major minerals and an example of a food that contains each.
9. Name three trace minerals and an example of a food that contains each.
10. List and discuss the different types of fats.
11. List and discuss some of the recommended nutritional modifications for both gaining muscle and losing fat.

Activities

General Nutrition

A. Determine the RMR for an athlete of your choice using the Harris-Benedict, Cunningham, and Mifflin-St. Jeor equations
B. Determine the following using the RMR determined from each the Harris-Benedict, Cunningham, and Mifflin-St. Jeor equations:
   I. Exercise Energy Expenditure for each PAL category (i.e., sedentary, low active, active, very active)
   II. TEF and TDEE for each PAL category
   III. Assign an appropriate activity level, then use Table 7.7 to calculate daily protein intake requirements

Name	Claire		Name	Ethan
Gender	Female		Gender	Male
Weight (lb)	167		Weight (lb)	189
Height (in)	62		Height (in)	73
Age (years)	43		Age (years)	22
% Body Fat	37		% Body Fat	17

References

Dunford, M., & Doyle, A. (2015). *Nutrition for sport and exercise*. (3rd Ed). Boston, MA: Cengage.

Grosvenor, M., & Smolin, L. (2012). *Visualizing nutrition: everyday choices*. (2nd Ed). New York, NY: John Wiley & Sons, Inc.

Institute of Medicine. (2005). *Dietary reference intakes for energy, carbohydrate, fiber, fat, fatty acid, cholesterol, protein and amino acids*. Retrieved from http://www.nap.edu/read/10490/chapter/1

Rosenbloom, C., & Coleman, E. (2012). *Sports nutrition: a practice manual for professionals*. (5th Ed). Chicago, IL: Academy of Nutrition and Dietetics.

The Academy of Nutrition and Dietetics, Dietitians of Canada, and American College of Sports Medicine. (2016). Nutrition and athletic performance. *Medicine & Science in Sports & Exercise, 48*(3), 543–568. doi: 10.1249/MSS.0000000000000852.

U. S. Department of Agriculture. (2015). *Composition of foods raw, processed, prepared. USDA national nutrient database for standard reference, release 28 (2015). Documentation and user guide*. Retrieved from https://www.ars.usda.gov/northeast-area/beltsville-md/beltsville-human-nutrition-research-center/nutrient-data-laboratory/docs/sr28-download-files/

Williams, M. (2007). *Nutrition for health, fitness, & sport*. New York, NY: McGraw Hill.

Sports Nutrition

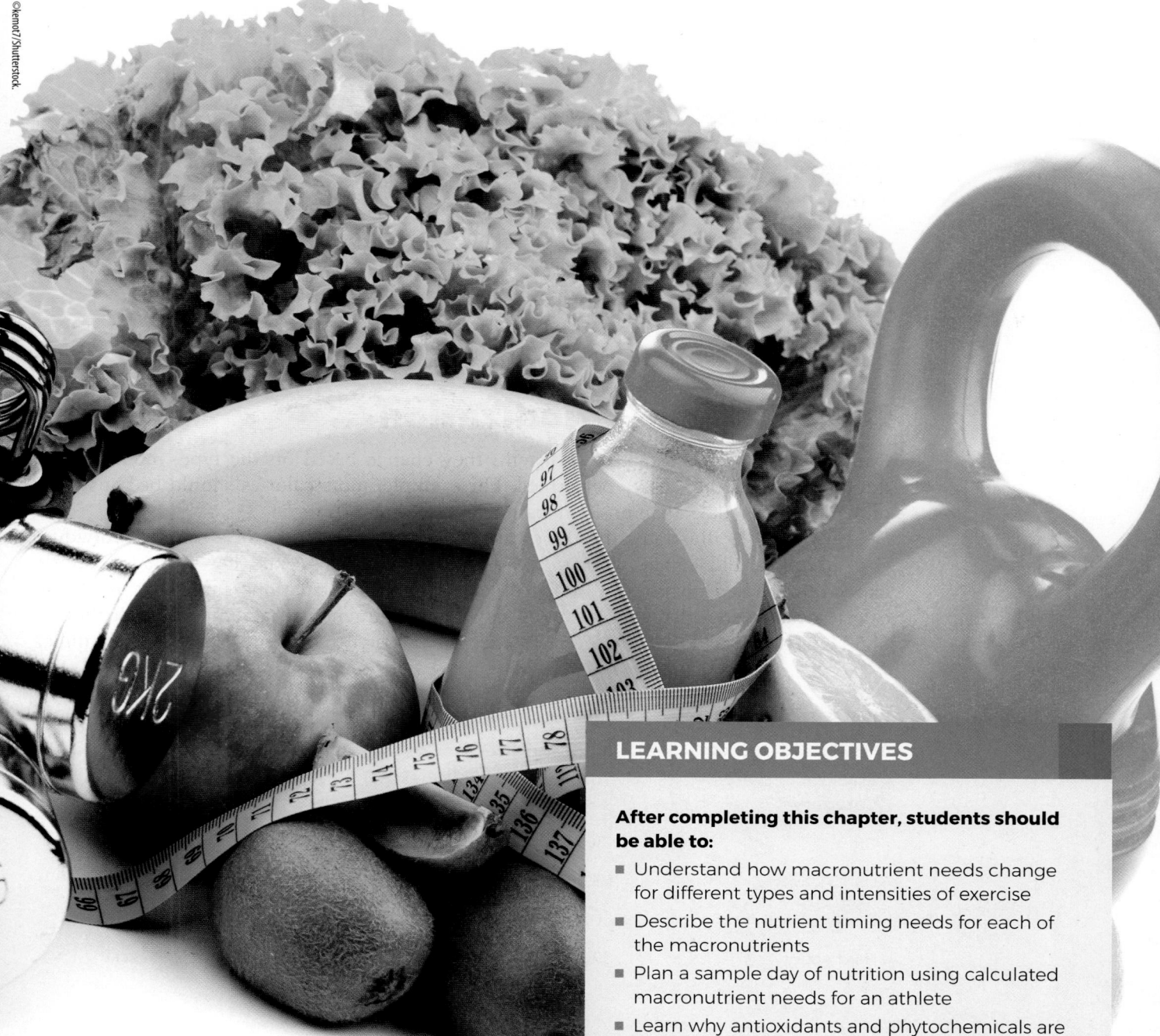

LEARNING OBJECTIVES

After completing this chapter, students should be able to:

- Understand how macronutrient needs change for different types and intensities of exercise
- Describe the nutrient timing needs for each of the macronutrients
- Plan a sample day of nutrition using calculated macronutrient needs for an athlete
- Learn why antioxidants and phytochemicals are important for health and performance

Introduction

Macronutrient recommendations are broad and fit the needs for most Americans. Although the recommendations for athletes generally fall within these ranges, they are often modified to better align with the specific nutritional requirements of the physical activity performed. In this chapter, you will learn the protein (PRO) and carbohydrate (CHO) recommendations for various types of athletes. And although fat is an important part of a healthy diet, there are no specific fat intake recommendations to enhance exercise performance. Research suggests that an athlete should consume at least 20% of his or her total calories from fat, but not more than 35% of their total calories from fat for performance (Rosenbloom & Coleman, 2012; Thomas, Erdman & Burke, 2016).

TABLE 8.1 lists the recommended macronutrient distribution ranges for endurance athletes, strength athletes, and athletes who regularly perform both endurance and strength training (aka mixed athletes).

TABLE 8.1 Sport-Specific Acceptable Macronutrient Distribution Ranges (AMDR)

Athlete Type	CHO	PRO	FAT
Endurance Athlete	55–65%	15–25%	20–30%
Mixed Athlete	50–55%	20–25%	25–30%
Strength Athlete	45–50%	20–30%	20–30%

Daily Caloric Periodization

Daily caloric needs are rarely consistent; they change based on the type, intensity, and duration of physical activity performed. For example, more calories should be consumed on hard training days than on light training or off days.

TABLE 8.2 illustrates the daily caloric periodization needs of a sample individual (i.e., a 25-year-old female who is 5'5" and weighs 150 lbs.) and her estimated caloric expenditure based on physical activity. The following calculations show how her daily caloric needs were calculated for an off day with the intended macronutrient distribution of 50% CHO, 25% PRO, and 25% FAT. Once the caloric needs are determined, the number

TABLE 8.2 Daily Caloric Periodization Based on Activity

Physical Activity Category	Total Kcal	CHO (50%)	PRO (25%)	FAT (25%)
Off	2165 kcal	1083 kcal	541 kcal	541 kcal
Light Activity	2593 kcal	1297 kcal	648 kcal	648 kcal
Moderate Activity	3026 kcal	1513 kcal	757 kcal	757 kcal
Hard Activity	3804 kcal	1902 kcal	951 kcal	951 kcal

of grams of each macronutrient must be established and the nutrition facts panel can help select appropriate foods.

- **CHO:** 2165 kcal × 0.50 = 1083 kcal (1083/4 = 270 g carbohydrate/day)
- **PRO:** 2165 kcal × 0.25 = 541 kcal (541/4 = 135 g protein/day)
- **FAT:** 2165 kcal × 0.25 = 541 kcal (541/9 = 60 g fat/day)

Carbohydrates and Exercise

Carbohydrates are the body's preferred source of energy. Individuals performing a light activity such as walking may only need 3–5 g/kg/day, whereas most athletes will need 5–8 g/kg/d on normal training days and up to 10–12 g/kg for endurance athletes or heavy competition days (Rosenbloom & Coleman, 2012; Thomas, Erdman & Burke, 2016).

Nutrient Timing for Carbohydrates

Carbohydrate Recommendations Prior to Exercise

Research has repeatedly demonstrated that carbohydrate consumption is crucial prior to workouts, particularly high-intensity workouts. However, there has been debate whether you can train your body to be more metabolically efficient at burning fat. While research in this area is still growing, current evidence suggests that the higher the intensity of the workout the more beneficial carbohydrates are for performance. Athletes who are going to run a race, do sprints, or participate in stop-and-go sports will clearly benefit from consuming adequate amounts of carbohydrate before exercise. The recommended intake of carbohydrates is 1–4 grams per kilogram body weight 1–4 hours prior to exercise. The intake should reduce gradually as the athlete approaches the time of the actual practice or competition. Intakes, however, will vary depending on individual tolerance. Some individuals will digest food more quickly than others and will need higher carbohydrate intake. An individual who commonly gets hungry or fatigued during workouts would be an example of someone who should eat closer to the higher end of the range prior to exercise. Individuals who often feel as if they are full, digest food slowly, or are nervous should consume the lower end of the range. In addition, higher amounts of carbohydrates will be needed for competition and high-intensity training days than low-intensity training days.

Carbohydrate Recommendations During Exercise

TABLE 8.3 indicates the recommended amount of carbohydrate intake based on the type and duration of physical activity. Carbohydrate needs can also vary based on environmental conditions and fitness level.

TABLE 8.3 Carbohydrate Recommendations During Exercise

Type of Activity	Recommended Carbohydrate Intake
Low, moderate intensity or <45 min	Water, carbohydrate not typically needed
High intensity 45–75 min	4–12 oz. of a sports drink
Endurance, intermittent, high-intensity 1–2 hours	30–60 g carbs/hour or (0.5 – 1.0 g/kg)
Endurance/ultra endurance 2–3+ hours	Up to 90 g carbs/hour

Data from from Rosenbloom CA and Coleman EJ. (2012). *Sports Nutrition A Practice Manual for Professionals*. 5th Edition. Chicago, IL: Academy of Nutrition and Dietetics.

Carbohydrate Recommendations Post Exercise

- Consume 1.0–1.2 g carbohydrate/kg/hr for the first 4 hours if competing again within 8 hours. If not competing again, 0.3g/kg of carbohydrate/kg body weight immediately after exercise is recommended to aid recovery.
- Consume medium to fast digesting carbohydrates after exercise for quick absorption (Rosenbloom & Coleman, 2012; Thomas, Erdman & Burke, 2016).

FAQ

Is it possible to gain muscle and lose fat at the same time?

This is a very popular and much debated topic among strength and conditioning professionals. Some experts argue that it is impossible to accomplish both goals simultaneously because the body must be in a completely different state to accomplish either goal. Specifically, the body must be in a caloric surplus (aka hypercaloric) state in order to gain weight (muscle) and a caloric deficit (aka hypocaloric) state in order to lose weight. The following formula is used to establish a weight range, using desired body fat goals. Here, FM stands for "fat mass" and FFM stands for "fat free mass."

Calculate Target Weight: Target Body Weight = Current FFM / 1 – (% Desired body fat)

For someone who wants to gain 5 lbs of lean muscle mass, the formula would be modified

Target Body Weight = Current FFM + 5 lb / 1 – (% Desired body fat)

FM = Current weight × Current body fat %

FFM = Current weight – FM Fat mass

Example:

A 189-lb male athlete wants to gain 5 lbs of lean mass but lower his body fat from 17% to 12–14% body fat.

Target Body Weight = Current FFM + 5 lb / 1 – (% Desired body fat)

FM = 189 lbs × 0.17% = 32 lbs fat

FFM = 189 lbs – 32 lbs = 157 lbs

Target Body Weight = 157 lbs + 5 lbs / 1 – (12% Desired body fat)

162/ 1 – 0.12 = 162/0.88 = 184 lbs for 12% body fat

162/ 1 – 0.14 or 162/0.86 = 188 lbs for 14% body fat

Plan:

To obtain this goal of increasing 5 lbs of lean muscle mass, a plan should be developed to assist with gaining 0.5 lbs per week by achieving caloric needs. Macronutrient intake should be balanced and meet the needs of the activity, meals, and snacks should be consumed every 3–4 hours. Reevaluate every 4 weeks, until goal body fat is achieved. Develop a maintenance plan once goals are met (Rosenbloom & Coleman, 2012).

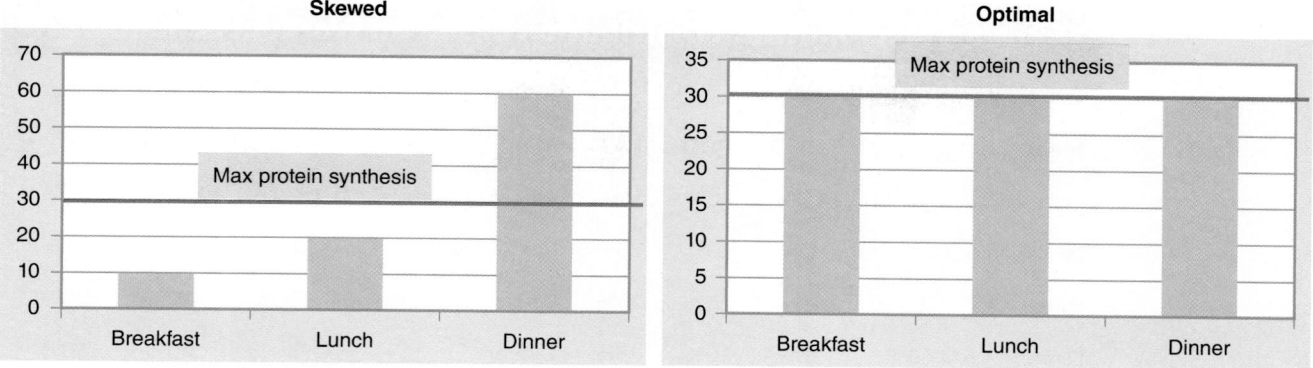

FIGURE 8.1 Typical Skewed and Optimal Pattern of Protein Consumption

Protein and Performance

Daily Nutrition

In addition to daily caloric periodization, athletes should also vary the macronutrient distribution ranges based both on exercise intensity and the time that physical activity is performed. It is best to consume higher carbohydrate and protein percentages and lower fat percentages on hard workout days then on light training days

Athletes should be concerned with both the total amount of protein intake per day and the amount consumed at each meal. They should consume 20-30 grams of protein at each meal (i.e., breakfast, lunch, dinner) in order to maximize muscle protein synthesis (Thomas, Erdman & Burke, 2016). **FIGURE 8.1** describes the typical skewed and optimal pattern of protein consumption (Campbell, n.d.).

Nutrient Timing

Research has demonstrated that consuming protein (0.5–1.0 g/kg of body weight) along with carbohydrates post exercise is beneficial for enhanced muscle recovery (Al-Masri & Bartlett, 2011; Thomas, Erdman & Burke, 2016). However, the research on protein before or during exercise is less clear. There may be some benefit to providing a small amount of protein (2% or approximately 3–5 g/hr.) during exercise to aid in recovery; however, protein intake during exercise has not been linked to enhanced performance (Al-Masri & Bartlett, 2011; Thomas, Erdman & Burke, 2016).

Daily Periodization

TABLE 8.4 on the next page provides macronutrient distribution recommendations based on when workouts are performed during the day. Specific macronutrient distribution recommendations are provided for morning, lunch, and evening workouts as well as off days. Some basic scientific principles are also included in these guidelines. For example, fat percentage intake is kept lower before workouts, while carbohydrate percentage intake is higher since carbohydrate, not fat, serves as the primary source of energy during physical activity. Fat also takes longer to break down and, if consumed before activity, will not yet be available as an energy source. Additionally, protein is incorporated post workout and evenly distributed throughout the day in order to promote the greatest anabolic effect.

TABLE 8.4 Macronutrient Distribution Based On Workout Schedule

Training Day (A.M. Workout)

Meal	CHO	PRO	FAT
Pre Workout	20%	20%	5%
Post Workout	25%	20%	20%
Lunch	30%	20%	25%
Dinner	20%	20%	25%
Bedtime Meal	5%	20%	25%

Training Day (Lunchtime Workout)

Meal	CHO	PRO	FAT
Breakfast	20%	20%	20%
Pre-Workout	15%	20%	10%
Lunch / Post Workout	30%	20%	20%
Dinner	30%	20%	30%
Bedtime Meal	5%	20%	20%

Training Day (P.M. Workout)

Meal	CHO	PRO	FAT
Breakfast	20%	20%	25%
Lunch	20%	20%	20%
Pre Workout	20%	20%	10%
Post Workout / Dinner	20%	20%	20%
Post-Post Workout	20%	20%	25%

Off Day (No Training)

Meal	CHO	PRO	FAT
Breakfast	20%	20%	20%
Snacks	20%	20%	20%
Lunch	20%	20%	20%
Dinner	20%	20%	20%
Bedtime Meal	20%	20%	20%

Meal Planning

Using the macronutrient distribution ranges, you should try to construct a daily meal plan based on the timing and intensity of the day's workout.

For example, **TABLE 8.5** illustrates a potential meal plan for the example of a light training day, requiring 2593 kcal (see Table 8.2). This plan could be further broken down into grams per macronutrient if using a Nutrition Facts panel, thereby making it easier to find food sources to meet individual needs.

TABLE 8.5 Sample Macronutrient Breakdown for a Light Activity Day

Light Activity Training Day (A.M. Workout)

Meal	CHO		PRO		FAT	
Pre Workout	20%	259 kcal	10%	65 kcal	5%	65 kcal
Post Workout	25%	324 kcal	25%	162 kcal	20%	130 kcal
Lunch	30%	389 kcal	20%	130 kcal	25%	162 kcal
Dinner	20%	259 kcal	25%	162 kcal	25%	162 kcal
Bedtime Meal	5%	65 kcal	20%	130 kcal	25%	162 kcal

Other Nutritional Considerations

Anti-Inflammation Foods

There are many reasons why inflammation occurs in the body including disease, infection, stress, and as a response to help heal injury. It is important for athletes, and those in physically demanding professions, to train appropriately and provide the body with the necessary food it needs for recovery and repair.

More research is needed in order to make specific recommendations on reducing excess inflammation with diet (Grosvenor & Smolin, 2012; Rosenbloom & Coleman, 2012). However, in addition to eating a well-balanced diet with adequate fiber, other common suggestions include consuming fish, omega-3 fatty acids, antioxidants, phytochemicals, and certain spices.

Fish and Omega-3 Fatty Acids

Consuming fish is recommended because it provides the body with fat soluble vitamins and also provides the body with omega-3 fatty acids (long-chain polyunsaturated fatty acids). The typical American diet is too high in omega-6 fatty acids (a family of pro-inflammatory and anti-inflammatory polyunsaturated fatty acids) and low in omega 3s. Foods that provide omega-3s include mackerel, tuna, salmon, walnuts, and flaxseed.

Omega-3 supplements are often recommended since most individuals do not eat the recommended three servings of fish per week. However, excessive amounts of omega-3s in the diet can actually increase inflammation.

Antioxidants & Phytochemicals

An antioxidant is a molecule or compound that inhibits oxidation (a reaction that occurs when oxygen combines with molecules in food to produce energy, water, and carbon dioxide). Antioxidants are often taken to prevent exercise-induced oxidative stress, which causes muscle fatigue and soreness. Many experts believe that eating a diet high in antioxidants will lead to improved recovery, muscle function, and performance. However, research has shown that these benefits are best seen from foods rather than supplements. The bioavailability (proportion of a consumed substance that enters circulation) of supplements is unknown and research indicates that taking large amounts of antioxidants may actually inhibit exercise-induced adaptations (Grosvenor & Smolin, 2012).

Phytochemicals are compounds that are not essential for life but are thought to function similarly and synergistically with antioxidants and may be beneficial for health (Grosvenor & Smolin, 2012; Rosenbloom & Coleman, 2012). There are thousands of phytochemicals and the most researched group are the flavonoids (Dunford & Doyle, 2015;

Omega-3 fatty acids: Unsaturated fatty acid, mainly found in fish oils, that have three double bonds within the hydrocarbon chain.

Omege-6 fatty acids: Family of pro-inflammatory and anti-inflammatory polyunsaturated fatty acids that have a final carbon-carbon double bond in the sixth bond (counting from the methyl end).

Antioxidant: Substance that removes potentially damaging oxidizing agents in the body.

Oxidation: Reaction that occurs when oxygen combines with molecules in food to produce energy, water, and carbon dioxide.

Bioavailability: Proportion of a drug or other substance that enters circulation that is able to have an active effect.

Phytochemical: Biologically active compounds found in plants.

TABLE 8.6 Common Antioxidants & Food Sources

Antioxidants	Food Sources
Vitamin C	Citrus fruits, leafy greens, berries
Vitamin E	Nuts, sunflower seeds, wheat germ
Vitamin A	Orange colored fruits and vegetables, leafy greens
Selenium	Egg yolk, beef, chicken, seafood, whole grains
Manganese	Seafood, nuts, seeds, whole grains, beans, leafy greens
Zinc	Oysters, beef, crab, fortified cereal, lobster

Data from Grovsner, Rosenbloom and Dunford.

TABLE 8.7 Phytochemicals and Food Sources

Phytochemicals	Food Sources
Flavonoids	Red, purple, and yellow pigmented foods: apple, citrus fruit, purple grapes, berries, onions
Phytoestrogens	Soybeans
Carotenoids	Yellow, orange fruits and vegetables: carrots, cantaloupe and leafy greens
Resveratrol	Red wine, peanuts, grapes
Anthocyanins	Blueberries, blackberries, plums, cranberries, raspberries, strawberries, tart cherries, beets

Data from Grovsner, Rosenbloom and Dunford.

Rosenbloom & Coleman, 2012). **TABLE 8.6** provides some examples of antioxidants and **TABLE 8.7** gives examples of some phytochemicals and the foods that contain them.

Spices

Spices can be added to everyday foods for an anti-inflammatory boost. Spices have antioxidant properties and many of them block inflammatory **cytokines** (substances secreted by immune system cells that affect other cells) and enzymes, which can result in less pain and fewer negative side effects that accompany inflammation. In one report, when sorted by antioxidant content, clove had the highest mean antioxidant value, followed by peppermint, allspice, cinnamon, oregano, thyme, sage, and rosemary (Benzie & Wachtel-Galor, 2011). **TABLE 8.8** lists some spices that have anti-inflammatory properties as well as food recommendations to combine them with.

Cytokines: Substances secreted by immune system cells that have an effect on other cells within the body.

TABLE 8.8 Spices and Usage Suggestions

Spices	Add To
Cinnamon	Oatmeal, baked goods, hot beverages
Cayenne	Sauces, marinades, rubs
Garlic	Any main dish or sauté with vegetables
Ginger	Tea, sweet or savory dishes
Turmeric	Curries, Indian dishes

Assessment and Application

Summary

- Macronutrient needs change depending on the type, intensity, and duration of exercise.
- Carbohydrates are the preferred source of fuel during exercise.
- To promote muscle anabolism, 20-30g of protein should be consumed several times throughout the day rather than all at once.
- Recovery meals should include a balance of carbohydrate and protein.
- Although it is possible to gain some muscle and lose some fat, it is less than optimal to try and accomplish both at the same time.
- Vitamins A, C, and E are a few of the antioxidants thought to help reduce muscle damage from oxidative stress from exercise.
- Spices can be added to many foods to block inflammatory cytokines.

Knowledge Check

1. List and discuss the nutrient timing recommendations for carbohydrates for pre-exercise, during exercise, and post exercise.
2. List the recommended protein intake for various types of athletes.
3. What are the protein recommendations after exercise?
4. Discuss the likelihood of gaining muscle and losing fat at the same time.
5. Discuss why antioxidant consumption may be beneficial for an athlete.
6. Of all the macronutrients, which one varies the most between an endurance and strength athlete?
7. Name three modifications an athlete could make to incorporate more antioxidants and phytochemicals into his or her diet.
8. Name two ways you would modify an athlete's eating schedule if he or she worked out in the morning versus the evening.
9. If a marathoner took 3 hours to complete the course, how many carbohydrates should he or she aim to consume during the event (provide a range)?
10. Name two ways an athlete could incorporate spices into his or her daily intake.
11. Name one way that nutrition aids muscle anabolism.

Activities

Sports Nutrition

A. Determine the AMDR for Claire as a predominantly endurance athlete.
B. Calculate how many grams of each macronutrient she should consume per day based on her recommended AMDR.
C. Determine the AMDR for Ethan as a predominantly strength athlete.
D. Calculate how many grams of each macronutrient he should consume per day based on his recommended AMDR.

References

Al-Masri L., & Bartlett, S. (2011). *100 Questions & answers about sports nutrition and exercise.* Burlington, MA: Jones & Bartlett.

Benzie F. F., Wachtel-Galor S. (2011). *Herbal medicine: biomolecular and clinical aspects.* (2nd ed.). Boca Raton, FL:CRC Press/Taylor & Francis.

Campbell, B. (n.d). Protein needs for athletes. NSCA Hot Topic Series. Retreived from: http://fitlabs.ru/wp-content/uploads/2017/05/Protein-Needs.pdf?x60603

Dunford, M., & Doyle, A. (2015). *Nutrition for sport and exercise.* (3rd Ed). Boston, MA: Cengage.

Grosvenor, M., & Smolin, L. (2012). *Visualizing nutrition: everyday choices.* (2nd Ed). New York, NY: John Wiley & Sons, Inc.

Rosenbloom, C. A., & Coleman E. J. (2012). *Sports Nutrition: a practice manual for professionals.* 5th Edition. Chicago, IL: Academy of Nutrition and Dietetics.

Thomas, D. T., Erdman, K. A., & Burke, L. M. (2016). American College of Sports Medicine joint position statement. Nutrition and athletic performance. *Medicine & Science in Sports & Exercise, 48*(3), 543–568.

Fad Diets and Supplements

LEARNING OBJECTIVES

After completing this chapter, students should be able to:

- Identify a fad diet
- Name an advantage and a disadvantage of common fad diets
- Define an ergogenic aid
- Name two nutrition-based ergogenic aids
- Evaluate a dietary supplement

Introduction

Fad diets are weight-loss programs or the use of supplements that promise to deliver fast results with minimal effort. Often, they are unsuccessful, too hard to maintain, and are typically unbalanced, which leads to nutrient deficiencies. The weight loss associated with fad diets is usually due to water and glycogen loss, which is counterproductive to athletic performance since it causes dehydration and the early onset of fatigue. Some of the long-term risks associated with fad diets include dehydration, **proteolysis** (loss of muscle protein), hypotension, and possible liver and/or kidney failure. Although fad diets sound appealing, as time is always an issue, their claims are rarely supported by scientific research and therefore not worth the risk.

Fad Diets

A sure way to recognize a **fad diet**, compared with a healthy dietary approach to weight loss, is by one or more of the following characteristics:

- A recommendation to eliminate or limit certain foods or food groups
- Weekly weight loss claims that are greater than 1–2 lbs per week
- A claim that you do not need to modify your current diet or food choices in order to lose weight
- A requirement that you buy their meals or shakes in order to be successful
- The use of non-peer reviewed studies to substantiate their claims

Some of the current fad diets include Atkins or similar ketosis diets, paleo, gluten-free, and vegetarian/vegan.

Atkins/Ketosis/Low Carb Diet

The effectiveness of low-carbohydrate diets likely has more to do with a temporary decrease in water weight than with reduced carbohydrate intake. When individuals significantly decrease their carbohydrate intake, they deplete their glycogen reserves, which are stored in the muscle along with water, and, therefore, quickly lose pounds due to reduced body water. However, once carbohydrates are reintroduced, they rapidly begin to store more water and regain the weight.

All of these diets promote eating a high-fat diet to lose weight. Some reports indicate success losing weight in the short term; however, long-term results vary. There are some medical concerns related to the high saturated fat, high triglyceride content and heart health. The other, more practical, problem with these diets is that they are hard to follow and often lack many important nutrients. Often, these diets require eating less than 50 grams of carbohydrates per day (which equates to less than three pieces of fruit per day). Since most foods contain some carbohydrates, people are likely losing weight on these diets because they are reducing their carbohydrate consumption, which in turn reduces their daily caloric intake and glycogen stores. In other words, they are losing weight because they ate fewer calories, not because carbohydrates are making them fat. In addition, research shows that although weight was lost, the majority of it was typically water and lean mass, not body fat (Williams, 2007).

Carbohydrates are the preferred energy source for your brain and muscles. When you consume a very low carbohydrate diet, your body produces **ketones** (an organic compound made when fats are broken down for energy) to help supply your brain and body with fuel. This only happens if the diet is consistently low in carbohydrates. Although often marketed as a benefit to performance, in most cases, the body's burning of ketones instead of carbohydrates is not a benefit. Individuals feel sluggish and tired, especially at first, although many claim that the sluggish feeling diminishes and actually improves over time. Even so, this is not feasible for the long term but, more importantly, research has not proven that low

Proteolysis: Breakdown of proteins or peptides into amino acids by enzymes.

Fad diet: A diest that promises quick weight loss through unhealthy and unbalanced dietary means.

Ketones: Organic compound containing a carbonyl group bonded to two hydrocarbon groups formed when fats (instead of carbohydrates) are broken down for energy.

carbohydrate diets are effective for most sports or high-intensity activities. In fact, current research suggests that any sport requiring a sprint, stop-and-go activity, or maintaining a high VO$_2$max would be better suited with carbohydrates being the primary source of energy.

Paleo Diet

The paleo diet appears to be healthy as it incorporates good high-quality foods such as nuts, seeds, eggs, fruits, vegetables, and grass-fed beef. While that part of the plan is reasonable, it can pose a significant financial strain on those on a tight budget. It is also very low in carbohydrate food choices, which does not benefit active populations and may hinder athletic performance. Additionally, a paleo diet eliminates some nutrient-dense foods including sweet potatoes, dairy, beans, and legumes, which have many health benefits. If someone were to follow a well-balanced diet, not excluding major food groups such as starches, whole grains, and dairy, all the foods in the paleo diet could be incorporated into a healthy, balanced diet.

Gluten-Free Diet

A gluten-free diet is one that excludes **gluten**, a protein found in wheat, rye, and barley. This type of diet is not meant to be a weight loss tool; however, many Americans use it as one. Certain subsets of the population, particularly those with **Celiac disease**, a disease in which the small intestine is hypersensitive to gluten thereby leading to issues with digestion, should follow a gluten-free diet. Others may have gastrointestinal issues that led them to follow a gluten-free diet. These cases are very difficult to assess since there are many different causes of gastrointestinal distress. Therefore, it is best to visit a physician to figure out the cause of the problem, while a registered dietitian can help find foods to include or avoid in order to manage symptoms. For example, if a person increases his or her fiber intake too quickly, he or she may have negative side effects. Others may not tolerate different types of sugars such as fructose, which is common in many baked goods. Still others may experience bloating if they eat too much carbohydrate at one time. All of these situations can lead some individuals to experiment with a gluten-free diet. Since there are a number of medical conditions that can lead to GI distress, it is best to first find out the cause of the problem, rather than just assuming one does not tolerate gluten.

There is no need or benefit to follow a gluten-free diet as a weight loss plan. It is just as easy to overeat gluten-free foods as it is to eat those that contain gluten. Also, if you are eliminating gluten, you are also likely reducing or eliminating whole grains, which are a good source of fiber, iron, and B vitamins. Anyone following this diet must be aware of the risks and should be sure to eat a good variety of foods to make up for those nutrients they may potentially be lacking.

Vegetarian/Vegan Diet

A **vegetarian** or **vegan** diet, if done correctly, can be incorporated into a healthy lifestyle. However, it should not be implemented solely for the purpose of losing weight. Many people think that just because they are eating salads or a plate of vegetables as meals, they are eating healthy and will lose weight. While vegetables are an important part of a healthy diet, vegetables are not the only aspect to consider when making healthy dining choices. They do not provide a lot of calories; therefore, individuals attempting to "eat healthy" and eat a plain salad for lunch with no dressing may end up ravenously hungry later in the day and overeat, either on snacks or at the next meal. The opposite problem can also occur. Specifically, salads can have a lot of calories, especially some of the loaded salads offered at restaurants. In some cases, these salads could contain over 1000 calories and may not be any healthier than the other alternatives.

Vegetarian diets can be a viable option and meet one's dietary needs if all other food groups are included. For example, protein can be found in whole grains, beans, legumes, eggs, and dairy. Vegans may have a hard time getting certain vitamins and/or minerals

Gluten: Gluten (derived from the Latin word glue) is a mixture of proteins found in wheat, rye, and barley that gives elasticity to dough, helping it rise, and gives the final product a chewy texture. It can also be found in products such as vitamin and nutrient supplements, lip balms, and certain medicines. It is important to note that less than 1% of the general population has Celiac disease (autoimmune disorder of the small intestines), which would require a gluten-free diet.

Celiac disease: A disease in which the small intestine is hypersensitive to gluten thereby leading to issues with digestion.

Vegetarian: Someone who does not eat any meat, poultry, game, fish, shellfish or by-product of animal slaughter.

Vegan: The strictest form of vegetarianism. Vegans not only exclude animal flesh but also dairy, eggs, and animal-derived ingredients.

naturally in their diet (e.g., vitamin B$_{12}$) and thus may need to take a supplement and follow-up with their healthcare provider to ensure they do not develop any nutrient deficiencies. Individuals following a vegetarian or vegan diet who do not take precautions are at the highest risk for nutritional deficiencies.

Intermittent Fasting

Another common fad is **intermittent fasting**. According to its proponents, intermittent fasting is not a diet per se but, rather, a new pattern of eating. There are different approaches to intermittent fasting: some eat one day and skip the next and others fast for 12 hours per day. The benefits and risks of fasting vary depending on how much caloric restriction is involved. In some cases, the goal is to keep the total number of calories consumed per day the same, which may be difficult for some people.

The theory behind intermittent fasting is that the body is in a higher fat-burning state while fasting compared with when food is consumed on a more frequent basis. There is some research, which indicates that intermittent fasting may have some benefits for obese individuals (Anton et al, 2017). However, there are limited data available when it comes to intermittent fasting among healthy individuals. In fact, research conducted on athletes shows a decline in their performance levels when in a fasting or low-energy state. In addition, there are several other problems, particularly for individuals who are working out and putting high demands on their bodies, as intermittent fasting can decrease performance levels. Since the body responds to the physiological stimulus provided, anything that reduces one's ability to train hard, in terms of volume and intensity, will diminish the key physiological adaptations associated with training (Israetel, Case & Hoffmann, n.d.).

Moreover, the recovery period is a critical time for muscle growth and repair and keeping the body in a state of starvation for long periods of time by means of fasting can cause the body to find other sources of fuel. Most commonly, the body obtains this fuel by breaking down muscle to provide energy via **gluconeogenesis**. As a result, the body will be in a catabolic state and reduce the benefits of training instead of stimulating muscle anabolism that occurs when the body is not fasted.

Nutritional Ergogenic Aids

An **ergogenic aid** is any method or product used to enhance mental and physical performance or recovery. This section will be divided into nutrition supplements, which are mostly food items and dietary supplements. Dietary supplements are not regulated by the Food and Drug Administration (FDA) and may or may not contain the active ingredients listed on the label. They may also contain illegal ingredients not listed on the label.

Products discussed here, for the most part, will contain a **Nutrition Facts label** instead of a **Supplement Facts label**. Products with a Nutrition Facts label are regulated by the FDA, meaning that the products must contain the active ingredient listed and are less likely to be cross-contaminated with illegal components. While safer, these products may still pose some risk. For example, they may contain high amounts of caffeine or **proprietary blends** (a list of ingredients for a product formula specific to a particular manufacturer). The products may also include herbs that are not regulated by any federal agency. Herbs may interfere with medications or have unknown side effects. Many energy drinks contain herbal forms of caffeine, in addition to the caffeine listed.

Often when the term "proprietary blend" is used, the amounts of the ingredients are not included and could be dangerously high. Some caffeinated and herbal supplements, such as ephedra, were banned because of the number of heart-related deaths that occurred in young, healthy athletes. **FIGURE 9.1** and **FIGURE 9.2** show examples of Supplement Facts and Nutrition Facts labels. It is also important to review the list of ingredients as well as all additives that are listed below the macronutrients and micronutrients.

Intermittent fasting: Specific dietary strategy that requires an intentional abstention from food, drink, or both, for a period of time for the primary purpose of losing weight.

Gluconeogenesis: Formation of glucose from precursors other than carbohydrates (e.g., amino acids, glycerol from fats, or lactate produced by muscle during anaerobic glycolysis).

Ergogenic aid: Any method or product used to enhance mental and physical performance or recovery.

Nutrition Facts label: Lists nutrients supplied and is based on a daily diet of 2000 kilocalories (kcal). The label was mandated by the 1990 Nutrition Labeling and Education Act (NEA).

Supplement Facts label: Lists the names and quantities of dietary ingredients present in the product, the serving size, and the servings per container.

Proprietary blends: A list of ingredients for a product formula specific to a particular manufacturer.

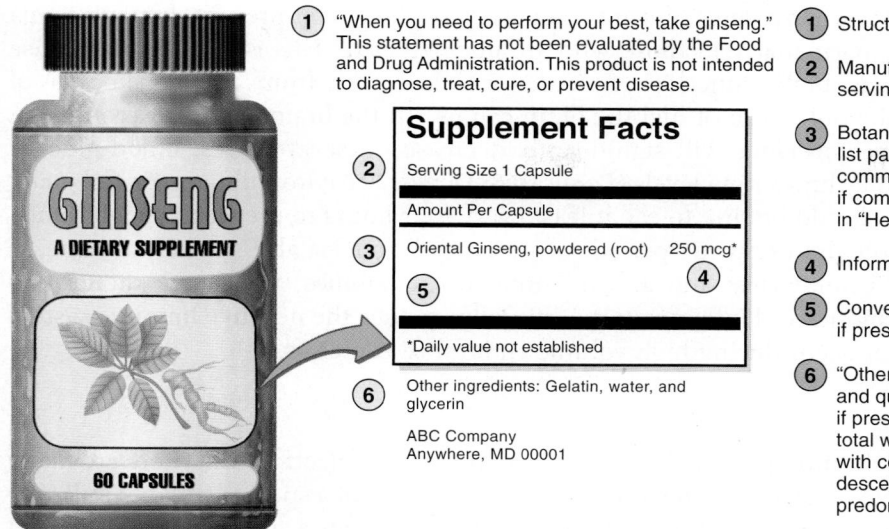

FIGURE 9.1 Supplement Facts Label

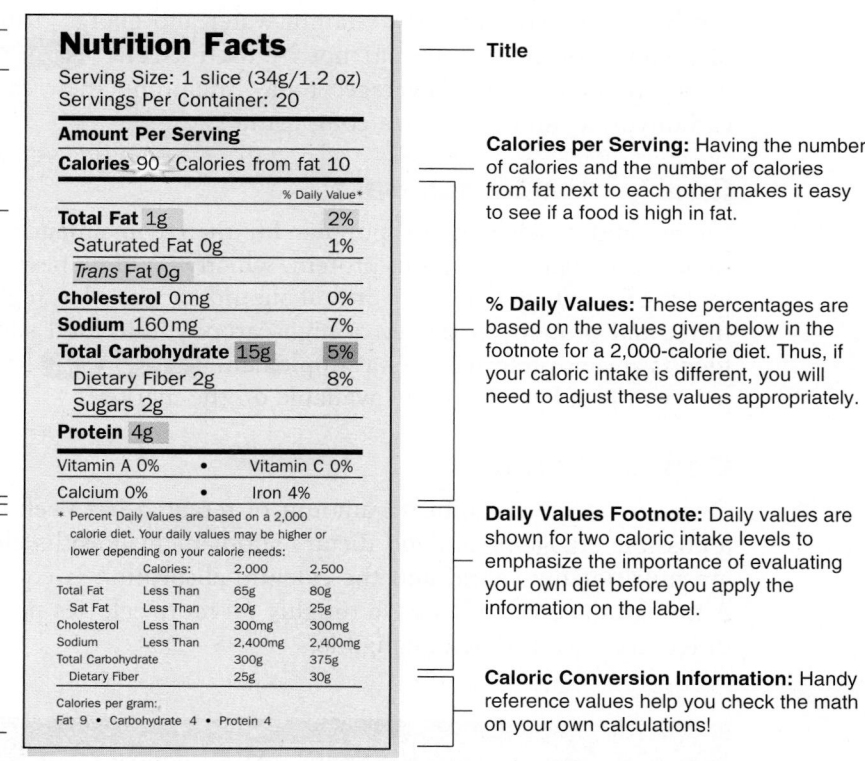

FIGURE 9.2 Nutrition Facts Label

Common Nutritional Ergogenic Aids

Carbohydrates are considered an ergogenic aid. Often, individuals will "carb-load" to top off their glycogen stores before a big game or event. Carbohydrates have been shown to enhance muscle and liver glycogen, thereby delaying fatigue. Adequate carbohydrate intake is also important due to its influence on the central nervous system (CNS) to delay fatigue. The CNS is driven by neurotransmitters such as serotonin and dopamine, which can help lower perceived exertion (Rosenbloom & Coleman, 2012).

The intake of carbohydrates during exercise also helps to prevent hypoglycemia (low blood sugar), particularly in those who are under fueled. This is important because hypoglycemia affects brain function. Glucose, which comes from the breakdown of carbohydrates, is the only form of fuel the brain can use. If the brain lacks fuel, confusion often sets in and performance will significantly decrease; in severe cases, blood glucose levels can drop to life-threatening levels (Dunford & Doyle, 2015; Rosenbloom & Coleman, 2012). Individuals should be sure to eat at least every four hours to prevent hypoglycemia.

Ingesting carbohydrates during periods of prolonged exercise also appears to increase blood neutrophils, monocytes, and anti-inflammatory cytokines, which are thought to decrease stress hormones and inflammation. This helps reduce the negative immune system responses that often occur during high volume endurance exercises.

Sports Drinks

Sports drinks by definition provide fluids, carbohydrates, and electrolytes. There are many other types of beverages available that do not meet the criteria of a sports drink but still may be confused as being one. The optimum carbohydrate content for a sports drink is between 6–8% or 14–19 grams per 8-oz. serving. If the carbohydrate concentration is much higher, it might cause gastrointestinal distress, diarrhea, and dehydration.

Drinks containing any additives such as herbs, creatine, gingko, or ephedra should not be consumed. Similarly, vitamin water and energy drinks do not meet the definition of a sports drink and should not be used as one. **TABLE 9.1** compares some of the more common sports beverages today, including their carbohydrate content, source of carbohydrate, and electrolyte composition.

Energy and Snack Bars

Energy and snack bars are popular for their convenience; however, not all bars are the same. Some bars are high in protein, which would be best consumed post exercise. Those looking for energy before a workout should choose a bar higher in carbohydrates and lower in fat and protein, or opt for a high-carbohydrate food such as a bagel. When available, food is always preferred over a supplement. **TABLE 9.2** lists some of the different pre and post workout bars currently available on the market.

Chocolate Milk

Over the years, a significant amount of research has been conducted on flavored milk as a possible ergogenic aid and dietary supplement. Results clearly show that flavored milks are nutritionally sound and the calcium absorption is equivalent to that of regular milk. Although flavored milks have roughly 60 more calories per serving than regular milk, the difference is considered negligible.

TABLE 9.1 Sports Drink Comparison

Name	% CHO	Sodium	Potassium	Source of Carbohydrate
Gatorade	6%	110	30	Sucrose, Glucose & Fructose
Powerade	6%	100	23	High Fructose Corn Syrup
Accelerade	6.2%	120	15	Sucrose, fructose, maltodextrin (also has 4g protein)
Skratch Labs	4%	120	20	Cane Sugar and Dextrose
Cytomax	6%	55	30	Maltodextrin, fructose, dextrose

TABLE 9.2 Pre- and Post-Workout Bars	
Pre-Workout Bars	**Post-Workout Bars**
Nature Valley Granola Bars	Honey Stinger Protein Bar
Fig Bars	Gatorade Protein Bar
Nutrigrain Bars	Cliff Builders Bar
Kashi Bars	Nature Valley Protein Bar

The benefits of flavored milk as a recovery beverage is well supported in the literature. Numerous studies have shown that chocolate milk, with its high carbohydrate and moderate protein intake, is an ideal post-workout recovery beverage and superior to most other high-carbohydrate recovery beverages with the same number of calories (Dunford & Doyle, 2015; Rosenbloom & Coleman, 2012). One study, using collegiate soccer players, compared chocolate milk with another high-carbohydrate recovery beverage. Although there were no statistical differences in terms of performance, post-exercise soreness, or mental/physical fatigue, the chocolate milk group had significantly lower levels of blood creatine kinase levels (which is a biomarker of muscle tissue damage) (Gilson et al, 2010).

The benefits of flavored milk extend well beyond recovery. Consumption aids with rehydration and provides a variety of essential nutrients needed after strenuous exercise. Additionally, chocolate milk is likely the most cost-effective post workout beverage on the market.

Dietary Supplements

Protein Shakes

There are many types of protein shakes. There are also many types of protein: whey, casein, soy, egg, and pea are the most common currently used. Whey is known for being quickly absorbed, whereas casein and soy are more slowly digested. Casein and soy are thought to be beneficial before an overnight fast to promote muscle **anabolism** (synthesis of complex molecules from simpler ones) and prevent **catabolism** (breakdown of complex molecules into simpler ones). Whey protein is often recommended immediately after a workout for faster absorption by the body (Dunford & Doyle, 2015; Rosenbloom & Coleman, 2012). There has been an increase in adding pea protein to bars and sports products, which may be a good source of protein for those who prefer non-meat or dairy sources. However, the bioavailability is not as high for vegetables sources. Therefore, those obtaining protein primarily from vegetable sources will need to consume slightly more to absorb enough.

Anabolism: Synthesis of complex molecules from simpler ones.

Catabolism: Breakdown of complex molecules from simpler ones.

The amount of protein in a supplement does not have to be excessive to produce results. Twenty to thirty grams of protein per shake is recommended. For reference, a 4 oz. piece of chicken breast (roughly the size of the palm of your hand) also contains roughly 28 grams of protein. Recent research suggests eating 20–30 grams of protein 5–6 times per day is the most efficient way to promote muscle anabolism and prevent muscle catabolism (Thomas, Erdman & Burke, 2016). **TABLE 9.3** on the next page lists potential pros and cons of the different types of protein.

Branched Chain Amino Acids

Branched Chain Amino Acids (BCAA) supplementation has been thought to reduce muscle protein breakdown, change neurotransmitter function to delay mental fatigue, and spare glycogen (although in most studies, glycogen was not spared without the addition of carbohydrates). BCAA have also been thought to lower perceived effort of physical activity.

TABLE 9.3 Potential Pros and Cons of the Different Types of Protein

Protein Type	Pro	Con
Whey Protein	Digests quickly, contains all essential amino acids; thought to be useful for muscle growth. Contains high amount of leucine for recovery	Many forms, costlier than food sources
Casein	Digested slowly; contains all essential amino acids	Slow for post workout recovery
Soy	Has cardiovascular benefits; contains all essential amino acids	High **phytoestrogens** (an estrogen occurring naturally in legumes)
1 Egg	Contains all essential amino acids	Contains 15 mg cholesterol per egg

Phytoestrogens: Plant-derived compounds found in a wide variety of foods, most notably soy.

Tryptophan: An essential amino acid and precursor of serotonin.

Serotonin: A neurotransmitter involved in sleep, depression, memory, and other neurological processes.

As far as neurotransmitter function is concerned, BCAA are thought to keep **tryptophan** (an essential amino acid and precursor of serotonin) levels low in the brain, therefore, preventing a rise in **serotonin** (a neurotransmitter that is involved in sleep, depression, memory, and other neurological processes). Increased serotonin levels are thought to cause fatigue by depressing the CNS. Although there are several proposed benefits of BCAA, current research only supports the decreased perception of exertion and decreased central fatigue. No performance benefits have been seen yet in regard to fueling (Rosenbloom & Coleman, 2012).

Creatine

Creatine is one of the most used and most researched supplements on the market and is naturally found in meat and fish. It is also produced in the kidney and liver and stored in the muscle. Consumption of creatine increases its concentration in muscle, which serves to regenerate adenosine triphosphate (ATP). The theory behind creatine supplementation is that it increases the phosphocreatine levels within the muscle. This increases the amount of available ATP during intense exercise, thereby improving strength, power, and slows the onset of fatigue. Creatine usage became popular in the 1990s for enhancing athletic performance and building lean body mass. Research on creatine shows:

- Increased muscle hypertrophy independent of training (due to intramuscular water retention)
- Increased ability to perform more reps per set
- Increased recovery ability between sets
- Improved total and maximal force in repetitive isometric muscle contractions
- Improved muscle strength and endurance in isotonic strength tests
- Improved muscular force/torque and endurance in isokinetic strength tests

However, not everyone who takes creatine will experience favorable results. In fact, research shows that although some users were classified as high responders (strong effect), others were classified as non-responders (no effect).

There are a few different proposed loading schedules for creatine. Some sport nutritionists recommend that creatine supplementation be cycled (e.g., 2 months on / 1 month off), whereas others endorse supplementation year round. Here is a proposed cycled supplementation plan:

- Loading Phase (1 week): 0.3 g/kg
- Maintenance Phase (3–5 weeks): 0.03 g/kg
- Non-Loading Maintenance (4–6 weeks): 0.045 g/kg

Those using creatine should be prepared for water weight fluctuation associated with its use. The average individual needs to replace about 2 grams of creatine per day to maintain normal creatine and creatine phosphate levels. This can be done through diet. However, vegetarians may consume as little as 0 grams per day of creatine, whereas meat eaters can consume 1-2 grams per day through food. Meats are the highest source of creatine in the diet (The National Standard Research Collaboration, n.d.).

Caffeine

Caffeine is an **alkaloid** (any class of nitrogenous organic compounds of plant origin that have pronounced physiological actions in humans) that has a very potent stimulating effect on the body's CNS and metabolism. Caffeine is thought to be a beneficial ergogenic aid because it blocks **adenosine** (a nucleoside involved in the energy metabolism of cells), increases neural activity and alertness, and subsequently decreases perceived level of effort. Caffeine is most beneficial in endurance events where exercise is performed at 70–80% VO$_2$max. The benefits occur at rather low doses and levels above 5mg/kg do not offer any additional benefit. In general, 400mg/day is thought to be safe for most people. Research on caffeine shows:

- Increased motivation for training
- Increased pain tolerance during training
- Increased ability to maintain performance during high-volume training sessions
- Improved (albeit slight) fat-burning ability
- Reduced appetite

There are some risks with caffeine usage that include dizziness or gastrointestinal distress, particularly if taken on an empty stomach. The rate of entry of caffeine into the blood depends on the product ingested. Caffeine from caffeinated beverages (e.g., coffee, tea, soft drinks) enters the bloodstream through the stomach and is generally absorbed with 45 minutes. Caffeine from caffeinated gum bypasses the stomach and enters the bloodstream via the membranes of the mouth and is generally absorbed in as little as 10 minutes. The **half-life** (time taken for the potency of an ingested drug to fall to half its original value) of caffeine is approximately five hours; however, that time can be reduced significantly based on a number of factors such as age, liver function, certain medications, and pregnancy.

Caffeine is generally recognized as safe up to 400mg/day for most people. However, caffeine supplements often contain higher doses than typical caffeinated beverages such as coffee or tea. Also, many supplements have added herbals that increase the caffeine content that the consumer may not be aware of. Caffeine supplements, including energy drinks, should be avoided or used with caution because the majority of adverse events and fatalities occur when caffeine is mixed with other compounds or consumed in amounts greater than 400mg/day (Department of Health and Human Services & Department of Agriculture, 2015). **TABLE 9.4** on the next page lists common sources of caffeine and their associated amounts.

Probiotics/Prebiotics

Probiotics are live microorganisms thought to increase the number of healthy bacteria in the gut, thereby reducing GI issues and respiratory illness. Further research needs to be done on the pros and cons of probiotics; however, currently, the benefits—particularly for those with GI issues (e.g., gas, diarrhea, or constipation)—appear to outweigh the risks.

Probiotics are now being added to different foods such as yogurt and are also sold as supplements. However, there are many different strands of bacteria and supplements may not include many of the strands. It is important to know why someone is taking a probiotic to ensure that it has the effective strand for their symptoms.

Prebiotics are also becoming more popular. They are plant fibers that feed the healthy bacteria already in our gut in order to promote further healthy growth. **FIGURE 9.3** on the next page is an example showing one of the many probiotic products that are commercially available.

Alkaloid: Any class of nitrogenous organic compounds of plant origin that have pronounced physiological actions in humans.

Adenosine: A nucleoside involved in the energy metabolism of cells.

Half-life: Time taken for the radioactivity of a specified isotope to fall to half of its original value.

Probiotics: Live microorganisms thought to increase the healthy bacteria in the gut, thereby reducing GI issues, and respiratory illness.

Prebiotics: Plant fibers that feed the healthy bacteria already in the gut to promote further healthy bacterial growth.

TABLE 9.4 Common Sources of Caffeine

Product	Amount	Caffeine (mg)
Brewed Coffee	12 oz	200
Expresso	1 oz	40
Dunkin Donuts	12 oz	156
Starbucks	12 oz	260
Brewed Tea	12 oz	80
Starbucks Iced Green Tea	12 oz	80
Coke	12 oz	35
Diet Coke	12 oz	45
Mountain Dew	12 oz	54
Diet Mountain Dew	12 oz	55
5-hour Energy	2 oz	138
Monster	16 oz	160
Red Bull	8.3 oz	80
Redline RTD	8 oz	250
Rockstar	8 oz	80
Vault	20 oz	118
Excedrin	2 tablets	130
NoDoz	1 tablets	200
Chocolate Bar	100 g	12-15

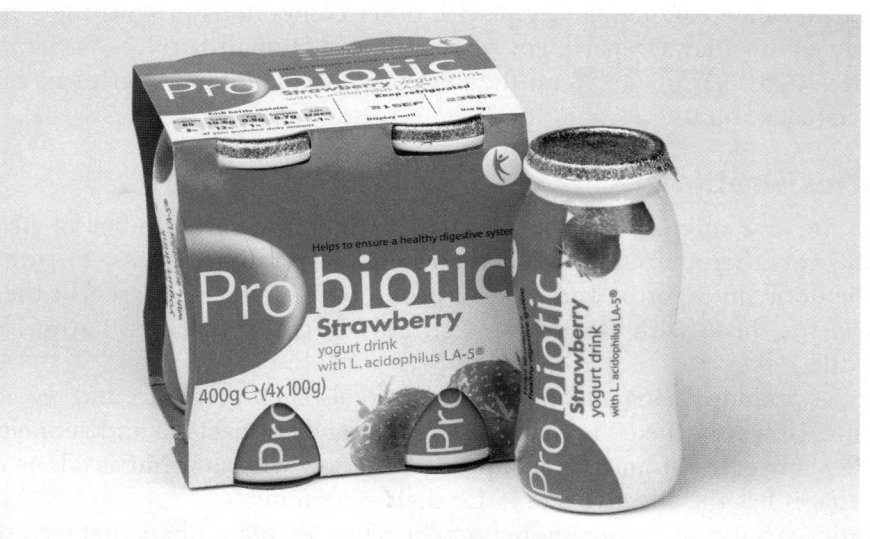

FIGURE 9.3 Sample Probiotic Product

© Pablo Paul / Alamy Stock Photo.

When should I select a supplement?

It is always best to obtain nutrients from food because it contains other components such as phytochemicals that help absorb the nutrients. However, in certain situations, such as a clinical deficiency diagnosed by a doctor or possibly a food allergy, a dietary supplement may be a good idea. Common supplements include Omega-3 fatty acids and vitamin D that are not present in a lot of food sources. Iron may also be needed in certain populations that have a high incidence of iron deficiency anemia (however, iron should not be taken without monitoring by a doctor). And although protein supplements are not necessary, they are convenient. Therefore, individuals may opt for a supplement if they cannot have a meal within an hour of a workout or competition.

Supplement Safety

There are a few ways to make an educated decision about supplement use in terms of their product safety. Third-party testing is one of the best ways and is done to check if the active ingredient is actually in the supplement. Some tests also check for illegal or non-reported ingredients. However, keep in mind that even if a product has one of these symbols indicating third-party testing, it could still test positive for illegal substances because of cross contamination or other reasons. If the test of a supplement comes back positive for an illegal substance, the consumer will have to pay the consequences, not the manufacturer. Depending on the individual situation, this could mean losing one's job or being banned from sports participation.

The distinctive U.S. Pharmacopeia Convention (USP) verified mark is awarded to dietary supplement products that successfully undergo and meet their stringent requirements. This symbol ensures that the active ingredient listed is in the product. Testing is voluntary and the manufacturer pays to display the USP mark on their product. When choosing a multi-vitamin, it would be wise to choose a product with this symbol. For more information on USP products, visit www.USP.org/.

The National Sanitation Foundation (NSF) Certified for Sport has an online directory of certified products. It can be searched by product name, company name, and nutrient or supplement type, goal, or mode of consumption. This directory does not recommend taking supplements; however, supplements are ranked in terms of their risk. Explanations for the rankings are also included. For more information on NSF-certified products, visit www.NSFSport.com/listings /certified_products.asp.

ConsumerLab.com (www.ConsumerLab.com) is an independent, third-party group started in 1999 that tests commercially available supplements. It publishes product reviews online that incorporate their test findings and product comparisons. It also offers a Quality Certification Program—approved products may carry the CL Seal for a limited period of time. Third-party testing is the best way consumers currently have to determine if a supplement contains its listed ingredients and is free of contamination.

On the next page, the USP Verified Mark is shown in **FIGURE 9.4**; the NSF mark is shown in **FIGURE 9.5**; and the ConsumerLab.com seal is shown in **FIGURE 9.6**.

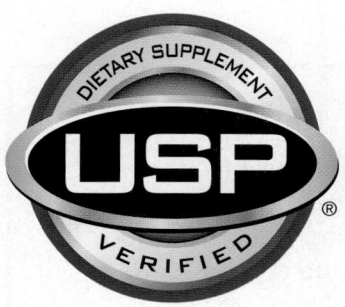

FIGURE 9.4 U.S. Pharmacopeia Convention

Used with permissions from U.S. Pharmacopeial Convention (USP).

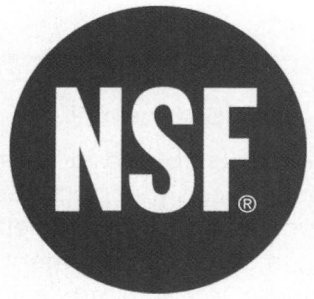

FIGURE 9.5 National Sanitation Foundation

Reproduced with permission from NSF International.

FIGURE 9.6 ConsumerLab.com Seal

Courtesy of ConsumerLab.com

Putting it all Together

When it comes to overall health, body composition, and performance, you cannot overlook a poor diet. Your foundation is based on the fuel you put into your body. The first step is to find the right caloric balance for your performance needs and goals.

The second step is to determine the appropriate macronutrient breakdown to meet the demand of your physical activities. When determining your food sources for those macronutrients, it is important to consume a variety of foods in order to obtain all the micronutrients you need to function and not have any vitamin or mineral deficiencies.

The next step is nutrient timing. If you are not getting enough calories, nutrient timing will not be as relevant because you will already be at a disadvantage.

Finally, if the goal is to maximize your athletic potential/performance, supplements have been shown to provide a small benefit for some. However, it is not necessary to take dietary supplements in order to gain an advantage. Most supplements do not offer anything that you cannot get from food. Foods provide the same benefits at a much lower cost and risk. If an athlete wants to take a supplement, it is important to research the product before taking it to minimize the risk of taking a contaminated supplement, which could lead to a positive drug test or a life-threatening situation.

Assessment and Application

Summary

- Fad diets are weight-loss programs or supplements that promise to deliver fast results with minimal effort.
- An ergogenic aid is any method or product used to enhance mental and physical performance or recovery
- Sports drinks provide fluids, carbohydrates, and electrolytes.
- BCAA supplementation has been thought to decrease muscle protein breakdown, change neurotransmitter function to delay mental fatigue, and spare glycogen
- Caffeine is thought to be a beneficial ergogenic aid because it blocks adenosine, increases alertness, and subsequently decreases the perceived level of effort.
- Third-party testing ensures that the active ingredient of a supplement is actually in the product.

Knowledge Check

1. Define and discuss the different type of fad diets.
2. Define and differentiate a Nutrition Facts label and a Supplement Facts label.
3. Define and discuss proprietary blend.
4. List and discuss some common nutritional ergogenic aids.
5. List and discuss the pros and cons associated with the different types of protein.
6. Define and discuss BCAA.
7. List and discuss some of the reported benefits associated with creatine supplementation.
8. List and discuss some of the reported benefits associated with caffeine supplementation.
9. Define and differentiate probiotics and prebiotics.
10. Describe and differentiate the USP, NSF, and Consumer Lab.

Activities

Fad Diets and Supplements

A. In order to lose weight, Claire has recently started a vegan diet. Conversely, in order to gain weight, Ethan has started a high-protein diet. Discuss some of the potential concerns associated with fad dieting and provide some basic dietary strategies that each could employ in order to achieve their respective goals.

B. Which dietary supplement(s), if any, would you recommend Claire and Ethan take in order to help them achieve their goals and explain why you chose it.

References

Anton, S. D., Moehl, K., Donahoo, W. T., Marosi, K., Lee, S. A., Mainous, A. G. 3rd, Mattson M. P. (2017). Flipping the metabolic switch: understanding and applying the health benefits of fasting. *Obesity*. October 31. doi: 10.1002/oby.22065.

Department of Health and Human Services and Department of Agriculture. *2015–2020 Dietary guidelines for americans*. (8th Ed.). December 2015. Available at http://health.gov/dietaryguidelines/2015/guidelines/

Dunford, M., & Doyle, A. (2015). *Nutrition for sport and exercise*. (3rd Ed). Boston, MA: Cengage.

Gilson, S. F., Saunders, M. J., Moran, C. W., Moore, R. W., Womack, C. J., & Todd, M. K. (2010). Effects of chocolate milk consumption on markers of muscle recovery following soccer training: a randomized cross-over study. *Journal of the International Society of Sports Nutrition*, 7(19). doi: 10.1186/1550-2783-7-19

Israetel, M., Case, J., & Hoffmann, J. *The renaissance diet: A scientific approach to getting leaner and building muscle*. [E-Book]. Retrieved from https://renaissanceperiodization.com/shop/the-renaissance-diet/.

Rosenbloom, C., & Coleman, E. (2012). *Sports nutrition: a practice manual for professionals*. (5th Ed). Chicago, IL: Academy of Nutrition and Dietetics.

The National Standard Research Collaboration (n.d.). *Drugs and supplements: creatine*. Retrieved from http://www.mayoclinic.org/drugs-supplements/creatine/background/hrb-20059125

Thomas, D. T., Erdman, K. A., & Burke, L. M. (2016). American College of Sports Medicine joint position statement. Nutrition and athletic performance. *Medicine & Science in Sports & Exercise, 48*(3), 543–568.

Williams, M. (2007). *Nutrition for health, fitness, & sport*. New York, NY: Mc-Graw Hill.

Appendix A

Nutritional Value of Selected Foods

Once you know your Total Daily Energy Expenditure (TDEE), or the number of calories you should be consuming per day, the next step is to design a dietary plan. This can be done in a couple of different ways. One approach is to record everything that you eat in a day and then assess where you are in terms of calories consumed and macronutrient distribution (i.e., CHO %, PRO %, and FAT %). The second approach is to build a dietary plan from scratch (using **Appendix B**) to ensure that you are meeting the targeted intake of daily calories and macronutrient distribution. Since caloric needs are based partially on physical activity, it may be necessary to develop separate dietary plans for off days, light-activity days, moderate-activity days, and hard-activity days.

Regardless of the approach taken, this Appendix can help. The information presented herein provides all of the necessary data to evaluate or select foods in order to ensure that the desired number of calories and micronutrient distribution are met. If a food item is not listed in the Appendix, nutritional information can be found either on the food's nutrition label or online (e.g., ChooseMyPlate.gov).

Assume that your pre-workout meal on a light-activity day calls for 389 kcal, with macronutrient distribution of 20% CHO, 10% PRO, and 5% FAT. This equates to 259 kcal of CHO, 65 kcal of PRO, and 65 kcal of FAT. And say that the following is what you actually ate.

- Half of a multigrain bagel = 97.605 kcal (195.21 ÷ 2), which equates to 76.9 kcal of CHO, 16.04 kcal of PRO, and 4.5 kcal of FAT*
- 1 cup non-fat vanilla yogurt = 191.1 kcal, which equates to 167 kcal of CHO, 28.8 kcal of PRO, and 0 kcal of FAT*
- 1 cup raw blueberries = 84.36 kcal, which equates to 85.8 kcal of CHO, 4.4 kcal of PRO, and 4.41 kcal of FAT*
- Total Kcal: 373, with macronutrient distribution of 85 % CHO, 13% PRO, and 2% FAT

Using the Appendix, we see that our pre-workout meal was quite close in terms of the desired number of calories; however, it was way off in terms of macronutrient distribution. As can be seen from this example, designing the perfect dietary plan can be challenging and time-consuming, but even then, it is necessary for many individuals looking to achieve their dietary goals (e.g., losing weight, gaining weight, maintaining weight).

---

*Note that in order to calculate the calories (kcal) from grams, the number of grams of a particular food item is multiplied by 4 for CHO and PRO and by 9 for FAT.

Food Description	Measure	Weight (g)	Kcal per serving (g)	Protein per serving (g)
Breads, Cereals, Grains, Starch				
Bagels, cinnamon-raisin	1 mini bagel (2.5"dia)	26.00	71.24	2.55
Bagels, egg	1 oz	28.35	78.81	3.01
Bagels, multigrain	1 piece, bagel	81.00	195.21	8.02
Bagels, oat bran	1 mini bagel (2.5"dia)	26.00	66.30	2.78
Bagels, plain, enriched, without calcium proportionate (including onion, poppy, sesame)	1 oz	28.35	77.96	2.98
Bagels, wheat	1 bagel	98.00	245.00	10.00
Bagels, whole grain white	1/2 piece bagel	43.00	109.65	4.00
Biscuits, plain or buttermilk, frozen, baked	1 oz	28.35	95.82	1.76
Bread sticks, plain	1 cup, small pieces	46.00	189.52	5.52
Bread stuffing, bread, dry mix	1 oz	28.35	109.43	3.12
Bread, French	1 oz	28.35	77.11	3.05
Bread, wheat, toasted	1 oz	28.35	88.74	3.67
Bread, cornbread, dry mix, unenriched (including corn muffin mix)	1 oz	28.35	118.50	1.98
Bread, cracked-wheat	1 oz	28.35	73.71	2.47
Bread, French or Vienna, whole wheat	1 slice	48.00	114.72	4.00
Bread, multi-grain (including whole-grain)	1 oz	28.35	75.13	3.79
Bread, naan, plain, commonly prepared, refrigerated	1 piece	90.00	261.90	8.66
Bread, pita, white, enriched	1 pita, large	60.00	165.00	5.46
Bread, pita, whole-wheat	1 pita, large	64.00	167.68	6.27
Bread, potato	1 slice	32.00	85.12	4.00
Bread, pumpernickel	1 oz	28.35	70.88	2.47
Bread, Raisin, enriched, toasted	1 oz	28.35	84.20	2.44
Bread, reduced calorie, oat bran	1 oz	28.35	56.98	2.27
Bread, rye	1 oz	28.35	73.43	2.41
Bread, wheat bran	1 oz	28.35	70.31	2.49
Bread, white, commonly prepared, toasted	1 oz	28.35	82.22	2.55
Cereals ready-to-eat, Cascadian Farm, Cinnamon Crunch	3/4 cup	27.00	109.89	1.54
Cereals ready-to-eat, Cascadian Farm, Honey Nut O's	1 cup	30.00	111.30	2.49
Cereals ready-to-eat, chocolate-flavored frosted puffed corn	1 cup	30.00	121.50	1.00
Cereals ready-to-eat, General Mills, Apple Cinnamon Chex	3/4 cup	31.00	126.48	1.45
Cereals ready-to-eat, General Mills, Cheerios	1 cup	28.00	105.28	3.39
Cereals ready-to-eat, General Mills, Chocolate Lucky Charms	3/4 cup	28.00	106.68	1.57

Carbohydrate per serving (g)	Sugar per serving (g)	Fiber per serving (g)	Total fat per serving (g)	Saturated fat per serving (g)	Mono fat per serving (g)	Poly fat per serving (g)
14.35	1.55	0.60	0.44	0.07	0.05	0.17
15.03	0.00	0.65	0.60	0.12	0.12	0.18
38.45	7.01	5.02	1.00	0.00	0.25	0.57
13.86	0.42	0.94	0.31	0.05	0.06	0.13
15.14	0.00	0.65	0.45	0.06	0.04	0.20
47.91	6.00	4.02	1.50	0.00	0.28	0.92
23.44	4.00	2.02	0.00	0.00	0.00	0.00
15.27	0.99	0.37	3.13	0.48	1.32	1.18
31.46	0.58	1.38	4.37	0.65	1.64	1.67
21.60	2.34	0.91	0.96	0.24	0.42	0.20
14.71	1.31	0.62	0.69	0.15	0.10	0.24
15.81	1.82	1.33	1.21	0.28	0.29	0.49
19.70	0.00	1.84	3.46	0.88	1.90	0.48
14.03	0.00	1.56	1.11	0.26	0.54	0.19
23.57	0.00	2.02	0.50	0.00	0.09	0.28
12.29	1.81	2.10	1.20	0.25	0.22	0.53
45.39	3.20	1.98	5.09	1.25	1.62	1.89
33.42	0.78	1.32	0.72	0.10	0.06	0.32
35.77	1.84	3.90	1.09	0.09	0.16	0.48
15.06	3.00	2.02	1.00	0.00	0.00	0.00
13.47	0.15	1.84	0.88	0.12	0.26	0.35
16.13	1.75	1.33	1.36	0.33	0.71	0.21
11.71	1.00	3.40	0.91	0.13	0.19	0.47
13.69	1.09	1.64	0.94	0.18	0.37	0.23
13.55	2.74	1.13	0.96	0.22	0.46	0.18
15.45	1.76	0.82	1.13	0.22	0.23	0.59
22.03	8.37	2.97	2.30	0.27	1.54	0.41
24.93	7.44	2.55	0.99	0.18	0.39	0.30
26.16	13.11	1.14	1.05	0.29	0.62	0.07
25.67	8.06	0.62	2.00	0.00	1.42	0.47
20.50	1.22	2.63	1.88	0.42	0.67	0.68
23.63	10.30	1.48	1.23	0.17	0.59	0.45

(continues)

Food Description	Measure	Weight (g)	Kcal per serving (g)	Protein per serving (g)
Breads, Cereals, Grains, Starch (*continued*)				
Cereals ready-to-eat, General Mills, Cinnamon Toast Crunch	3/4 cup	31.00	127.10	1.69
Cereals ready-to-eat, General Mills, Cocoa Puffs	3/4 cup	27.00	103.41	1.51
Cereals ready-to-eat, General Mills, Cookie Crisp	3/4 cup	26.00	98.80	1.35
Cereals ready-to-eat, General Mills, Corn Chex	1 cup	31.00	114.70	1.98
Cereals ready-to-eat, General Mills, Fiber One 80 Calories, Choc Squares	3/4 cup	30.00	75.90	0.99
Cereals ready-to-eat, General Mills, Fiber One Bran Cereal	1/2 cup	30.00	62.10	1.98
Cereals ready-to-eat, General Mills, Fiber One, Nutty Clusters & Almonds	1 cup	55.00	191.40	4.35
Cereals ready-to-eat, General Mills, Frosted Cheerios	3/4 cup	27.00	101.52	2.43
Cereals ready-to-eat, General Mills, Frosted Toast Crunch	3/4 cup	30.00	123.00	1.56
Cereals ready-to-eat, General Mills, Honey Nut Cheerios	3/4 cup	28.00	105.28	2.48
Cereals ready-to-eat, General Mills, Honey Nut Clusters	1 cup	57.00	213.18	4.39
Cereals ready-to-eat, General Mills, Kix	1.25 cup	30.00	107.10	2.31
Cereals ready-to-eat, General Mills, Lucky Charms	3/4 cup	27.00	102.60	2.07
Cereals ready-to-eat, General Mills, Multi Grain Cheerios, Peanut Butter	3/4 cup	28.00	109.20	1.90
Cereals ready-to-eat, General Mills, Oatmeal Crisp, Crunchy Almond	1 cup	60.00	234.00	5.93
Cereals ready-to-eat, General Mills, Oatmeal Crisp, Hearty Raisin	1 cup	62.00	230.64	5.27
Cereals ready-to-eat, General Mills, Raisin Nut Bran	3/4 cup	49.00	180.32	4.01
Cereals ready-to-eat, General Mills, Reese's Puffs	3/4 cup	29.00	119.77	1.97
Cereals ready-to-eat, General Mills, Rice Crunchins	3/4 cup	21.00	80.01	1.00
Cereals ready-to-eat, General Mills, Total Raisin Bran	1 cup	53.00	165.36	2.97
Cereals ready-to-eat, Health Valley, Fiber 7 Flakes	3/4 cup	31.00	109.43	4.48
Cereals ready-to-eat, Kashi Organic Promise, Berry Fruitful	29 biscuits	55.00	174.90	5.89
Cereals ready-to-eat, Kashi Organic Promise, Strawberry Fields	1 cup	55.00	196.90	5.17
Cereals ready-to-eat, Kashi, Organic Promise Autumn wheat	29 biscuits	54.00	182.52	6.48
Cereals ready-to-eat, Kellogg's, Frosted Mini-Wheats, Maple & Brown Sugar, Bite Sze	25 biscuits	55.00	193.05	4.79
Cereals ready-to-eat, Kellogg, Kellogg's All-Bran Bran Buds	1/3 cup	30.00	77.10	2.67

Carbohydrate per serving (g)	Sugar per serving (g)	Fiber per serving (g)	Total fat per serving (g)	Saturated fat per serving (g)	Mono fat per serving (g)	Poly fat per serving (g)
24.18	9.39	2.11	3.18	0.30	1.53	0.65
22.60	10.04	1.54	1.40	0.27	0.46	0.57
21.97	9.05	1.33	1.14	0.21	0.36	0.44
26.35	3.44	1.46	0.74	0.12	0.19	0.40
25.20	5.19	10.56	0.87	0.27	0.21	0.33
25.29	0.30	13.86	0.69	0.12	0.15	0.39
43.73	12.16	10.01	3.74	0.38	1.82	0.94
21.55	8.64	2.03	1.27	0.30	0.46	0.48
23.58	8.76	1.47	3.03	0.30	2.01	0.66
22.31	9.21	1.99	1.40	0.15	0.31	0.29
48.56	14.14	3.59	1.14	0.29	0.11	0.23
24.85	2.93	2.64	1.04	0.17	0.30	0.38
21.84	9.76	1.35	1.36	0.24	0.43	0.42
22.96	9.10	1.68	1.73	0.25	0.76	0.64
46.85	13.73	4.92	4.01	0.66	1.86	1.32
50.10	16.92	4.65	2.35	0.50	0.81	0.93
39.20	13.97	5.98	2.60	0.49	0.98	0.98
21.92	10.24	1.36	3.22	0.61	1.36	1.07
17.00	2.00	1.01	0.50	0.00	0.00	0.00
40.70	17.12	4.82	0.85	0.21	0.16	0.42
24.23	6.20	4.37	0.44	0.08	0.08	0.19
41.91	8.03	5.78	0.72	0.11	0.11	0.28
45.93	11.28	2.75	0.39	0.06	0.06	0.11
42.66	6.70	6.05	0.76	0.16	0.11	0.49
46.59	12.49	5.67	0.83	0.22	0.11	0.44
24.30	8.01	12.75	0.75	0.15	0.15	0.45

(continues)

Food Description	Measure	Weight (g)	Kcal per serving (g)	Protein per serving (g)
Breads, Cereals, Grains, Starch (*continued*)				
Cereals ready-to-eat, Kellogg, Kellogg's All-Bran Complete wheat Flakes	3/4 cup	29.00	94.83	2.96
Cereals ready-to-eat, Kellogg, Kellogg's All-Bran original	1/2 cup	31.00	80.29	4.07
Cereals ready-to-eat, Kellogg, Kellogg's Apple Jacks	1 cup	28.00	105.00	1.43
Cereals ready-to-eat, Kellogg, Kellogg's Cocoa Krispies	3/4 cup	31.00	120.59	1.43
Cereals ready-to-eat, Kellogg, Kellogg's Cracklin' Oat Bran	3/4 cup	49.00	193.55	4.51
Cereals ready-to-eat, Kellogg, Kellogg's Crispix	1 cup	29.00	109.62	1.91
Cereals ready-to-eat, Kellogg, Kellogg's Froot Loops	1 cup	29.00	108.75	1.54
Cereals ready-to-eat, Kellogg, Kellogg's Frosted Mini-Wheats, Bite Size	21 biscuits	54.00	189.00	4.96
Cereals ready-to-eat, Kellogg, Kellogg's Frosted Rice Krispies	3/4 cup	30.00	115.20	1.29
Cereals ready-to-eat, Kellogg, Kellogg's Honey Crunch Corn Flakes	3/4 cup	30.00	115.50	2.04
Cereals ready-to-eat, Kellogg, Kellogg's low fat Granola with Raisins	2/3 cup	60.00	228.60	5.40
Cereals ready-to-eat, Kellogg, Kellogg's Mueslix	2/3 cup	55.00	195.25	4.73
Cereals ready-to-eat, Kellogg, Kellogg's Raisin Bran	1 cup	59.00	187.62	4.55
Cereals ready-to-eat, Kellogg, Kellogg's Rice Krispies Treats Cereal	3/4 cup	30.00	118.50	1.29
Cereals ready-to-eat, Kellogg, Kellogg's Special K Chocolatey Strawberry	3/4 cup	29.00	106.72	2.00
Cereals ready-to-eat, Kellogg, Kellogg's Special K Red Berries	1 cup	31.00	110.98	1.95
Cereals ready-to-eat, Kellogg, Kellogg's, Raisin Bran Crunch	1 cup	53.00	187.62	3.49
Cereals ready-to-eat, Kellogg, Special K, Fruit & Yogurt	3/4 cup	32.00	117.44	2.27
Cereals ready-to-eat, Kellogg's Cinnamon Jacks	1 cup	28.00	111.16	1.65
Cereals ready-to-eat, Kellogg's Frosted Mini-wheats, Big Bite	7 biscuit	58.00	203.00	5.34
Cereals ready-to-eat, Kellogg's Krave Double Chocolate Cereal	3/4 cup	30.00	119.10	2.13
Cereals ready-to-eat, Kellogg's, Special K Protein Plus	3/4 cup	32.00	114.88	9.98
Cereals ready-to-eat, Malt-O-Meal, Berry Colossal Crunch	3/4 cup	30.00	118.80	1.26
Cereals ready-to-eat, Malt-O-Meal, Coco-Roos	3/4 cup	30.00	116.70	1.02
Cereals ready-to-eat, Malt-O-Meal, Colossal Crunch	3/4 cup	30.00	120.30	1.09
Cereals ready-to-eat, Malt-O-Meal, Honey Graham Squares	3/4 cup	30.00	119.40	1.34

Carbohydrate per serving (g)	Sugar per serving (g)	Fiber per serving (g)	Total fat per serving (g)	Saturated fat per serving (g)	Mono fat per serving (g)	Poly fat per serving (g)
23.66	5.45	5.02	0.73	0.12	0.12	0.38
23.01	4.86	9.08	1.52	0.34	0.28	0.62
24.70	12.24	2.60	0.95	0.53	0.17	0.25
27.25	11.97	0.43	0.84	0.65	0.09	0.03
34.45	13.72	6.22	6.91	3.04	2.40	1.37
25.29	3.71	0.29	0.23	0.06	0.06	0.09
25.52	12.09	2.70	0.99	0.52	0.17	0.26
45.04	10.96	5.83	0.86	0.22	0.11	0.48
27.39	12.06	0.15	0.12	0.03	0.03	0.03
26.10	9.90	1.02	0.57	0.09	0.30	0.18
48.06	16.74	4.44	3.12	0.72	1.32	0.96
41.20	13.81	4.24	2.97	0.33	1.38	0.76
45.60	18.47	6.73	1.60	0.28	0.20	0.56
25.68	8.88	0.12	1.26	0.27	0.36	0.06
24.16	8.29	2.76	1.13	0.87	0.06	0.17
27.00	9.21	2.64	0.40	0.09	0.09	0.16
45.00	18.66	4.24	0.95	0.21	0.16	0.37
27.30	10.27	2.59	0.93	0.45	0.03	0.10
23.24	9.49	2.52	2.18	0.36	0.92	0.76
48.37	11.77	6.26	0.93	0.23	0.12	0.52
22.77	10.89	3.18	3.36	0.78	0.84	1.56
19.39	6.50	2.66	0.83	0.16	0.10	0.51
25.97	12.50	0.54	1.25	0.36	0.38	0.30
26.03	14.43	0.99	1.38	0.77	0.27	0.17
24.48	12.75	0.51	1.58	0.67	0.44	0.21
22.40	9.81	1.32	2.99	0.45	0.94	1.13

(continues)

Food Description	Measure	Weight (g)	Kcal per serving (g)	Protein per serving (g)
Breads, Cereals, Grains, Starch (*continued*)				
Cereals ready-to-eat, Malt-O-Meal, Honey Nut Scooters	1 cup	30.00	116.10	2.58
Cereals ready-to-eat, Malt-O-Meal, Oat Blenders with Honey & Almonds	3/4 cup	30.00	113.70	2.34
Cereals ready-to-eat, Malt-O-Meal, Raisin Bran Cereal	1 cup	59.00	201.78	4.50
Cereals ready-to-eat, Malt-O-Meal, Tootie Fruities	1 cup	32.00	125.12	1.50
Cereals ready-to-eat, oat bran Flakes, Health Valley	1 cup	50.00	190.00	5.00
Cereals ready-to-eat, Post Bran Flakes	3/4 cup	30.00	98.40	2.97
Cereals ready-to-eat, Post Great grains Banana Nut Crunch	1 cup	59.00	230.10	5.78
Cereals ready-to-eat, Post, Cocoa Pebbles	3/4 cup	29.00	115.13	1.39
Cereals ready-to-eat, Post, Fruity Pebbles	3/4 cup	27.00	108.54	1.25
Cereals ready-to-eat, Post, Honey Bunches Of Oats, Honey Roasted	3/4 cup	30.00	120.30	2.14
Cereals ready-to-eat, Post, Honey Bunches Of Oats, with Almonds	3/4 cup	32.00	130.88	2.46
Cereals ready-to-eat, Post, Honeycomb Cereal	1.5 cup	32.00	126.08	1.92
Cereals ready-to-eat, Post, Waffle Crisp	1 cup	30.00	117.00	1.98
Cereals ready-to-eat, Quaker Whole Hearts Oat Cereal	3/4 cup	28.00	105.28	2.14
Cereals ready-to-eat, Quaker, Cap'n Crunch	3/4 cup	27.00	107.46	1.19
Cereals ready-to-eat, Quaker, Cap'n Crunch with Crunchberries	3/4 cup	26.00	103.22	1.16
Cereals ready-to-eat, Quaker, Cap'n Crunch's Peanut Butter Crunch	3/4 cup	27.00	112.59	1.92
Cereals ready-to-eat, Quaker, Honey Graham Oh's	3/4 cup	27.00	111.24	1.06
Cereals ready-to-eat, Quaker, King Vitaman	1.5 cup	31.00	118.11	1.99
Cereals ready-to-eat, Quaker, low fat 100% Natural Granola with Raisins	2/3 cup	55.00	213.40	4.63
Cereals ready-to-eat, Quaker, Oatmeal Squares	1 cup	56.00	212.24	6.37
Cereals ready-to-eat, Quaker, Quaker Crunchy Bran	3/4 cup	27.00	89.37	1.72
Cereals ready-to-eat, Quaker, Quaker Granola with Oats, Wheat & Raisins	1/2 cup	51.00	210.12	4.93
Cereals ready-to-eat, Quaker, Quaker Oat Cinnamon Life	3/4 cup	32.00	119.68	2.92
Cereals ready-to-eat, Quaker, Quaker Oat Life, plain	3/4 cup	32.00	119.68	3.19
Cereals ready-to-eat, Quaker, Shredded wheat, Bagged Cereal	3 biscuits	63.00	219.24	7.08
Cereals, Malt-O-Meal, Maple & Brown Sugar Hot Wheat Cereal, dry	1/4 cup	45.00	165.60	3.97
Cereals, Quaker, Hominy Grits, white, regular, dry	1/4 cup	41.00	148.01	3.61

Carbohydrate per serving (g)	Sugar per serving (g)	Fiber per serving (g)	Total fat per serving (g)	Saturated fat per serving (g)	Mono fat per serving (g)	Poly fat per serving (g)
23.89	8.99	1.89	1.35	0.19	0.33	0.40
23.18	6.08	1.83	1.46	0.19	0.68	0.41
47.42	19.49	6.02	1.10	0.25	0.21	0.54
27.50	14.50	0.70	1.02	0.22	0.47	0.31
39.00	11.00	4.00	1.50	0.50	0.35	0.45
24.15	5.58	5.49	0.63	0.12	0.09	0.36
41.83	10.33	6.61	5.19	0.65	2.23	2.03
24.85	10.38	0.46	1.19	1.04	0.06	0.03
23.25	9.26	0.22	1.09	0.97	0.04	0.03
24.36	5.94	1.26	1.64	0.19	0.85	0.39
25.47	6.40	1.76	2.34	0.26	1.28	0.67
27.72	10.08	1.02	0.94	0.41	0.19	0.29
24.90	10.41	1.32	1.50	0.27	0.51	0.51
22.43	6.03	2.55	1.57	0.23	0.75	0.41
23.09	11.97	0.68	1.38	0.90	0.17	0.20
22.34	11.49	0.68	1.26	0.80	0.16	0.20
21.24	9.01	0.73	2.49	1.06	0.71	0.58
22.59	11.67	0.57	2.06	1.54	0.19	0.19
25.99	6.28	1.05	1.07	0.49	0.20	0.35
44.31	14.11	5.28	3.04	0.53	1.40	0.79
43.55	9.35	4.65	2.70	0.49	0.89	0.85
22.59	5.58	4.13	1.10	0.55	0.21	0.33
38.08	12.56	4.79	5.29	0.57	2.99	1.22
25.29	8.06	2.02	1.31	0.25	0.44	0.42
24.88	6.22	2.11	1.42	0.27	0.47	0.45
51.04	0.51	7.43	1.27	0.26	0.19	0.77
36.23	12.60	0.81	0.21	0.04	0.02	0.09
32.47	0.26	0.66	0.66	0.06	0.12	0.21

(continues)

Food Description	Measure	Weight (g)	Kcal per serving (g)	Protein per serving (g)
Breads, Cereals, Grains, Starch (*continued*)				
Cereals, Quaker, Instant Grits, Butter Flavor, dry	1 packet	28.00	103.32	2.27
Cereals, Quaker, Instant Grits, Ham N Cheese Flavor, dry	1 packet	28.00	99.40	3.00
Cereals, Quaker, Instant Oatmeal, Fruit & Cream variant, dry	1 packet	35.00	132.65	2.91
Cereals, Quaker, Instant Oatmeal, Raisin and Spice, dry	1 packet	43.00	154.80	3.92
Cereals, Quaker, Quaker Multigrain Oatmeal, dry	1/2 cup	40.00	133.60	5.06
Cereals, Quaker, Quick Oats, dry	1/2 cup	40.00	148.40	5.48
Corn flour, whole-grain, white	1 cup	117.00	422.37	8.11
Corn flour, yellow, masa, enriched	1 cup	114.00	413.82	9.64
Corn grain, white	1 cup	166.00	605.90	15.64
Cornmeal, Degermed, unenriched, white	1 cup	157.00	580.90	11.16
Cornmeal, whole-grain, white	1 cup	122.00	441.64	9.91
Cracker meal	1 oz	28.35	108.58	2.64
Crackers, Cheese, Red Fat	1 serving	30.00	125.40	3.00
Crackers, Cheese, sandwich-type with cheese filling	6 crackers	39.00	191.10	3.48
Crackers, cheese, whole grain	55 pieces	31.00	127.72	2.98
Crackers, flavored, fish-shaped	10 goldfish	5.20	24.08	0.53
Crackers, Water Biscuits	4 crackers	14.00	53.76	1.00
Crackers, Melba Toast, plain, without salt	0.5 oz	14.20	55.38	1.72
Crackers, multigrain	4 crackers	14.00	67.48	0.99
Crackers, Saltines, low sodium (including Oyster, Soda, Soup)	0.5 oz	14.20	59.78	1.35
Crackers, Saltines, whole wheat (including multi-grain)	1 serving	14.00	55.72	1.00
Crackers, standard snack-type, with whole wheat	5 crackers	15.00	69.45	1.09
Crackers, Toast Thins, low sodium	1 serving	31.00	137.02	2.00
Crackers, wheat, regular	16 crackers	34.00	154.70	2.48
Crackers, whole grain, sandwich-type, with peanut butter filling	6 crackers	43.00	199.95	6.07
Crackers, whole-wheat	1 serving	28.00	119.56	2.96
Croutons, seasoned	0.5 oz	14.20	66.03	1.53
English muffins, plain, enriched, without calcium proportionate (including sourdough)	1 oz	28.35	66.62	2.18
English muffins, wheat	1 oz	28.35	63.22	2.47
English muffins, whole grain white	1 muffin	57.00	139.65	4.00
Garlic bread, frozen	1 slice, presliced	43.00	150.50	3.59
Keebler, Toasteds, Buttercrisps Crackers	5 crackers	16.00	79.20	0.88

Carbohydrate per serving (g)	Sugar per serving (g)	Fiber per serving (g)	Total fat per serving (g)	Saturated fat per serving (g)	Mono fat per serving (g)	Poly fat per serving (g)
20.95	0.25	1.32	1.58	0.72	0.26	0.14
19.90	0.75	1.18	1.31	0.30	0.63	0.29
26.40	10.94	2.10	2.23	0.46	0.73	0.47
32.54	15.33	2.49	1.72	0.26	0.51	0.54
29.05	0.98	4.76	1.09	0.18	0.24	0.45
27.27	0.57	3.76	2.75	0.44	0.79	0.92
89.91	0.75	8.54	4.52	0.64	1.19	2.06
87.31	0.00	7.30	4.21	0.61	1.14	1.97
123.27	0.00	0.00	7.87	1.11	2.08	3.59
124.74	2.53	6.12	2.75	0.35	0.61	1.30
93.81	0.78	8.91	4.38	0.62	1.16	2.00
22.94	0.09	0.74	0.48	0.08	0.04	0.20
20.46	0.00	0.99	3.50	1.00	0.64	1.58
22.92	4.81	0.74	9.52	1.88	5.58	0.91
17.76	0.00	1.98	4.97	0.99	2.48	0.99
3.41	0.06	0.16	0.92	0.11	0.54	0.20
10.19	0.00	0.99	1.00	0.00	0.57	0.34
10.88	0.00	0.89	0.45	0.06	0.11	0.18
9.46	1.68	0.49	2.86	0.46	0.70	1.65
10.56	0.32	0.41	1.26	0.28	0.32	0.58
9.56	0.00	0.94	1.50	0.00	0.39	1.01
10.26	1.56	0.74	2.68	0.65	0.68	1.19
20.97	4.00	3.01	5.00	1.00	1.02	2.67
24.05	5.26	2.35	5.58	1.09	1.18	2.88
23.47	4.05	4.04	9.11	1.95	4.20	1.93
19.47	0.33	2.88	3.96	0.58	0.91	1.94
9.02	0.63	0.71	2.60	0.75	1.35	0.34
13.04	0.00	0.77	0.51	0.07	0.09	0.25
12.70	0.44	1.30	0.57	0.08	0.08	0.24
28.60	1.00	2.00	1.00	0.00	0.00	0.00
17.94	1.59	1.08	7.14	2.27	2.01	2.34
10.40	1.34	0.29	3.79	0.64	0.93	2.19

(continues)

Food Description	Measure	Weight (g)	Kcal per serving (g)	Protein per serving (g)
Breads, Cereals, Grains, Starch (continued)				
Keebler, Toasteds, Wheat Crackers	5 crackers	16.00	74.56	1.33
Keebler, Zesta, Saltines with Whole Wheat	5 crackers	15.00	62.40	1.26
Keebler, Zesta, Saltines, original	5 crackers	15.00	62.70	1.23
Kellogg, Kellogg's Eggo, Buttermilk Pancake	3 pancakes	116.00	284.20	6.15
Kellogg's, Simply Eggo, original	2 waffles	70.00	205.80	4.34
Kellogg's, Special K, Multigrain Crackers	24 crackers	30.00	120.30	2.70
Macaroni & cheese, box mix with cheese sauce, prepared	1 cup, prepared	189.00	309.96	12.63
Macaroni, vegetables, enriched, dry	1 cup, spiral shaped	84.00	308.28	11.04
Muffins, blueberry, dry mix	1 serving	43.00	125.99	1.50
Muffins, oat bran	1 oz	28.35	76.55	1.98
Muffins, wheat bran, dry mix	1 oz	28.35	112.27	2.01
Noodles, egg, dry, enriched	1 cup	38.00	145.92	5.38
Noodles, egg, dry, Unenriched	1 cup	38.00	145.92	5.38
Oat flour, part debranned	1 cup	104.00	420.16	15.25
Oats	1 cup	156.00	606.84	26.35
Pancakes, buttermilk, prepared from recipe	1 oz	28.35	64.35	1.93
Pancakes, plain, dry mix, complete, prepared	1 oz	28.35	55.00	1.47
Pancakes, whole-wheat, dry mix, incomplete, prepared	1 oz	28.35	58.97	2.41
Pasta, cooked, enriched, with added salt	1 cup, spaghetti not packed	124.00	194.68	7.19
Pasta, cooked, unenriched, with added salt	1 cup, spaghetti not packed	124.00	194.68	7.19
Pasta, dry, enriched	1 cup, spaghetti	91.00	337.61	11.87
Pasta, whole-wheat, dry	1 cup, spaghetti	91.00	320.32	12.62
Potato, yellow fleshed, hash brown, shredded, salt added In processing, frozen, unprepared	3 oz	85.00	68.85	1.73
Potatoes, hash brown, refrigerated, unprepared	1 cup, unprepared	159.00	133.56	2.78
Potatoes, mashed, ready-to-eat	1 cup	229.00	242.74	4.51
Potatoes, yellow fleshed, French fries, frozen, unprepared	3 oz	85.00	137.70	2.10
Rice & Wheat Cereal Bar	1 bar	22.00	89.98	2.00
Rice Crackers			0.00	0.00
Rice flour, white, unenriched	1 cup	158.00	578.28	9.40
Rice Mix, Cheese flavor, dry mix, unprepared	1/4 cup, dry rice mix	57.00	206.34	5.00
Rice Mix, White & Wild, flavored, unprepared	1/4 cup dry rice mix and 4 tsp seasoning mix	57.00	202.35	6.00

Carbohydrate per serving (g)	Sugar per serving (g)	Fiber per serving (g)	Total fat per serving (g)	Saturated fat per serving (g)	Mono fat per serving (g)	Poly fat per serving (g)
10.58	1.44	0.64	3.20	0.51	0.80	1.82
11.27	0.32	0.48	1.44	0.21	0.36	0.87
11.42	0.24	0.38	1.35	0.20	0.33	0.83
44.78	11.60	1.16	9.28	1.51	2.32	5.10
30.31	4.13	0.91	7.63	1.96	1.40	3.43
22.62	6.24	2.58	2.82	0.42	0.66	1.47
43.66	2.97	2.27	9.43	3.09	4.19	1.97
62.90	0.00	3.61	0.87	0.13	0.10	0.36
26.23	14.07	0.60	1.40	0.50	0.30	0.56
13.69	2.33	1.30	2.10	0.31	0.48	1.17
20.70	0.00	0.00	3.40	0.83	1.82	0.54
27.08	0.71	1.25	1.69	0.45	0.48	0.51
27.08	0.71	1.25	1.69	0.45	0.48	0.51
68.33	0.83	6.76	9.48	1.67	2.98	3.46
103.38	0.00	16.54	10.76	1.90	3.40	3.95
8.14	0.00	0.00	2.64	0.52	0.67	1.27
10.40	0.00	0.37	0.71	0.14	0.25	0.23
8.33	0.00	0.79	1.84	0.50	0.49	0.68
37.93	0.69	2.23	1.15	0.22	0.16	0.40
37.93	0.69	2.23	1.15	0.22	0.44	0.40
67.95	2.43	2.91	1.37	0.25	0.16	0.51
66.77	2.49	8.37	2.67	0.39	0.33	1.03
15.28	0.20	1.70	0.06	0.01	0.00	0.00
30.46	1.45	2.86	0.13	0.00	0.00	0.00
30.43	4.03	4.35	11.47	6.03	2.83	1.57
21.26	0.31	1.87	4.96	1.21	0.00	0.00
16.00	7.00	0.40	2.00	0.00	1.44	0.45
0.00	0.00	0.00	0	0.00	0.00	0.00
126.61	0.19	3.79	2.24	0.61	0.70	0.60
42.11	3.00	1.03	2.00	1.00	0.43	0.38
43.40	1.00	1.03	0.50	0.00	0.10	0.32

(continues)

Food Description	Measure	Weight (g)	Kcal per serving (g)	Protein per serving (g)
Breads, Cereals, Grains, Starch (*continued*)				
Rice noodles, dry	2 oz	57.00	207.48	3.39
Rice, brown, long-grain, raw	1 cup	185.00	678.95	13.95
Rice, brown, medium-grain, raw	1 cup	190.00	687.80	14.25
Rice, white, long-grain, regular, raw, unenriched	1 cup	185.00	675.25	13.19
Rice, white, medium-grain, raw, enriched	1 cup	195.00	702.00	12.89
Rolls, dinner, plain, commonly prepared (including Brown-n-Serve)	1 roll	28.00	86.80	3.04
Rolls, dinner, wheat	1 roll	28.00	76.44	2.41
Rolls, French	1 oz	28.35	78.53	2.44
Rolls, hamburger or hot dog, plain	1 roll	44.00	122.76	4.30
Rolls, hamburger or hot dog, whole wheat	1 roll	56.00	150.64	6.93
Rolls, hamburger, whole grain white, calcium-fortified	1 roll	43.00	109.65	4.00
Rolls, Pumpernickel	1 medium	36.00	99.36	3.89
Rye grain	1 cup	169.00	571.22	17.47
Spaghetti, protein-fortified, dry, enriched	2 oz	57.00	213.18	12.41
Spaghetti, Spinach, cooked	1 cup	140.00	182.00	6.41
Spanish Rice Mix, dry mix, prepared (with Canola/Vegetable Oil)	1 cup	198.00	247.50	6.47
Sunshine, Krispy, Soup & Oyster Crackers (large)	16 crackers	15.00	62.40	1.29
Sweet Potato Puffs, frozen, unprepared	3 oz	85.00	136.85	1.16
Sweet potatoes, French fries, frozen as packaged, salt added	12 fries	51.00	92.82	1.10
Waffle, buttermilk, frozen, ready-to-heat, toasted	1 oz	28.00	86.52	2.08
Waffles, plain, frozen, ready-to-heat, toasted	1 oz	28.35	88.45	2.04
Waffles, whole wheat, low-fat, frozen, ready-to-heat	2 waffles	70.00	179.90	5.00
Wheat flour, white, all-purpose, enriched, unbleached	1 cup	125.00	455.00	12.91
Wild rice, cooked	1 cup	164.00	165.64	6.54
Yellow rice with seasoning, dry packet mix, unprepared	2 oz	57.00	195.51	4.00
Fruits and Vegetables				
Apples (raw), Fuji (with skin)	1 cup, sliced	109.00	68.67	0.22
Apples (raw), Red Delicious (with skin)	1 cup, sliced	109.00	64.31	0.29
Applesauce (canned, sweetened, with salt)	1 cup	255.00	193.80	0.46
Applesauce (canned, unsweetened, without added vitamin C)	1 cup	244.00	102.48	0.41

Carbohydrate per serving (g)	Sugar per serving (g)	Fiber per serving (g)	Total fat per serving (g)	Saturated fat per serving (g)	Mono fat per serving (g)	Poly fat per serving (g)
45.70	0.07	0.91	0.32	0.09	0.10	0.09
141.06	1.22	6.66	5.92	1.09	1.95	1.85
144.72	0.00	6.46	5.10	1.02	1.84	1.82
147.91	0.22	2.41	1.22	0.33	0.38	0.33
154.71	0.00	2.73	1.13	0.31	0.35	0.30
14.57	1.55	0.56	1.81	0.39	0.53	0.70
12.88	0.46	1.06	1.76	0.42	0.87	0.31
14.23	0.09	0.91	1.22	0.27	0.56	0.24
22.05	3.20	0.79	1.72	0.37	0.33	0.78
25.16	3.32	3.42	2.45	0.52	0.40	0.99
20.00	4.00	0.99	1.50	0.50	0.24	0.53
18.67	0.14	1.94	1.0	0.18	0.22	0.43
128.20	1.66	25.52	2.75	0.33	0.35	1.30
37.42	0.00	1.37	1.27	0.19	0.15	0.56
36.61	0.00	0.00	0.88	0.13	0.10	0.36
45.03	3.54	2.97	4.71	0.77	1.65	1.72
11.42	0.36	0.39	1.40	0.24	0.32	0.78
26.11	6.50	1.62	3.04	0.26	0.00	0.00
18.15	6.58	2.91	4.55	0.59	1.89	1.46
13.55	1.23	0.73	2.66	0.64	1.48	0.43
13.97	1.42	0.68	2.72	0.46	1.39	0.62
34.41	3.00	3.01	2.50	0.50	0.50	1.00
95.39	0.34	3.38	1.22	0.19	0.11	0.52
35.00	1.20	2.95	0.56	0.08	0.08	0.35
42.57	1.00	1.03	1.00	0.00	0.25	0.47
16.59	12.73	2.29	0.20	0.00	0.00	0.00
15.33	11.42	2.51	0.22	0.00	0.00	0.00
50.77	0.00	3.06	0.46	0.08	0.02	0.14
27.50	22.91	2.68	0.24	0.02	0.00	0.03

(continues)

Food Description	Measure	Weight (g)	Kcal per serving (g)	Protein per serving (g)
Fruits and Vegetables (*continued*)				
Apricot Nectar (canned, with vitamin C)	1 cup	251.00	140.56	0.93
Apricots (canned, heavy syrup, drained)	1 cup, halves	219.00	181.77	1.40
Apricots (raw)	1 cup, halves	155.00	74.40	2.17
Artichokes (Globe or French) (raw)	1 artichoke, medium	128.00	60.16	4.19
Asparagus (raw)	1 cup	134.00	26.80	2.95
Avocados (raw), all common variants	1 cup, cubes	150.00	240.00	3.00
Bananas (raw)	1 cup, mashed	225.00	200.25	2.45
Beet greens (cooked, boiled, drained, with salt)	1 cup, 1" pieces	144.00	38.88	3.70
Beets (raw)	1 cup	136.00	58.48	2.19
Blackberries (raw)	1 cup	144.00	61.92	2.00
Blueberries (dried, sweetened)	1/4 cup	40.00	126.80	1.00
Blueberries (raw)	1 cup	148.00	84.36	1.10
Broccoli, Chinese (cooked)	1 cup	88.00	19.36	1.00
Broccoli flower clusters (raw)	1 cup, flowerets	71.00	19.88	2.12
Broccoli (raw)	1 cup, chopped	91.00	30.94	2.57
Broccoli Stalks (raw)	1 stalk	114.00	31.92	3.40
Brussels Sprouts (raw)	1 cup	88.00	37.84	2.97
Burdock Root (cooked, boiled, drained, with salt)	1 cup	125.00	110.00	2.61
Butterbur (cooked, boiled, drained, with salt)			0.00	0.00
Cabbage, common, fresh harvest (raw)	1/2 cup, shredded	35	8.40	0.42
Cabbage (raw)	1 cup, chopped	89	22.25	1.14
Cabbage, red (raw)	1 cup, chopped	89	27.59	1.27
Carrots, baby (raw)	1 large	15	5.25	0.10
Carrots (raw)	1 cup, chopped	128	52.48	1.19
Cauliflower, green (raw)	1 cup	64	19.84	1.89
Cauliflower (raw)	1 cup, chopped	107	26.75	2.05
Cherries, Sour, Red (raw)	1 cup, without pits	155	77.50	1.55
Cherries, sweet (canned, pitted, heavy syrup, drained)	1 cup	179	148.57	1.31
Cherries, Tart (dried, sweetened)	1/4 cup	40	133.20	0.50
Clementines (raw)	1 fruit	74	34.78	0.63
Collards (raw)	1 cup, chopped	36	11.52	1.09
Corn, sweet, white (raw)	1 ear, small	73	62.78	2.35
Corn, sweet, yellow (raw)	1 cup	145	124.70	4.74
Cranberries (dried, sweetened)	1/4 cup	40	123.20	0.07
Cranberries (raw)	1 cup, chopped	110	50.60	0.51
Cucumber, with peel (raw)	1/2 cup, slices	52	7.80	0.34
Dates, Medjool	1 date, pitted	24	66.48	0.43

Carbohydrate per serving (g)	Sugar per serving (g)	Fiber per serving (g)	Total fat per serving (g)	Saturated fat per serving (g)	Mono fat per serving (g)	Poly fat per serving (g)
36.12	33.23	1.51	0.23	0.02	0.10	0.04
46.67	40.84	5.91	0.24	0.02	0.10	0.05
17.24	14.32	3.10	0.60	0.04	0.26	0.12
13.45	1.27	6.91	0.19	0.05	0.01	0.08
5.20	2.52	2.81	0.16	0.05	0.00	0.07
12.80	0.99	10.05	21.99	3.19	14.70	2.72
51.39	27.52	5.85	0.74	0.25	0.07	0.16
7.86	0.86	4.18	0.29	0.04	0.05	0.10
13.00	9.19	3.81	0.23	0.04	0.04	0.08
13.84	7.03	7.63	0.71	0.02	0.07	0.40
32.00	27.00	3.00	1.00	0.08	0.16	0.52
21.45	14.74	3.55	0.49	0.04	0.07	0.22
3.35	0.74	2.20	0.63	0.10	0.04	0.29
3.59	1.05	1.63	0.25	0.04	0.02	0.12
6.04	1.55	2.37	0.34	0.04	0.01	0.03
5.97	0.00	0.00	0.40	0.06	0.03	0.19
7.88	1.94	3.34	0.26	0.05	0.02	0.13
26.44	4.44	2.25	0.18	0.00	0.00	0.00
0.00	0.00	0.00	0.00	0.00	0.00	0.00
1.88	0.00	0.81	0.06	0.01	0.00	0.03
5.16	2.85	2.22	0.09	0.03	0.02	0.02
6.56	3.41	1.87	0.14	0.02	0.01	0.07
1.24	0.71	0.44	0.02	0.00	0.00	0.01
12.26	6.07	3.58	0.31	0.05	0.02	0.15
3.90	1.94	2.05	0.19	0.03	0.02	0.09
5.32	2.04	2.14	0.30	0.14	0.04	0.03
18.88	13.16	2.48	0.47	0.11	0.13	0.14
37.72	28.96	4.12	0.38	0.07	0.09	0.10
32.18	26.86	1	0.29	0.06	0.07	0.08
8.89	6.79	1.26	0.11	0.00	0.00	0.00
1.95	0.17	1.44	0.22	0.02	0.01	0.07
13.88	2.35	1.97	0.86	0.13	0.25	0.41
27.12	9.08	2.90	1.96	0.47	0.63	0.71
33.12	29.02	2.12	0.44	0.04	0.12	0.07
13.17	4.70	3.96	0.14	0.01	0.02	0.06
1.89	0.87	0.26	0.06	0.02	0.00	0.02
17.99	15.95	1.61	0.04	0.00	0.00	0.00

(continues)

Fruits and Vegetables (*continued*)

Food Description	Measure	Weight (g)	Kcal per serving (g)	Protein per serving (g)
Eggplant (raw)	1 cup, cubes	82	20.50	0.80
Figs (raw)	1 large	64	47.36	0.48
Garlic (raw)	1 cup	136	202.64	8.65
Grapefruit juice, pink (raw)	1 cup	247	96.33	1.24
Grapefruit (raw), pink, red, and white, all areas	1 cup, sections with juice	230	73.60	1.45
Grapes, American type (slip skin) (raw)	1 cup	92	61.64	0.58
Grapes, red or green (European type, such as Thompson seedless, raw)	1 cup	151	104.19	1.09
Guava nectar (canned, with added vitamin C)	1 cup	251	158.13	0.23
Guavas, Common (raw)	1 cup	165	112.20	4.21
Horned Melon (Kiwano)	1 cup	233	102.52	4.15
Jackfruit (canned, syrup pack)	1 cup, drained	178	163.76	0.64
Kale (raw)	1 cup	16	7.84	0.68
Kiwifruit, Zespri Sungold (raw)	1 fruit	81	51.03	0.83
Leeks, bulb and lower-leaf portion (freeze-dried)	1 tbsp	0.2	0.64	0.03
Lemons (raw, without peel)	1 cup, sections	212	61.48	2.33
Lettuce, Butterhead (including Boston and Bibb types) (raw)	1 cup, shredded or chopped	55	7.15	0.74
Lettuce, Cos or Romaine (raw)	1 cup, shredded	47	7.99	0.58
Lettuce, red leaf (raw)	1 cup, shredded	28	4.48	0.37
Limes (raw)	1 fruit	67	20.10	0.47
Mango (dried, sweetened)			0.00	0.00
Mangos (raw)	1 cup, pieces	165	99.00	1.35
Melons, Cantaloupe (raw)	1 cup, balls	177	60.18	1.49
Melons, Honeydew (raw)	1 cup, diced	170	61.20	0.92
Mushroom, white (raw)	1 cup, pieces or slices	70	15.40	2.16
Mushrooms, brown, Italian, or Crimini (raw)	1 cup, whole	87	19.14	2.18
Mushrooms, Chanterelle (raw)	1 cup	54	20.52	0.80
Mushrooms, Enoki (raw)	1 large	5	1.85	0.13
Mushrooms, Maitake (raw)	1 cup, diced	70	21.70	1.36
Mushrooms, Morel (raw)	1 cup	66	20.46	2.06
Mushrooms, Portabella (raw)	1 cup, diced	86	18.92	1.81
Mushrooms, Shiitake (raw)	1 piece, whole	19	6.46	0.43
Mushrooms, white (raw)	1 cup, pieces or slices	70	15.40	2.16
Mustard greens (cooked, boiled, drained, with salt)	1 cup, chopped	140	36.40	3.58
Naranjilla (lulo; pulp, freezed, unsweetened)	1 cup, thawed	120	30.00	0.53
Nectarines (raw)	1 cup, slices	143	62.92	1.52

Carbohydrate per serving (g)	Sugar per serving (g)	Fiber per serving (g)	Total fat per serving (g)	Saturated fat per serving (g)	Mono fat per serving (g)	Poly fat per serving (g)
4.82	2.89	2.46	0.15	0.03	0.01	0.06
12.28	10.41	1.86	0.19	0.04	0.04	0.09
44.96	1.36	2.86	0.68	0.12	0.01	0.34
22.72	0.00	0.00	0.25	0.03	0.03	0.06
18.58	16.05	2.53	0.23	0.03	0.03	0.06
15.78	14.95	0.83	0.32	0.10	0.01	0.09
27.33	23.37	1.36	0.24	0.08	0.01	0.07
40.79	32.50	2.51	0.15	0.05	0.05	0.03
23.63	14.72	8.91	1.57	0.45	0.14	0.66
17.61	0.00	0.00	2.94	0.00	0.00	0.00
42.61	0.00	1.60	0.25	0.00	0.00	0.00
1.40	0.36	0.58	0.15	0.01	0.01	0.05
12.79	9.96	1.13	0.23	0.05	0.02	0.09
0.15	0.00	0.02	0.00	0.00	0.00	0.00
19.76	5.30	5.94	0.64	0.08	0.02	0.19
1.23	0.52	0.61	0.12	0.02	0.00	0.06
1.55	0.56	0.99	0.14	0.02	0.01	0.08
0.63	0.13	0.25	0.06	0.00	0.00	0.02
7.06	1.13	1.88	0.13	0.01	0.01	0.04
0.00	0.00	0.00	0.00	0.00	0.00	0.00
24.72	22.54	2.64	0.63	0.15	0.23	0.12
14.44	13.91	1.59	0.34	0.09	0.01	0.14
15.45	13.80	1.36	0.24	0.06	0.01	0.10
2.28	1.39	0.70	0.24	0.04	0.00	0.11
3.74	1.50	0.52	0.09	0.01	0.00	0.04
3.70	0.63	2.05	0.29	0.00	0.00	0.00
0.39	0.01	0.14	0.01	0.00	0.00	0.00
4.88	1.45	1.89	0.13	0.02	0.02	0.06
3.37	0.40	1.85	0.38	0.04	0.03	0.29
3.33	2.15	1.12	0.30	0.05	0.02	0.10
1.29	0.45	0.48	0.09	0.00	0.00	0.00
2.28	1.39	0.70	0.24	0.04	0.00	0.11
6.31	1.97	2.80	0.66	0.02	0.15	0.06
7.08	4.49	1.32	0.26	0.00	0.00	0.00
15.09	11.28	2.43	0.46	0.04	0.13	0.16

(continues)

Fruits and Vegetables (*continued*)

Food Description	Measure	Weight (g)	Kcal per serving (g)	Protein per serving (g)
Okra (cooked, boiled, drained, with salt)	1/2 cup, slices	80	17.60	1.50
Okra (raw)	1 cup	100	33.00	1.93
Olives, Jumbo-Super Colossal, (ripe, canned)	1 super colossal	15	12.15	0.15
Olives, small-extra large (ripe, canned)	1 tbsp	8.4	9.66	0.07
Onions (raw)	1 cup, chopped	160	64.00	1.76
Onions, sweet (raw)	1 serving	148	47.36	1.18
Onions, Welsh (raw)			0.00	0.00
Oranges (raw, with peel)	1 cup	170	107.10	2.21
Papayas (raw)	1 cup, 1" pieces	145	62.35	0.68
Parsley (freeze-dried)	1 tbsp	0.4	1.08	0.13
Parsnips (cooked, boiled, drained, with salt)	1/2 cup, slices	78	55.38	1.03
Passion-Fruit, Granadilla, Purple (raw)	1 cup	236	228.92	5.19
Peaches (canned, heavy dyrup, drained)	1 cup	222	159.84	1.15
Peaches, yellow (raw)	1 cup, slices	154	60.06	1.40
Pears (canned, heavy syrup, drained)	1 cup	201	148.74	0.48
Pears (raw)	1 cup, slices	140	79.80	0.50
Pepper, banana (raw)	1 cup	124	33.48	2.06
Peppers, hot chili, green (raw)	1 pepper	45	18.00	0.90
Peppers, hot chili, red (raw)	1 pepper	45	18.00	0.84
Peppers, jalapeno (raw)	1 cup, sliced	90	26.10	0.82
Peppers, sweet, yellow (raw)	1 pepper, large	186	50.22	1.86
Peppers, sweet, green (raw)	1 cup, chopped	149	29.80	1.28
Pickle relish, hamburger	1 tbsp	15	19.35	0.09
Pickles, cucumber, dill or kosher dill	1 spear, small	35	4.20	0.18
Pickles, Cucumber, sweet (Includes Bread & Butter Pickles)	1 cup, chopped	160	145.60	0.93
Pineapple, all variants (raw)	1 cup, chunks	165	82.50	0.89
Plums (dried), Prunes, (uncooked)	1 cup, pitted	174	417.60	3.79
Plums (raw)	1 cup, sliced	165	75.90	1.16
Pokeberry shoots, Poke (raw)	1 cup	160	36.80	4.16
Pomegranates (raw)	1/2 cup	87	72.21	1.45
Potatoes, Flesh and skin (raw)	1/2 cup, diced	75	57.75	1.54
Potatoes, hash brown (freezed, plain, unprepared)	1/2 cup	105	86.10	2.16
Potatoes, mashed, home-prepared (whole milk added)	1 cup	210	174.30	4.01
Potatoes, mashed, prepared from granules, without milk, whole milk and margarine	1 cup	210	226.80	4.31
Potatoes, red, flesh and skin (raw)	1/2 cup, diced	75	52.50	1.42

Carbohydrate per serving (g)	Sugar per serving (g)	Fiber per serving (g)	Total fat per serving (g)	Saturated fat per serving (g)	Mono fat per serving (g)	Poly fat per serving (g)
3.61	1.92	2.00	0.17	0.04	0.02	0.04
7.45	1.48	3.20	0.19	0.03	0.02	0.03
0.84	0.00	0.38	1.03	0.14	0.76	0.09
0.53	0.00	0.27	0.90	0.12	0.66	0.08
14.94	6.78	2.72	0.16	0.07	0.02	0.03
11.17	7.43	1.33	0.12	0.00	0.00	0.00
0.00	0.00	0.00	0.00	0.00	0.00	0.00
26.35	0.00	7.65	0.51	0.06	0.09	0.10
15.69	11.34	2.47	0.38	0.12	0.10	0.08
0.17	0.00	0.13	0.02	0.00	0.00	0.00
13.27	3.74	3.12	0.23	0.04	0.09	0.04
55.18	26.43	24.54	1.65	0.14	0.20	0.97
40.91	32.55	2.66	0.40	0.03	0.10	0.15
14.69	12.92	2.31	0.39	0.03	0.10	0.13
38.35	33.00	5.43	0.36	0.02	0.07	0.08
21.32	13.65	4.34	0.20	0.03	0.12	0.13
6.63	2.42	4.22	0.56	0.06	0.03	0.30
4.26	2.30	0.68	0.09	0.01	0.00	0.05
3.96	2.39	0.68	0.20	0.02	0.01	0.11
5.85	3.71	2.52	0.33	0.08	0.03	0.10
11.76	0.00	1.68	0.39	0.06	0.00	0.00
6.91	3.58	2.53	0.25	0.09	0.01	0.09
5.17	0.00	0.48	0.08	0.01	0.04	0.02
0.84	0.37	0.35	0.11	0.03	0.00	0.04
33.84	29.23	1.60	0.66	0.11	0.01	0.17
21.65	16.25	2.31	0.20	0.01	0.02	0.07
111.15	66.35	12.35	0.66	0.15	0.09	0.11
18.84	16.37	2.31	0.46	0.03	0.22	0.07
5.92	0.00	2.72	0.64	0.00	0.00	0.00
16.27	11.89	3.48	1.02	0.10	0.08	0.07
13.12	0.62	1.58	0.07	0.02	0.00	0.03
18.61	0.00	1.47	0.65	0.17	0.01	0.28
36.90	3.11	3.15	1.20	0.63	0.26	0.14
30.24	0.00	4.62	10.35	2.70	4.29	2.86
11.93	0.97	1.28	0.11	0.03	0.00	0.04

(continues)

Food Description	Measure	Weight (g)	Kcal per serving (g)	Protein per serving (g)
Fruits and Vegetables (*continued*)				
Potatoes, russet, flesh and skin (raw)	1/2 cup, diced	75	59.25	1.61
Potatoes, white, flesh and skin (raw)	1/2 cup, diced	75	51.75	1.26
Prickly pears (raw)	1 cup	149	61.09	1.09
Prune juice (canned)	1 cup	256	181.76	1.56
Prunes (canned, heavy syrup pack, solids, and liquids)	1 cup	234	245.70	2.04
Pumpkin (raw)	1 cup, 1" cubes	116	30.16	1.16
Radishes (raw)	1 cup, slices	116	18.56	0.79
Raisins, seedless	1 cup, packed	165	493.35	5.07
Raspberries (raw)	1 cup	123	63.96	1.48
Shallots (freeze-dried)	1 tbsp	0.9	3.13	0.11
Soybeans, green (cooked, boiled, drained, with salt)	1 cup	180	253.80	22.23
Spinach (raw)	1 cup	30	6.90	0.86
Squash, summer, all variants (raw)	1 cup, sliced	113	18.08	1.37
Squash, zucchini, baby (raw)	1 large	16	3.36	0.43
Strawberries (raw)	1 cup, halves	152	48.64	1.02
Succotash, corn and limas (raw)			0.00	0.00
Swamp Cabbage, Skunk Cabbage (raw)	1 cup, chopped	56	10.64	1.46
Sweet potato (cooked, candied, home-prepared)	1 piece	105	172.20	0.93
Sweet potato, unprepared (raw)	1 cup, cubes	133	114.38	2.09
Tangerines, Mandarin Oranges (raw)	1 cup, sections	195	103.35	1.58
Tomatillos (raw)	1 medium	34	10.88	0.33
Tomatoes, green (raw)	1 cup	180	41.40	2.16
Tomatoes, orange (raw)	1 cup, chopped	158	25.28	1.83
Tomatoes, red, ripe (cooked)	1 cup	240	43.20	2.28
Tomatoes, red, ripe, year-round average (raw)	1 cup, cherry tomatoes	149	26.82	1.31
Tomatoes (sun-dried)	1 cup	54	139.32	7.62
Tomatoes, yellow (raw)	1 cup, chopped	139	20.85	1.36
Turnip greens (cooked, boiled, drained, with salt)	1 cup, chopped	144	28.80	1.64
Turnips (raw)	1 cup, cubes	130	36.40	1.17
Watermelon (raw)	1 cup, balls	154	46.20	0.94
Yam (raw)	1 cup, cubes	150	177.00	2.30
Milk and Dairy Products				
Butter, with salt	1 pat	5.00	35.85	0.04
Butter, without salt	1 pat	5.00	35.85	0.04
Cheese, American, nonfat or fat-free	1 serving	19.00	23.94	4.00
Cheese, blue	1 oz	28.35	100.08	6.07

Carbohydrate per serving (g)	Sugar per serving (g)	Fiber per serving (g)	Total fat per serving (g)	Saturated fat per serving (g)	Mono fat per serving (g)	Poly fat per serving (g)
13.55	0.47	0.98	0.06	0.02	0.00	0.03
11.78	0.86	1.80	0.08	0.02	0.00	0.03
14.26	0.00	5.36	0.76	0.10	0.11	0.32
44.67	42.11	2.56	0.08	0.01	0.05	0.02
65.05	0.00	8.89	0.47	0.04	0.30	0.10
7.54	3.20	0.58	0.12	0.06	0.02	0.01
3.94	2.16	1.86	0.12	0.04	0.02	0.06
130.65	97.66	6.10	0.76	0.10	0.08	0.06
14.69	5.44	7.99	0.80	0.02	0.08	0.46
0.73	0.34	0.14	0.00	0.00	0.00	0.00
19.89	0.00	7.56	11.52	1.33	2.18	5.42
1.09	0.13	0.66	0.12	0.02	0.00	0.05
3.79	2.49	1.24	0.20	0.05	0.02	0.10
0.50	0.00	0.18	0.06	0.01	0.00	0.03
11.67	7.43	3.04	0.46	0.02	0.07	0.24
0.00	0.00	0.00	0.00	0.00	0.00	0.00
1.76	0.00	1.18	0.11	0.00	0.00	0.00
33.73	28.61	2.20	3.72	2.28	0.93	0.21
26.76	5.56	3.99	0.07	0.02	0.00	0.02
26.01	20.63	3.51	0.60	0.08	0.12	0.13
1.99	1.34	0.65	0.35	0.05	0.05	0.14
9.18	7.20	1.98	0.36	0.05	0.05	0.15
5.02	0.00	1.42	0.30	0.04	0.04	0.12
9.62	5.98	1.68	0.26	0.04	0.04	0.11
5.80	3.92	1.79	0.30	0.04	0.05	0.12
30.11	20.30	6.64	1.60	0.23	0.26	0.60
4.14	0.00	0.97	0.36	0.05	0.06	0.15
6.28	0.76	5.04	0.33	0.08	0.02	0.13
8.36	4.94	2.34	0.13	0.01	0.01	0.07
11.63	9.55	0.62	0.23	0.02	0.06	0.08
41.82	0.75	6.15	0.26	0.06	0.01	0.11
0.00	0.00	0.00	4.06	2.57	1.05	0.15
0.00	0.00	0.00	4.06	2.52	1.17	0.15
2.00	1.00	0.00	0.00	0.00	0.00	0.00
0.66	0.14	0.00	8.15	5.29	2.21	0.23

(continues)

Milk and Dairy Products (*continued*)

Food Description	Measure	Weight (g)	Kcal per serving (g)	Protein per serving (g)
Cheese, Brie	1 oz	28.35	94.69	5.88
Cheese, Cheddar	1 cup, diced	132.00	533.28	30.19
Cheese, Colby	1 cup, diced	132.00	520.08	31.36
Cheese, cottage, creamed, large or small Curd	4 oz	113.00	110.74	12.57
Cheese, cream	1 tbsp	14.50	50.75	0.89
Cheese, Feta	1 cup, crumbled	150.00	396.00	21.32
Cheese, Fontina	1 cup, diced	132.00	513.48	33.79
Cheese, Goat, Soft Type	1 oz	28.35	74.84	5.25
Cheese, Gouda	1 oz	28.35	100.93	7.07
Cheese, Gruyere	1 oz	28.35	117.09	8.45
Cheese, Limburger	1 cup	134.00	438.18	26.87
Cheese, Mexican, Blend, Red Fat	1 oz	28.35	79.95	7.00
Cheese, Monterey	1 cup, diced	132.00	492.36	32.31
Cheese, Mozzarella, whole milk	1 cup, shredded	112.00	336.00	24.83
Cheese, Muenster	1 cup, diced	132.00	485.76	30.90
Cheese, Parmesan, Grated	1 cup	100.00	420.00	28.42
Cheese, Parmesan, Hard	1 oz	28.35	111.13	10.14
Cheese, Provolone	1 cup, diced	132.00	463.32	33.77
Cheese, Ricotta, part skim milk	1/2 cup	124.00	171.12	14.12
Cheese, Romano	1 oz	28.35	109.71	9.02
Cheese, Swiss	1 cup, diced	132.00	518.76	35.59
Coconut milk, canned	1 cup	226.00	445.22	4.57
Coconut milk, raw	1 cup	240.00	552.00	5.50
Cream, fluid, half and half	1 fl oz	30.20	37.15	0.95
Cream, sour, cultured	1 tbsp	12.00	23.76	0.29
Cream, whipped, ceam topping, pressurized	1 cup	60.00	154.20	1.92
Eggnog	1 cup	254.00	223.52	11.56
Ice Creams, Breyers, All Natural Light French Chocolate	1/2 cup	68.00	136.68	3.60
Ice Creams, Breyers, All Natural Light Mint Chocolate Chip	1/2 cup	68.00	133.28	3.19
Ice Creams, Breyers, All Natural Light Vanilla Chocolate Strawberry	1/2 cup	68.00	109.48	3.19
Ice Cream, soft serve, chocolate	1/2 cup	86.00	190.92	3.53
Kraft Free Singles American Nonfat Cheese Product	1 slice	21.00	31.08	4.77
Milk Shakes, thick chocolate	1 fl oz	28.40	33.80	0.87

Carbohydrate per serving (g)	Sugar per serving (g)	Fiber per serving (g)	Total fat per serving (g)	Saturated fat per serving (g)	Mono fat per serving (g)	Poly fat per serving (g)
0.13	0.13	0.00	7.85	4.94	2.27	0.23
4.08	0.63	0.00	43.97	24.90	12.20	1.88
3.39	0.69	0.00	42.39	26.69	12.25	1.26
3.82	3.02	0.00	4.86	1.94	0.88	0.14
0.80	0.55	0.00	4.99	2.93	1.29	0.22
6.14	6.14	0.00	31.92	22.42	6.93	0.89
2.05	2.05	0.00	41.10	25.34	11.47	2.18
0.00	0.00	0.00	5.98	4.13	1.36	0.14
0.63	0.63	0.00	7.78	4.99	2.20	0.19
0.10	0.10	0.00	9.17	5.36	2.85	0.49
0.66	0.66	0.00	36.52	22.44	11.53	0.66
0.97	0.16	0.00	5.50	3.28	1.42	0.21
0.90	0.66	0.00	39.97	25.17	11.55	1.19
2.45	1.15	0.00	25.03	14.73	7.36	0.86
1.48	1.48	0.00	39.65	25.23	11.50	0.87
13.91	0.07	0.00	27.84	15.37	7.13	1.39
0.91	0.23	0.00	7.32	4.65	2.13	0.16
2.82	0.74	0.00	35.14	22.54	9.76	1.02
6.37	0.38	0.00	9.81	6.11	2.87	0.32
1.03	0.21	0.00	7.64	4.85	2.22	0.17
1.90	0.00	0.00	40.91	24.06	10.62	1.77
6.35	0.00	0.00	48.21	42.75	2.05	0.53
13.30	8.02	5.28	57.22	50.74	2.43	0.63
1.43	1.25	0.00	3.14	2.12	1.00	0.17
0.56	0.41	0.00	2.32	1.22	0.55	0.10
7.49	4.80	0.00	13.33	8.30	3.85	0.50
20.45	20.45	0.00	10.64	6.58	3.31	0.50
20.18	16.35	0.68	4.95	2.91	0.00	0.00
19.31	17.26	0.41	4.82	3.05	0.00	0.00
17.72	15.28	0.27	2.96	1.84	0.00	0.00
19.09	18.20	0.60	11.18	6.42	3.00	0.40
2.46	1.41	0.04	0.21	0.15	0.00	0.00
6.01	5.92	0.09	0.77	0.48	0.22	0.03

(continues)

Food Description	Measure	Weight (g)	Kcal per serving (g)	Protein per serving (g)
Milk and Dairy Products (*continued*)				
Milk Shakes, thick vanilla	1 fl oz	28.40	31.81	1.10
Milk, buttermilk, fluid, cultured, lowfat	1 cup	245.00	98.00	8.11
Milk, chocolate, lowfat, with added vitamins A & D	1 cup	250.00	155.00	8.65
Milk, canned, evaporated, with added vitamin D and without added vitamin A	1 fl oz	31.50	42.21	2.15
Milk, dry, nonfat, instant, with added vitamins A & D	1 cup	68.00	243.44	23.87
Milk, dry, whole, with added vitamin D	1/4 cup	32.00	158.72	8.42
Milk, lowfat, fluid, 1% milkfat, with added nonfat milk solids, vitamins A & D	1 cup	245.00	105.35	8.53
Milk, Red Fat, Fluid, 2% milkfat, protein-fortified, with added vitamins A & D	1 cup	246.00	137.76	9.72
Silk Soy Yogurt, Black Cherry	1 container	170.00	149.60	4.00
Silk Soy Yogurt, Blueberry	1 container	170.00	149.60	4.00
Silk Soy Yogurt, Key Lime	1 container	170.00	149.60	4.00
Silk Soy Yogurt, Peach	1 container	170.00	159.80	4.00
Silk Soy Yogurt, Plain	1 container	227.00	149.82	5.99
Sour cream, reduced fat	1 tbsp	12.00	21.72	0.84
Soymilk (all flavors), Lowfat, with added calcium, vitamins A & D	1 cup	243.00	104.49	4.01
Yogurt, chocolate, nonfat milk	1 container	170.00	190.40	6.00
Yogurt, fruit, lowfat, 10 grams of protein per 8 oz	1 container	170.00	173.40	7.43
Yogurt, frozen, flavors other than chocolate, lowfat			0.00	0.00
Yogurt, Greek, fruit, whole milk			0.00	0.00
Yogurt, Greek, plain, lowfat	1 container	200.00	146.00	19.90
Yogurt, Greek, strawberry, lowfat	1 container	150.00	154.50	12.26
Yogurt, Greek, vanilla, lowfat			0.00	0.00
Yogurt, plain, lowfat, 12 grams protein per 8 oz	1 container	170.00	107.10	8.93
Yogurt, vanilla, nonFat	1 cup	245.00	191.10	7.20
Meat, Fish, Beans, and Other Proteins				
Almond butter, plain, with salt	1 tbsp	16.00	98.24	3.35
Almonds, dry roasted, with salt	1 cup, whole kernels	138.00	825.24	28.92
Bacon, turkey, low sodium	1 serving	15.00	37.95	2.00
Bass, striped, raw	3 oz	85.00	82.45	15.07
Beans, sdzuki, mature seeds, cooked, boiled, without salt	1 cup	230.00	294.40	17.30
Beans, baked, canned, plain or vegetarian	1 cup	254.00	238.76	12.07
Beans, black turtle, mature seeds, cooked, boiled, with salt	1 cup	185.00	240.50	15.13

Carbohydrate per serving (g)	Sugar per serving (g)	Fiber per serving (g)	Total fat per serving (g)	Saturated fat per serving (g)	Mono fat per serving (g)	Poly fat per serving (g)
5.04	5.04	0.00	0.86	0.54	0.25	0.03
11.74	11.74	0.00	2.16	1.34	0.62	0.08
24.65	24.85	0.25	2.50	1.46	1.35	0.24
3.16	3.16	0.00	2.38	1.45	0.74	0.08
35.49	35.49	0.00	0.49	0.32	0.13	0.02
12.29	12.29	0.00	8.55	5.36	2.54	0.21
12.18	0.00	0.00	2.38	1.48	0.69	0.09
13.51	12.94	0.00	4.87	3.03	1.41	0.18
29.00	19.99	1.02	2.01	0.00	0.00	0.00
29.00	21.00	1.02	2.01	0.00	0.00	0.00
30.01	21.00	1.02	2.01	0.00	0.00	0.00
31.99	25.01	1.02	2.01	0.00	0.00	0.00
22.00	12.01	0.91	4.00	0.50	0.00	0.00
0.84	0.04	0.00	1.69	1.04	0.49	0.06
17.50	8.51	1.94	1.51	0.00	0.50	1.00
40.00	25.45	2.04	0.00	0.00	0.00	0.00
32.39	32.39	0.00	1.84	1.18	0.50	0.05
0.00	0.00	0.00	0.00	0.00	0.00	0.00
0.00	0.00	0.00	0.00	0.00	0.00	0.00
7.88	7.12	0.00	3.84	2.46	0.97	0.15
17.84	16.85	1.50	3.86	2.40	0.98	0.17
0.00	0.00	0.00	0.00	0.00	0.00	0.00
11.97	11.97	0.00	2.64	1.70	0.72	0.07
41.75	14.41	0.00	0.00	0.00	0.00	0.00
3.01	1.00	1.65	8.88	1.05	5.19	2.18
28.99	6.71	15.04	72.51	5.65	45.64	17.88
0.72	0.00	0.00	3.00	1.00	1.29	0.64
0.00	0.00	0.00	1.98	0.43	0.56	0.67
56.97	0.00	16.79	0.23	0.08	0.02	0.05
53.70	20.22	10.41	0.94	0.18	0.24	0.31
45.05	0.59	15.36	0.65	0.16	0.06	0.28

(continues)

Meat, Fish, Beans, and Other Proteins (*continued*)

Food Description	Measure	Weight (g)	Kcal per serving (g)	Protein per serving (g)
Beans, French, mature seeds, cooked, boiled, with salt	1 cup	177.00	228.33	12.48
Beans, Great Northern, mature seeds, cooked, boiled, with salt	1 cup	177.00	208.86	14.74
Beans, kidney, all types, mature seeds, raw	1 cup	184.00	612.72	43.39
Beans, navy, mature seeds, raw	1 cup	208.00	700.96	46.45
Beans, pinto, mature seeds, raw	1 cup	193.00	669.71	41.34
Beans, Shellie, canned, solids, and Liquids	1 cup	245.00	73.50	4.31
Beans, small white, mature seeds, cooked, boiled, with salt	1 cup	179.00	254.18	16.06
Beans, snap, green, raw	1 cup, 0.5 pieces	100.00	31.00	1.83
Beans, white, mature seeds, raw	1 cup	202.00	672.66	47.19
Beans, yellow, mature seeds, cooked, boiled, with salt	1 cup	177.00	254.88	16.21
Beef sausage, pre-cooked	1 serving	48.00	194.40	7.44
Beef, chuck, short ribs, boneless, 0" fat, choice, cooked, braised	3 oz	85.00	212.50	24.51
Beef, shoulder steak, boneless, lean only, 0" fat, choice, grill	3 oz	85.00	151.30	24.26
Beef, brisket, whole, lean, all grades, raw	1 oz	28.35	43.94	5.87
Beef, bottom sirloin, tri-tip roast, lean, 0" fat, select, raw	3 oz	85.00	109.65	18.14
Beef, chuck, undiluted boiled pot roast or steak, boneless, lean, 0" fat, choice, raw	3 oz	85.00	123.25	18.01
Beef, cured, corned beef, brisket, raw	1 oz	28.35	56.13	4.16
Beef, cured, pastrami	1 package, 2.5 oz	71.00	104.37	15.48
Beef, cured, sausage, cooked, smoked	1 sausage	43.00	134.16	6.07
Beef, flank, steak, lean and lat, 0" fat, all grades, raw	3 oz	85.00	131.75	18.04
Beef, grass-fed, ground, raw	1 serving	85.00	168.30	16.51
Beef, ground, 70% lean meat / 30% fat, loaf, cooked, baked	3 oz	85.00	204.85	20.29
Beef, ground, 75% lean meat / 25% fat, patty, cooked, broiled	3 oz	85.00	237.15	21.73
Beef, ground, 85% lean meat / 15% fat, patty, cooked, broiled	3 oz	85.00	212.50	22.04
Beef, ground, 90% lean meat / 10% fat, raw	4 oz	113.00	198.88	22.60
Beef, ground, 93% lean meat / 7% fat	4 oz	113.00	171.76	23.56
Beef, ground, 95% lean meat / 5% fat, raw	4 oz	113.00	154.81	24.19
Beef, loin, top loin steak, boneless, lip off, lean and fat, 0" fat, choice, raw	3 oz	85.00	145.35	18.86

Carbohydrate per serving (g)	Sugar per serving (g)	Fiber per serving (g)	Total fat per serving (g)	Saturated fat per serving (g)	Mono fat per serving (g)	Poly fat per serving (g)
42.52	0.00	16.64	1.35	0.15	0.09	0.80
37.33	0.00	12.39	0.80	0.25	0.04	0.33
110.42	4.10	45.82	1.53	0.22	0.12	0.84
126.36	8.07	31.82	3.12	0.35	0.27	1.82
120.72	4.07	29.92	2.37	0.45	0.44	0.79
15.17	1.54	8.33	0.47	0.06	0.03	0.27
46.20	0.00	18.62	1.15	0.30	0.10	0.49
6.97	3.26	2.70	0.22	0.05	0.01	0.11
121.75	4.26	30.70	1.72	0.44	0.15	0.74
44.75	0.60	18.41	1.91	0.49	0.17	0.82
0.01	0.00	0.00	18.03	7.25	7.87	0.49
0.00	0.00	0.00	12.71	3.59	8.31	0.69
0.00	0.00	0.00	5.31	2.21	2.76	0.35
0.00	0.00	0.00	2.09	0.73	0.98	0.07
0.00	0.00	0.00	3.58	1.28	1.82	0.17
0.33	0.00	0.00	5.53	2.35	2.75	0.27
0.04	0.00	0.00	4.22	1.34	2.04	0.15
0.26	0.07	0.00	4.13	1.90	1.50	0.10
1.04	0.00	0.00	11.57	4.92	5.58	0.45
0.00	0.00	0.00	6.09	2.53	2.49	0.24
0.00	0.00	0.00	10.82	4.53	4.08	0.45
0.00	0.00	0.00	13.06	5.16	6.22	0.35
0.00	0.00	0.00	16.04	6.16	7.33	0.44
0.00	0.00	0.00	13.10	5.01	5.67	0.41
0.00	0.00	0.00	11.30	4.44	4.74	0.39
0.00	0.00	0.00	7.91	3.25	3.24	0.33
0.00	0.00	0.00	5.65	2.47	2.25	0.29
0.00	0.00	0.00	7.79	3.22	3.68	0.43

(continues)

Food Description	Measure	Weight (g)	Kcal per serving (g)	Protein per serving (g)
Meat, Fish, Beans, and Other Proteins (*continued*)				
Beef, rib eye steak/roast, bone-In, lip-on, lean, 1/8" fat, all grades, raw	3 oz	85.00	141.10	18.04
Beef, rib, shortribs, lean only, choice, raw	1 oz	28.35	49.05	5.40
Beef, rib, whole lean and fat, 1/8" fat, select, raw	1 oz	28.35	81.65	4.75
Beef, round, bottom round, roast, lean, 1/8" fat, all grades, cooked	1 oz	28.35	46.21	7.94
Beef, round, top round, steak, lean, 1/8" fat, all grades, cooked, broiled	1 oz	28.35	52.45	9.02
Beef, shank crosscuts, lean, 1/4" fat, choice, raw	1 oz	28.35	36.29	6.17
Beef, shoulder top blade steak, boneless, lean, 0" fat, all grades, raw	3 oz	85.00	118.15	17.31
Beef, short loin, porthouse steak, lean and fat, 1/8" fat, all grades, raw	3 oz	85.00	181.90	17.42
Beef, tenderloin, lean and fat, 1/8" fat, prime, raw	1 oz	28.35	77.68	5.15
Beef, top sirloin, steak, lean and fat, 0" fat, all grades, cooked, broiled	3 oz	85.00	180.20	24.93
Beerwurst, beer salami, pork	1 slice	23.00	54.74	3.28
Beef, chuck, clod, top and center, steak, lean and fat, 0" fat, all grades, raw	3 oz	85.00	119.85	17.57
Beef, chuck, shoulder clod, top and center, steak, lean and fat, 0" fat, select, raw	3 oz	85.00	119.00	17.96
Blood sausage	4 slices	100.00	379.00	14.60
Bluefish, raw	1 fillet	150.00	186.00	30.06
Bologna, beef	1 slice	30.00	89.70	3.27
Bratwurst beef & pork smoked	2 1/3 oz	66.00	196.02	8.05
Broadbeans (fava beans), mature seeds, cooked, boiled, with salt	1 cup	170.00	187.00	12.92
Butterfish, raw	1 fillet	32.00	46.72	5.53
Carp, raw	3 oz	85.00	107.95	15.16
Cashew Nuts, dry roasted, with salt	1 cup, halves and whole	137.00	786.38	20.97
Catfish, Channel, cooked, breaded and fried	1 fillet	87.00	199.23	15.74
Catfish, Channel, farmed, cooked, dry heat	1 fillet	143.00	205.92	26.37
Caviar, black and red, granular	1 tbsp	16.00	42.24	3.94
Chestnuts, European, roasted	1 cup	143.00	350.35	4.53
Chicken breast, oven-roasted, fat-free, sliced	2 slices	42.00	33.18	7.05
Chicken breast, tenders, breaded, uncooked	1 piece	15.00	39.45	2.21
Chicken breast, deli, rotisserie seasoned, sliced, prepackaged	1 slice	12.00	11.76	2.09
Chicken patty, frozen, cooked	1 patty	60.00	172.20	8.91

Carbohydrate per serving (g)	Sugar per serving (g)	Fiber per serving (g)	Total fat per serving (g)	Saturated fat per serving (g)	Mono fat per serving (g)	Poly fat per serving (g)
0.00	0.00	0.00	7.68	3.01	3.51	0.37
0.00	0.00	0.00	2.89	1.23	1.24	0.11
0.00	0.00	0.00	6.79	2.80	2.93	0.24
0.00	0.00	0.00	1.62	0.56	0.68	0.07
0.00	0.00	0.00	1.55	0.53	0.65	0.07
0.00	0.00	0.00	1.09	0.36	0.50	0.04
0.00	0.00	0.00	5.46	2.32	2.80	0.31
0.00	0.00	0.00	11.95	5.08	5.57	0.56
0.00	0.00	0.00	6.19	2.54	2.63	0.25
0.00	0.00	0.00	8.22	3.19	3.37	0.31
0.47	0.00	0.00	4.32	1.44	2.07	0.54
0.00	0.00	0.00	5.00	1.69	2.50	0.34
0.00	0.00	0.00	4.68	1.52	1.64	0.29
1.29	1.29	0.00	34.50	13.40	15.90	3.46
0.00	0.00	0.00	6.36	1.37	2.69	1.59
1.29	0.62	0.00	7.84	3.15	3.66	0.35
1.32	0.00	0.00	17.38	4.01	5.28	1.04
33.41	3.09	9.18	0.68	0.11	0.13	0.28
0.00	0.00	0.00	2.57	1.08	1.08	0.19
0.00	0.00	0.00	4.76	0.92	1.98	1.22
44.79	6.86	4.11	63.50	12.55	37.42	10.74
6.99	0.00	0.61	11.60	2.86	4.88	2.89
0.00	0.00	0.00	10.28	2.27	4.45	1.94
0.64	0.00	0.00	2.86	0.65	0.74	1.18
75.73	15.16	7.29	3.15	0.59	1.09	1.24
0.91	0.04	0.00	0.16	0.05	0.05	0.03
2.25	0.06	0.17	2.36	0.49	0.97	0.50
0.35	0.09	0.00	0.22	0.07	0.09	0.05
7.70	0.00	0.18	11.75	2.20	5.00	2.88

(continues)

Meat, Fish, Beans, and Other Proteins (*continued*)

Food Description	Measure	Weight (g)	Kcal per serving (g)	Protein per serving (g)
Chicken, broilers or fryers, drumstick, meat and skin, cooked, roasted	1 drumstick, with skin	105.00	200.55	24.52
Chicken, broilers or fryers, leg, meat and skin, cooked, roasted	3 oz	85.00	156.40	20.43
Chicken, broilers or fryers, light meat, meat and skin, cooked, fried, batter	1 unit	113.00	313.01	26.61
Chicken, broilers or fryers, wing, meat only, cooked, fried	1 unit	12.00	25.32	3.62
Chicken, cornish game hens, meat only, cooked, roasted	3 oz	85.00	113.90	19.81
Chicken, roasting, meat only, raw	3 oz	85.00	94.35	17.28
Chicken, skin (drumsticks and thighs), raw	1 oz	28.35	124.74	2.72
Chickpeas (garbanzo beans, Bengal gram), mature seeds, raw	1 cup	200.00	756.00	40.94
Chili with beans, canned	1 cup	256.00	263.68	15.67
Chorizo, pork and beef	1 oz	28.35	128.99	6.83
Clam, mixed species, raw	3 oz	85.00	73.10	12.47
Cod, Atlantic, raw	3 oz	85.00	69.70	15.14
Cowpeas, common, mature seeds, cooked, boiled, with salt	1 cup	171.00	198.36	13.22
Crab, Alaska King, raw	3 oz	85.00	71.40	15.55
Crab, blue, raw	3 oz	85.00	73.95	15.35
Crab, queen, raw	3 oz	85.00	76.50	15.73
Crayfish, mixed species, wild, raw	3 oz	85.00	65.45	13.57
Croaker, Atlantic, raw	1 fillet	79.00	82.16	14.05
Crustaceans, shrimp, raw	3 oz	85.00	72.25	17.09
Cusk, raw	1 fillet	122.00	106.14	23.17
Cuttlefish, mixed species, raw	3 oz	85.00	67.15	13.80
Drum, freshwater, raw	3 oz	85.00	101.15	14.91
Duck, wild, breast, meat only, raw	1 unit	73.00	89.79	14.49
Egg, white, dried	1 oz	28.00	106.96	22.71
Egg, white, raw, fresh	1 large	33.00	17.16	3.60
Egg, whole, cooked, hard-boiled	1 cup, chopped	136.00	210.80	17.11
Egg, whole, cooked, poached	1 large	50.00	71.50	6.26
Egg, whole, cooked, scrambled	1 large	61.00	90.89	6.09
Falafel, home-prepared	1 patty	17.00	56.61	2.26
Fish, cod, Pacific, raw	1 fillet	116.00	80.04	17.71
Fish, mahi-mahi, raw	3 oz	85.00	72.25	15.73
Fish, pollock, Alaska, raw	1 fillet	77.00	43.12	9.39

Carbohydrate per serving (g)	Sugar per serving (g)	Fiber per serving (g)	Total fat per serving (g)	Saturated fat per serving (g)	Mono fat per serving (g)	Poly fat per serving (g)
0.00	0.00	0.00	10.66	2.88	4.36	2.19
0.00	0.00	0.00	7.64	2.08	3.03	1.58
10.74	0.00	0.00	17.45	4.66	7.20	4.07
0.00	0.00	0.00	1.10	0.30	0.37	0.25
0.00	0.00	0.00	3.29	0.84	1.05	0.80
0.00	0.00	0.00	2.30	0.57	0.71	0.57
0.22	0.00	0.00	12.54	3.43	5.38	2.57
125.90	21.40	24.40	12.08	1.21	2.75	5.46
33.89	4.22	8.45	9.63	2.90	4.10	0.64
0.53	0.00	0.00	10.85	4.08	5.22	0.98
3.03	0.00	0.00	0.82	0.16	0.10	0.16
0.00	0.00	0.00	0.57	0.11	0.08	0.20
35.50	5.64	11.12	0.91	0.24	0.08	0.38
0.00	0.00	0.00	0.51	0.08	0.07	0.11
0.03	0.00	0.00	0.92	0.19	0.16	0.33
0.00	0.00	0.00	1.00	0.12	0.22	0.36
0.00	0.00	0.00	0.81	0.14	0.15	0.25
0.00	0.00	0.00	2.50	0.86	0.91	0.37
0.00	0.00	0.00	0.43	0.09	0.07	0.13
0.00	0.00	0.00	0.84	0.16	0.11	0.34
0.70	0.00	0.00	0.60	0.10	0.07	0.11
0.00	0.00	0.00	4.19	0.95	1.86	0.98
0.00	0.00	0.00	3.10	0.96	0.88	0.42
2.18	1.51	0.00	0.00	0.00	0.00	0.00
0.24	0.23	0.00	0.06	0.00	0.00	0.00
1.52	1.52	0.00	14.43	4.44	5.54	1.92
0.36	0.19	0.00	4.74	1.56	1.82	0.95
0.98	0.85	0.00	6.70	2.03	2.71	1.48
5.41	0.00	0.00	3.03	0.41	1.73	0.71
0.00	0.00	0.00	0.48	0.10	0.08	0.19
0.00	0.00	0.00	0.60	0.16	0.10	0.14
0.00	0.00	0.00	0.32	0.10	0.06	0.15

(continues)

Food Description	Measure	Weight (g)	Kcal per serving (g)	Protein per serving (g)
Meat, Fish, Beans, and Other Proteins (*continued*)				
Fish, salmon, sockeye, raw	1 oz, boneless	28.35	37.14	6.31
Fish, tilapia, raw	1 fillet	116.00	111.36	23.29
Fish, trout, brook, raw, New York State	1 filet	149.00	163.90	31.63
Fish, tuna, light, canned In water, drained solids	1 oz	28.35	24.38	5.51
Flatfish (flounder and sole species), raw	1 oz, boneless	28.35	19.85	3.52
Frankfurter, beef, pork, and turkey, fat-free	1 frank	57.00	62.13	7.13
Frankfurter, turkey	1 oz	28.35	63.22	3.47
Frijoles Rojos Volteados (refried beans, red, canned)	1 cup	233.00	335.52	11.65
Game meat, deer, raw	1 oz	28.35	34.02	6.51
Gefiltefish, commercial, sweet recipe	1 piece	42.00	35.28	3.81
Goose, domesticated, meat and skin, raw	3 oz	85.00	315.35	13.48
Ground turkey, 85% lean, 15% fat, raw	1 patty	85.00	153.00	14.37
Ground turkey, 93% lean, 7% fat, raw	1 oz	28.35	42.53	5.31
Grouper, mixed species, raw	3 oz	85.00	78.20	16.47
Haddock, raw	3 oz	85.00	62.90	13.87
Halibut, Atlantic and Pacific, raw	3 oz	85.00	77.35	15.78
Ham honey smoked cooked	1.94 oz	55.00	67.10	9.86
Ham, sliced, prepackaged, deli meat (96% fat free, water added)	1 slice	13.00	13.91	2.19
Hazeleanuts or filberts	1 cup, chopped	115.00	722.20	17.19
Herring, Atlantic, raw	1 oz, boneless	28.35	44.79	5.09
Herring, Pacific, raw	3 oz	85.00	165.75	13.93
Hickorynuts, dried	1 cup	120.00	788.40	15.26
Hummus, commercial	1 tbsp	15.00	24.90	1.19
Hyacinth beans, mature seeds, raw	1 cup	210.00	722.40	50.19
Kielbasa, fully cooked, grilled	3 oz	85.00	286.45	10.58
Lamb, domestic, foreshank, lean, 1/4" fat, choice, raw	1 oz	28.35	34.02	5.98
Lentils, pink or red, raw	1 cup	192.00	687.36	45.91
Lentils, raw	1 cup	192.00	675.84	47.29
Lima beans, large, mature seeds, raw	1 cup	178.00	601.64	38.20
Liverwurst Spread	1/4 cup	55.00	167.75	6.81
Lobster, northern, raw	1 lobster	150.00	115.50	24.78
Lotus seeds, raw	1 oz	28.35	25.23	1.17
Luncheon meat, pork with ham, minced, canned, including Spam (Hormel)	2 oz	56.00	176.40	7.50
Lupins, mature seeds, raw	1 cup	180.00	667.80	65.11
Macadamia nuts, dry roasted, with salt	1 cup, whole or halves	132.00	945.12	10.28

Carbohydrate per serving (g)	Sugar per serving (g)	Fiber per serving (g)	Total fat per serving (g)	Saturated fat per serving (g)	Mono fat per serving (g)	Poly fat per serving (g)
0.00	0.00	0.00	1.33	0.23	0.39	0.32
0.00	0.00	0.00	1.97	0.68	0.58	0.42
0.00	0.00	0.00	4.07	0.89	1.21	1.15
0.00	0.00	0.00	0.27	0.06	0.03	0.08
0.00	0.00	0.00	0.55	0.13	0.15	0.11
6.39	0.00	0.00	0.91	0.29	0.42	0.20
1.08	0.34	0.00	4.90	1.14	1.63	1.12
36.05	0.00	10.95	16.15	2.16	3.91	10.20
0.00	0.00	0.00	0.69	0.27	0.19	0.13
3.11	0.00	0.00	0.73	0.17	0.35	0.12
0.00	0.00	0.00	28.58	8.31	15.10	3.20
0.00	0.00	0.00	10.66	2.90	3.87	2.96
0.00	0.00	0.00	2.36	0.62	0.81	0.72
0.00	0.00	0.00	0.87	0.20	0.17	0.27
0.00	0.00	0.00	0.38	0.08	0.05	0.14
0.00	0.00	0.00	1.13	0.25	0.40	0.25
4.00	0.00	0.00	1.30	0.48	0.68	0.13
0.09	0.00	0.00	0.53	0.16	0.21	0.08
19.21	4.99	11.16	69.86	5.13	52.50	9.11
0.00	0.00	0.00	2.56	0.58	1.06	0.60
0.00	0.00	0.00	11.80	2.77	5.84	2.06
21.90	0.00	7.68	77.24	8.45	39.13	26.26
2.14	0.00	0.90	1.44	0.22	0.61	0.54
127.55	0.00	53.76	3.55	0.60	0.16	1.50
4.28	2.03	0.00	25.23	8.41	10.68	4.58
0.00	0.00	0.00	0.93	0.33	0.37	0.09
121.15	0.00	20.74	4.17	0.73	0.96	2.18
121.63	3.90	20.54	2.04	0.30	0.37	1.01
112.82	15.13	33.82	1.23	0.29	0.11	0.55
3.24	0.91	1.38	14.00	5.46	6.76	1.33
0.00	0.00	0.00	1.13	0.27	0.33	0.44
4.90	0.00	0.00	0.15	0.02	0.03	0.09
2.58	0.00	0.00	14.90	5.59	7.56	1.13
72.67	0.00	34.02	17.53	2.08	7.09	4.39
16.94	5.46	10.56	100.43	15.77	78.24	1.98

(continues)

Food Description	Measure	Weight (g)	Kcal per serving (g)	Protein per serving (g)
Meat, Fish, Beans, and Other Proteins (*continued*)				
Macaroni and cheese loaf, chicken, pork, and beef	1 slice	38.00	86.64	4.47
Mackerel, Atlantic, raw	1 fillet	112.00	229.60	20.83
Meatballs, frozen, Italian style	3 oz	85.00	243.10	12.24
Milkfish, raw	3 oz	85.00	125.80	17.45
Mixed nuts, dry roasted, with peanuts, with salt	1 cup	137.00	813.78	23.70
Monkfish, raw	3 oz	85.00	64.60	12.31
Mori-Nu, tofu, silken, firm	1 slice	84.00	52.08	5.80
Mothbeans, mature seeds, raw	1 cup	196.00	672.28	44.96
Mullet, striped, raw	1 oz	28.35	33.17	5.49
Mung beans, mature seeds, raw	1 cup	207.00	718.29	49.39
Mussel, blue, raw	1 cup	150.00	129.00	17.85
New England brand sausage, pork, beef	1 slice	23.00	37.03	3.97
Nuts, almonds, oil roasted, lightly salted	1 cup, whole kernels	157.00	952.99	33.33
Nuts, pilinuts, dried	1 cup	120.00	862.80	12.96
Nuts, pine nuts, dried	1 cup	135.00	908.55	18.48
Nuts, waleanuts, dry roasted, with salt added	1 oz	28.00	180.04	4.00
Ocean perch, Atlantic, raw	1 oz, boneless	28.35	22.40	4.34
Octopus, common, raw	3 oz	85.00	69.70	12.67
Oyster, eastern, wild, raw	6 medium	84.00	42.84	4.80
Oyster, pacific, raw	1 medium	50.00	40.50	4.73
Pastrami, beef, 98% fat-Free	6 slices	57.00	54.15	11.17
Pastrami, turkey	2 slices	57.00	79.23	9.29
Peanut butter, chunk style, with salt	2 tbsp	32.00	188.48	7.70
Peanut butter, smooth style, with salt	2 tbsp	32.00	191.36	7.11
Peanuts, all types, dry-roasted, with salt	1 oz	28.35	166.41	6.90
Peanuts, all types, dry-roasted, without salt	1 cup	146.00	857.02	35.55
Peas, split, mature seeds, cooked, boiled, with salt	1 cup	196.00	227.36	16.35
Pecans	1 cup, chopped	109.00	753.19	10.00
Perch, mixed species, raw	1 fillet	60.00	54.60	11.63
Pheasant, raw, meat and skin	3 oz	85.00	153.85	19.30
Pigeon peas, mature seeds, raw	1 cup	205.00	703.15	44.49
Pike, northern, raw	3 oz	85.00	74.80	16.37
Pike, walleye, raw	3 oz	85.00	79.05	16.27
Pistachio nuts, raw	1 cup	123.00	688.80	24.80
Polish sausage, pork	3 oz	85.00	277.10	11.99
Pollock, Atlantic, raw	3 oz	85.00	78.20	16.52
Pompano, Florida, raw	1 oz, boneless	28.35	46.49	5.24

Carbohydrate per serving (g)	Sugar per serving (g)	Fiber per serving (g)	Total fat per serving (g)	Saturated fat per serving (g)	Mono fat per serving (g)	Poly fat per serving (g)
4.42	0.00	0.00	5.68	2.13	2.89	0.63
0.00	0.00	0.00	15.56	3.65	6.11	3.75
6.85	2.95	1.96	18.88	6.48	7.81	2.84
0.00	0.00	0.00	5.72	1.41	2.19	1.56
34.73	6.58	12.33	70.49	8.91	43.01	14.75
0.00	0.00	0.00	1.29	0.29	0.20	0.52
2.02	1.07	0.08	2.27	0.34	0.45	1.25
120.58	0.00	0.00	3.16	0.71	0.25	1.47
0.00	0.00	0.00	1.07	0.32	0.31	0.20
129.62	13.66	33.74	2.38	0.72	0.33	0.79
5.54	0.00	0.00	3.36	0.64	0.76	0.91
1.11	0.00	0.00	1.74	0.59	0.84	0.17
27.76	7.14	16.49	86.62	6.60	54.63	21.23
4.78	0.00	0.00	95.46	37.42	44.67	9.13
17.66	4.85	5.00	92.30	6.61	25.33	46.00
5.00	1.00	1.99	17.00	1.50	2.34	12.37
0.00	0.00	0.00	0.44	0.08	0.13	0.09
1.87	0.00	0.00	0.88	0.19	0.14	0.20
2.28	0.52	0.00	1.44	0.40	0.21	0.44
2.48	0.00	0.00	1.15	0.26	0.18	0.45
0.88	0.00	0.00	0.66	0.00	0.32	0.02
1.90	1.90	0.06	3.54	0.80	1.10	0.81
6.90	2.69	2.56	15.98	2.43	7.40	4.46
7.14	3.36	1.60	16.44	3.30	8.30	4.01
6.03	1.39	2.38	14.08	2.19	7.42	2.77
31.04	7.15	12.26	72.50	11.28	38.22	14.27
40.20	5.68	16.27	0.76	0.11	0.16	0.32
15.11	4.33	10.46	78.45	6.74	44.47	23.56
0.00	0.00	0.00	0.55	0.11	0.09	0.22
0.00	0.00	0.00	7.90	2.30	3.67	1.00
128.70	0.00	30.75	3.05	0.68	0.02	1.67
0.00	0.00	0.00	0.59	0.10	0.13	0.17
0.00	0.00	0.00	1.04	0.21	0.25	0.38
33.42	9.42	13.04	55.74	7.27	28.61	17.69
1.39	0.00	0.00	24.41	8.78	11.49	2.62
0.00	0.00	0.00	0.83	0.11	0.10	0.41
0.00	0.00	0.00	2.68	0.99	0.73	0.32

(continues)

Food Description	Measure	Weight (g)	Kcal per serving (g)	Protein per serving (g)
Meat, Fish, Beans, and Other Proteins (*continued*)				
Pork sausage, link or patty, unprepared	1 link	25.00	72.00	3.85
Pork, bacon, rendered fat, cooked	3 oz	85.00	763.30	0.06
Pork, cured, ham (water added), rump, bone-in, lean, heated, roasted	3 oz	85.00	102.85	18.20
Pork, fresh, ground, raw	1 oz	28.35	74.56	4.79
Pork, fresh, Belly, raw	1 oz	28.35	146.85	2.65
Pork, fresh, leg, whole, lean and fat, raw	1 oz	28.35	69.46	4.94
Pork, fresh, loin, whole, lean and fat, raw	3 oz	85.00	168.30	16.78
Pork, fresh, shoulder, whole, lean and fat, raw	1 oz	28.35	66.91	4.87
Pout, ocean, raw	3 oz	85.00	67.15	14.14
Pumpkin and squash seeds, whole, roasted, without salt	1 cup	64.00	285.44	11.87
Quail, meat and skin, raw	1 quail	109.00	209.28	21.40
Refried beans, canned, fat-free	1 cup	231.00	182.49	12.34
Roast beef, deli style	1 slice, oval	9.30	10.70	1.73
Rockfish, Pacific, mixed species, raw	3 oz	85.00	76.50	15.61
Roe, mixed species, raw	1 tbsp	14.00	20.02	3.12
Roughy, orange, raw	3 oz	85.00	64.60	13.95
Ruffed grouse, breast meat, skinless, raw	4 oz	113.00	126.56	29.31
Sablefish, raw	3 oz	85.00	165.75	11.40
Salami Italian pork	1 oz	28.00	119.00	6.08
Salmon, Atlantic, wild, raw	3 oz	85.00	120.70	16.86
Sardine, Pacific, canned in tomato sauce, drained solid, with Bone	1 cup	89.00	164.65	18.57
Sausage, chicken, beef, pork, skinless, smoked	1 link	84.00	181.44	11.42
Sausage, Italian, pork, raw	1 link	113.00	390.98	16.10
Scallop, mixed species, raw	1 unit, 2 large or 5 small	30.00	20.70	3.62
Sea bass, mixed species, raw	1 fillet	129.00	125.13	23.77
Seatrout, mixed species, raw	3 oz	85.00	88.40	14.23
Seeds, Flaxseed	1 tbsp, whole	10.30	55.00	1.88
Seeds, sunflower seed kernels from shell, dry roasted, with salt added	1 cup	128.00	698.88	24.74
Smoked link sausage, pork	1 link	68.00	210.12	8.15
Snapper, mixed species, raw	3 oz	85.00	85.00	17.43
Soy protein isolate	1 oz	28.35	94.97	25.04
Soybeans, mature seeds, raw	1 cup	186.00	829.56	67.87
Spiny Lobster, mixed species, raw	3 oz	85.00	95.20	17.51
Squid, mixed species, raw	1 oz, boneless	28.35	26.08	4.42

Carbohydrate per serving (g)	Sugar per serving (g)	Fiber per serving (g)	Total fat per serving (g)	Saturated fat per serving (g)	Mono fat per serving (g)	Poly fat per serving (g)
0.23	0.23	0.00	6.20	1.89	2.46	1.11
0.00	0.00	0.00	84.58	27.19	35.22	8.95
0.74	0.71	0.00	3.03	1.07	1.37	0.33
0.00	0.00	0.00	6.01	2.23	2.68	0.54
0.00	0.00	0.00	15.03	5.48	7.00	1.60
0.00	0.00	0.00	5.35	1.85	2.38	0.57
0.00	0.00	0.00	10.69	3.71	4.77	1.14
0.00	0.00	0.00	5.10	1.77	2.27	0.54
0.00	0.00	0.00	0.77	0.27	0.28	0.03
34.40	0.00	11.78	12.42	2.35	3.86	5.66
0.00	0.00	0.00	13.13	3.68	4.56	3.25
31.19	1.41	10.86	1.04	0.21	0.10	0.66
0.06	0.03	0.00	0.34	0.12	0.14	0.03
0.00	0.00	0.00	1.14	0.29	0.33	0.34
0.21	0.00	0.00	0.90	0.20	0.23	0.37
0.00	0.00	0.00	0.60	0.01	0.20	0.09
0.00	0.00	0.00	0.99	0.15	0.05	0.15
0.00	0.00	0.00	13.01	2.72	6.85	1.74
0.34	0.34	0.00	10.36	3.67	5.10	1.01
0.00	0.00	0.00	5.39	0.83	1.79	2.16
0.48	0.38	0.09	9.30	2.39	4.29	1.88
6.80	1.60	0.00	12.01	4.03	6.02	0.71
0.73	0.00	0.00	35.40	12.74	16.20	4.55
0.95	0.00	0.00	0.15	0.04	0.01	0.04
0.00	0.00	0.00	2.58	0.66	0.55	0.96
0.00	0.00	0.00	3.07	0.86	0.75	0.62
2.97	0.16	2.81	4.34	0.38	0.78	2.96
19.60	3.49	11.52	63.74	6.68	12.17	42.09
0.64	0.64	0.00	19.20	6.33	7.62	2.47
0.00	0.00	0.00	1.14	0.24	0.21	0.39
0.00	0.00	0.00	0.96	0.12	0.18	0.47
56.10	13.63	17.30	37.09	5.36	8.19	20.93
2.07	0.00	0.00	1.28	0.20	0.23	0.50
0.87	0.00	0.00	0.39	0.10	0.03	0.15

(continues)

Food Description	Measure	Weight (g)	Kcal per serving (g)	Protein per serving (g)
Meat, Fish, Beans, and Other Proteins (*continued*)				
Sturgeon, mixed species, raw	3 oz	85.00	89.25	13.72
Sucker, white, raw	3 oz	85.00	78.20	14.25
Sunfish, pumpkin seed, raw	1 fillet	48.00	42.72	9.31
Swordfish, raw	3 oz	85.00	122.40	16.71
Tilefish, raw	3 oz	85.00	81.60	14.88
Tofu, dried-frozen (Koyadofu)	1 piece	17.00	81.09	8.92
Tofu, Fried	1 oz	28.35	76.55	5.34
Trout, mixed species, raw	1 fillet	79.00	116.92	16.41
Tuna salad	3 oz	85.00	158.95	13.63
Tuna, fresh, bluefin, raw	3 oz	85.00	122.40	19.83
Tuna, fresh, yellowfin, raw	1 oz, boneless	28.35	30.90	6.92
Turbot, European, raw	3 oz	85.00	80.75	13.64
Turkey white rotisserie deli cut	1.69 oz	48.00	53.76	6.48
Turkey bacon, unprepared	1 serving	14.00	31.64	2.23
Turkey breast, low salt, prepackaged or deli, luncheon meat	1 slice	28.00	30.52	6.11
Turkey from whole, light meat, raw	1 serving	85.00	96.90	20.11
Turkey from whole, dark meat, meat only, raw	1 serving	85.00	91.80	18.09
Turkey sausage, fresh, raw	1 serving	57.00	88.35	10.71
Turkey, breast, from whole bird, meat only, raw	4 oz	114.00	129.96	26.97
Turkey, Drumstk, from whole bird, meat only, raw	3 oz	85.00	92.65	20.11
Turkey, wing, from whole bird, meat only, raw	3 oz	85.00	96.90	20.11
Veal, breast, fat, cooked	1 oz	28.35	147.70	2.66
Veal, breast, plate half, boneless, lean and fat, cooked, braised	3 oz	85.00	239.70	22.04
Veal, Leg (top round), lean, raw	1 oz	28.35	30.33	6.03
Veal, loin, lean, raw	3 oz	85.00	96.90	18.57
Veal, shank (fore and hind), lean, raw	1 oz	28.35	30.62	5.47
Veggie burgers or soyburgers unprepared	1 pattie	70.00	123.90	10.99
Waleanuts, black, dried	1 cup, chopped	125.00	773.75	30.08
Whey, acid, dried	1 cup	57.00	193.23	6.69
Whey, sweet, dried	1 cup	145.00	511.85	18.75
whitefish, mixed species, raw	3 oz	85.00	113.90	16.23
Whiting, mixed species, raw	1 fillet	92.00	82.80	16.85
Winged beans, mature seeds, raw	1 cup	182.00	744.38	53.96
Wolffish, Atlantic, raw	3 oz	85.00	81.60	14.88
Yardlong beans, mature seeds, raw	1 cup	167.00	579.49	40.63
Yellowtail, mixed species, raw	3 oz	85.00	124.10	19.67

Carbohydrate per serving (g)	Sugar per serving (g)	Fiber per serving (g)	Total fat per serving (g)	Saturated fat per serving (g)	Mono fat per serving (g)	Poly fat per serving (g)
0.00	0.00	0.00	3.43	0.78	1.65	0.59
0.00	0.00	0.00	1.97	0.38	0.60	0.69
0.00	0.00	0.00	0.34	0.07	0.06	0.12
0.00	0.00	0.00	5.65	1.36	2.53	0.97
0.00	0.00	0.00	1.96	0.37	0.49	0.51
1.71	0.00	1.22	5.16	0.75	1.14	2.91
2.51	0.77	1.11	5.72	0.83	1.26	3.23
0.00	0.00	0.00	5.22	0.91	2.57	1.18
8.00	0.00	0.00	7.87	1.31	2.45	3.50
0.00	0.00	0.00	4.17	1.07	1.36	1.22
0.00	0.00	0.00	0.14	0.05	0.03	0.04
0.00	0.00	0.00	2.51	0.64	0.52	0.75
3.70	1.92	0.19	1.44	0.06	0.28	0.18
0.26	0.00	0.00	2.37	0.63	0.87	0.66
0.98	0.98	0.14	0.23	0.06	0.07	0.05
0.12	0.04	0.00	1.26	0.25	0.22	0.22
0.13	0.09	0.00	2.13	0.58	0.64	0.52
0.27	0.00	0.00	4.61	1.12	1.50	1.36
0.16	0.06	0.00	1.69	0.33	0.30	0.29
0.12	0.04	0.00	1.26	0.25	0.22	0.22
0.12	0.04	0.00	1.26	0.25	0.22	0.22
0.00	0.00	0.00	15.12	6.07	7.49	0.81
0.00	0.00	0.00	16.11	6.32	7.74	1.04
0.00	0.00	0.00	0.50	0.15	0.16	0.05
0.00	0.00	0.00	2.47	0.95	1.15	0.16
0.00	0.00	0.00	0.80	0.21	0.28	0.09
9.99	0.75	3.43	4.41	1.01	1.24	1.42
11.98	1.38	8.50	74.16	4.35	19.30	45.55
41.87	41.87	0.00	0.31	0.19	0.08	0.01
107.97	107.97	0.00	1.55	0.99	0.43	0.05
0.00	0.00	0.00	4.98	0.77	1.70	1.83
0.00	0.00	0.00	1.21	0.23	0.26	0.39
75.91	0.00	47.14	29.70	4.19	10.94	7.88
0.00	0.00	0.00	2.03	0.31	0.71	0.72
103.39	0.00	18.37	2.19	0.57	0.19	0.94
0.00	0.00	0.00	4.45	1.09	1.69	1.21

Food Description	Measure	Weight (g)	Kcal per serving (g)	Protein per serving (g)
Fats, Oils, and Sweets				
Animal fat, bacon grease	1 tsp	4.30	38.57	0.00
Cake, angel food, commonly prepared	1 piece	28.00	72.24	1.65
Cake, boston crm pie, commonly prepared	1 oz	28.35	71.44	0.68
Cake, cherry fudge with chocolate frosting	1 oz	28.35	74.84	0.68
Cake, chocolate, prepared from recipe without frosting	1 piece	95.00	352.45	5.04
Cake, gingerbread, dry mix	1 oz	28.35	123.89	1.25
Cake, pound, commonly prepared, other than all butter, enriched	1 piece	30.00	116.70	1.56
Cake, pudding-type, chocolate, dry mix	1 oz	28.35	110.85	1.30
Cake, white, prepared from recipe without frosting	1 piece	74.00	264.18	4.00
Cake, yellow, commonly prepared, with chocolate frosting, in-store bakery	1 piece	144.00	545.76	4.55
Cheesecake commonly prepared	1 oz	28.35	91.00	1.56
Coffeecake, cinnamon with crumb topping, commonly prepared, enriched	1 oz	28.35	118.50	1.93
Cookies, brownies, commonly prepared	1 oz	28.35	114.82	1.36
Cookies, butter, commonly prepared, enriched	1 oz	28.35	132.39	1.73
Cookies, chocolate chip, refrigerated dough	1 serving	33.00	148.83	1.31
Cookies, gingersnaps	1 oz	28.35	117.94	1.59
Cookies, graham crackers, plain or honey (including cinnamon)	1 oz	28.35	121.91	1.90
Cookies, oatmeal, commonly prepared, regular	1 oz	28.35	127.58	1.76
Cookies, peanut butter, commonly prepared, regular	1 oz	28.35	134.10	2.53
Cookies, raisin, soft-type	1 oz	28.35	113.68	1.16
Cookies, shortbread, commonly prepared, plain	1 oz	28.35	145.72	1.52
Cookies, sugar, commonly prepared, regular (including vanilla)	1 oz	28.35	131.54	1.52
Danish pastry, cheese	1 oz	28.35	106.03	2.27
Desserts, apple crisp, prepared-from-recipe	1/2 cup	141.00	227.01	2.47
Desserts, pudding, chocolate, dry mix, regular	1 package	99.00	358.38	2.57
Doughnuts, cake-type, chocolate, sugared or glazed	1 oz	28.35	118.22	1.28
Doughnuts, cake-type, plain, sugared or glazed	1 oz	28.35	120.77	1.47
Dressing, honey mustard, fat-free	2 tbsp	30.00	50.70	0.32
Fish oil, salmon	1 tbsp	13.60	122.67	0.00
Fish oil, sardine	1 tbsp	13.60	122.67	0.00
Margarine, regular, 80% fat, composite, stick, with salt	1 tbsp	14.00	100.38	0.02
Margarine-like spread, Smart Balance HeartRight Light Buttery Spread	1 tbsp	14.00	47.18	0.00

Carbohydrate per serving (g)	Sugar per serving (g)	Fiber per serving (g)	Total fat per serving (g)	Saturated fat per serving (g)	Mono fat per serving (g)	Poly fat per serving (g)
0.00	0.00	0.00	4.28	1.68	1.93	0.48
16.18	0.00	0.42	0.22	0.03	0.02	0.10
12.16	10.24	0.40	2.41	0.69	1.29	0.29
10.77	9.34	0.14	3.54	1.44	1.25	0.66
50.73	0.00	1.52	14.35	5.16	5.74	2.62
21.15	13.22	0.48	3.91	0.98	2.21	0.51
15.75	0.00	0.30	5.37	1.39	2.98	0.68
22.73	11.21	0.65	2.31	0.57	0.79	0.64
42.33	26.26	0.59	9.18	2.42	3.93	2.33
79.72	56.48	2.16	25.56	8.34	10.39	6.81
7.23	6.18	0.11	6.38	2.81	2.45	0.45
13.24	0.00	0.57	6.61	1.64	3.68	0.88
18.12	10.38	0.60	4.62	1.20	2.54	0.64
19.53	5.74	0.23	5.33	3.13	1.57	0.28
20.14	12.55	0.50	7.04	2.77	3.44	0.72
21.80	5.65	0.62	2.78	0.69	1.52	0.39
22.02	7.04	0.96	3.01	0.46	0.71	1.53
19.48	6.99	0.79	5.13	1.28	2.84	0.72
16.49	8.10	0.60	6.75	1.91	3.06	1.02
19.28	13.48	0.34	3.86	0.98	2.17	0.50
18.08	6.14	0.37	7.43	2.30	1.90	2.36
19.09	7.74	0.37	5.54	2.17	1.98	1.06
10.55	1.97	0.28	6.21	1.93	3.21	0.73
43.48	27.75	1.97	4.84	0.97	1.88	1.61
88.41	42.45	4.46	2.08	1.22	0.70	0.08
16.27	9.05	0.62	5.64	1.45	3.20	0.70
14.40	0.00	0.43	6.49	1.68	3.60	0.82
11.53	5.33	0.36	0.44	0.10	0.21	0.09
0.00	0.00	0.00	13.60	2.70	3.95	5.48
0.00	0.00	0.00	13.60	4.07	4.60	4.33
0.10	0.00	0.00	11.30	2.13	5.44	3.40
0.28	0.00	0.00	5.10	1.41	1.92	1.35

(continues)

Fats, Oils, and Sweets (*continued*)

Food Description	Measure	Weight (g)	Kcal per serving (g)	Protein per serving (g)
Margarine-like, margarine-butter blend, soybean oil and butter	1 tbsp	14.10	102.51	0.04
Margarine-like, vegetable oil-butter spread, tub, with salt	1 tbsp	14.00	50.68	0.14
Oil, almond	1 tbsp	13.60	120.22	0.00
Oil, avocado	1 tbsp	14.00	123.76	0.00
Oil, canola	1 tbsp	14.00	123.76	0.00
Oil, cocnt	1 tbsp	13.60	121.31	0.00
Oil, cocoa butter	1 tbsp	13.60	120.22	0.00
Oil, hazelnut	1 tbsp	13.60	120.22	0.00
Oil, industrial, canola for salads, woks and light frying	1 tbsp	13.60	120.22	0.00
Oil, olive, salad or cooking	1 tbsp	13.50	119.34	0.00
Oil, Pam Cooking Spray, original	1 spray	0.30	2.38	0.00
Oil, peanut, salad or cooking	1 tbsp	13.50	119.34	0.00
Oil, poppyseed	1 tbsp	13.60	120.22	0.00
Oil, sesame, salad or cooking	1 tbsp	13.60	120.22	0.00
Oil, sunflower, linoleic (less than 60%)	1 tbsp	13.60	120.22	0.00
Pie crust, standard-type, dry mix, prepared, baked	1 piece	20.00	100.20	1.34
Pie crust, standard-type, frozen, ready-to-bake, enriched	1 piece	18.00	82.26	1.11
Pie, apple, commonly prepared, enriched flour	1 oz	28.35	67.19	0.54
Pie, banana cream, prepared from mix, no-bake type	1 oz	28.35	71.16	0.96
Pie, blueberry, commonly prepared	1 oz	28.35	65.77	0.51
Pie, cherry, commonly prepared	1 oz	28.35	73.71	0.57
Pie, coconut creme, commonly prepared	1 oz	28.35	84.48	0.60
Pie, lemon meringue, commonly prepared	1 oz	28.35	75.98	0.43
Pie, peach	1 oz	28.35	63.50	0.54
Pie, pumpkin, commonly prepared	1 oz	28.35	68.89	1.11
Pie, vanilla cream, prepared from recipe	1 oz	28.35	78.81	1.36
Puddings, banana, dry mix, inst	1 package	99.00	363.33	0.00
Puddings, chocolate, ready-to-eat	1 oz	28.35	40.26	0.59
Puddings, coconut cream, dry mix, regular	1 package	88.00	381.92	0.88
Puddings, lemon, dry mix, instant	1 package	99.00	374.22	0.00
Puddings, rice, dry mix, prepared with 2% milk	1/2 cup	128.00	142.08	4.21
Puddings, tapioca, ready-to-eat, fat free	1 container	112.00	105.28	1.61
Puddings, vanilla, dry mix, instant, prep with whole milk	1/2 cup	142.00	161.88	3.83

Carbohydrate per serving (g)	Sugar per serving (g)	Fiber per serving (g)	Total fat per serving (g)	Saturated fat per serving (g)	Mono fat per serving (g)	Poly fat per serving (g)
0.11	0.00	0.00	11.33	2.00	4.27	3.41
0.14	0.00	0.00	5.60	1.01	2.58	1.76
0.00	0.00	0.00	13.60	1.12	9.51	2.37
0.00	0.00	0.00	14.00	1.62	9.88	1.89
0.00	0.00	0.00	14.00	1.03	8.86	3.94
0.00	0.00	0.00	13.47	11.22	0.86	0.23
0.00	0.00	0.00	13.60	8.12	4.47	0.41
0.00	0.00	0.00	13.60	1.01	10.61	1.39
0.00	0.00	0.00	13.60	1.06	8.32	3.59
0.00	0.00	0.00	13.50	1.86	9.85	1.42
0.06	0.00	0.00	0.24	0.02	0.15	0.07
0.00	0.00	0.00	13.50	2.28	6.24	4.32
0.00	0.00	0.00	13.60	1.84	2.68	8.49
0.00	0.00	0.00	13.60	1.93	5.40	5.67
0.00	0.00	0.00	13.60	1.37	6.17	5.45
10.08	0.00	0.36	6.08	1.54	3.46	0.77
8.75	0.67	0.45	4.69	1.47	2.19	0.57
9.64	4.44	0.45	3.12	1.08	1.24	0.62
8.96	0.00	0.17	3.66	1.96	1.29	0.22
9.89	2.80	0.28	2.84	0.48	1.20	1.00
11.28	4.05	0.23	3.12	0.73	1.65	0.58
10.57	5.25	0.37	4.71	1.98	2.06	0.44
13.38	6.76	0.34	2.47	0.50	0.76	1.03
9.33	4.60	0.23	2.84	0.43	1.20	1.06
9.87	5.35	0.51	2.76	0.56	1.30	0.50
9.24	3.59	0.17	4.08	1.14	1.71	0.97
91.77	75.80	0.00	0.59	0.09	0.14	0.35
6.52	4.87	0.00	1.30	0.36	0.77	0.03
72.02	70.88	1.41	10.00	10.00	0.00	0.00
94.45	0.00	0.00	0.69	0.10	0.28	0.25
26.64	0.00	0.13	2.09	1.24	0.56	0.08
23.87	15.88	0.00	0.39	0.14	0.01	0.00
27.97	25.60	0.00	4.12	2.47	1.19	0.21

(continues)

Food Description	Measure	Weight (g)	Kcal per serving (g)	Protein per serving (g)
Fats, Oils, and Sweets (*continued*)				
Salad dressing, 1000 island, commercial, regular	1 tbsp	16.00	60.64	0.17
Salad dressing, blue or roquefort cheese, low calorie	1 tbsp	15.00	14.85	0.77
Salad dressing, caesar dressing, regular	1 tbsp	14.70	79.67	0.32
Salad dressing, French dressing, commercial, regular	1 tbsp	16.00	73.12	0.12
Salad dressing, Italian dressing, commercial, regular	1 tbsp	14.70	35.28	0.06
Salad dressing, ranch dressing, regular	1 tbsp	15.00	64.50	0.20
Salad dressing, sesame seed dressing, regular	1 tbsp	15.00	66.45	0.47
Shortening, household, partially hydrogenated soybean-cottonseed	1 tbsp	12.80	113.15	0.00
Strudel, apple	1 oz	28.35	77.68	0.94
Sugars, brown	1 tsp, unpacked	3.00	11.40	0.00
Sugars, granulated	1 packet	2.80	10.84	0.00
Sugars, powdered	1 cup, unsifted	120.00	466.80	0.00
Syrups, table blends, cane and 15% maple	1 cup	315.00	875.70	0.00
Toppings, butterscotch or caramel	2 tbsp	41.00	88.56	0.50
Toppings, strawberry	2 tbsp	42.00	106.68	0.08
Vegetable oil spread, 60% fat, stick/tub/bottle, without salt	1 tbsp	14.00	74.62	0.02
Vegetable oil spread, unspecified oils, approximately 37% fat, with salt	1 tbsp	14.90	50.51	0.08

Carbohydrate per serving (g)	Sugar per serving (g)	Fiber per serving (g)	Total fat per serving (g)	Saturated fat per serving (g)	Mono fat per serving (g)	Poly fat per serving (g)
2.34	2.43	0.13	5.61	0.81	1.26	2.92
0.44	0.42	0.00	1.08	0.39	0.27	0.36
0.49	0.41	0.07	8.50	1.29	1.99	4.83
2.49	2.55	0.00	7.17	0.90	1.35	3.36
1.78	1.58	0.00	3.10	0.43	0.83	1.58
0.89	0.70	0.00	6.68	1.04	1.38	3.87
1.29	1.25	0.15	6.78	0.93	1.79	3.77
0.00	0.00	0.00	12.80	3.20	5.70	3.34
11.65	7.30	0.62	3.18	0.58	0.93	1.51
2.94	2.91	0.00	0.00	0.00	0.00	0.00
2.80	2.79	0.00	0.00	0.00	0.00	0.00
119.72	117.37	0.00	0.00	0.00	0.00	0.00
218.99	214.83	0.32	0.32	0.06	0.10	0.16
23.37	23.37	0.00	0.00	0.00	0.00	0.00
27.85	11.50	0.29	0.04	0.00	0.01	0.02
0.12	0.00	0.00	8.37	1.69	2.71	3.71
0.10	0.00	0.00	5.63	1.29	2.08	1.85

Appendix B

Developing a Sample Meal Plan

Step 1

Using **Table 7.1**, calculate your Resting Metabolic Rate (RMR).

Gender:		Age (years):
Weight (kg):		**Height (cm):**
Fat Free Mass (FFM; kg):		**Date:**

RMR Equation	For Males	For Females
Harris–Benedict	66.4730 + (13.7516 × Weight) + (5.0033 × Height) − (6.7750 × Age) 66.4730 + (13.7516 × ____) + (5.0033 × ____) − (6.7750 × ____) = _____	665.09550 + (9.563 × Weight) + (1.8496 × Height) − (4.6756 × Age) 665.09550 + (9.563 × ____) + (1.8496 × ____) − (4.6756 × ____) = _____
Cunningham	500 + (22 × FFM) 500 + (22 × ____) = _____	500 + (22 × FFM) 500 + (22 × ____) = _____
Mifflin–St. Jeor	(10 × Weight) + (6.25 × Height) − (5 × Age) + 5 (10 × ____) + (6.25 × ____) − (5 × ____) + 5 = _____	(10 × Weight) + (6.25 × Height) − (5 × Age) − 161 (10 × ____) + (6.25 × ____) − (5 × ____) − 161 = _____

Step 2

Using **Table 7.2**, select the appropriate Physical Activity Category (PAC), and associated Physical Activity Level (PAL), to calculate your predicted Exercise Energy Expenditure (EEE).

PAC	PAL Coefficient	Exercise Energy Expenditure (EEE)
Sedentary	1.25	EEE = RMR (_____) × 1.25 = _____
Low Activity	1.50	EEE = RMR (_____) × 1.50 = _____
Active	1.75	EEE = RMR (_____) × 1.75 = _____
Very Active	2.20	EEE = RMR (_____) × 2.20 = _____

Step 3

Calculate the Thermal Effect of Food (TEF) and Total Daily Energy Expenditure (TDEE).

$$\text{TEF} = \text{EEE} (\underline{\hspace{2cm}}) \times 0.10 = \underline{\hspace{2cm}} \quad (\textit{round to the nearest 100 kcal})$$

$$\text{TDEE} = \text{EEE} (\underline{\hspace{2cm}}) + (\text{TEF}) (\underline{\hspace{2cm}}) = \underline{\hspace{2cm}}$$

Remember, if your goal is to

- Lose weight: Subtract between 250–500 kcal from your TDEE
- Gain weight: Add between 250–500 kcal from your TDEE
- Maintain weight: Consume the same number of kcal as your TDEE

Step 4

Using **Table 8.1**, select the appropriate Acceptable Macronutrient Distribution Range (AMDR).

AMDR Recommendation	CHO	PRO	FAT
Institute of Medicine (IOM)	45–65%	10–35%	20–35%
Endurance Athlete	55–65%	15–25%	20–30%
Mixed Athlete	50–55%	20–25%	25–30%
Strength Athlete	45–50%	20–30%	20–30%

Desired CHO %	Desired PRO %	Desired FAT %

Step 5

Multiply your TDEE from Step 3 by your desired CHO, PRO, and FAT % from Step 4 to determine the exact number of calories you should be consuming for each macronutrient per day.

	TDEE	Desired %	(TDEE x Desired %) =
CHO			
PRO			
FAT			

Step 6

Using **Tables 8.4** and **8.5**, select the appropriate Macronutrient Distribution based off your workout schedule then calculate the number of calories (kcal) required for each macronutrient per meal.

	CHO %	CHO Kcal	PRO %	PRO Kcal	FAT %	FAT Kcal
Meal 1						
Meal 2						
Meal 3						
Meal 4						
Meal 5						

Step 7

Using **Appendix A**, select appropriate food items to match the distribution requirements for each macronutrient per meal.

Meal 1

	Recommended Kcal	Actual Kcal	Serving Size	Quantity	Food Description
CHO					
PRO					
FAT					

Meal 2

	Recommended Kcal	Actual Kcal	Serving Size	Quantity	Food Description
CHO					
PRO					
FAT					

Meal 3

	Recommended Kcal	Actual Kcal	Serving Size	Quantity	Food Description
CHO					
PRO					
FAT					

Meal 4

	Recommended Kcal	Actual Kcal	Serving Size	Quantity	Food Description
CHO					
PRO					
FAT					

Meal 5

	Recommended Kcal	Actual Kcal	Serving Size	Quantity	Food Description
CHO					
PRO					
FAT					

Remember, to calculate **Actual Kcal**

- For CHO: Multiply number of grams by 4
- For PRO: Multiply number of grams by 4
- For FAT: Multiply number of grams by 9

Step 8

Repeat **Steps 1–7**, as may be necessary, to accommodate different training days (i.e., off days, light days, active days, and very active days) and workout schedules (i.e., morning workout, lunchtime workout, evening workout).

Glossary of Terms

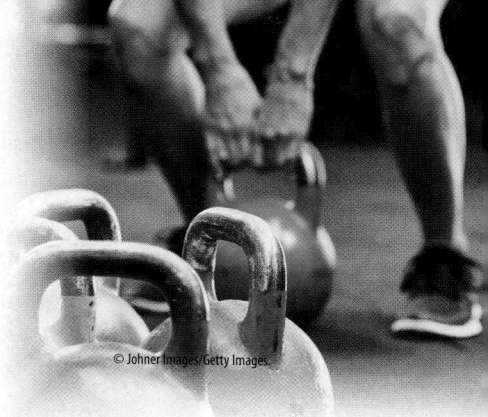

© Johner Images/Getty Images.

1-Repetition maximum (1RM): Greatest amount of weight that can be lifted for one repetition.

2-for-2 Rule: Progression recommendation in strength training requiring weight be added when you can perform two or more repetitions over the assigned repetition goal in the last set for two consecutive workouts.

Actin: A cellular protein found in microfilaments that is active in muscular contraction, cellular movement, and maintenance of cell shape.

Active rest: A means of recovery during or post workout that involves either stretching or exercising at lower intensity.

Adenosine: A nucleoside involved in the energy metabolism of cells.

Adenosine diphosphate (ADP): A nucleotide composed of adenosine and two phosphate groups that is formed as an intermediate between ATP and AMP and that is reversibly converted to ATP by the addition of a high-energy phosphate group.

Adenosine triphosphate (ATP): Principal molecule for storing and transferring energy in cells.

Aerobic activity: Any form of sustained *exercise* (e.g., jogging, rowing, swimming, or cycling) that stimulates and strengthens the heart and lungs thereby improving the body's utilization of oxygen.

Aerobic metabolism: Means of producing energy through the combustion of carbohydrates, amino acids, and fats in the presence of oxygen.

Agonist muscle: Most skeletal muscle is arranged in opposing pairs. The contracting muscle is the agonist muscle during an exercise.

Air displacement plethysmography (aka BodPod): A method that uses air displacement to determine body volume in order to calculate percent body fat.

Alkaloid: Any class of nitrogenous organic compounds of plant origin that have pronounced physiological actions in humans.

Alveoli: The tiny air sacs within the lungs that allow for rapid gaseous exchange.

Amino acids: Amino acids are the building blocks of proteins. The body absorbs amino acids through the small intestine into the blood.

Amortization phase: One of the three plyometric phases of movement that occurs between the concentric and eccentric phases and is considered to be the most crucial phase in the body's ability to produce power.

Anabolism: Synthesis of complex molecules from simpler ones.

Anaerobic metabolism: Means of producing energy through the combustion of carbohydrates in the absence of oxygen.

Android: Apple-shaped fat distribution mainly around the trunk and upper body, such as the abdomen, chest, shoulder, and neck.

Angle of pennation: An angle formed between the orientation of the muscle fibers and the long axis of its tendon.

Antagonist muscle: Most skeletal muscle is arranged in opposing pairs. The contracting muscle is the agonist muscle during an exercise. The antagonist muscle is the opposite (opposing) the agonist muscle.

Anthropometry: Study of the measurements and proportions of the human body.

Antioxidant: Substance that removes potentially damaging oxidizing agents in the body.

Appendicular skeleton: Bones that comprise the limbs as well as shoulder and pelvic girdles.

Arterial system: A system of arteries and arterioles that carry oxygenated blood away from the heart.

Arteriole: A small diameter blood vessel in the microcirculation that extends and branches out from an artery and leads to capillaries.

Arteries: Large diameter blood vessels that carries blood from the heart to another part of the body.

Arthritis: Painful inflammation and/or stiffness of the joints.

Assistance exercise: Recruit smaller muscle areas, involve only one primary joint, and are considered less important to improving sport performance.

Atrium: Either of the two upper chambers of the heart that receive blood from the veins and in turn push it into the ventricles.

Axial skeleton: Bones that comprise the skull and vertebral column.

Balance: The ability to stay upright or stay in control of body movement; coordination is the ability to move two or more body parts under control, smoothly and efficiently. There are two types of balance: static and dynamic.

Beta oxidation: Catabolic process by which fatty acid molecules are broken down in the mitochondria to form acetyl-CoA and enter the Krebs cycle.

Bioavailability: Proportion of a drug or other substance that enters circulation that is able to have an active effect.

Bioelectrical impedance (BIA): A method of estimating percent body fat that uses a painless electrical current to determine the amount of fat mass and fat-free mass within the body.

Bioenergetics: Study of the transformation of energy in living organisms.

Biological age: Subjective age based on an individual's development.

Body composition: Any method of measure used to describe the percentages of fat, bone, water and muscle.

Body composition assessment (BCA): method (e.g., circumference measurements, skin-folds) used to estimate a person's percent body fat.

Body mass index (BMI): A weight-to-height ratio, calculated by dividing weight in kilograms by the square of height in meters, which is used as an indicator of obesity and underweight.

Bronchi: Either of the two main branches of the trachea leading into the lungs where they divide into smaller branches (bronchioles).

Bronchioles: Tiny branch of air tubes within the lungs that connect the bronchi to the alveoli (air sacs).

Caloric density: Refers to the calorie content of food. Examples of calorie dense (in contrast to nutrient dense) foods include potato chips, desserts, and candy.

Capillaries: Tiny blood vessels that facilitate the exchange of oxygen, nutrients, hormones, and other substances between the blood and the interstitial fluid in the various tissues of the body.

Carbohydrate: One of the three essential macronutrients, along with fats and protein, used as an energy source by the body. Carbohydrates come in simple forms such as sugars and in complex forms such as starches and fiber. The body breaks down most sugars and starches into glucose, which the body uses to fuel the cells. Complex carbohydrates are derived from plants.

Carbonic anhydrase: An enzyme that catalyzes the decomposition of carbonic acid into carbon dioxide and water, facilitating transfer of carbon dioxide from tissues to blood and from blood to alveolar air.

Cardiac Output: The amount of blood the heart pumps through the circulatory system in a minute. Stroke volume and the heart rate determine cardiac output.

Cardiovascular fitness: Ability of the heart and lungs to supply oxygen to the working muscle tissues as well as the ability of the muscles to use that oxygen to produce energy for movement.

Cartilaginous joints: Joint covered with cartilage to allow movement between bones.

Catabolism: Breakdown of complex molecules from simpler ones.

Catecholamines: Class of aromatic amines (organic compound derived from ammonia) that includes neurotransmitters such as epinephrine and dopamine.

Celiac disease: A disease in which the small intestine is hypersensitive to gluten thereby leading to issues with digestion.

Cholesterol: Cholesterol is a waxy, fat-like substance found in all cells of the body. The body needs some cholesterol to make hormones, vitamin D, and substances that help in digestion. The body can manufacture all the cholesterol it needs; however, cholesterol can also be found in food (animal products). High levels of cholesterol in the blood can increase the risk of heart disease.

Chronological age: Number of years that an individual has lived.

Circuit training: A form of conditioning or resistance training that incorporates both strength building and muscular endurance. A "circuit" is one completion of all prescribed exercises in the program.

Circumference measurements (aka girth measurements): A method used to assess body composition that involves taking measurements at various sites in order to predict percent body fat.

Closed kinetic chain (CKC): Exercises where the hand (for arm movement) or foot (for leg movement) are fixed, cannot move, and remains in constant contact with an immobile surface, usually the ground or base of a machine (e.g., leg press).

Cluster sets: Sets that incorporate intra-set rest periods that allow for better manipulation of volume and intensity.

Collagen: Main structural protein found in connective tissue.

Complex carbohydrates: Excess glucose linked together for storage.

Complex training: A form of conditioning that combines resistance training with plyometric training.

Compound set: A compound set involves sequentially performing two different exercises for the same muscle group.

Concentric contraction: A type of muscle activation that increases tension on a muscle as it shortens.

Cool-down: Easy exercise completed immediately after more intense activity to allow the body to gradually transition to a resting or near-resting state.

Core exercise: Recruit one or more large muscle areas, involve two or more primary joints, and receive priority because of their direct application to the sport.

Corticosteriod injection: A shot used to provide short-term pain relief and reduce swelling and inflammation in a joint, tendon, or bursa.

Cortisol: A glucocorticoid produced by the adrenal cortex that mediates various metabolic processes, has anti-inflammatory and immosuppressive properties.

Counter-movements: Movement in which the athlete begins from an upright standing position, initiates a downward movement by flexing the knees and hips, then immediately extends the knees and hips again to jump vertically off the ground.

Creatine kinase: An enzyme that when elevated in the blood is a marker of damaged tissue in either the brain, skeletal muscle, or heart.

Creatine phosphate (CP): A phosphate group found in muscle cells that stores phosphates to provide energy for muscular contraction.

Crepitus: Any grinding, creaking, cracking, grating, crunching, or popping sound that occurs when moving a joint.

Criterion performance standards: Use normative data that ranks individuals against an established standard (e.g., pass/fail cut-off score).

Cytokines: Substances secreted by immune system cells that have an effect on other cells within the body.

Deload: A short planned period of recovery. A typical deload period will last a week.

Detraining: Physiological adaptations associated with chronic exercise are not permanent. Once the stimulus is reduced or eliminated, the biological system(s) will revert back to pre-training levels.

Dietary supplements: A dietary supplement is a product taken to supplement the diet and typically contain one or more of the following ingredients vitamins, minerals, herbs or other botanicals (of or pertaining to plants), amino acids, as well as various other substances. Supplements are not required to go through the testing of effectiveness and safety that drugs do.

Diffusion: The passive movement of molecules (e.g., oxygen, carbon dioxide) along a concentration gradient traveling from regions of higher to regions of lower concentration.

Directed adaptation: A fundamental principle to exercise programming that states that in order to get better at something, you must train it over and over.

Disaccharide: Two monosaccharides linked together.

Distal attachment: An attachment that is situated far from the point of attachment to the body.

Dual energy x-ray absorptiometry (DEXA): A method of estimating percent body fat that uses two x-ray beams of different energy levels to determine fat mass, lean mass, and muscle mass.

Duration: Amount of time spent exercising within a specific training session.

Dyspnea: Difficult or labored breathing.

Eccentric contraction: A type of muscle activation that increases tension on a muscle as it lengthens.

Eccentric training: A strength training technique which exaggerates the lengthening phase of a movement and allows for 30–40 percent more weight to be lifted than can be done concentrically (muscle shortening phase). (Also known as negative training).

Ectomorph: Body type that is lean and delicate.

Elasticity: Ability of connective tissue to return to its original length after a passive stretch.

Electrolytes: Electrolytes are minerals found in the body fluids. They include sodium, potassium, magnesium, and chloride. When you are dehydrated, your body does not have enough fluid and electrolytes.

Electron transport chain (ETC): A series of complexes that transfer electrons from electron donors to electron acceptors and couples with the transfer of protons across a membrane.

Endergonic reaction: A reaction that requires energy to be driven.

Endomorphic: Body type that is round and with a high proportion of body fat.

Exercise energy expenditure: Amount of energy expended during physical activity (e.g., endurance training, strength training).

Ergogenic aid: Any method or product used to enhance mental and physical performance or recovery.

Essential amino acids (aka indispensable amino acids): Amino acids that must be consumed in the diet because the body cannot make them.

Excess post-exercise oxygen consumption (EPOC): A measurably increased rate of oxygen intake following strenuous activity intended to erase the body's "oxygen deficit".

Exercise economy: Relates to the quantity of oxygen (ml/kg/min) required to move at a given speed or generate a specific amount of power and influenced by a number of factors including: neuro-muscular co-ordination, percentage of type I muscle fibers, elastic energy storage, and joint stability and flexibility.

Exergonic reaction: A reaction that loses energy as a result of the reaction.

Fad diets: Diets that promises quick weight loss through unhealthy and unbalanced dietary means.

Fartlek: Swedish for "speed play", is a form of endurance training that combines long slow distance (LSD) with interval training.

Fast glycolysis: Method of providing energy for activities of short duration (i.e., 10–30 seconds), that replenishes very quickly and produces 2 ATP molecules per glucose molecule.

Fast-Twitch Fiber: A type of muscle fiber that is composed of strong, rapidly contracting fibers, adapted for high-intensity, low-endurance activities.

Fat: Along with carbohydrates and protein, fat is one of the three major sources of energy in the diet. Fat contains 9 calories per gram, which is more than twice that provided by carbohydrates or protein (4 calories per gram). Due to its high caloric content, a high intake of fat increases the risk for obesity. Fat is used to help insulate the body as well aid in the absorption of certain vitamins.

Fatigue management: After several weeks of hard training, recovery becomes incomplete as fatigue accumulates over time thereby requiring an intentional decrease in training volume and/or intensity.

Fatty acids: Fatty acids are a major component of fats and are used by the body for energy and tissue development.

Feasibility: Practicality of a test in terms of cost, man-power, equipment, and space.

Fiber: Fiber is a carbohydrate substance found in plants. Fiber helps you feel full faster and stay full longer – which can help in terms of weight control. Fiber also aids in digestion and helps prevent constipation.

Fiber type transition: Adaptation of specific muscle fibers (typically the intermediate muscle fibers) to become more aerobic or anaerobic in nature as a result of training.

Fibrosis: Process in which fibrous connective tissue starts to replace degenerating muscle fibers.

Fibrous joints: Form of articulation in which bones are connected by a fibrous tissue. Fibrous joints have no joint cavity and movement is minimal or nonexistent.

Field test: A test used to assess ability that is performed away from the laboratory and does not require extensive training or expensive equipment to administer.

First-class lever: A situation when a lever has the fulcrum in the middle with a muscle attachment on one side and the load (resistance) on the other.

Fitness test: A series of exercises designed to assess fitness (e.g., endurance, strength, agility, etc.).

Fitness trident: Depicts the three most important components of fitness and foundation of any strength and conditioning program. Specifically: strength, endurance, and mobility.

Flavin adenine dinucleotide (FADH): One of two redox cofactors created during the Krebs cycle that is used during the electron transport chain to produce energy (ATP).

Flexibility: Range of motion of the joints or the ability of the joints to move freely through their entire range of motion.

Frequency: Number of times one exercises within a specified period of time.

Fulcrum: The point on which a level rests or pivots.

Genetic potential: Theoretical optimum performance capability which an individual could achieve in a specific activity, after an ideal upbringing, nutrition, and training.

Gluconeogenesis: Formation of glucose from precursors other than carbohydrates (e.g., amino acids, glycerol from fats, or lactate produced by muscle during anaerobic glycolysis).

Gluten: Gluten (derived from the Latin word glue) is a mixture of proteins found in wheat, rye, and barley which gives elasticity to dough, helping it rise, and gives the final product a chewing texture. It can also be found in products such as vitamin and nutrient supplements, lip balms, and certain medicines. It is important to note that less than 1% of the general population has Celiac disease (autoimmune disorder of the small intestines) which would require a gluten-free diet.

Glycemic index: Instead of counting the total amount of carbohydrates in foods in their unconsumed state, Glycemic Index (GI) measures the actual impact of these foods on blood sugar. Foods are ranked as being very low, low, medium, or high in their GI value. Low-GI diets have been associated with decreased risk of cardiovascular disease, type 2 diabetes, metabolic syndrome, stroke, depression, chronic kidney disease, formation of gall stones, neural tube defects, formation of uterine fibroids, and cancers of the breast, colon, prostate, and pancreas.

Glycemic load: Takes into account the number of grams of carbohydrate in a food to determine how quickly the food raises blood glucose levels. It can be calculated by multiplying the glycemic index of the food by the grams of carbohydrate in a serving of that food, divided by 100.

Glycogen: Storage form of carbohydrates in skeletal muscles and the liver.

Glycolysis: Process in cell metabolism by which carbohydrates and sugars, especially glucose, are broken down to produce ATP and pyruvic acid.

Golgi tendon organ: Proprioceptive sensory receptor organ that senses changes in muscle tension.

Gynoid: Pear-shaped fat distribution pattern mainly around the lower upper body, such as the hips, thighs, and butt.

Half-life: Time taken for the radioactivity of a specified isotope to fall to half of its original value.

Heme: Non-protein part of hemoglobin found in animal products.

Hemoglobin: The oxygen-carrying pigment and predominate protein found in red blood cells.

Henneman's size principle: Under load, motor units are recruited from smallest to largest.

Herniated disk: A rupture of the annulus fibrosis (fibrocartilagenous material that surrounds the intervertebral disk) enabling the nucleus pulposus (gelatinous substance in the center portion of the intervertebral disk) to extrude through the fibers.

High-intensity interval training: A form of interval training that alternates short periods of intense anaerobic exercise with less-intense recovery periods.

High-tension exercises: Exercises in which one tenses a specific muscle then moves that muscle against tension as if simulating that a heavy weight were being lifted.

Hypertrophy: A method of strength training intended to induce muscle growth.

Hypoglycemia: Low blood sugar condition that occurs when the level of glucose in the blood drops below normal.

Hypoxia training: a type of training that uses a specially designed mask or device to reduce the amount of oxygen being taken in by the lungs and/or being delivered to the working muscles. In theory, doing so allows the body to become more efficient at consuming, delivering, and utilizing oxygen.

Incontinence: Lack of voluntary control over urination or defecation.

Indispensable amino acids: Amino acids that must consumed in the diet because they can not be manufactured in the human body.

Individuality: Genetics plays a major role in how fast and to what degree one will respond to a particular training program.

Inferior attachment: An attachment that is situated closer to or towards the feet.

Injury analysis: Part of the needs analysis that evaluates common sites for joint and muscle injuries as well as causative factors.

Intensity: Amount of effort or work that must be invested into a specific training session.

Intermediate fibers (aka fast oxidative-glycolytic fibers): Fast twitch muscle fibers that have been converted via endurance training. These fibers are slightly larger in diameter, have more mitochondria, greater blood supply, and more fatigue resistance than typical fast twitch fibers.

Intermittent fasting: Specific dietary strategy that requires an intentional abstention from food, drink, or both, for a period of time for the primary purpose of losing weight.

Interval training: A form of endurance training that involves high-intensity intervals (typically 3–5 minutes in duration) close to VO_2max.

Ischemia: Inadequate blood supply to an organ (especially the heart) or part of the body.

Isokinetic contraction: Muscular contraction that occurs at a constant speed. A piece of equipment called an Isokinetic Dynamometer is used to measure the (constant) speed of isokinetic muscle contraction.

Isometric contraction: A type of strength training in which the joint angle and muscle length do not change during contraction (as compared to isotonic contractions).

Isotonic contraction: Muscular contraction against resistance in which the length of the muscle changes. Isotonic movements are either concentric or eccentric.

Joint: Point of articulation between two or more bones.

Ketones: Organic compound containing a carbonyl group bonded to two hydrocarbon groups formed when fats (instead of carbohydrates) are broken down for energy.

Lactate: Byproduct of glucose utilization by muscle cells during anaerobic glycolysis.

Lactate threshold: The intensity of exercise at which lactate begins to accumulate in the blood at a faster rate than it can be removed.

Linear periodization: Traditional model with gradual progressive increases in intensity over time.

Load: Amount of weight assigned to an exercise set.

Long slow distance (LSD) training: A form of continuous training performed at a constant pace of low to moderate intensity over an extended distance or duration.

Macronutrient: Type of food (e.g., fat, protein, carbohydrate) required in large amounts in the human diet.

Magnetic resonance imaging (MRI): A procedure that uses magnetism, radio waves, and a computer to create pictures from inside the body.

Maximal lactate steady state (MLSS): Highest blood lactate concentration and work load that can be maintained over time without a continual blood lactate accumulation.

Mesocycle: One of the three cycles of traditional periodization and represents a specific block of training designed to accomplish a particular training goal. Mesocylces typically last a month but can range anywhere from 2 weeks to several months.

Mesomorph: Body type that is compact and muscular.

Metabolic equivalent (MET): A MET also is defined as oxygen uptake in ml/kg/min with one MET equal to the oxygen cost of sitting quietly, equivalent to 3.5 ml/kg/min.

Metabolism: Metabolism is the total processes (both anabolic and catabolic) used by the body to get or make energy from food.

Microcycle: The shortest of the three cycles of traditional periodization and typically lasts about a week.

Micronutrient: Type of food (e.g., vitamins, minerals) required in trace amounts in the human diet.

Minerals: Consist of inorganic elements found in foods that are essential to certain metabolic functions. Examples include sodium, potassium, chloride, calcium, phosphate, sulfate, magnesium, iron, copper, zinc, manganese, iodine, selenium, and molybdenum.

Minute ventilation: Amount of air (in liters) that a person breathes per minute. Minute ventilation is calculated by multiplying respiratory rate and tidal volume (normal volume of air displaced between normal inhalation and exhalation).

Mobility: Degree to which a joint is allowed to move before being restricted by surrounding tissue.

Monosaccharide: Single sugar unit, such as glucose.

Monounsaturated fat: Type of fat found in avocados, canola oil, nuts, olives and olive oil, and seeds. Monounsaturated fats (aka "healthy fats") are thought to help lower cholesterol and reduce heart disease risk. However, monounsaturated fat has the same number of calories as other types of fat and may contribute to weight gain if eaten in excess.

Motor neuron: A nerve cell (neuron) whose cell body is located in the spinal cord and whose fiber (axon) projects outward from the spinal cord to innervate and control muscle cells.

Motor unit: Physiological unit comprised of a motor neuron and the skeletal muscle fibers innervated by that motor neuron's axonal terminals.

Movement analysis: Part of the needs analysis that evaluates body and limb movement and muscular involvement of the sport.

Muscles of expiration: Muscles that depress the ribcage during exhalation.

Muscles of inspiration: Muscles that elevate the ribcage during inhalation.

Muscle spindle: A sensory organ located within the muscle that is sensitive to the stretch of the muscle.

Myofibril: Long, cylindrical organelle in striated muscle cells, composed mainly of actin and myosin filaments, that run the entire length of the cell.

Myoglobin: An iron-containing protein found in muscle fibers that combines with oxygen released by red blood cells and transfers it to the mitochondria of muscle cells to produce energy.

Myosin: Globulin that combines with actin to form actomyosin (protein complex in muscle fibers that shortens when stimulated and causes muscle contractions).

Myosin heavy chain (MHC): Portion of the myosin filament responsible for muscle contraction. There are three types of MHC (i.e., type I, IIa, IIx), each with a different contractile speed. MHC IIx has the fastest contractile speed (and is called fast-twitch), whereas MHC I has the slowest (and is called slow-twitch).

Near-infrared interactance (NIR): A method of estimating percent body fat that uses near infrared light to differentiate between fat mass and fat-free mass within the body.

Needs analysis: A two-stage process in developing a strength and conditioning program to include an evaluation of the sport and an assessment of the athlete.

Neuromuscular junction: A chemical synapse (junction) formed by the contact between the presynaptic terminal of a motor neuron and the postsynaptic membrane of a muscle fiber.

Nicotinamide adenine dinucleotide (NADH): One of two redox cofactors created during the Krebs cycle that is used during the electron transport chain to produce energy (ATP).

Non-linear periodization: An alternative method that involves large fluctuations in load and volume assignments.

Normative performance standards: Use normative data derived from a sample of participants in order to rank individual performance. (e.g., Outstanding = Performance above or equal to the top 10 percentile).

Nutrient density: Refers to food choices based off the nutrients they provide (e.g., vitamins, minerals, fiber). Examples of nutrient dense foods include milk, vegetables, protein foods, and grains.

Nutrition facts label: Lists nutrients supplied and is based on a daily diet of 2,000 kilocalories (kcal). The label was mandated by the 1990 Nutrition Labeling and Education Act (NEA).

Objectivity: Degree to which a test is free from individual bias.

Olympic lifting: Type of strength (power) training in which athletes attempt to lift near maximum loads that are mounted on barbells.

Omega-3 fatty acids: Unsaturated fatty acid, mainly found in fish oils, that have three double bonds within the hydrocarbon chain.

Omege-6 fatty acids: Family of pro-inflammatory and anti-inflammatory polyunsaturated fatty acids that have a final carbon-carbon double bond in the sixth bond (counting from the methyl end).

Open kinetic chain (OKC): Exercises that are performed where the hand or foot are free to move (e.g., dumbbell lateral raises).

Overload: Greater than normal stress (load) is required in order for training adaptations to occur. These adaptations lead to increased athletic performance in terms of speed, strength, power, endurance, etc.

Overtraining: The point where a person displays a decrease in performance and/or plateauing as a result of consistently performing at a level or training load that exceeds their recovery capacity.

Oxidation: Reaction that occurs when oxygen combines with molecules in food to produce energy, water, and carbon dioxide.

Oxygen debt: Period of time after high intensity exercise when the demand for oxygen is greater than the supply.

Oxygen deficit: Difference between the oxygen required and what is actually taken in during about of high intensity exercise.

Pace/tempo training: A form of endurance training that uses intensities at or slightly higher than race pace intensity.

Peaking: The traditional approach to periodization divides training into various periods to include preparation, competition, and transition periods. As the competition draws closer, training becomes more specific and intense. This buildup to in training intensity prior to competition is referred to as "peaking".

Peak height velocity (PHV): Period of adolescent maturation where the maximum rate of growth occurs.

Peak weight velocity: Period of adolescent maturation associated with a rapid increase in body weight due to significant increases in the amount of muscle and bone mass.

Pennate muscle: Muscle fibers that are obliquely aligned with its tendon.

Percent daily value (DV): An area on the nutrition facts label that helps consumers determine the level of various nutrients in a standard serving of food. DV are based on an intake of 2000 calories.

Perimysium: Thin layer of connective tissue that surrounds each individual muscle fiber.

Periodization: A form of strength training that uses a strategic implementation of training phases (e.g., hypertrophy, strength, power). These phases periodically increase and decrease both volume and intensity in order to prevent overtraining and maximize gains.

Phasic muscles: Extensor muscles that tend to get weaker with age.

Phosphagen system: Fastest method to resynthesize ATP used for all-out exercise lasting up to about 10 seconds. However, since there is a limited amount of stored CP and ATP in the muscle, fatigue occurs rapidly.

Physiological analysis: Part of the needs analysis that evaluates the strength, power, size, and muscular endurance priorities of the sport.

Phytochemical: Biologically active compounds found in plants.

Phytoestrogens: Plant derived compounds found in a wide variety of foods, most notably soy.

Pilates: A system of exercises using a special apparatus intended to improve physical strength, flexibility, and posture, and enhance mental awareness.

Piriformis syndrome: An uncommon neuromuscular disorder caused when the piriformis muscle compresses the sciatic nerve.

Plasticity: Ability of connective tissue to assume a new or greater length after a passive stretch.

Plyometrics: A form of conditioning in which muscles exert maximum force in short intervals of time with the goal of increasing muscular power.

Polysaccharide: Several monosaccharides linked together.

Polyunsaturated fat: Type of fat that is liquid at room temperature. There are two types of polyunsaturated fatty acids (PUFAs).

Post-activation potentiation: A theory that purports that the contractile history of a muscle influences the mechanical performance of subsequent muscle contractions.

Power exercise: Structural exercises that are performed very quickly or explosively.

Prebiotics: Plant fibers that feed the healthy bacteria already in the gut to promote further healthy bacterial growth.

Prehab: Series of exercises and activities that if performed regularly will help to improve athletic performance and reduce the risk of injury.

Pre-exhaustion: Reverse exercise arrangement where the athlete purposely fatigues a large muscle group as a result of performance of a single-joint exercise prior to a multi-joint exercise involving the same muscle.

Pre-stretch: To extend a limb or body part to its full length or range of motion.

Probiotics: Live microorganisms thought to increase the healthy bacteria in the gut, thereby reducing GI issues, and respiratory illness.

Progression: Periodic increases in training variables (e.g., load, intensity, duration, frequency) in order for improvements to continue over time.

Progressive overload: Gradual increase in volume, intensity, frequency, or time in order to prevent training plateaus and achieve the targeted goal.

Proprietary blends: A list of ingredients for a product formula specific to a particular manufacturer.

Proprioreceptors: Specialized sensory receptors located within joints, muscles, and tendons that detect pressure and tension and relay that information to the brain.

Protein: An essential macronutrient, along with carbohydrates and fat, the body needs for good health. Proteins are made up of essential and nonessential amino acids. The body manufactures 13 nonessential amino acids, which aren't available from food.

Proteolysis: Breakdown of proteins or peptides into amino acids by enzymes.

Proximal attachment: An attachment that is situated close to the point of attachment to the body.

Qigong: A Chinese system of physical exercises and breathing control similar to tai chi.

Range of motion (ROM): Measurement of movement around a specific joint or body part.

Rate of perceived exertion (RPE): A method of measuring physical activity intensity level based on how hard you feel like your body is working.

Recovery: Time required between exercise sessions to allow the body to repair and replenish depends on the type and intensity of the exercise performed.

Referred pain: Pain that is felt in a part of the body other than its actual source.

Reliability: Degree of consistency or repeatability of a test.

Repetition (rep): A complete motion of a particular exercise or movement pattern.

Repetition maximum: The maximum amount of weight that can be lifted within a specified repetition range.

Repetition training: A form of endurance training that uses high-intensity intervals (typically 30–90 seconds in duration) at intensities greater than VO2max.

Residual volume: Volume of air remaining in the lungs after maximal expiration.

Resting metabolic rate (RMR): Energy expended to maintain life. RMR makes up 70–75% of our total daily energy expenditure.

Rest-pause technique: A method that involves stopping during the completion of a set, resting for a short period and then continuing on with the set.

Sarcomere: Fundamental unit of muscle structure, comprised of actin and myosin filaments, responsible for muscle contraction.

Sarcopenia: Age related loss of skeletal muscle mass and strength.

Sarcoplasm: The colorless material comprising the living cell, excluding the nucleus.

Satiety: Feeling of being full.

Saturated fat: Type of fat that is solid at room temperature. Saturated fat is found in full-fat dairy products (e.g., butter, cheese, cream, ice cream, and whole milk), coconut oil, lard, palm oil, ready-to-eat meats, and the skin and fat of chicken and turkey, among other foods. Saturated fats have the same number of calories as other types of fat, and may contribute to weight gain if eaten in excess.

Second-class lever: A situation when a lever has the fulcrum on one side with the muscle attachment on the other side and the load in the middle.

Serotonin: A neurotransmitter involved in sleep, depression, memory, and other neurological processes.

Set: A group of repetitions sequentially per-formed before the athlete stops to rest.

Skinfolds: A method of body composition that uses the thickness of skin at various sites in order to predict percent body fat.

Sliding-filament theory: Actin (thin) filaments of muscle fibers slide past the myosin (thick) filaments during muscle contraction.

Slow glycolysis: Method of providing energy for activities of relatively short duration (i.e., 2–3 minutes), that replenishes quickly and produces 2 ATP molecules per glucose molecule.

Slow-twitch fiber: A type of muscle fiber that develops less tension more slowly than a fast-twitch fiber but is more fatigue resistant due to its high oxygen content and enzyme activity.

Specificity: Training should be relevant to the activity the individual is training for in order to produce the desired training effect.

Spinal stenosis: An abnormal narrowing of the spinal canal, which may occur in any of the regions of the spine, resulting in a neurological deficit. Symptoms include pain, numbness, loss of motor control, and paraesthesia (tingling or pricking sensation caused by pressure on or damage to peripheral nerves).

Stability: Ability to maintain or control joint movement or position.

Stabilizer muscle: A muscle that contracts with no significant movement to maintain posture or fixate a joint.

Starch: Storage form of carbohydrates in plants.

Stimulus-recovery-adaptation (SRA): Physiological adaptations take place during recovery, not training. As a result, frequency recommendations for each of the different types of exercise types should be based off the amount of time required to recover.

Strength training (aka Resistance training): Type of physical exercise specializing in the use of resistance in order to improve the strength, anaerobic endurance, and size of skeletal muscle.

Stretch reflex: A muscle contraction in response to stretching which provides automatic regulation of skeletal muscle length.

Stretch-shortening cycle (SSC): An active stretch (eccentric contraction) of a muscle followed by an immediate shortening (concentric contraction) of that same muscle.

Stroke volume: Amount of blood ejected from the left ventricle in one contraction.

Structural exercise: Exercises that load the spine directly or indirectly.

Subcutaneous fat: Fat stored below the dermis layer of the skin and is not necessarily hazardous to your health.

Subjectivity: Degree to which a test is influenced by individual bias.

Superior attachment: An attachment that is situated closer to or towards the head of the body.

Super set: A superset involves two sequentially performed exercises that stress two opposing muscles or muscle areas (i.e., an agonist and its antagonist).

Supplement facts label: Lists the names and quantities of dietary ingredients present in the product, the serving size, and the servings per container.

Synergist muscle: A muscle that assists another muscle to accomplish a movement.

Synovial joints: Joint that has fibrous capsule surrounding the articulating surfaces of adjoining bones and is filled with synovial fluid.

Tai chi: An ancient Chinese form of exercise that was originally created as a fighting art. The words Tai Chi Chuan loosely translate to mean supreme ultimate exercise or skill.

Talk test: A simple way to measure exercise intensity. In general, during moderate-intensity activity you can talk, but not sing. During vigorous-intensity activity, you will not be able to say more than a few words without pausing for a breath.

Tapering: Practice of reducing exercise volume (40-50%), while maintaining exercise intensity, in the days just prior to competition to ensure adequate recovery.

Target muscle: The primary muscle intended to train or exercise.

Technical error of measurement (TEM): Variability in the measured scores taken on the same subjects at multiple sessions.

Thermic effect of food (TEF): Calories burned to digest food and accounts for roughly 10% of the total calories burned in a day.

Third-class lever: A situation when a lever has the fulcrum on one side, the load on the other side and the muscle attachment in the middle.

Total daily energy expenditure: The total amount of calories an individual burns in a day.

Tonic muscles: Flexor muscles that tend to get tighter with age.

Trachea: A large membranous tube reinforced by rings of cartilage that extends from the larynx to the bronchial tubes and conveys air to and from the lungs.

Training age: Number of years that an individual has spent training and participating in various sports.

Trans fat: Type of fat that is created when liquid oils are changed into solid fats, like shortening and some margarines. This is done to make food last longer without going bad. Trans fat are found in crackers, cookies, and snack foods. Trans fat are believed to raise LDL (bad) cholesterol and lower HDL (good) cholesterol.

Treadmill tempo run: New type of pace/tempo training aimed at targeting a desired run time for a specific race distance (e.g., 1.5-miles).

Triglycerides: Triglycerides are a type of fat found in the blood. High levels of triglycerides may increase the risk of coronary artery heart disease, especially in women.

Troponin: Globular protein complex involved in muscle contraction and occurs with tropomyosin in the thin filaments of muscle tissue.

Tropomyosin: Protein involved in muscle contraction that is related to myosin and occurs together with troponin in the thin filaments of muscle tissue.

Tryptophan: An essential amino acid and precursor of serotonin.

Underwater weighing (aka hydrostatic weighing): A method that uses the displacement of water in order to determine body volume and calculate percent body fat.

Undulating (non-linear) periodization: An alternative method that involves large fluctuations in load and volume assignments.

Valgus: Form deficiency caused by the oblique displacement of a limb away from the midline of the body.

Validity: Degree to which a test measures what it is supposed to measure, and is the most important characteristic of testing.

Variation: Periodic rotation of exercises in order to prevent training plateaus and/or overtraining.

Varus: Form deficiency caused by the oblique displacement of a limb towards the midline of the body.

Vegan: The strictest form of vegetarianism. Vegans not only exclude animal flesh, but also dairy, eggs, and animal-derived ingredients.

Vegetarian: Someone who does not eat any meat, poultry, game, fish, shellfish or by-product of animal slaughter.

Vein: A large diameter blood vessel that carries blood low in oxygen content from the body back to the heart.

Venous return: Rate of blood flow back to the heart.

Venous system: A system composed of veins and venules that returns deoxygenated blood back to the heart.

Ventricle: Either of the two lower chambers of the heart that receive blood from the atria and in turn push it into the arteries.

Venule: A small diameter blood vessel that connects the capillaries to the veins.

Visceral fat: Unseen fat stored around your organs and is linked to several metabolic disorders and diseases.

Vitamins: Various organic substances, either found in food or produced by the body, that are essential in minute quantities and act as coenzymes/precursors of coenzymes in the regulation of certain metabolic processes. Vitamins do not provide energy or serve as building units.

VO2max: Maximum amount of oxygen that an individual can utilize during intense or maximal exercise. It is measured as milliliters of oxygen used in one minute per kilogram of body weight (ml/kg/min).

Volume: The total amount of weight lifted in a training session.

Yoga: A Hindu spiritual and ascetic discipline that includes breath control, simple meditation, and the adoption of specific bodily postures used for health and relaxation.

Waist circumference: Measurement taken around the abdomen at the level of the umbilicus used as a screen for certain weight-related health risks.

Waist-to-hip ratio (WHR): An indicator of health risk that is calculated by dividing the waist measurement by the hip measurement.

Warm-up: Gradual increase in exercise intensity intended to prepare the body for the more intense and demanding activity to follow.

Index

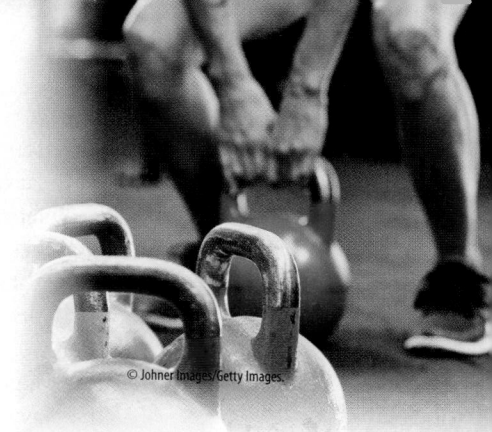

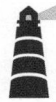

World Headquarters
Jones & Bartlett Learning
5 Wall Street
Burlington, MA 01803
978-443-5000
info@jblearning.com
www.jblearning.com

Jones & Bartlett Learning books and products are available through most bookstores and online booksellers. To contact Jones & Bartlett Learning directly, call 800-832-0034, fax 978-443-8000, or visit our website, www.jblearning.com.

Substantial discounts on bulk quantities of Jones & Bartlett Learning publications are available to corporations, professional associations, and other qualified organizations. For details and specific discount information, contact the special sales department at Jones & Bartlett Learning via the above contact information or send an email to specialsales@jblearning.com.

Production Credits

VP, Product Management: David D. Cella
Director of Product Management: Cathy L. Esperti
Product Manager: Sean Fabery
Product Assistant: Hannah Dziezanowski
Director of Vendor Management: Amy Rose
Vendor Manager: Molly Hogue
Director of Marketing: Andrea DeFronzo
VP, Manufacturing and Inventory Control: Therese Connell
Composition: SourceHOV LLC

Project Management: SourceHOV LLC
Cover Design: Kristin E. Parker
Rights & Media Specialist: Merideth Tumasz
Media Development Editor: Troy Liston
Cover Image (Title Page, Part Opener, Chapter Opener): © Johner Images/Getty Images
Printing and Binding: LSC Communications
Cover Printing: LSC Communications

Library of Congress Cataloging-in-Publication Data
Names: Peterson, David D. 1972- author. | Rittenhouse, Melissa A., author.
Title: A practical guide to personal conditioning / David D. Peterson and Melissa A. Rittenhouse.
Description: Burlington, MA : Jones & Bartlett Learning, [2019] | Includes bibliographical references and index.
Identifiers: LCCN 2017050080 | ISBN 9781284240191 (pbk. : alk. paper)
Subjects: LCSH: Physical fitness–Physiological aspects. | Exercise–Physiological aspects. | Nutrition.
Classification: LCC RA781 .P488 2019 | DDC 613.7–dc23 LC record available at https://lccn.loc.gov/2017050080

6048

Printed in the United States of America
22 21 20 19 18   10 9 8 7 6 5 4 3 2 1

A PRACTICAL GUIDE TO

Personal
CONDITIONING

DAVID D. PETERSON, EdD, CSCS*D

Assistant Professor of Kinesiology
Cedarville University
Cedarville, OH

MELISSA A. RITTENHOUSE, PhD, RD, CSSD

Nutrition/Exercise Scientist
Henry M. Jackson Foundation for the Advancement of Military Medicine
Private Practice Dietitian
Bethesda, MD

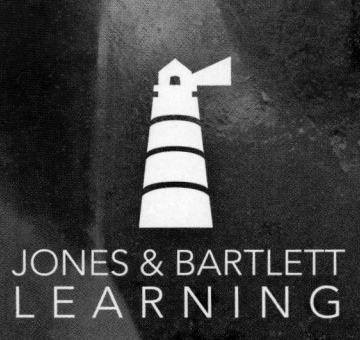

JONES & BARTLETT
LEARNING

Contents

Preface

The annual Office for National Statistics (ONS) *Blue Book* publication contains the estimates of the domestic and national product, income and expenditure of the United Kingdom.

The presentation of accounts is based on the *European System of Accounts 1995* (ESA95), which is itself based on the *System of National Accounts 1993* (SNA93). The SNA93 has been adopted world wide.

Quarterly estimates

Quarterly estimates of the main components of the National Accounts for the last few years are published in ONS *First Releases* and, in more detail with commentary, in the *United Kingdom Economic Accounts* (UKEA).

A number of long run quarterly and annual estimates consistent with the *Blue Book* are available in the on-line publication *Economic & Labour Market Review (ELMR)*. The latest estimates are also given in summary form in the *Monthly Digest of Statistics* and the quarterly income, capital and financial accounts for each sector are published regularly in *Financial Statistics*.

ONS data and publications website (www.ons.gov.uk)

Users can download time series, cross-sectional data and metadata from across the Government Statistical Service (GSS) using the site search and index functions from the homepage. Many datasets can be downloaded, in whole or in part, and directory information for all GSS statistical resources can be consulted, including censuses, surveys, periodicals and enquiry services. Information is posted as PDF electronic documents or in XLS and CSV formats, compatible with most spreadsheet packages.

Time series data

The Time series data facility on the website provides access to around 40,000 time series, of primarily macro-economic data, drawn from the main tables in a range of our major economic and labour market publications. Users can download complete releases, or view and download customised selections of individual time series.

National Statistics data

All data in the Blue Book are 'National Statistics', are fully compliant with the National Statistics Code of Practice and carry the National Statistics kitemark.

Comments and enquiries

ONS looks forward to receiving comments on its publications.

Suggestions for improvements or alterations to the *Blue Book* can be sent in writing to:

John Dye

Blue Book Editor

GE107

Office for National Statistics

1 Myddelton Street

LONDON EC1R 1UW

Tel: 020 7014 2088 Fax: 020 7014 2453

Email: gdp@ons.gsi.gov.uk

Enquiries regarding National Accounts should be directed to the following:

National accounts:
Jon Beadle 020 7014 2084
(jon.beadle@ons.gsi.gov.uk)

Sector and financial accounts:
Michael Rizzo 020 7014 2082
(michael.rizzo@ons.gsi.gov.uk)

Household final consumption expenditure:
Ann Harris 020 7014 2116
(ann.harris@ons.gsi.gov.uk)

General government and public sector:
David Vincent 020 7014 2125
(david.vincent@ons.gsi.gov.uk)

Gross capital formation:
Neil Wilson 020 7014 2107
(neil.wilson@ons.gsi.gov.uk)

Exports and imports of goods:
Caroline Lakin 020 7014 2020
(caroline.lakin@ons.gsi.gov.uk)

Exports and imports of services:
Tom Orford 020 7014 2027
(tom.orford@ons.gsi.gov.uk)

Gross value added by industry:
Bruce Omundsen 01633 456406
(bruce.omundsen@ons.gsi.gov.uk)

Input–Output supply and use tables/Production accounts:
Alex Clifton-Fearnside 020 7014 2078
(alex.clifton-fearnside@ons.gsi.gov.uk)

Households and NPISH sector:
Ann Harris 020 7014 2116
(ann.harris@ons.gsi.gov.uk)

Non-financial corporations:
Julian Collins 020 7014 2014
(julian.collins@ons.gsi.gov.uk)

Financial corporations:
Richard Dagnall 020 7014 2011
(richard.dagnall@ons.gsi.gov.uk)

Rest of the world:
John Bundey 020 7014 2002
(john.bundey@ons.gsi.gov.uk)

Capital stock and non-financial balance sheets:
Neil Wilson 020 7014 2107
(neil.wilson@ons.gsi.gov.uk)

Environmental accounts:
Donna Livesey 01633 455814
(donna.livesey@ons.gsi.gov.uk)

The *Blue Book* is a collaborative effort. ONS is grateful for the assistance provided by the various government departments and organisations that have contributed to this book.

An introduction to the United Kingdom National Accounts

The *Blue Book* presents the full set of economic accounts, or National Accounts, for the United Kingdom. These accounts are compiled by the Office for National Statistics (ONS). They record and describe economic activity in the United Kingdom and as such are used to support the formulation and monitoring of economic and social policies.

This edition of the *Blue Book* presents estimates of the UK domestic and national product, income and expenditure covering the calendar years 1999–2007. The tables of the main aggregates are extended to cover 1993–1998 on a consistent basis. Data for 2007 are not yet available for the production account, the generation of income account, Input-Output Supply and Use Tables and for the full detailed industrial analysis of gross value added and its income components.

The accounts are based on the European System of Accounts 1995 (ESA95),[1] itself based on the System of National Accounts 1993 (SNA93),[2] which is being adopted by national statistical offices throughout the world. The UK National Accounts have been based on the ESA95 since September 1998. The 1998 edition of the *Blue Book* explains the main changes; a more detailed explanation of changes can be found in *Introducing the ESA95 in the UK*.[3] A detailed description of the structure for the accounts is provided in a separate National Statistics publication *UK National Accounts Concepts, Sources and Methods*.[4]

This introduction gives a brief overview of the accounts, explains their framework and sets out the main changes included in this edition of the *Blue Book*. Definitions of terms used throughout the accounts are included in the glossary. Explanations of more specific concepts are provided within the relevant parts.

The *Blue Book* comprises five parts:

Part 1 provides a summary of the UK National Accounts along with explanations and tables that cover the main national and domestic aggregates, for example gross domestic product (GDP) at current market prices and chained volume measures and the GDP deflator; gross value added (GVA) at basic prices; gross national income (GNI); gross national disposable income (GNDI); and where appropriate their equivalents net of capital consumption; population estimates; employment estimates and GDP per head; and the UK summary accounts (the goods and services account, production accounts, distribution and use of income accounts and accumulation accounts). It also includes details of revisions to the data.

Part 2 includes Input-Output Supply and Use Tables and analyses of gross value added at current market prices and chained volume measures, capital formation and employment, by industry.

Part 3 provides a description of the institutional sectors as well as explaining different types of transactions, the sequence of the accounts and the balance sheets. Explanation is also given of the statistical adjustment items needed to reconcile the accounts. This part comprises the fullest available set of accounts showing transactions by sectors and appropriate sub-sectors of the economy (including the rest of the world).

Part 4 covers other additional analyses. It includes tables showing the percentage growth rates of the main aggregates and supplementary tables for capital consumption, gross fixed capital formation, capital stock, non-financial balance sheets, public sector data, and GNI and GNP consistent with the ESA79 compiled for EU budgetary purposes.

Part 5 covers environmental accounts.

Overview of the accounts

In the UK priority is given to the production of a single estimate of GDP using the income, production and expenditure data. The income analysis is available at current prices, expenditure is available at both current prices and chained volume measures and value added on a quarterly basis is compiled in chained volume measures only. Income, capital and financial accounts are also produced for each of the institutional sectors: non-financial corporations, financial corporations, general government and the households and non-profit institutions serving households sectors. The accounts are fully integrated, but with a statistical discrepancy, known as the statistical adjustment, shown for each sector account (which reflects the difference between the sector net borrowing or lending from the capital account and the identified borrowing or lending in the financial accounts which should theoretically be equal). Financial transactions and balance sheets are also produced for the rest of the world sector in respect of its dealings with the UK.

Summary of Changes

The main structural change introduced in this edition of the *Blue Book* is the introduction of a revised method for the allocation of 'financial intermediation services indirectly measured' (FISIM). Further information on this method can

1

be found in Chapter one of this publication, and the data in table 1.8. In addition, this year has seen the reintroduction of annual supply and use tables in Chapter two after a temporary suspension in 2007 to allow for the first stage of National Accounts modernisation.

The basic framework of the UK National Accounts

The accounting framework provides for a systematic and detailed description of the UK economy. It includes the sector accounts, which provide, by institutional sector, a description of the different stages of the economic process from production through income generation, distribution and use of income to capital accumulation and financing; and the Input-Output framework, which describes the production process in more detail. It contains all the elements required to compile aggregate measures such as GDP, gross national income (previously known as gross national product), saving and the current external balance (the balance of payments). The economic accounts provide the framework for a system of volume and price indices, so that chained volume measures of aggregates such as GDP can be produced. It should be noted that, in this system, value added, from the production approach, is measured at basic prices (including other taxes *less* subsidies on production but not on products) rather than at factor cost (which excludes all taxes *less* subsidies on production). The system also encompasses measures of population and employment.

The whole economy is subdivided into institutional sectors. For each sector, current price accounts run in sequence from the production account through to the balance sheet.

The accounts for the whole UK economy and its counterpart, the rest of the world, follow a similar structure to the UK sectors, although several of the rest of the world accounts are collapsed into a single account because they can never be complete when viewed from a UK perspective.

The table numbering system is designed to show the relationships between the UK, its sectors and the rest of the world. A three part numbering system (for example, 5.2.1) has been adopted for the accounts drawn directly from the ESA95. The first two digits denote the sector; the third digit denotes the ESA account. In this way for example, table 5.2.1 is the central government production account, table 5.3.1 is the local government production account and table 5.3.2 is the local government generation of income account. Not all sectors can have all types of account, so the numbering is not necessarily consecutive within each sector's chapter. For the rest of the world, the identified components of accounts 2–6 inclusive are given in a single account numbered 2. The UK whole economy accounts consistent with the ESA95 are given in section 1.6 as a time series and in section 1.7 in detailed matrix format with all sectors, the rest of the world, and the UK total identified.

The ESA95 code for each series is shown in the left hand column. The ESA95 codes use the prefix 'S' for the classification of institutional sectors. The ESA95 classification of transactions and other flows comprises transactions in products (prefix P), distributive transactions (prefix D), transactions in financial instruments (prefix F) and other accumulation entries (prefix K). Balancing items are classified using the prefix B. Within the financial balance sheets, financial assets/liabilities are classified using the prefix AF and non-financial assets/ liabilities using the prefix AN.

What is an account? What is its purpose?

An account records and displays all of the flows and stocks for a given aspect of economic life. The sum of resources is equal to the sum of uses with a balancing item to ensure this equality. Normally the balancing item will be an economic measure which is itself of interest.

By employing a system of economic accounts we can build up accounts for different areas of the economy which highlight, for example, production, income and financial transactions. In many cases these accounts can be elaborated and set out for different institutional units and groups of units (or sectors). Usually a balancing item has to be introduced between the total resources and total uses of these units or sectors and, when summed across the whole economy, these balancing items constitute significant aggregates. Table A below provides the structure of the accounts and shows how GDP estimates are derived as the balancing items.

The integrated economic accounts

The integrated economic accounts of the UK provide an overall view of the economy. The sequence of accounts is shown in Figure 1 below. Figure 1 presents a summary view of the accounts, balancing items and main aggregates and shows how they are expressed.

The accounting structure is uniform throughout the system and applies to all units in the economy, whether they are institutional units, sub-sectors, sectors or the whole economy, though some accounts (or transactions) may not be relevant for some sectors.

The accounts are grouped into four main categories: goods and services account, current accounts, accumulation accounts and balance sheets.

The goods and services account (Account 0)

The goods and services account is a transactions account which balances total resources, from output and imports, against the uses of these resources in consumption, investment, inventories and exports. Because the resources are simply balanced with the uses, there is no balancing item. The goods and services account is discussed in detail in chapters 3 and 12 of *UK National Accounts Concepts, Sources and Methods*.[4]

Current accounts: the production accounts and the distribution of income accounts

Current accounts deal with production, distribution of income and use of income.

The production account (Account I)

The production account displays the transactions involved in the generation of income by the activity of producing goods and services. In this case the balancing item is value added (B.1). For the nation's accounts, the balancing item (the sum of value added for all industries) is, after the addition of taxes less subsidies on products, gross domestic product (GDP) at market prices or net domestic product when measured net of capital consumption. The production accounts are also shown for each institutional sector.

The production accounts are discussed in detail in Chapters 4 and 13 of *Concepts, Sources and Methods*.[4]

Distribution and use of income account (Account II)

The distribution and use of income account shows the distribution of current income (in this case value added) carried forward from the production account, and has as its balancing item saving (B.8), which is the difference between income (disposable income) and expenditure (or final consumption). There are three sub-accounts which break down the distribution of income into the primary distribution of income, the secondary distribution of income and the redistribution of income in kind.

Primary incomes are those that accrue to institutional units as a consequence of their involvement in production, or their ownership of productive assets. They include property income (from lending or renting assets) and taxes on production and imports, but exclude taxes on income or wealth, social contributions or benefits and other current transfers. The primary distribution of income shows the way these are distributed among institutional units and sectors. The primary distribution account is itself divided into two sub-accounts – the generation and the allocation of primary incomes – but the further breakdown in the ESA95 of the allocation of primary income account into an entrepreneurial income account and an allocation of other primary income account has not been adopted in the UK..

The secondary distribution of income account shows how the balance of primary incomes for an institutional unit or sector is transformed into its disposable income by the receipt and payment of current transfers (excluding social transfers in kind). A further two sub-accounts – the use of disposable income and the use of adjusted disposable income – look at the use of income for either consumption or saving. These accounts are examined in detail in Chapters 5 and 14 of *Concepts, Sources and Methods*.[4]

Aggregated across the whole economy the balance of the primary distribution of income provides national income (B.5) (which can be measured net or gross), the balance of the secondary distribution of income in kind provides national disposable income (B.6), and the balance of the use of income accounts provides national saving (B.8). These are shown in Figure 1.

The accumulation accounts (Accounts III and IV)

The accumulation accounts cover all changes in assets, liabilities and net worth (the difference for any sector between its assets and liabilities). The accounts are structured to allow various types of change in these elements to be distinguished.

The first group of accounts covers transactions which would correspond to all changes in assets/liabilities and net worth which result from transactions for example, savings and voluntary transfers of wealth (capital transfers). These accounts are the capital account and financial account which are distinguished in order to show the balancing item net lending/borrowing (B.9).

The second group of accounts relates to changes in assets, liabilities and net worth due to other factors (for example the discovery or re-evaluation of mineral reserves, or the reclassification of a body from one sector to another). Within this second group, the other changes in assets accounts, has not been implemented in the UK except for the general government financial account (see tables 11.4–11.6).

Capital account (Account III.1)

The capital account concerns the acquisition of non-financial assets (some of which will be income creating and others which are wealth only) such as fixed assets or inventories, financed out of saving, and capital transfers involving the redistribution of wealth. Capital transfers include, for example, capital grants from private corporations to public corporations (for example, private sector contributions to the extension of the Jubilee line). This account shows how saving finances investment in the economy. In addition to gross fixed capital formation and changes in inventories, it shows the redistribution of capital assets between sectors of the economy and the rest of the world. The balance on the capital account, if negative, is designated net borrowing, and measures the net amount a unit or sector is obliged to borrow from others; if positive the balance is described as net lending, the amount the UK or a sector has available to lend to others. This balance is also referred to as the financial surplus or deficit and the net aggregate for the five sectors of the economy equals net lending/borrowing from the rest of the world.

Financial account (Account III.2)

The financial account shows how net lending and borrowing are achieved by transactions in financial instruments. The net

A UK summary accounts, 2006

Total economy: all sectors and the rest of the world

£ million

		RESOURCES						USES		TOTAL
		UK total economy S.1	Non-financial corporations S.11	Financial corporations S.12	General government S.13	Households & NPISH S.14+S.15	Not sectorised S.N	Rest of the world S.2	Goods & services	
	Current accounts									
I	**PRODUCTION / EXTERNAL**									
0	**ACCOUNT OF GOODS AND SERVICES**									
P.7	Imports of goods and services							419 588		419 588
P.6	Exports of goods and services								376 384	376 384
P.1	Output at basic prices	2 384 827	1 516 232	170 837	318 890	378 868				2 384 827
P.2	Intermediate consumption								1 207 595	1 207 595
D.21-D.31	Taxes less subsidies on products	144 628					144 628			144 628
II.1.1	**GENERATION OF INCOME**									
B.1g	**Gross domestic product, value added at market prices**	**1 321 860**	**714 508**	**89 529**	**160 371**	**212 824**	**144 628**			**1 321 860**
B.11	External balance of goods and services							43 204		43 204
II.1.2	**ALLOCATION OF PRIMARY INCOME**									
D.1	Compensation of employees	714 751				714 751		1 803		716 554
D.21-D.31	Taxes less subsidies on products	140 132			140 132			4 496		144 628
D.29-D.39	Other taxes less subsidies on production	14 518	16 109	1 578	–	-3 169		3 220		14 518
B.2g	Operating surplus, gross	368 310	246 788	36 628	12 931	71 963				368 310
B.3g	Mixed income, gross	78 908				78 908				78 908
di	Statistical discrepancy between income components and GDP	–						–		–
D.4	Property income	680 377	106 500	405 561	10 901	157 415		226 606		906 983
II.2	**SECONDARY DISTRIBUTION OF INCOME**									
B.5g	National income, balance of primary incomes, gross	1 330 681	184 547	21 061	151 310	973 763	–			1 330 681
D.5	Current taxes on income, wealth etc	223 718			223 718			464		224 182
D.61	Social contributions	202 405	3 425	87 845	110 621	514		–		202 405
D.62	Social benefits other than social transfers in kind	225 891				225 891		1 737		227 628
D.7	Other current transfers	219 890	8 368	37 409	115 059	59 054		23 459		243 349
II.3	**REDISTRIBUTION OF INCOME IN KIND**									
B.6g	Disposable income, gross	1 320 024	146 890	37 211	283 480	852 443	–			1 320 024
D.63	Social transfers in kind	205 324				205 324				205 324
II.4	**USE OF INCOME**									
B.7g	Adjusted disposable income, gross	1 320 024	146 890	37 211	110 365	1 025 558	–			1 320 024
B.6g	Disposable income, gross	1 320 024	146 890	37 211	283 480	852 443	–			1 320 024
P.4	Actual final consumption								1 132 537	1 132 537
P.3	Final consumption expenditure								1 132 537	1 132 537
D.8	Adjustment for change in households' net equity in pension funds	31 714				31 714		-9		31 705
	Accumulation accounts									
III.1.1	**CHANGE IN NET WORTH DUE TO SAVING AND CAPITAL TRANSFERS**									
B.8g	Saving, gross	187 496	146 890	5 506	-2 189	37 289	–			187 496
B.12	Current external balance							45 031		45 031
D.9	Capital transfers receivable	31 464	8 122	446	14 652	8 244		2 426		33 890
D.9	Capital transfers payable	-30 497	-630	-446	-24 689	-4 732		-3 393		-33 890
III.1.2	**ACQUISITION ON NON-FINANCIAL ASSETS** **Changes in liabilities and net worth**									
B.10.1.g	Changes in net worth due to saving and capital transfers	188 463	154 382	5 506	-12 226	40 801	–	44 064		232 527
P.51	Gross fixed capital formation								227 920	227 920
-K.1	(Consumption of fixed capital)									
P.52	Changes in inventories								4 322	4 322
P.53	Acquisitions less disposals of valuables								285	285
K.2	Acquisitions less disposals of non-produced non-financial assets									
de	Statistical discrepancy between expenditure components and GDP								–	–
III.2	**FINANCIAL ACCOUNT**									
B.9	**Net lending(+) / net borrowing(-)**	-44 056	27 728	-3 275	-34 866	-33 643	–	44 056		–
	Changes in liabilities									
F.2	Currency and deposits	791 056	–	785 662	5 394			278 416		1 069 472
F.3	Securities other than shares	255 677	11 961	202 988	39 621	1 107		108 052		363 729
F.4	Loans	433 114	151 059	148 132	1 356	132 567		131 207		564 321
F.5	Shares and other equity	89 242	6 937	82 305		–		93 837		183 079
F.6	Insurance technical reserves	62 000		62 000						62 000
F.7	Other accounts payable	78 331	5 021	35 177	1 953	36 180		1 639		79 970

A UK summary accounts, 2006

Total economy: all sectors and the rest of the world

continued   £ million

		USES						RESOURCES	TOTAL	
		UK total economy	Non-financial corporations	Financial corporations	General government	Households & NPISH	Not sector-ised	Rest of the world	Goods & services	TOTAL
		S.1	S.11	S.12	S.13	S.14+S.15	S.N	S.2		
	Current accounts									
I	**PRODUCTION / EXTERNAL**									
0	**ACCOUNT OF GOODS AND SERVICES**									
P.7	Imports of goods and services								419 588	419 588
P.6	Exports of goods and services							376 384		376 384
P.1	Output at basic prices								2 384 827	2 384 827
P.2	Intermediate consumption	1 207 595	801 724	81 308	158 519	166 044			1 207 595	1 207 595
D.21-D.31	Taxes *less* subsidies on products								144 628	144 628
B.1g	**Gross domestic product, value added at market prices**	**1 321 860**	**714 508**	**89 529**	**160 371**	**212 824**	**144 628**			**1 321 860**
B.11	External balance of goods and services							43 204		43 204
II.1.1	**GENERATION OF INCOME**									
D.1	Compensation of employees	715 496	451 611	51 323	147 440	65 122		1 058		716 554
D.21-D.31	Taxes *less* subsidies on products	144 628					144 628			144 628
D.29-D.39	Other taxes *less* subsidies on production	17 738			17 738			3 220		14 518
B.2g	Operating surplus, gross	368 310	246 788	36 628	12 931	71 963				368 310
B.3g	Mixed income, gross	78 908				78 908				78 908
di	Statistical discrepancy between income components and GDP	–					–			–
II.1.2	**ALLOCATION OF PRIMARY INCOME**									
D.4	Property income	669 535	168 741	421 128	30 392	49 274		237 448		906 983
B.5g	National income, balance of primary incomes, gross	1 330 681	184 547	21 061	151 310	973 763	–			1 330 681
II.2	**SECONDARY DISTRIBUTION OF INCOME**									
D.5	Current taxes on income, wealth etc	223 533	37 183	15 475	1 075	169 800		649		224 182
D.61	Social contributions	202 349				202 349		56		202 405
D.62	Social benefits other than social transfers in kind	227 628	3 425	56 140	167 053	1 010				227 628
D.7	Other current transfers	229 051	8 842	37 489	149 100	33 620		14 298		243 349
B.6g	Disposable income, gross	1 320 024	146 890	37 211	283 480	852 443	–			1 320 024
II.3	**REDISTRIBUTION OF INCOME IN KIND**									
B.7g	Adjusted disposable income, gross	1 320 024	146 890	37 211	110 365	1 025 558	–			1 320 024
D.63	Social transfers in kind	205 324			173 115	32 209				205 324
II.4	**USE OF INCOME ACCOUNT**									
B.6g	Disposable income, gross									
P.4	Actual final consumption	1 132 537			112 554	1 019 983				1 132 537
P.3	Final consumption expenditure	1 132 537			285 669	846 868				1 132 537
D.8	Adjustment for change in households' net equity in pension funds	31 705		31 705						31 705
B.8g	Saving, gross	187 496	146 890	5 506	-2 189	37 289	–			187 496
B.12	Current external balance							45 031		45 031
	Accumulation accounts									
III.1.1	**CHANGE IN NET WORTH DUE TO SAVING AND CAPITAL TRANSFERS**									
D.9	Capital transfers receivable									
D.9	Capital transfers payable									
B.10.1.g	Changes in net worth due to saving and capital transfers	188 463	154 382	5 506	-12 226	40 801	–	44 064		232 527
III.1.2	**ACQUISITION OF NON-FINANCIAL ASSETS**									
	Changes in assets									
P.51	Gross fixed capital formation	227 920	121 173	8 650	23 667	74 430				227 920
-K.1	(Consumption of fixed capital)	-147 858	-80 360	-5 944	-12 931	-48 623				-147 858
P.52	Changes in inventories	4 322	4 142	199	-4	-15				4 322
P.53	Acquisitions less disposals of valuables	285	-42	-74	14	387				285
K.2	Acquisitions less disposals of non-produced non-financial assets	-8	1 381	6	-1 037	-358		8		–
de	Statistical discrepancy between expenditure components and GDP	–					–			–
B.9	**Net lending(+) / net borrowing(-)**	-44 056	27 728	-3 275	-34 866	-33 643	–	44 056		–
III.2	**FINANCIAL ACCOUNT: changes in assets**									
F.1	Monetary gold and SDRs	47			47			-47		
F.2	Currency and deposits	734 994	64 725	583 092	6 913	80 264		334 478		1 069 472
F.3	Securities other than shares	194 952	6 513	197 815	2 245	-11 621		168 777		363 729
F.4	Loans	481 200	52 896	426 472	4 494	-2 662		83 121		564 321
F.5	Shares and other equity	115 613	76 443	57 566	-2 541	-15 855		67 466		183 079
F.6	Insurance technical reserves	60 826	1 371	144	61	59 250		1 174		62 000
F.7	Other accounts receivable	79 913	5 254	40 887	2 897	30 875		57		79 970
dB.9f	Statistical discrepancy between non-financial and financial transactions	-2 181	-4 496	7 013	-658	-4 040	–	2 181		–

Figure 1   Synoptic presentation of the accounts, balancing items and main aggregates

Accounts	Full sequence of accounts for institutional sectors			Balancing items	Main aggregates [1]
Current accounts	I.	Production account		B.1 Value added	Domestic product (GDP/NDP)
	II.	Distribution and use of income accounts			
		II.1. Primary distribution of income accounts	II.1.1. Generation of income account	B.2 Operating surplus B.3 Mixed income	
			II.1.2. Allocation of primary income account	B.5 Balance of primary incomes	National income (GNI, NNI)
		II.2. Secondary distribution of income account		B.6 Disposable income	National disposable income
		II.3. Redistribution of income in kind account		B.7 Adjusted disposable income	
		II.4. Use of income account			
		II.4.1. Use of disposable income account		B.8 Saving	National saving
		II.4.2. Use of adjusted disposable income account			
Accumulation accounts	III.	Accumulation accounts			
		III.1. Capital account		B.10.1 (Changes in net worth, due to saving and capital transfers) B.9 Net lending/Net borrowing	
		III.2. Financial account		B.9 Net lending/Net borrowing	
Balance sheets	IV.	Financial balance sheets	IV.3. Closing balance sheet	B.90 Financial net worth	
Transaction accounts					
Goods and services account	0	Goods and services account			National expenditure
Rest of the world account (external transactions account)					
Current accounts	V.	Rest of the world account	V.I. External account of goods and services	B.11 External balance of goods and services	External balance of goods and services
			V.II. External account of primary income and current transfers	B.12 Current external balance	Current external balance
Accumulation accounts		V.III. External accumulation accounts	V.III.1. Capital account	B.10.1 (Changes in net worth due to current external balance and capital transfers) B.9 Net lending/Net borrowing	
			V.III.2. Financial account	B.9 Net lending/Net borrowing	Net lending/Net borrowing of the nation
Balance sheets		V.IV. External assets and liabilities account	V.IV.3. Closing balance sheet	B.90 Net worth	
Balance sheets				B.10 Changes in net worth B.90 Net worth	

1/ Most balancing items and aggregates may be calculated gross or net.

acquisitions of financial assets are shown separately from the net incurrence of liabilities. The balancing item is again net lending or borrowing.

In principle net lending or borrowing in the capital account should be identical to net lending or borrowing on the financial account. However in practice, because of errors and omissions, this identity is very difficult to achieve for the sectors and the economy as a whole. The difference is known as the statistical discrepancy (previously known as the balancing item).

The balance sheet (Account IV)

The second group of accounts within the accumulation accounts completes the full set of accounts in the system. These include the balance sheets and a reconciliation of the changes that have brought about the change in net worth between the beginning and the end of the accounting period.

The opening and closing balance sheets show how total holdings of assets by the UK or its sectors match total liabilities and net worth (the balancing item). In detailed presentations of the balance sheets the various types of asset and liability can be shown. Changes between the opening and closing balance sheets for each group of assets and liabilities result from transactions and other flows recorded in the accumulation accounts, or reclassifications and revaluations. Net worth equals changes in assets less changes in liabilities..

Rest of the world account (Account V)

This account covers the transactions between resident and non-resident institutional units and the related stocks of assets and liabilities. The rest of the world plays a similar role to an institutional sector and the account is written from the point of view of the rest of the world. This account is discussed in detail in chapter 24 of *Concepts, Sources and Methods*.[4]

Satellite accounts

Satellite accounts are accounts which involve areas or activities not dealt with in the central framework above, either because they add additional detail to an already complex system or because they actually conflict with the conceptual framework. The UK has begun work on a number of satellite accounts and one such – the UK environmental accounts – links environmental and economic data in order to show the interactions between the economy and the environment. Summary information from the environmental accounts is presented in part 5. More detailed information on the environmental accounts is available from the National Statistics website at www.statistics.gov.uk/environmentalaccounts.

Some definitions

The text within Sections 1-3 explains the sources and methods used in the estimation of the UK economic accounts, but it is

sensible to precede them with an explanation of some of the basic concepts and their 'UK specific' definitions, namely:

- the limits of the UK national economy: economic territory, residency and centre of economic interest

- economic activity: what production is included – the production boundary

- what price is used to value the products of economic activity

- estimation or imputation of values for non-monetary transactions

- the rest of the world: national and domestic

A full description of the accounting rules is provided in Chapter 2 of *Concepts, Sources and Methods*.[4]

The limits of the national economy: economic territory, residence and centre of economic interest

The economy of the United Kingdom is made up of institutional units (see chapter 10 of *Concepts, Sources and Methods*[4]) which have a centre of economic interest in the UK economic territory. These units are known as resident units and it is their transactions which are recorded in the UK National Accounts. The definitions of these terms are given below:

The UK economic territory is made up of:

- Great Britain and Northern Ireland (the geographic territory administered by the UK government within which persons, goods, services and capital move freely)

- any free zones, including bonded warehouses and factories under UK customs control

- the national airspace, UK territorial waters and the UK sector of the continental shelf

It excludes the offshore islands, the Channel Islands and the Isle of Man, which are not part of the United Kingdom or members of the European Union.

Within the ESA95 the definition of economic territory also includes:

- territorial enclaves in the rest of the world (like embassies, military bases, scientific stations, information or immigration offices, aid agencies, etc., used by the British government with the formal political agreement of the governments in which these units are located)

but excludes:

- any extra territorial enclaves (that is, parts of the UK geographic territory like embassies and US military bases used by general government agencies of other countries, by the institutions of the European Union or by international organisations under treaties or by agreement)

Centre of economic interest and residency

An institutional unit has a centre of economic interest and is a resident of the UK when, from a location (for example, a dwelling, place of production or premises) within the UK economic territory, it engages and intends to continue engaging (indefinitely or for a finite period; one year or more is used as a guideline) in economic activities on a significant scale. It follows that if a unit carries out transactions on the economic territory of several countries it has a centre of economic interest in each of them (for example, BP has an interest in many countries where it is involved in the exploration and production of oil and gas). Ownership of land and structures in the UK is enough to qualify the owner to have a centre of interest here.

Within the definition given above resident units are households, legal and social entities such as corporations and quasi corporations (for example, branches of foreign investors), non-profit institutions and government. Also included here however are so called 'notional residents'.

Travellers, cross border and seasonal workers, crews of ships and aircraft and students studying overseas are all residents of their home countries and remain members of their households. However an individual who leaves the UK for a year or more (except students and patients receiving medical treatment) ceases to be a member of a resident household and becomes a non-resident even on home visits.

Economic activity: what production is included?

As GDP is defined as the sum of all economic activity taking place in UK territory, having defined the economic territory it is important to be clear about what is defined as economic activity. In its widest sense it could cover all activities resulting in the production of goods or services and so encompass some activities which are very difficult to measure. For example, estimates of smuggling of alcoholic drink and tobacco products, and the output, expenditure and income directly generated by that activity, have been included since the 2001 edition of the *Blue Book*.

In practice a 'production boundary' is defined, inside which are all the economic activities taken to contribute to economic performance. This economic production may be defined as activity carried out under the control of an institutional unit that uses inputs of labour or capital and goods and services to produce outputs of other goods and services. These activities range from agriculture and manufacturing through service producing activities (for example, financial services and hotels and catering) to the provision of health, education, public administration and defence; they are all activities where an output is owned and produced by an institutional unit, for which payment or other compensation has to be made to enable a change of ownership to take place. This omits purely natural processes.

The decision whether to include a particular activity within the production boundary takes into account the following:

- does the activity produce a useful output?

- is the product or activity marketable and does it have a market value?

- if the product does not have a meaningful market value can a market value be assigned (that is, can a value be imputed)?

- would exclusion (or inclusion) of the product of the activity make comparisons between countries or over time more meaningful?

In practice the ESA95 production boundary can be summarised as follows:

The production of all goods whether supplied to other units or retained by the producer for own final consumption or gross capital formation, and services only in so far as they are exchanged in the market and/or generate income for other economic units.

For households this has the result of including the production of goods on own-account, for example the produce of farms consumed by the farmer's own household (however, in practice produce from gardens or allotments has proved impossible to estimate in the United Kingdom so far). The boundary excludes the production of services for own final consumption (household domestic and personal services like cleaning, cooking, ironing and the care of children and the sick or infirm). Although the production of these services does take considerable time and effort, the activities are self-contained with limited repercussions for the rest of the economy and, as the vast majority of household domestic and personal services are not produced for the market, it is very difficult to value the services in a meaningful way.

What price is used to value the products of economic activity?

In the UK a number of different prices may be used to value inputs, outputs and purchases. The prices are different depending on the perception of the bodies engaged in the transaction, that is, the producer and user of a product will usually perceive the value of the product differently, with the result that the output prices received by producers can be distinguished from the prices paid by purchasers.

These different prices – purchasers' (or market) prices, basic prices and producers' prices – are looked at in turn below. They differ as a result of the treatment of taxes less subsidies on products, and trade and transport margins. Although the factor cost valuation (see explanation in Part 1) is not required under the SNA93 or the ESA95, ONS will continue to provide figures for gross value added at factor cost for as long as customers continue to find this analysis useful.

Basic prices

These prices are the preferred method of valuing output in the accounts. They reflect the amount received by the producer for a unit of goods or services, *minus* any taxes payable, and plus any subsidy receivable on that unit as a consequence of production or sale (that is, the cost of production including subsidies). As a result the only taxes included in the price will be taxes on the output process – for example business rates and vehicle excise duty – which are not specifically levied on the production of a unit of output. Basic prices exclude any transport charges invoiced separately by the producer. When a valuation at basic prices is not feasible then producers' prices may be used.

Producers' prices

Producers' prices equal basic prices plus those taxes paid per unit of output (other than taxes deductible by the purchaser, such as VAT, invoiced for output sold) less any subsidies received per unit of output.

Purchasers' or Market prices

These are the prices paid by the purchaser and include transport costs, trade margins and taxes (unless the taxes are deductible by the purchaser).

Purchasers' prices equal producers' prices plus any non-deductible VAT or similar tax payable by the purchaser plus transport costs paid separately by the purchaser and not included in the producers' price.

'Purchaser's prices' are also referred to as 'market prices', for example 'GDP at market prices'.

The rest of the world: national and domestic

Domestic product (or income) includes production (or primary incomes generated and distributed) resulting from all activities taking place 'at home' or in the UK domestic territory. This will include production by any foreign owned company in the United Kingdom but exclude any income earned by UK residents from production taking place outside the domestic territory. Thus gross domestic product is also equal to the sum of primary incomes distributed by resident producer units.

The definition of gross national income can be introduced by considering the primary incomes distributed by the resident producer units above. These primary incomes, generated in the production activity of resident producer units, are distributed mostly to other residents' institutional units. For example, when a resident producer unit is owned by a foreign company, some of the primary incomes generated by the producer unit are likely to be paid abroad. Similarly, some primary incomes generated in the rest of the world may go to resident units. Thus, when looking at the income of the nation, it is necessary to exclude that part of resident producers' primary income paid

abroad, but include the primary incomes generated abroad but paid to resident units; that is,

Gross domestic product (or income)

>   *less*

>   primary incomes payable to non-resident units

>   *plus*

>   primary incomes receivable from the rest of the world

>   *equals*

>   Gross national income

Thus gross national income (GNI) at market prices is the sum of ,gross primary incomes receivable by resident institutional units/sectors.

National income includes income earned by residents of the national territory, remitted (or deemed to be remitted in the case of direct investment) to the national territory, no matter where the income is earned; that is,

Real GDP (chained volume measures)

>   *plus*

>   trading gain

>   *equals*

>   Real gross domestic income (RGDI)

Real gross domestic income (RGDI)

>   *plus*

>   real primary incomes receivable from abroad

>   *less*

>   real primary incomes payable abroad

>   *equals*

>   Real gross national income (real GNI)

Real GNI (chained volume measures)

>   *plus*

>   real current transfers from abroad

>   *less*

>   real current transfers abroad

>   *equals*

>   Real gross national disposable income (real GNDI)

Receivables and transfers of primary incomes, and transfers to and from abroad are deflated using the index of gross domestic final expenditure.

Gross domestic product: the concept of net and gross

The term gross refers to the fact that when measuring domestic production we have not allowed for an important phenomenon: capital consumption or depreciation. Capital goods are different from the materials and fuels used up in the production process because they are not used up in the period of account but are instrumental in allowing that process to take place. However, over time capital goods do wear out or become obsolete and in this sense gross domestic product does not give a true picture of value added in the economy. In other words, in calculating value added as the difference between output and costs we should include as a current cost that part of the capital goods used up in the production process; that is, the depreciation of the capital assets.

Net concepts are net of this capital depreciation, for example:

Gross domestic product

minus

consumption of fixed capital

equals

Net domestic product

However, because of the difficulties in obtaining reliable estimates of the consumption of fixed capital (depreciation), gross domestic product remains the most widely used measure of economic activity.

Symbols and conventions used

Symbols

In general, the following symbols are used:

..   not available

-   nil or less than £500,000

£ billion denotes £1,000 million.

Sign conventions

Resources and Uses

Increase shown positive

Decrease shown negative

Capital account

Liabilities, net worth and Assets:

Increase shown positive

Decrease shown negative

Financial account

Assets: net acquisition shown positive

net disposal shown negative

Liabilities: net acquisition shown positive

net disposal shown negative

Balance sheet

Assets and liabilities each shown positive

Balance shown positive if net asset, negative if net liability

References

1. *Eurostat (1995) European System of Accounts 1995 (ESA95)*. ISBN 92 827 7954 8

2. UN, OECD, IMF, EU (1993) *System of National Accounts 1993 (SNA93)*. ISBN 92 1 161352 3

3. Office for National Statistics (1998) *Introducing the ESA95* in the UK. ISBN 0 11 621061 3. The Stationery Office: London.

4. Office for National Statistics (1998) *National Accounts Concepts, Sources and Methods*. ISBN 0 11 621062. The Stationery Office: London.

Articles

Akritidis L (2002) Accuracy assessment of National Accounts statistics. *Economic Trends*, No. 589.

Baxter M (1998) Developments in the measurement of general government output. *Economic Trends*, No. 537.

Fletcher D and Williams M (2002) Index of Production redevelopment. *Economic Trends,* No. 587.

Jenkinson G (1997) Quarterly integrated economic accounts – The United Kingdom approach. *Economic Trends*, No. 520.

Jones G (2000) The development of the annual business inquiry. *Economic Trends*, No. 564.

Powell M and Swatch N (2002) An investigation into the coherence of deflation methods in the National Accounts. *Economic Trends*, No. 588.

Pritchard A (2003) Understanding government output and productivity. *Economic Trends*, No. 596.

Ruffles D, Tily G, Caplan D and Tudor S (2003) VAT missing trader intra-community fraud: The effect on balance of payments statistics and UK National Accounts. *Economic Trends*, No. 597.

Sheerin C (2002) UK Material Flow Accounting. *Economic Trends*, No. 583.

Skipper H (2005) Early estimates of GDP: information content and forecasting methods. *Economic Trends*, No. 617.

Soo A and Charmokly Z (2003) The application of annual chain-linking to the Gross National Income system. *Economic Trends,* No. 593.

Tuke A and Beadle J (2003) The effect of annual chain-linking on Blue Book 2002 annual growth estimates. *Economic Trends*, No. 593.

Calendar of economic events: 1980–2007

1980

Jan	Steel strike begins
Mar	Medium Term Financial Strategy announced
Jun	Britain becomes a net exporter of oil
	Agreement to reduce UK's budget contribution to EEC
Oct	Dollar exchange rate peaks at $2.39 per £
Nov	Ronald Reagan elected US President

1981

Jan	Bottom of worst post-War slump in Britain
Feb	The Times sold to Rupert Murdoch
Mar	Budget announces windfall tax on banks
Jul	Cuts in university spending announced
Aug	Minimum Lending Rate (MLR) suspended

1982

Feb	Laker Airlines collapses
Mar	British naval task force sent to Falklands
Jun	Ceasefire in Falklands
Jul	Hire purchase controls abolished
Aug	Barclays Bank starts opening on Saturdays
Sep	Unemployment reaches 3 million
Nov	Channel 4 Television begins transmission

1983

Jun	£450m EC budget rebate granted to UK
Jul	£500m public spending cuts announced
Sep	3% target set for public sector pay
Oct	European Parliament freezes budget rebate

1984

Mar	Miners' strike begins
Jun	Robert Maxwell buys Daily Mirror
Jun	Fontainebleau Summit agrees permanent settlement of UK's contribution to EEC
Oct	Bank of England rescues Johnson Matthey
Nov	British Telecom plc privatised
Dec	Agreement to hand over Hong Kong to China in 1997

1985

Jan	FT Index reaches 1,000 for the first time
Mar	End of year long miners' strike
	Dollar exchange rate bottoms out at $1.05/£
Dec	NatWest, Barclays and Lloyds Banks announce 'free banking'

1986

Jan	Michael Heseltine resigns from Government over Westland Helicopters affair
Feb	Single European Act signed
Mar	Budget cuts basic rate of income tax to 29% and introduces Personal Equity Plans (PEPs)
	Greater London Council abolished
Apr	Chernobyl nuclear reactor disaster
	Bus services deregulated
	The Independent newspaper founded
Nov	'Big Bang' deregulates dealing in the City
Dec	British Gas privatisation

1987

Jan	Prosecutions for insider dealing in Guinness case
	British Airways privatisation
Mar	Budget reduces basic rate of tax to 27%
Oct	"Hurricane" strikes Britain
	'Black Monday': collapse of stock market

1988

Mar	Budget reduces basic rate of tax to 25%; top rate to 40%
	BL sold to BMW
Jun	Barlow-Clowes collapses
Jul	Piper Alpha oil rig disaster
Sep	Worst ever UK trade deficit announced
Nov	George Bush elected US President
Dec	Salmonella outbreak in Britain

1989

Mar	Exon Valdez oil spillage disaster in Alaska

Apr   Chinese authorities quell dissidents in Tiananmen Square

Jul   Blue Arrow report from DTI

Oct   Nigel Lawson resigns as Chancellor

Nov   Ford takes over Jaguar

     Fall of Berlin Wall

1990

Mar   Budget introduces tax exempt savings accounts (TESSAs)

Apr   BSE ('mad cow disease') identified

     New Education Act brings in student loans

     Community Charge ('poll tax') introduced

Aug   Kuwait invaded by Iraq

Oct   Official reunification of Germany

     UK enters Exchange Rate Mechanism

Nov   John Major replaces Mrs Thatcher as PM

     Privatisation of electricity boards

1991

Jan   NHS internal market created

     Gulf War begins

Feb   Gulf War ends

Mar   Air Europe collapses

     Budget restricts mortgage interest relief to basic rate: Corporation Tax reduced and VAT increased

Jul   BCCI closed by Bank of England

Nov   Maastricht agreement signed with UK opt-outs

Dec   Mikhail Gorbachev replaced by Boris Yeltsin as President of the Soviet Union

1992

Jan   Russia agrees to join the IMF

Feb   'Delors Package' raises EC's spending limits to 1.37% of GDP to aid poorer member states

Mar   Budget raises lower rate of income tax to 20%

     Midland Bank agrees merger with Hong Kong and Shanghai Bank

Apr   Conservatives win General Election

May   Swiss vote in a referendum to join the IMF and IBRD

     Reform of EC Common Agricultural Policy agreed, switching from farm price support to income support

Sep   'Black Wednesday': UK leaves Exchange Rate Mechanism

Oct   North American Free Trade Agreement (NAFTA) signed

Nov   Bill Clinton defeats George Bush in US presidential election

Dec   Plan for National Lottery announced

1993

Jan   Council Tax announced as replacement for Community Charge

     University status given to polytechnics

Mar   Budget imposes VAT on domestic fuel

Nov   Parliament votes to relax Sunday trading rules

     First autumn Budget cuts public expenditure and increases taxes

Dec   Uruguay Round of tariff reductions approved

1994

Jan   European Economic Area formed linking EU and EFTA

Apr   Eurotunnel opens

Aug   IRA ceasefire begins

Oct   Brent Walker leisure group collapses

Nov   First draw of National Lottery

Dec   Coal industry privatised

1995

Jan   EU expanded to include Sweden, Finland and Austria

     World Trade Organisation succeeds GATT

Feb   Barings Bank collapses

Sep   Net Book Agreement suspended

1996

Jan   Gilt 'repo' market established

Mar   Rebates worth £1billion paid to electricity consumers after break up of National Grid

May   Railtrack privatised, reducing public service borrowing requirement by £1.1 billion

Aug   CREST clearing system initiated

Sep   Privatisation of National Power and PowerGen reduces PSBR by further £1.0 billion

1997

Apr   Alliance and Leicester Building Society converts to bank

May   Labour Party wins General Election

Chancellor announces operational independence for the Bank of England, decisions on interest rates to be taken by a new Monetary Policy Committee

Jun   Halifax Building Society converts to a bank

Norwich Union floated on the stock market

Jul   Gordon Brown presents his first Budget, setting inflation target of 2.5%

Woolwich Building Society converts to a bank

Bristol and West Building Society converts to a bank

Aug   Stock market falls in Far East, Hang Seng Index ending 20% lower than a year earlier

Economic and financial crisis in Russia

Dec   The first instalment of the windfall tax on utilities (£2.6 billion) is paid

1998

Apr   Sterling Exchange Rate Index hits its highest point since 1989

Mortgage payments rise as MIRAS is cut from 15% to 10%

The New Deal for the unemployed is introduced

Jun   The Bank of England's 'repo' rate is raised by 0.25% to a peak of 7.5%

Economic and Fiscal Strategy Report announces new format for public finances, distinguishing between current and capital spending

Aug   BP merges with Amoco to create the UK's largest company

Oct   The Working Time Directive, setting a 48-hour week, takes effect

Dec   The second instalment of the windfall tax on utilities (£2.6 billion) is paid

Ten of the eleven countries about to enter the euro harmonised interest rates at 3.0%

1999

Jan   Introduction of Euro currency

Mar   Allocation of new car registration letters switched from yearly in August to twice yearly

Budget, energy tax announced

Apr   Introduction of ISAs replaces PEPs and TESSAs

Introduction of national minimum wage

Advanced Corporation tax abolished

Jun   The Bank of England 'repo' rate reduced to low point of 5%

Nov   Jubilee Line extension completed

Dec   Pre-budget statement

Year 2000 preparations (Y2K)

2000

Jan   Confounding expectations, the millennium passed without any major problems

Feb   House price growth peaks at 15% in January and February

Oil price rises to highest level in ten years

The UK company Vodafone takes over the German company Mannesman for £113bn

Apr   Government announces issue of 3G mobile phone spectrum licenses

May   Share prices in so-called internet companies start falling

Competition commission finds that UK car prices high relative to EU prices

BMW sells Rover and Ford shuts Dagenham plant

June   Inward investment in the UK hits record levels, with a large proportion made up of take-over deals

July   Hauliers and farmers stage large scale protests over the price of fuel

Aug   European banking regulators investigate £117bn of new loans made to telecommunications companies, reflecting concerns that banks have overlent to the sector

Nov   George W Bush elected US President

Dec   US GDP growth slows sharply, following prolonged expansion

2001

Jan   The Federal Reserve cuts interest rates twice in one month, by 0.5% each time

Feb   The FTSE share price index falls below the symbolic 6000 points mark

Apr   It emerges that Japan's bad debt problems are even worse than feared

May   In the UK, business insolvencies are at a six year high

Jun   Pharmaceutical company Glaxo sheds 18,000 staff, 7% of its UK workforce

Sep   Terrorist attacks in United States. The World Trade Centre in New York is destroyed

Oct   The US attacks Afghanistan

Argentina devalues its currency and defaults on its debt of $155 billion, the biggest default in history

Railtrack collapses after the Government refuses to give further subsidies

Nov   Bank of England cuts interest rates from 4.5% to 4.0%

Dec   In the third quarter of 2001, US GDP shrinks for the first time in eight years

Enron, the 8th largest company in the United States, collapses leading to concerns about accountancy practices, banking involvement and financial market regulation

2002

Jan   Euro notes and coins enter circulation

Apr   UK tax rises announced to fund NHS

Jun   WorldCom collapsed – the biggest corporate failure in history

Network Rail took over the running of the railways

Aug   IMF announced a $30 billion loan for Brazil, its biggest ever bailout of a struggling economy

Oct   UK housing boom peaks as house price inflation reaches 30%

Nov   US Federal Reserve cuts rate to 1.25%, a 40 year low in reaction to fears that the economy is running out of steam

Slowing UK economy forces doubling of the estimate of public borrowing

Dec   ECB cuts interest rates for the first time in more than a year, from 2.75% to 2.5%

Stock markets around the world fell sharply over the second half of the year, with the FTSE100 dropping below 4000

2003

Jan   Sweden pushes back its preferred date of euro entry from early 2005 to 2006

The FTSE 100 drops by nearly 50% since its peak in 1999, reaching its lowest level since 1995

UK economic growth at its lowest level since 1992, at 1.8% per annum

UK manufacturing jobs fall to their lowest level since records began

Feb   UK interest rates reduced by 0.25% to 3.75% due to weak internal and external demand

Mar   Iraq war begins

Jul   UK interest rates reduced by 0.25% to 3.5%, its nadir since May 1954, due to weak demand

Nov   UK interest rates raised by 0.25% to 3.75%

2004

Feb   UK interest rates raised by 0.25% to 4.0%

Mar   Gordon Brown delivers his eighth Budget statement

May   UK Interest rates rise 0.25% to 4.25%

Price of oil breaches $40 barrier

Petrol prices reach 80p a litre

June Federal Reserve of US raises interest rates by 0.25% to 1.25%

UK Interest rates rise 0.25% to 4.5%

July Gordon Brown releases 2004–05 Spending Review

Atkinson Review of gov't output measurement published

Aug   Bank of England raises interest rates 0.25% to 4.75%

Nov   George Bush wins US election

2005

Jan   Sir Tony Atkinson presents his report on the 'Measurement of government output and productivity in the National Accounts'

Mar   Federal Reserve Committee raises interest rates by 0.25% to 2.75%

May   Labour win general election

June Oil reaches near $60 a barrel – due to proposed strike in Norway

July G8 Summit in Gleneagles, Scotland

UK wins right to host Olympics in 2012

Aug   Bank of England cuts interest rates by 0.25% to 4.5%

Hurricane Katrina hits the US

US crude oil prices breach $70 a barrel

Oct   UK House price inflation hits 9 year low of 2.2% in October according to ODPM

Dec   ECB raises interest rates by 0.25% to 2.5%

Fed raises interest rates for the 13th consecutive time by 0.25% to 4.25%

2006

Jan   Ukraine / Russia gas dispute leads to cuts in gas supplies to Europe

Fed raises interest rates by 0.25% to 4.50%

Mar   ECB raises interest rates by 0.25% to 2.5%

FTSE breaks 6000 barrier

Gordon Brown delivers Budget statement

Fed raises interest rates by 0.25% to 4.75%

May   Fed raises interest rates by 0.25% to 5.00%

Oil prices have rise above $73 a barrel

State pension age to rise to 68 from 2044

June   Oil reaches $74 a barrel in response Iran nuclear dispute

ECB raises interest rates by 0.25% to 2.75%

Fed raises interest rates by 0.25% to 5.25%

July   Israel–Lebanon conflict pushes barrel of oil to $78 a barrel

Japan's Central Bank raises interest rate form 0.0% to 0.25% – the first increase in six years

G8 summit held in Russia

Aug   Bank of England raises Interest rates by 0.25% to 4.75%

ECB raises interest rates by 0.25% to 3.00%

Sep   At $64.55, Oil prices fell to their lowest level since the end of March

Greece announces 25 per cent increase in annual GDP after a new GDP calculation is applied

Oct   ECB lifts repo rate by 25 basis points to 3.25%

World output increased by 5.2% in the year to the second quarter

Nov   Bank of England raises Interest rates by 0.25% to 5.00%

Dec   The pound surges against the dollar – Sterling is at its highest level since Black Wednesday

The European Central Bank increase interest rates by 25 basis points to 3.5%

OPEC agrees to cut oil production from the 1st February 2007

2007

Jan   Bank of England raises Interest rates by 0.25% to 5.25%

The euro has displaced the US dollar as the world's leading currency in international bond markets

Feb   FTSE 100 hit a 6-year high after a flurry of takeover speculation

Mar   ECB lifts repo rate by 25 basis points to 3.75%

Apr   Sterling moves past the $2 mark for the first time since 1992

May   Bank of England raises Interest rates by 0.25% to 5.25%

Aug   The financial crisis began with Central banks intervening on a large scale as banks around the world stopped lending to each other

Sep   Oil hit a new record high of $93.80

Sterling rose to a 26 year high of $2.0694 against the dollar

Nov   Crude oil futures hit a record closing high, finishing above $98 a barrel

The three-month interbank interest rate hit 6.59 per cent

UK house prices recorded their biggest fall in 12 years

Dec   Bank of England cuts the rate of interest by 0.25% to 5.5%

The Federal Reserve cut interest rates by 0.25% to 4.25%

Main aggregates and summary accounts

Part 1

Chapter 1

National Accounts at a glance

Gross domestic product

In 2007 the output of the economy as measured by the chained volume measure of **gross domestic product** (GDP) was 3.0 per cent higher than in 2006, compared with a rise of 2.8 per cent in 2006 over 2005. The chained volume measure of GDP rose by 66.2 per cent between 1987 and 2007.

Money GDP (at current market prices) increased by 6.0 per cent between 2007 and 2006, compared to a 5.5 per cent increase in 2006 over 2005. Since 1987, money GDP has grown by a factor of 3.3.

Annual changes GDP chained volume measures

Percentage change

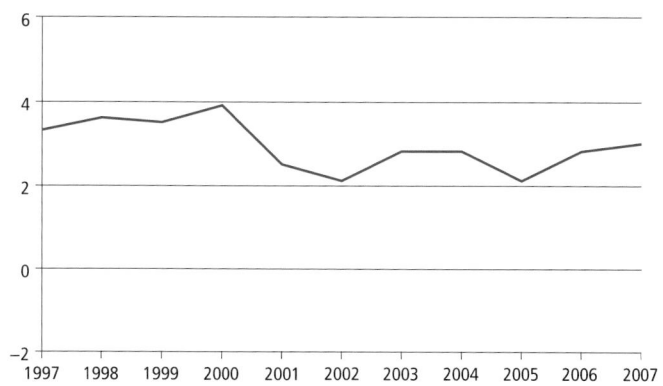

Gross domestic product deflator

This graph shows changes in the implied GDP deflator based on expenditure at market prices.

The annual rate of growth in the GDP expenditure deflator is 2.9 per cent in 2007 over 2006. This is the fourth consecutive year where growth of the GDP deflator has remained below 3.0 per cent.

Annual changes in the GDP market prices deflator

Percentage change

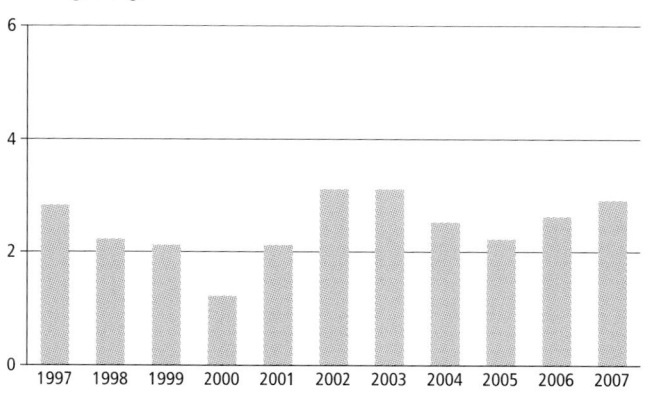

GDP: contribution of expenditure components to growth in 2007

The growth in real GDP of 3.0 per cent in 2007 can be split amongst the various expenditure components. This table shows what effect the change in each component would have had if all other components had remained unchanged. The rise in Household and NPISH final expenditure has been the strongest positive influence on growth. In contrast, net exports showed a negative influence on growth.

Contributions to annual growth in the chained volume measure of GDP, 2007

Component	Change in GDP	
	£m	%
Household and NPISH final expenditure	23,765	2.0
General government final expenditure	4,424	0.4
GFCF	15,042	1.2
Changes in inventories	2,274	0.2
Net exports	−9,176	−0.7
Other[1]	873	0.0
Total	37,201	3.0

1 Comprises acquisition of valuables and the statistical discrepancy between the expenditure measure and the average measure of GDP

Gross final expenditure at current prices: share by category of expenditure

Gross final expenditure (GFE) measures the sum of final uses of goods and services produced by, or imported to, the UK. In 2007, just under two-thirds of the total GFE was attributed to households and NPISH final consumption (49 per cent). Exports of goods and services accounted for around 20 per cent and the remainder was split between general government consumption (16 per cent) and gross capital formation (14 per cent).

GFE at current prices: share by category of expenditure

Per cent

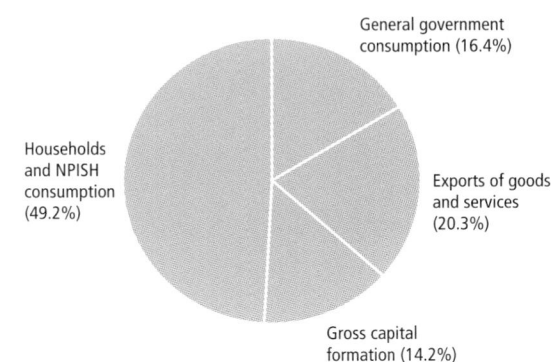

GDP at current prices: share by category of income

The income approach to GDP measures the income earned by individuals and corporations in the production of goods and services. In 2007, over half (53 per cent) of GDP at current market prices was accounted for by compensation of employees, which is largely comprised of wages and salaries. Total operating surplus, which includes corporations' gross trading profits accounted for just over one-fifth (22 per cent). Taxes and subsidies on production and imports, included to convert the estimate to market prices, accounted for 12 per cent of the remainder.

GDP at current market prices: share by category of income

Per cent

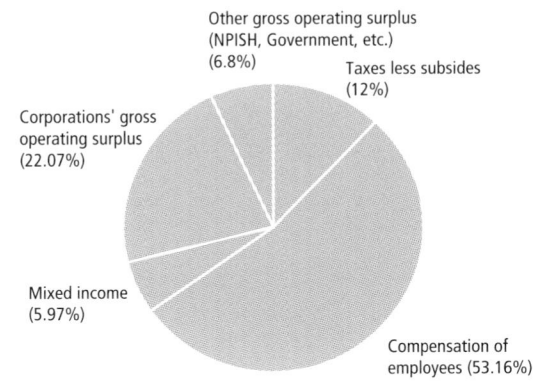

Gross value added at basic prices, by industry

In 2007 compared to 2006, the output of the production sector rose by 0.4 per cent, while the service sector rose by 3.7 per cent. The output of the agriculture, hunting, forestry and fishing sector fell by 0.8 per cent.

GVA at basic prices, by industry

Percentage change

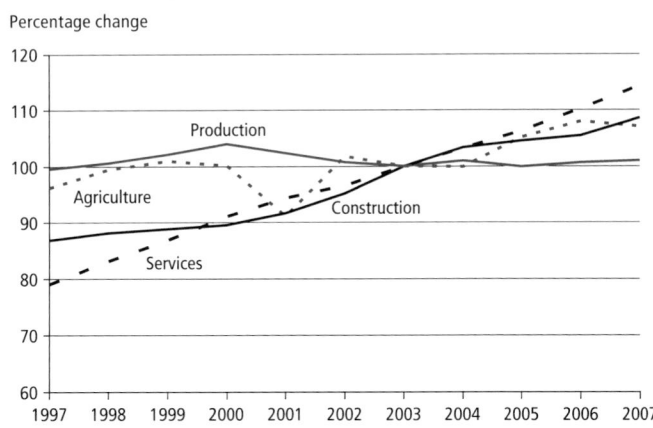

Gross value added at basic prices, by industry, 2003

In 2003, the latest base year, just over three quarters of total gross value added was from the services sector, compared to 18 per cent from the production sector. Most of the remainder was attributed to the construction sector.

Gross value added at basic prices, by industry, 2003

Percentage change

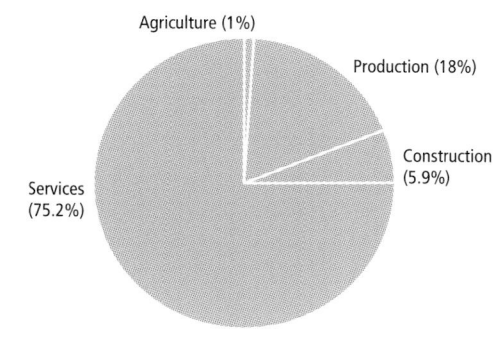

GDP per head

GDP chained volume measures per head rose by 4.2 per cent in 2007 compared to 2.3 per cent in 2006.

GDP per head

Percentage change

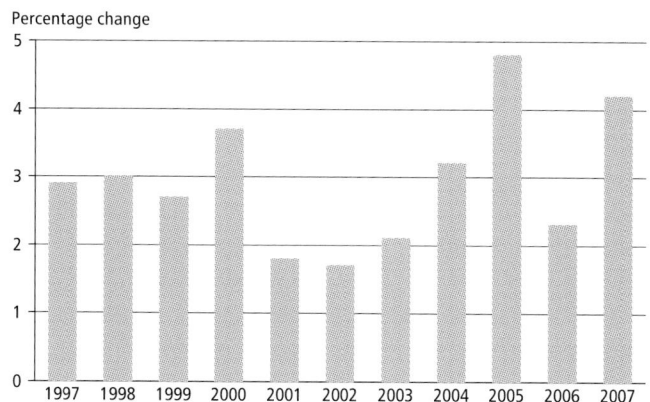

GDP and real household disposable income

Real household disposable income (RHDI) is the total resources available to the households sector after deductions. RHDI rose by 0.1 per cent in 2007, while the chained volume measure of GDP rose by 3.0 per cent.

Comparison of GDP and real household disposable income

Index 2003=100

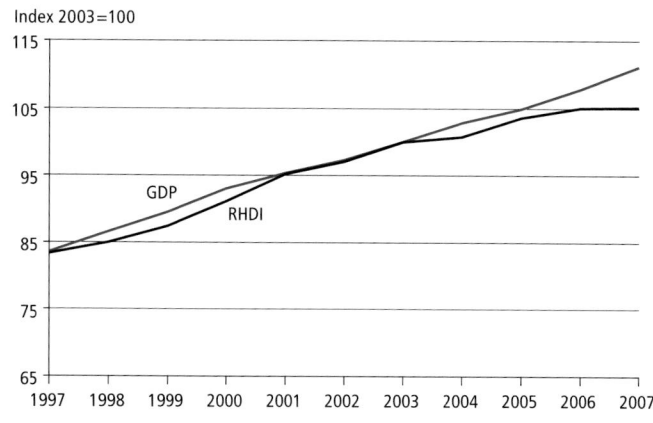

Main aggregates and summary accounts

UK GDP and national income
(Tables 1.1, 1.2, 1.3, 1.4)

Gross domestic product at current prices

The three approaches and the need for balancing

Gross Domestic Product (GDP) is arguably the most important aggregate or summary indicator for purposes of economic analysis and comparisons over time. It measures total domestic activity and can be defined in three different ways:

- GDP is the sum of gross value added of the institutional sectors or the industries *plus* taxes and *less* subsidies on products (which are not allocated to sectors and industries). It is also the balancing item in the total economy production account

- GDP is the sum of final uses of goods and services by resident institutional units (actual final consumption and gross capital formation), *plus* exports and *less* imports of goods and services

- GDP is the sum of uses in the total economy generation of income account (compensation of employees, taxes on production and imports *less* subsidies, gross operating surplus and gross mixed income of the total economy)

This is also the basis of estimating GDP. The use of three different methods which, as far as possible, use independent sources of information avoids sole reliance on one source and allows greater confidence in the overall estimation process.

The resulting estimates however, like all statistical estimates, contain errors and omissions; we obtain the best estimate of GDP (that is, the published figure) by reconciling the estimates obtained from all three approaches. On an annual basis this reconciliation is carried out through the construction of the Input-Output Supply and Use Tables for the years for which data are available, and for subsequent periods by carrying forward the level of GDP set by the annual balancing process by using the quarterly movements in production, income and expenditure indicators.

For years in which no input-output balance has been struck a statistical discrepancy exists between estimates of the total expenditure components of GDP and the total income components of GDP after the balancing process has been carried out. This statistical discrepancy is made up of two components which are shown in the accounts, namely:

- the statistical discrepancy (expenditure adjustment), which is the difference between the sum of the expenditure components and the definitive estimate of GDP, plus

- the statistical discrepancy (income adjustment), which is the difference between the sum of the income components and the definitive estimate of GDP (with sign reversed)

As outlined in the framework above, the different approaches to the measurement of GDP provide various breakdowns useful for a wide range of economic analyses. These approaches are described in more detail below.

The income approach

The income approach provides estimates of GDP and its 'income' component parts at current market prices. The sources and methods of this approach are described in detail in Chapter 14 of *Concepts, Sources and Methods*.[1]

As it suggests, the income approach adds up all income earned by resident individuals or corporations in the production of goods and services and is therefore the sum of uses in the generation of income account for the total economy (or alternatively the sum of primary incomes distributed by resident producer units).

However some types of income are not included – these are transfer payments like unemployment benefit, child benefit or state pensions. Although they do provide individuals with money to spend, the payments are made out of, for example, taxes and national insurance contributions. Transfer payments are a **redistribution** of existing incomes and do not themselves represent any addition to current economic activity. To avoid double counting, these transfer payments and other current transfers (for example, taxes on income and wealth) are excluded from the calculation of GDP although they are recorded in the secondary distribution of income account.

In the UK the income measure of GDP is obtained by summing together:

- gross operating surplus

- gross mixed income

- compensation of employees (wages and salaries and employers' social contributions)

- taxes on production and imports

   less any subsidies on production

Mixed income is effectively the operating surplus of unincorporated enterprises owned by households, which implicitly includes remuneration for work done by the owner or other members of the household. This remuneration cannot be identified separately from the return to the owner as entrepreneur.

As most of these incomes are subject to tax, the figures are usually obtained from data collected for tax purposes by HM Revenue & Customs. However, because there is some delay in providing good quality estimates by this method, other sources are used to provide initial estimates.

The operating surplus and mixed income are measures of profit that exclude any holding gains. (Holding gains result when, although no new goods or services have been produced, the value of inventories and fixed assets has increased simply as the result of an increase in the price of the item.)

National Statistics aims to cover the UK economy as comprehensively as possible. It is recognised that some income is not declared to the tax authorities, and to allow for this adjustments are routinely made to the GDP income measure. In 2006 the adjustment for undeclared income was about £22.5 billion, approximately 1.7 per cent of GDP.

Although the income approach cannot be used to calculate chained volume measures directly (because it is not possible to separate income components into prices and quantities in the same way as for goods and services) some estimates are obtained indirectly. The expenditure-based **GDP deflator at market prices** (also known as the **index of total home costs**) is used to deflate the current market price estimates to provide a chained volume measure of the total income component of GDP for balancing purposes.

Data on the income components can be found in Table 1.2.

The expenditure approach

The expenditure approach measures total expenditure on finished or final goods and services produced in the domestic economy or, alternatively, the sum of final uses of goods and services by resident institutional units **less** the value of imports of goods and services.

The total is obtained from the sum of final consumption expenditure by households, non-profit institutions serving households and government on goods and services, gross capital formation (capital expenditure on tangible and intangible fixed assets, changes in inventories and acquisitions **less** disposals of valuables) and net exports of goods and services.

This approach can be represented by the following equation:

$$GDP = C + G + I + X - M$$

Where: C = final consumption expenditure by households and NPISH sectors,

G = government consumption expenditure,

I = investment or gross capital formation,

X = exports and M = imports.

The data for these categories are estimated from a wide variety of sources including expenditure surveys, the government's internal accounting system, surveys of traders and the administrative documents used in the importing and exporting of some goods.

To avoid double counting in this approach it is important to classify consumption expenditures as either final or intermediate. **Final consumption** involves the consumption of goods purchased by or for the ultimate consumer or user. These expenditures are final because the goods are no longer part of the economic flow or being traded in the market place. **Intermediate consumption** on the other hand is consumption of goods and services which are used or consumed in the production process. Gross capital formation is treated separately from intermediate expenditure as the goods involved are not used up within the production process in an accounting period.

Exports include all sales to non-residents, and exports of both goods and services have to be regarded as final consumption expenditure, since they are final as far as the UK economy is concerned.

Imports of goods and services are deducted because although they are included directly or indirectly in final consumption expenditure they are not part of domestic production. What remains is what has been produced in the UK – gross domestic product using the expenditure approach.

Data on the current price expenditure components can be found in Table 1.2.

As well as GDP at current prices the expenditure approach is used to estimate chained volume measures of GDP. The chained volume measure shows the change in GDP **after** the effects of inflation have been removed (see 'UK GDP Chained Volume Measures' below).

GDP at market prices (£ million)

	Current prices	Chained volume measures
1995	733,266	894,988
1996	781,726	920,757
1997	830,094	951,208
1998	879,102	985,506
1999	928,730	1,019,735
2000	976,533	1,059,658
2001	1,021,828	1,085,745
2002	1,075,564	1,108,508
2003	1,139,746	1,139,746
2004	1,200,595	1,171,178
2005	1,252,505	1,195,276
2006	1,321,860	1,229,196
2007	1,401,042	1,266,397

The reference year for the chained volume measure series in this edition of the *Blue Book* is 2003; the chained volume measure of GDP for 2003 is referenced to, and therefore equal to, the annual current price estimate of GDP for 2003.

Two methods are used to remove the effects of inflation to obtain these chained volume measures. For some series, price indices for particular goods and services – such as components of the retail prices index (RPI) or the producer price index (PPI) – are used to 'deflate' the current price series. For other series, chained volume measures are assumed to be proportional to the volume of goods or services. Chained volume measures of GDP and its main expenditure components can be found in Table 1.3; the calculation of these chained volume measures are explained below

The production approach

The production approach to the estimation of GDP, which is also referred to as the output approach, looks at the contribution to production of each economic unit; that is the value (at basic prices) of their total output **less** the value of the inputs used up in the production process. The sum of these gross values added, **plus** taxes and **less** subsidies on products for all producers, is GDP at market prices: the production account balancing item. The following paragraphs give a brief overview of the methodology. It should be noted that the production approach concentrates on the basic price concept.

In theory, chained volume measures of value added should be estimated by double deflation; that is, deflating separately the inputs and the outputs of each economic unit (valued in chained volume measures) and then subtracting one from the other. But, because it is hard to get reliable information from companies, double deflation is only used in the estimation of output for the agriculture and electricity industries. So, for

most industries movements in the chained volume measures for gross value added are estimated by the use of output series. For industries whose outputs are goods, output can be estimated from the physical quantities of goods produced or from the value of output deflated by an index of price.

Apart from the use of output to estimate chained volume measures of Value Added, which accounts for around 80 per cent of the total of the production measure, a number of other kinds of indicator might be used as a proxy for the change in gross value added. For example, they may be estimated by changes in inputs, where the inputs chosen may be materials used, employment or some combination of these.

In the short-term it is reasonable to assume that movements in value added can be measured this way. However, changes in the ratio of output and inputs to gross value added can be caused by many factors: new production processes, new products made and inputs used; and changes in inputs from other industries will all occur over time. Aggregated over all industries the impact of these changes will be lessened. In the longer term all indicators are under constant review, with more suitable ones being used as they become available.

The estimate of gross value added for all industries (the proxy for the quarterly production measure of GDP) is finally obtained by combining or 'weighting together' the estimates for each industrial sector according to its relative importance (as established in the Input-Output Supply and Use Tables). For each year these weights are based on Input-Output data for the immediately preceding year, except for the most recent years where the weights are based on Input-Output data for 2003. This use of previous years' weights is a feature of the move to annual chain-linking, introduced in this edition of the *Blue Book* (see 'UK GDP Chained Volume Measures' below). Data can be found in Table 2.4.

Headline GDP

The chained volume measure of **gross domestic product at market prices** provide the key indicator of the state of the economy; this is sometimes called 'headline' GDP. The chained volume measure of **gross value added at basic prices** (GVA), another useful short-term indicator of growth in the economy, is the headline measure for the production approach. It is compiled in a way which is relatively free of short-term fluctuations due to uncertainties of timing. The construction of chained volume measures of **gross domestic product at factor cost** however, requires an adjustment for the relevant taxes and subsidies which can be subject to erratic changes. As a result the factor cost measure is less suitable as an indicator of short-term movements in the economy.

The figure below shows the distinction between market prices, basic prices and factor cost measures.

ESA95 code	
	Gross domestic product, at market prices
D.211	*Less* value added taxes (VAT) on products
D.212, D.214	*Less* other taxes on products (for example, alcohol duty)
D.31	*Plus* subsidies on products
	Gross value added, at basic prices
D.29	*less* taxes on production other than taxes on products (for example, business rates, vehicle excise duty paid by businesses and operating licences)
	Gross value added, at factor cost

GDP at market prices includes taxes on production, whilst GDP at basic prices includes only those taxes on production, such as business rates which are not taxes on products and GDP at factor cost excludes all taxes on production. A more detailed explanation of taxes follows.

Taxes

Taxes on production and imports including taxes on products (D.2), along with subsidies (D.3) (which can be regarded as negative taxes) make up the factor cost adjustment which represents the difference between GDP at market prices (sum of final expenditures) and GVA at factor cost (sum of incomes). This adjustment has to be added to the sum of incomes to obtain GDP at market prices. The basic price adjustment, which is the sum of **taxes on products** (D.21) *less* **subsidies on products** (D.31), is the difference between GVA at basic prices and GDP at market prices. Details of the taxes which comprise **taxes on production** are included in Table 11.1.

Taxes on production and imports (D.2) are taxes paid during the production or import of goods and services. They are paid irrespective of whether profits are made. They comprise taxes on products (D.21) and other taxes on production (D.29).

Taxes on products (D.21) are taxes paid per unit of good or service produced, sold, leased, transferred, exported or imported. They are included in the prices paid to suppliers of goods and services, so they are included in intermediate consumption at purchasers' prices (except for deductible VAT). Fuel duty is an example.

Deductible VAT differs from other **taxes on products**. It is levied like other **taxes on products** but producers are reimbursed by government for the amount they pay when goods and services are bought. Intermediate consumption at **purchasers' prices** is the price paid less deductible VAT refunded. The value of sales or production at **producers'**

prices also excludes any deductible VAT charged.

Suppliers are required to pay to government any **taxes on products** included in their prices. So the supplier's net revenue from selling the good is the selling price less the taxes on products included in the selling price. This is the **basic price**. It is the price at which market output is measured since it represents the producers' actual revenue.

Other taxes on production (D.29) are taxes which producers have to pay but they are not paid when goods and services are bought and so are not included in intermediate consumption. They are levied separately and are usually linked to the use of fixed capital or to the right to undertake certain regulated activities. Examples are non-domestic rates, vehicle excise duty, and various licence fees where the fee is much higher than the cost of administering the licence and so, in effect, is classified as taxation.

Other aggregates – Gross national disposable income

In the discussions so far we have yet to consider the measure which represents the total **disposable income** of the countrys' residents. Gross national income (GNI) represents the **total income** of UK residents and is the balancing item of the UK allocation of primary income account. It can also be derived from GDP by adding net employment income and net property income from the rest of the world. However there are two other areas which affect UK residents' command over resources.

First, there are flows into and out of the country which are not concerned with economic production. These are current transfers from abroad and current transfers paid abroad. They include transactions with the European Union, overseas aid and private gifts. An estimate of gross national disposable income (GNDI) is reached by adjusting GNI by the amount of net income received. GNI and GNDI are shown in Table 1.1.

Second, disposable income is affected by the terms of trade effect. Some of the expenditure by UK residents is on imported goods and services; some of the income earned by residents is from exports of goods and services. If UK export prices fall relative to the price of imports then the terms of trade effect would move against the UK; that is, residents would have to sell more exports to be able to continue to buy the same amount of imports. The purchasing power of UK residents would be diminished to this extent. Similarly, if UK export prices rose relative to prices of imports then the effect would be opposite: the purchasing power of residents would rise. An adjustment is made specifically for the terms of trade effect in calculating the chained volume measure of GNDI, also shown in Table 1.1.

UK GDP chained volume measures (Tables 1.1, 1.3, 1.4)

When looking at the change in the economy over time, the main concern is usually whether more goods and services are actually being produced now than at some time in the past. Over time, changes in current price GDP show changes in the monetary value of the components of GDP and, as these changes in value can reflect changes in both price and volume, it is difficult to establish how much of an increase in the series is due either to increased activity in the economy or to an increase in the price level. It is therefore useful to measure GDP in real terms (that is, excluding price effects) as well as at current prices. In most cases the revaluation of current price data to remove price effects (known as deflation) is carried out by using price indices such as component series of the retail prices index or producer price index to deflate current price series at a detailed level of disaggregation. In the 2003 edition of the Blue Book a new method of measuring GDP in real terms, **annual chain-linking**, was introduced to replace fixed base chain-linking which was used in previous editions of the *Blue Book*. The real GDP time series produced by annual chain-linking are referred to as **chained volume measures**.

In the UK economic accounts the expenditure approach is used to provide current price and chained volume measures of GDP. Because of the difficulties in accounting for changes in labour productivity it is not possible to obtain direct chained volume measures of GDP from the income data. However, an approximate aggregate measure is calculated by deflating the current price estimates using the GDP deflator derived from the expenditure measure for balancing purposes. The production measure of GDP is largely based on output measures.

The introduction of annual chain-linking

The fixed-base chain-linking method, which was used in editions of the *Blue Book* prior to 2003, produced 'constant price' estimates of GDP whereby the price structure prevailing in 1995 was used to compile data from 1994 onwards. For years prior to 1994 more appropriate pricing structures were used and, in order to link all of the 'constant price' estimates to produce continuous time series, a process of chain-linking was used whereby blocks of constant price data with different price bases were linked together. In the link years, figures were calculated with reference to two consecutive base years to obtain a linking factor so that the whole time series could be shown with reference to the latest base year. This system of fixed-base chain-linking is described in more detail at pages 36 to 38 of the 2002 edition of the *Blue Book*.

In the 2003 edition of the *Blue Book*, the fixed-base chain-linking method was replaced with an annual chain-linking

process which produces 'chained volume measures' of GDP. Chained volume measures are calculated by applying the price structure prevailing in the previous year for each year, except the most recent available years where chained volume measures are calculated by applying the price structure prevailing in 2003. The year 2003 is therefore the 'latest base year' for chained volume measures published in this edition of the *Blue Book*. Thus estimates for 2004 to 2007 inclusive are based on 2003 prices, estimates for 2003 are based on 2002 prices and so on. These 'previous years prices' data are chain-linked to produce continuous time series called 'chained volume measures', in a similar fashion to the fixed-based chain-linking described in the above paragraph.

These chained volume measure series are shown in £ million and referenced onto the 'latest base year' which is 2003 in this edition of the *Blue Book*. Current price data therefore equals chained volume measures annually in 2003. The process of annually chain-linking 'previous years prices' data onto a continuous time series referenced onto the latest base year results in a loss of additivity in the annual data prior to the latest base year. Thus chained volume measures prior to 2003 are non-additive in this edition of the *Blue Book*. Usually the the 'latest base year' and therefore the 'reference year' will move forward by one year. However, in the 2008 edition of the Blue Book, the 'latest base year' will continue to be 2003 due to the restrictions outlined above.

In the expenditure measure of GDP all of the components are annually chain-linked, as described above, and the chained volume measure of total GDP is aggregated from these. The output approach involves weighting together the detailed components using the contribution to current price GVA (or weight) in the immediately preceding year and annually chain-linking to produce a continuous time series. The application of annual chain-linking to the output measure of GDP is described in detail in an article published in the October 2001 edition of *Economic Trends*.[1]

Annual chain-linking provides more accurate measures of growth in the economy than that provided by the old method of fixed-base chain-linking because more up to date, and therefore more appropriate, price structures are used. The move to annual chain-linking is also consistent with international guidelines laid down in the *System for National Accounts 1993 (SNA93)*.

Index numbers and price indices

Some chained volume measure series are expressed as index numbers in which the series are simply scaled proportionately to a value of 100 in the reference year. These index numbers are volume indices of the 'base weighted' or 'Laspeyres' form.

(see chapter 2 of *Concepts, Sources and Methods*[2]) Aggregate price indices are of the 'Paasche' or 'current-weighted' form. They are generally calculated indirectly by dividing the current price value by the corresponding chained volume measure and multiplying by 100. Examples are the GDP deflator and the households' consumption deflator.

Value indices are calculated by scaling current price values proportionately to a value of 100 in the reference year. By definition such a value index, if divided by the corresponding volume index and multiplied by 100, will give the corresponding price index.

Population, employment and GDP per head (Table 1.5)

Population and employment data are supplementary to the system of accounts. The estimated population of the UK is as at 30 June and includes all those resident in the UK, whatever their nationality. They include members of both UK and non-UK armed forces and their dependants stationed in the UK and exclude members of H.M. armed forces stationed in the rest of the world. This is recognised as not being in strict accord with ESA95 requirements, which are for all UK armed forces and dependants, wherever stationed, to be included and all non-UK ones to be excluded. At present, this is the most appropriate estimate available; it is used to calculate GDP per head.

The total employment data are from the UK Labour Force Survey (LFS) which is recognised as the most appropriate source for coherent national aggregate labour market estimates. The LFS is a household survey which uses definitions which are consistent with the International Labour Organisation recommendations and have been adopted by all EU member countries. The coverage of the LFS is people living in private households and, from 1992, student halls of residence and NHS accommodation; it is not precisely consistent with either the home population data or the ESA95 requirements.

The employment data in the table are estimates of people according to their economic and employment status. They are not comparable with estimates of jobs, as shown in Table 2.5, as some people have more than one job. The total employment figures include people on government sponsored training and employment programmes and unpaid family workers.

UK summary accounts (Tables 1.6.0 – 1.6.9)

The UK summary accounts show the full set of accounts for the UK total economy. The accounts comprise the goods and services account, the production account, the distribution and use of income account and the accumulation accounts. The structure of the accounts is explained in the introduction.

UK summary accounts by sector (Tables 1.7.1 – 1.7.9)

The framework

As can be seen in Table 1.7, the UK sector accounts can be used to show the economic accounting framework in considerable detail by elaborating the accounts in three different dimensions:

- the institutional sectors
- the types of transaction
- the national and sector balance sheets

The institutional sectors

The first dimension involves the breakdown of the current account into institutional sectors grouped broadly according to their roles in the economy. Examples of these roles are: income distribution, income redistribution, private consumption, collective consumption, investment, financial intermediation, etc. Most units have more than one role but a natural classification is to distinguish between corporations, government and households. The rest of the world sector is also identified as having a role although it is obviously not part of the domestic economy.

The types of transaction

The second dimension is that of the type of transaction which relates to the particular account within which the transaction appears. These can be grouped broadly according to purpose, whether current, capital or financial.

Summary of the UK institutional sectors

Sectors and sub-sectors	ESA95	code
Non-financial corporations	**S.11**	
Public		S.11001
National private and foreign controlled		S.11002/3
Financial corporations	**S.12**	
Central bank		S.121
Other monetary financial institutions		S.122
Other financial intermediaries		S.123
Financial auxiliaries		S.124
Insurance corporations and pension funds		S.125
General government:	**S.13**	
Central government		S.1311
Local government		S.1313
Households	**S.14**	
Non-profit institutions serving households (NPISH)	**S.15**	
Rest of the world	**S.2**	

The balance sheets

To complete the full set of accounts the system includes balance sheets and a reconciliation of the changes that have brought about the change between the beginning and the end of the period. At present the UK does not compile the latter except for the general government sector which are available in the ONS Public sector finances release.

In theory the net lending or borrowing from the capital account for each sector should equal the net borrowing or lending from the financial account. In practice, because of errors and omissions in the accounts, a balance is rarely achieved and the difference is known as the **statistical discrepancy** although, across all accounts, when an Input-Output balance is available, these sum to zero. Consolidating the current and accumulation accounts would provide a balanced account which would look like many of the presentations of commercial accounts.

Assessment of Quality

ONS is committed to providing users with ways to assess the fitness for purpose of official statistics and has developed Quality Reports for key outputs in order to communicate quality information, as outlined in an article published in June 2005.[3] Quality Reports are structured around information on the six Eurostat dimensions of quality: relevance, accuracy, timeliness and punctuality, accessibility and clarity, comparability and coherence. The package considers both static and dynamic quality measures and where possible provides both qualitative and quantitative analysis. A dedicated area for Quality Information on Economic Statistics is available on the National Statistics website,[4] including a Summary Quality Report for GDP.[5]

In March 2008, ONS met a commitment made to monitor closely the quality of quarterly estimates during the modernisation of National Accounts. The article[6] was also in response to the Treasury Committee report on the ONS efficiency programme. In particular, tools for measuring the accuracy and coherence of the National Accounts were described.

Accuracy and reliability

One key aspect of quality for many users is accuracy. National Statistics strives to publish timely, consistent, and coherent estimates of GDP that accurately represent productive activity in the economy. The basis of these estimates is strengthened by the inter-relationships within the system, and the subsequent requirement that the many (and often independent) data sources are internally consistent. However, it remains very difficult to comment on the accuracy of GDP.

Estimates of GDP are built from numerous sources of information, including business surveys, household and other social surveys, administrative information and survey data from the Inland Revenue. Data is collected monthly, quarterly, annually and in some cases from ad hoc surveys. Some of the resulting estimates that feed into GDP will be firmly based whilst others may be weaker.

Assessing the accuracy of an estimate involves assessing the errors associated with that estimate. Sampling errors can be calculated for estimates derived from random samples. At present, sampling errors are calculated for several surveys that feed into GDP, but for other surveys there remain technical problems to be solved before reliable estimates of error can be formed. A program of work is currently underway which will lead to the publication of sampling errors for all major ONS business surveys.

In addition to sampling errors, accuracy is also affected by non-sampling errors such as limitations in coverage and measurement problems. Though there is limited information about non-sampling errors it is likely that for some surveys non-sampling errors are the more important source of error. Data validation by survey statisticians, additional consistency checks and the inclusion of coverage adjustments where survey sources are known to have shortcomings reduce non-sampling error and improve the quality of the accounts.

Even if the sampling and non-sampling errors of all individual data sources were known, the complexity of the process by which GDP is estimated is such that it would be difficult to build up an overall estimate of accuracy from the component series. The process of bringing together the three approaches to GDP into one measure, which uses detailed supply and demand balances, brings in extra information about the accuracy of the raw data and its consistency with other sources. This adds significantly to the accuracy of the overall estimate of GDP, but this cannot be measured scientifically.

One alternative approach to measuring the quality of GDP estimates is to use evidence from analyses of revisions to growth rates, outlined below. The purpose is to assess the reliability of GDP estimates, referring to the closeness of early estimates to subsequently estimated values.

Assessing the reliablity of the initial estimates of GDP

In order to achieve timeliness, National Accounts estimates are published first as preliminary quarterly estimates, approximately 25 days after the end of the quarter in question. Some components of this preliminary estimate contain a large proportion of estimation, as survey data available at this point is limited. An article in the April 2005 edition of *Economic Trends* provides analysis on the information content, and the proportion of model based forecasts at this and other early stages of the compilation process[7]. This preliminary estimate of growth is therefore often subject to revisions when more comprehensive data become available. Revisions are recorded for timely estimates and the initial results and future developments are described in an article in the October edition of *Economic & Labour Market Review*.[8] In addition, methodological changes in the National Accounts processes might lead to further revisions of the estimates. Looking at the size and direction of revisions is an important way of assessing the reliability of early estimates. This information is also used internally to guide the production of subsequent figures, but the historical level of revisions should not be used by users as a measure of the reliability of current estimates.

In revisions analysis, the revisions to initial estimates of growth rates of GDP are tested to discover if the mean revision is statistically significantly different from zero.

Following an announcement in the March 2004 edition of *Economic Trends*,[9] ONS now publishes information on revisions in the background notes of its First Releases. Text about possible future revisions is included, along with a table showing the mean revision over the last five years. A modified t-statistic is used to determine whether there is statistical evidence that this mean revision is statistically significantly different from zero (if the test is not significant this implies that the observed revisions might have occurred by chance). The table also shows the average absolute revision to the key variables over this period (the average size of revisions over the last five years) as a further indication of the reliability of the latest figures. A summary of the revisions analysis published to April 2005, and the user feedback received was published in May 2005.[10]

Following a second announcement, in *Economic Trends*[11] this revisions analysis is now supported by revisions triangles on the National Statistics website. These are spreadsheets that show how an estimate has evolved over time. The provision of these triangles allows users to produce their own revisions analysis and fully investigate the reliability of national accounts estimates. Revisions triangles are available for GDP and its key components at: www.statistics.gov.uk/statbase/Product. asp?vlnk=13560&More=n

More in-depth revisions analysis is published regularly by ONS in *Economic & Labour Market Review*. The latest results were published in November 2007,[12] following the 2007 *Blue Book* and relating to data from 1995 to 2004 (the latest data have been published in the last three *Blue Books*). It looks at revisions to estimates for quarterly GDP growth and its production, expenditure and income components, by stages of

the GDP compilation process, where different methods or different data are used at each stage. The stages are as follows:

- **Preliminary Estimate (M1)** – Month One, published around 25 days after the end of the quarter when the estimate is prepared on the basis of a limited proportion of survey data from short-term indicator surveys on the production side

- **UK Output, Income and Expenditure (M2)** – Month Two, published around 55 days after the end of the quarter when the estimate is based on more complete data on the production side, and early information from the expenditure and income approaches

- **Quarterly National Accounts (M3)** – Month Three, published around 85 days after the end of the quarter when fuller survey data for the components of each of the production (output), expenditure and income measures are available from short-term indicators and other surveys, but production remains the main source

- **Blue Book One (BB1)** – the first time the estimate appears in the *Blue Book*, typically after new and more comprehensive annual data sources have become available, around three to twelve months after publication of the corresponding M1 estimate

- **Blue Book Two (BB2)** – the stage at which Input-Output Supply and Use balancing is applied to the estimate for the first time, around twelve to eighteen months after it is first published. Due to the modernisation process, 2005 (in addition to 2006) was balanced for the first time this year using supply and use balancing

- **Post Blue Book Two (Post-BB2)** – the Input-Output Supply and Use balancing is run for the second time, and longer run methodological changes may be introduced to the current data and back series, including revised benchmark data. Due to the modernisation process, 2004 (and not 2005) was balanced for a second time this year using supply and use balancing

The breakdown by stage is outlined below.

Revisions at each stage of the quarterly constant price GDP growth estimate:

1995 Q1 – 2004 Q4	Mean Revision
Month Three (M3) *less* Month One (M1)	0.01
Blue Book One (BB1) *less* M3	0.04
Blue Book Two (BB2) *less* BB1	0.01
Post Blue Book Two (Post-BB2)	0.10*
Total revisions	0.15*

* Shows that the mean revision is statistically significant.

The results of the revisions analysis by stages showed that the only individual stage with a mean revision statistically significantly different from zero was post *Blue Book*.[2] A large proportion of the revisions occur at this later stage of the compilation process. These revisions in the later stages could be caused by changes in methodology. Revisions in the early stages would mostly be due to data replacing early forecasts and models, and more comprehensive data becoming available. Later stage revisions contribute to a total mean revision of 0.15 which is statistically significant.

The revisions analysis is also applied to the output, expenditure and income components of GDP. However, only some output components have been published at M1 during the period analysed, all expenditure components are not published until at least the Month Two (M2) stage and most income components are first published at M3 during this time period. Additionally the data for components was only available from 1996 at the earliest, which meant the data windows and revision periods differed from that analysed in the GDP revisions analysis.

Of the components, only revisions to gross fixed capital formation, imports and exports are statistically significant within expenditure. Further investigation of the components of imports and exports showed that the revisions followed a similar trend and thus offset each other to a certain extent. Revisions to Distribution, Hotels and Catering and Transport, Storage and Communication are significant within output, although revisions to services are not. There are no significant revisions to any of the income components.

Summary of the revisions to expenditure components

1996 Q1 – 2004 Q4	% of GDP (2003)	Mean Revision
Household Final Consumption Expenditure	62.8	0.00
Non-Profit Institutions Serving Households Final Consumption Expenditure	2.4	−0.41
General Government Final Consumption Expenditure	21.0	−0.06
Gross Capital Formation	16.1	1.16*
Total Exports	25.7	0.77*
Total Imports	−28.4	0.61*

* Shows that the mean revision is statistically significantly different from zero.

Summary of the revisions to output components

1996 Q1 – 2004 Q4	% of GVA (2003)	Mean Revision
Agriculture	1.0	0.40
Production	18.5	0.20
Construction	6.1	0.04
Services	74.4	0.16
Distribution, Hotels and Catering	15.3	0.28*
Transport, Storage and Communications	7.8	0.43*
Business Services and Finance	27.7	0.24
Government and Other Services	23.5	0.00

* Shows that the mean revision is statistically significant different from zero.

Summary of the revisions to income components

1996 Q1 – 2004 Q4	% of GVA (2003)	Mean Revision
Compensation employees	55.6	0.20
Public non-financial corporations	0.7	−2.03
Private non-financial corporations	18.2	0.25
Financial corporations	3.6	4.71
Other income	9.2	−1.56
Taxes on productsless subsidies	12.7	–

* Shows that the mean revision is statistically significant different from zero.

National Statistics regularly looks at revisions to initial estimates and although no correction factors are applied to data series, the information is used in the GDP balancing procedure to identify areas where improvements to early models might be made. Regular monitoring of the revisions to estimates continues, and the results are published in *Economic & Labour Market Review*.

Balances

Further assessment of the reliability of the consolidated economic and sector accounts can be gained by examination of the capital and financial accounts - which should, in theory, show a balance between the net lending/borrowing in the capital account and financial account for each sector. However, because of errors and omissions in the accounts, such a balance is rarely achieved. The resulting statistical discrepancy items required to equate these accounts are shown in this publication (see Table D at Part 3).

These discrepancies provide a measure of reliability as they reflect errors and omissions in the accounts. Some components of the accounts (for example, estimates for general government) provide excellent coverage and are very reliable whilst others (for example life insurance and pension funds) are less fully covered. A detailed table, which looks specifically at the reliability of components of the sector financial accounts, is published in *Financial Statistics Explanatory Handbook*. However, because of the many sources of information that feed into the economic accounts it is not possible to generalise these 'reliability measures' to the aggregate estimates.

Spurious accuracy and rounding to the nearest £ million

One final point must also be made about the reliability of the statistics. In most of the published tables no attempt is made to round estimates beyond the nearest £ million. In some instances this shows figures which appear to have more precision than evidence warrants.

The reasons for this presentation are as follows:

- rounded figures can distort differences over time or between items

- some of the estimates in the tables are fairly precise and, if such an estimate is small, rounding would unnecessarily distort what it shows; yet if such series were not rounded to the nearest £ million the major aggregates of which they are components would appear precise even though other components were heavily rounded

- not rounding beyond the nearest £ million aids users who prepare derived statistics, by avoiding the accumulation of rounding errors which can occur when a number of rounded numbers are manipulated

- in presenting numbers to the nearest £ million, the rounding is usually such that the components add to the total at current prices, so that the accounts balance. In particular the quarterly estimates, both before and after seasonal adjustment, add up to the calendar year totals. However, there are some small differences between the sum of component series and the total shown, due to rounding

Changes since last year's *Blue Book*

An analysis of revisions in current prices since last year's *Blue Book* is shown in Table B.

This is the first *Blue Book* in which a revised methodology for the output of financial intermediation services indirectly measured (FISIM) has been included.

Financial Intermediaries (FIs) charge explicit commissions and fees for their services to their customers, as well as implicit ones by paying or charging different rates of interest to borrowers and lenders. FIs pay lower rates of interest than would otherwise be the case to those that lend them money, and charge higher rates of interest to those who borrow from them. The resulting receipts of interest are used to offset their expenses and provide an operating surplus. This is reflected by the action of the FIs observed on the market: they do not charge customers individually for services provided, but benefit from the implicit margin between their interest rates on lending and deposit business. However, in this situation, the national accounts must use an indirect measure of the value of the services for which the FIs do not charge explicity called FISIM.

FISIM output generated by FIs is allocated between the various users of the service for which no explicit charges are made. Hence it is treated in national accounts as: intermediate consumption by businesses; final consumption by households, general government, and non-profit institutions serving households; and exports to non-residents.

There is also an estimate for imported FISIM, generated by the non-resident FIs, and allocated into intermediate and final consumption.

To calculate FISIM output and allocate it into the user sectors, detailed sectorised interest and stocks data on loans and deposits are required. The FISIM output series generated by banks and building societies are compiled differently for each of the two time periods:

- From 1999 onwards, the FISIM series were compiled by the Bank of England using detailed data sourced from its own specially designed enquiries

- Before 1998, the series were compiled by ONS using detailed stocks data sourced from the Bank of England. The required interest data were derived from the effective interest rates used elsewhere in the National Accounts

The remaining FISIM output generated by the other financial intermediaries and the FISIM import series were compiled by ONS using the ONS enquiries and the Balance of Payment statistics data sources.

See Akritidis[13] for a more detailed description of the methodology, an update and analysis of the results, and assessment of the impact of FISIM on GDP in both nominal and real terms. The data produced using these methods can be found in table 1.8 of this publication.

Apart from FISIM, the revisions to the aggregate GDP levels and growth from 2004 to 2006 follow the re-introduction of the supply use processes and the incorporation of annual benchmark survey estimates, especially the Annual business Inquiry. In *Blue Book* 2006, 2003 and 2004 were balanced. In this year's *Blue Book*, 2004 has been re-balanced and 2005 and 2006 have been balanced for the first time. More details can be found in chapter 2 of this publication.

B   Revisions since ONS Blue Book, 2007 edition

£ million

	1999	2000	2001	2002	2003	2004	2005	2006
National accounts aggregates								
At current prices								
Gross domestic product at market prices	16 785	17 602	18 531	19 771	21 501	16 299	18 529	22 238
less Basic price adjustment	–	–	–	–	–	–341	37	–35
Gross value added at basic prices	16 785	17 602	18 531	19 771	21 501	16 640	18 492	22 273
Expenditure components at current prices								
Domestic expenditure on goods and services at market prices								
Households	14 377	15 732	15 282	16 402	17 448	14 971	19 396	19 891
Non-profit making institutions serving households	311	362	391	454	483	–205	–1 183	–1 104
General government	132	121	81	113	120	1 061	–263	–1 143
Gross fixed capital formation	–	–	–	–	–	–1 588	–544	–6 831
Changes in inventories	–	–	–	–	–	–161	902	587
Acquisitions less disposals of valuables	–	–	–	–	–	–	–	240
Total exports	2 909	2 217	3 726	4 025	5 280	4 698	4 238	6 693
Statistical discrepancy (expenditure)	–	–	–	–	–	–	–1 243	–635
Total imports	944	830	949	1 223	1 830	2 477	2 774	–4 540
Income components at current prices								
Compensation of employeees	–	–	–	–	–	–618	–4 600	–5 791
Gross operating surplus								
Public non-financial corporations	–14	–12	–13	–71	–65	385	434	408
Private non-financial corporations	–6 815	–7 630	–7 905	–7 104	–7 854	–11 352	–11 954	–9 732
Financial corporations	999	–2 559	–277	–6 489	–8 201	–14 864	–7 397	–9 082
General government	–	–	–	–	–	–252	–431	–719
Household sector	–6 061	–4 788	–6 083	–6 897	–6 951	–7 527	–9 159	–10 462
Mixed income	–792	–874	–839	–804	–798	858	–817	44
Taxes on production and imports	–	–	–	–	–	123	229	–65
less subsidies	–	–	–	–	–	–619	–614	–480
Statistical discrepancy (income)	–	–	–	–	–	–	916	551

References

1   Tuke A and Reed G (2001) The Effects of Annual Chain-linking on the Output Measure of GDP. *Economic Trends* No. 575.

2   Office for National Statistics (1998) *National Accounts Concepts, Sources and Methods.* The Stationery Office; London.

3   Jenkinson G (2005) *Publishing Quality Information for National Accounts Outputs.*

4   Quality Information for Economic Statistics webpage, www.statistics.gov.uk/about_ns/economicstatistics_ qualityreports.asp

5   Robinson H (2005) *Summary Quality Report for GDP data releases.*

6   Meader R (2007) Revisions to Quarterly GDP Growth and its Components *Economic & Labour Market Review.* Vol 1 No. 11.

7   Skipper H (2005) Early estimates of GDP: information content and forecasting methods *Economic Trends* No. 617.

8   Mainwaring H and Skipper H (2007) GDP(O) Revisions analysis system: outline and indicative results *Economic & Labour Market Review* Vol. 1 No. 10.

9   Jenkinson G (2004) ONS Policy on Standards for Presenting Revisions Analysis in Time Series First Releases, *Economic Trends* No. 604.

10 George E and Obuwa D (2005) *Revisions Analysis Published by National Accounts: A Summary to April 2005.*

11 George E and Jenkinson G (2005) Publication of Revisions Triangles on the National Statistics Website *Economic Trends* No. 614.

12 Meader R and Tily G (2007) Revisions to Quarterly GDP Growth and its Components *Economic & Labour Market Review* Vol. 2 No. 1.

13 Akritidis L (2007) Improving the Measurement of Banking Services in the UK National Accounts *Economic & Labour Market Review* Vol 1 No 5.

Other articles

■ Jones F (1998) Rebasing the National Accounts *Economic Trends* No. 535.

■ Penneck S and Mahajan S (1999) Annual Coherence Adjustments in the National Accounts *Economic Trends* No. 551.

■ Brueton A (1999) The Development of Chain-Linked and Harmonised Estimates of GDP at Constant prices *Economic Trends* No. 552.

■ Andrews T (2000) Improvements to Economic Statistics *Economic Trends* No. 555.

■ Akritidis L (2002) Accuracy Assessment of National Accounts Statistics *Economic Trends* No. 589

■ Tuke A and Beadle J (2003) The effect of annual chain-linking on Blue Book 2002 annual growth estimates, *Economic Trends* No 593.

■ Ruffles D, Tily G, Caplan D and Tudor S (2003) VAT Missing Trader Intra-Community fraud: the effect on Balance of Payments statistics and UK National Accounts *Economic Trends* No. 597.

■ Tily G (2006) Improvements to timely measures of service sector output, *Economic Trends* No. 630.

■ For further reading, and access to all these articles see the National Statistics webpage dedicated to revisions analyisis at: www.statistics.gov.uk/about_ns/economic_revisions.asp

1.1 UK national and domestic product
Main aggregates: index numbers and values

Current prices and chained volume measures (Reference year 2003)

			1994	1995	1996	1997	1998	1999	2000
	INDICES (2003=100)								
	VALUES AT CURRENT PRICES								
B.1*g	Gross domestic product at current market prices ("money GDP")	YBEU	60.8	64.3	68.6	72.8	77.1	81.5	85.7
B.1g	Gross value added at current basic prices	YBEX	61.1	64.4	68.8	72.9	77.0	81.1	85.2
	CHAINED VOLUME MEASURES								
B.1*g	Gross domestic product at market prices	YBEZ	76.2	78.5	80.8	83.5	86.5	89.5	93.0
B.6*g	Gross national disposable income at market prices	YBFP	73.7	75.0	77.7	81.3	85.4	87.5	90.7
B.1g	Gross value added at basic prices	CGCE	76.6	78.7	80.9	83.6	86.8	89.9	93.4
	PRICES								
	Implied deflator of GDP at market prices	YBGB	79.8	81.9	84.9	87.3	89.2	91.1	92.2
	VALUES AT CURRENT PRICES (£ million)								
	Gross measures (before deduction of fixed capital consumption) at current market prices								
B.1*g	**Gross Domestic Product ("money GDP")**	YBHA	692 987	733 266	781 726	830 094	879 102	928 730	976 533
D.1+D.4	Employment, property and entrepreneurial income from the rest of the world (receipts *less* payments)	YBGG	1 351	−842	−2 367	324	11 803	−1 043	1 962
-D.21+D.31	Subsidies (receipts) *less* taxes (payments) on products from/to the rest of the world	−QZOZ	−3 349	−5 220	−3 116	−2 919	−3 651	−3 438	−4 098
+D.29-D.39	Other subsidies on production from/to the rest of the world	−IBJL	286	293	261	208	241	338	335
B.5*g	**Gross National Income (GNI)**	ABMX	691 275	727 497	776 504	827 707	887 495	924 587	974 732
D.5,6,7	Current transfers from the rest of the world (receipts *less* payments)	−YBGF	−2 127	−2 438	−1 686	−3 036	−4 764	−4 224	−6 016
B.6*g	**Gross National Disposable Income**	NQCO	689 148	725 059	774 818	824 671	882 731	920 363	968 716
	Adjustment to current basic prices								
B.1*g	**Gross Domestic Product (at current market prices)**	YBHA	692 987	733 266	781 726	830 094	879 102	928 730	976 533
-D.21 +D.31	Adjustment to current basic prices (*less* taxes *plus* subsidies on products)	−NQBU	−72 645	−79 331	−83 316	−90 570	−97 116	−105 956	−112 248
B.1g	**Gross Value Added (at current basic prices)**	ABML	620 342	653 935	698 410	739 524	781 986	822 774	864 285
-K.1	*Net measures (after deduction of fixed capital consumption) at current market prices*	−NQAE	−86 646	−89 130	−93 364	−95 179	−98 960	−105 507	−111 251
B.1*n	Net domestic product	NHRK	606 341	644 136	688 362	734 915	780 142	823 223	865 282
B.5*n	Net national income	NSRX	604 629	638 367	683 140	732 528	788 535	819 080	863 481
B.6*n	Net national disposable income	NQCP	602 502	635 929	681 454	729 492	783 771	814 856	857 465
	CHAINED VOLUME MEASURES (Reference year 2003, £ million)								
	Gross measures (before deduction of fixed capital consumption) at market prices								
B.1*g	**Gross Domestic Product**	ABMI	868 560	894 988	920 757	951 208	985 506	1 019 735	1 059 658
TGL	Terms of trade effect ("Trading gain or loss")	YBGJ	−17 687	−24 175	−20 699	−12 482	−10 083	−6 595	−10 361
GDI	Real gross domestic income	YBGL	850 873	870 813	900 058	938 726	975 423	1 013 140	1 049 297
D.1+D.4	Real employment, property and entrepreneurial income from the rest of the world (receipts *less* payments)	YBGI	1 659	−1 000	−2 724	365	13 072	−1 136	2 103
-D.21+D.31	Subsidies (receipts) *less* taxes (payments) on products from/to the rest of the world	−QZPB	−4 104	−6 185	−3 577	−3 291	−4 044	−3 745	−4 392
+D.29-D.39	Other subsidies on production from/to the rest of the world	−IBJN	350	347	300	234	267	368	359
B.5*g	**Gross National Income (GNI)**	YBGM	848 735	863 927	894 015	935 993	984 711	1 008 594	1 047 337
D.5,6,7	Real current transfers from the rest of the world (receipts *less* payments)	−YBGP	−2 608	−2 888	−1 936	−3 422	−5 276	−4 601	−6 448
B.6*g	**Gross National Disposable Income**	YBGO	846 131	861 042	892 086	932 573	979 432	1 003 991	1 040 885
	Adjustment to basic prices								
B.1*g	**Gross Domestic Product (at market prices)**	ABMI	868 560	894 988	920 757	951 208	985 506	1 019 735	1 059 658
-D.21 +D.31	Adjustment to basic prices (*less* taxes *plus* subsidies on products)	−NTAQ	−90 868	−96 324	−99 676	−103 014	−105 165	−107 873	−112 020
B.1g	**Gross Value Added (at basic prices)**	ABMM	777 889	798 860	821 280	848 400	880 567	912 134	947 927
-K.1	*Net measures (after deduction of fixed capital consumption) at market prices*	−CIHA	−96 635	−96 433	−98 885	−101 460	−105 466	−110 533	−114 722
B.5*n	Net national income at market prices	YBET	751 619	767 225	794 953	834 548	879 349	898 050	932 606
B.6*n	Net national disposable income at market prices	YBEY	749 030	764 353	793 050	831 140	874 071	893 453	926 150

1.1

UK national and domestic product
Main aggregates: index numbers and values

continued   **Current prices and chained volume measures (Reference year 2003)**

			2001	2002	2003	2004	2005	2006	2007
	INDICES (2003=100)								
	VALUES AT CURRENT PRICES								
B.1*g	Gross domestic product at current market prices ("money GDP")	YBEU	89.7	94.4	100.0	105.3	109.9	116.0	122.9
B.1g	Gross value added at current basic prices	YBEX	89.4	94.3	100.0	105.3	109.9	116.0	122.9
	CHAINED VOLUME MEASURES								
B.1*g	Gross domestic product at market prices	YBEZ	95.3	97.3	100.0	102.8	104.9	107.8	111.1
B.6*g	Gross national disposable income at market prices	YBFP	93.9	97.1	100.0	102.8	104.2	106.1	109.6
B.1g	Gross value added at basic prices	CGCE	95.5	97.2	100.0	102.7	104.9	107.9	111.1
	PRICES								
	Implied deflator of GDP at market prices	YBGB	94.1	97.0	100.0	102.5	104.8	107.5	110.6
	VALUES AT CURRENT PRICES (£ million)								
	Gross measures (before deduction of fixed capital consumption) at current market prices								
B.1*g	**Gross Domestic Product ("money GDP")**	YBHA	1 021 828	1 075 564	1 139 746	1 200 595	1 252 505	1 321 860	1 401 042
D.1+D.4	Employment, property and entrepreneurial income from the rest of the world (receipts *less* payments)	YBGG	9 425	18 286	17 523	17 830	21 872	10 097	8 606
-D.21+D.31	Subsidies (receipts) *less* taxes (payments) on products from/to the rest of the world	-QZOZ	-3 920	-2 890	-2 596	-1 234	-4 260	-4 496	-4 731
+D.29-D.39	Other subsidies on production from/to the rest of the world	-IBJL	582	519	592	592	3 408	3 220	2 943
B.5*g	**Gross National Income (GNI)**	ABMX	1 027 915	1 091 479	1 155 265	1 217 783	1 273 525	1 330 681	1 407 860
D.5,6,7	Current transfers from the rest of the world (receipts *less* payments)	-YBGF	-3 182	-6 500	-7 843	-9 645	-11 052	-10 657	-11 943
B.6*g	**Gross National Disposable Income**	NQCO	1 024 733	1 084 979	1 147 422	1 208 138	1 262 473	1 320 024	1 395 917
	Adjustment to current basic prices								
B.1*g	**Gross Domestic Product (at current market prices)**	YBHA	1 021 828	1 075 564	1 139 746	1 200 595	1 252 505	1 321 860	1 401 042
-D.21 +D.31	Adjustment to current basic prices (*less* taxes *plus* subsidies on products)	-NQBU	-114 234	-118 470	-124 738	-132 021	-137 384	-144 628	-153 321
B.1g	**Gross Value Added (at current basic prices)**	ABML	907 594	957 094	1 015 008	1 068 574	1 115 121	1 177 232	1 247 721
	Net measures (after deduction of fixed capital consumption) at current market prices								
-K.1		-NQAE	-115 796	-121 914	-125 603	-135 184	-138 520	-147 858	-158 143
B.1*n	Net domestic product	NHRK	906 032	953 650	1 014 143	1 065 411	1 113 985	1 174 002	1 242 899
B.5*n	Net national income	NSRX	912 119	969 565	1 029 662	1 082 599	1 135 005	1 182 823	1 249 717
B.6*n	Net national disposable income	NQCP	908 937	963 065	1 021 819	1 072 954	1 123 953	1 172 166	1 237 774
	CHAINED VOLUME MEASURES (Reference year 2003, £ million)								
	Gross measures (before deduction of fixed capital consumption) at market prices								
B.1*g	**Gross Domestic Product**	ABMI	1 085 745	1 108 508	1 139 746	1 171 178	1 195 276	1 229 196	1 266 397
TGL	Terms of trade effect ("Trading gain or loss")	YBGJ	-11 125	-3 696	–	690	-8 676	-9 628	-4 066
GDI	Real gross domestic income	YBGL	1 074 620	1 104 812	1 139 746	1 171 868	1 186 600	1 219 568	1 262 331
D.1+D.4	Real employment, property and entrepreneurial income from the rest of the world (receipts *less* payments)	YBGI	9 901	18 775	17 523	17 411	20 732	9 323	7 768
-D.21+D.31	Subsidies (receipts) *less* taxes (payments) on products from/to the rest of the world	-QZPB	-4 118	-2 967	-2 596	-1 205	-4 038	-4 151	-4 270
+D.29-D.39	Other subsidies on production from/to the rest of the world	-IBJN	611	533	592	578	3 230	2 973	2 656
B.5*g	**Gross National Income (GNI)**	YBGM	1 081 003	1 121 154	1 155 265	1 188 652	1 206 524	1 227 713	1 268 485
D.5,6,7	Real current transfers from the rest of the world (receipts *less* payments)	-YBGP	-3 342	-6 673	-7 843	-9 419	-10 476	-9 840	-10 779
B.6*g	**Gross National Disposable Income**	YBGO	1 077 665	1 114 481	1 147 422	1 179 233	1 196 048	1 217 873	1 257 706
	Adjustment to basic prices								
B.1*g	**Gross Domestic Product (at market prices)**	ABMI	1 085 745	1 108 508	1 139 746	1 171 178	1 195 276	1 229 196	1 266 397
-D.21 +D.31	Adjustment to basic prices (*less* taxes *plus* subsidies on products)	-NTAQ	-116 584	-121 657	-124 738	-128 532	-130 433	-133 633	-138 328
B.1g	**Gross Value Added (at basic prices)**	ABMM	969 279	986 849	1 015 008	1 042 646	1 064 843	1 095 563	1 128 069
-K.1	*Net measures (after deduction of fixed capital consumption) at market prices*	-CIHA	-118 072	-123 405	-125 553	-133 203	-133 706	-139 227	-144 976
B.5*n	Net national income at market prices	YBET	962 937	997 724	1 029 712	1 055 449	1 072 818	1 088 486	1 123 509
B.6*n	Net national disposable income at market prices	YBEY	959 613	991 053	1 021 869	1 046 030	1 062 342	1 078 646	1 112 730

1.2 UK gross domestic product and national income
Current prices

£ million

			1993	1994	1995	1996	1997	1998	1999	2000
	GROSS DOMESTIC PRODUCT									
	Gross domestic product: Output									
B.1g	Gross value added, at basic prices									
P.1	Output of goods and services	NQAF	1 164 069	1 245 161	1 332 337	1 427 240	1 510 279	1 596 283	1 683 788	1 777 360
-P.2	less intermediate consumption	−NQAJ	−576 795	−624 819	−678 402	−728 830	−770 755	−814 297	−861 014	−913 075
B.1g	**Total Gross Value Added**	**ABML**	**587 274**	**620 342**	**653 935**	**698 410**	**739 524**	**781 986**	**822 774**	**864 285**
D.211	Value added taxes (VAT) on products	QYRC	42 208	45 806	47 984	50 919	54 964	56 541	61 512	64 189
D.212,4	Other taxes on products	NSUI	30 853	33 507	38 068	39 972	43 076	46 999	50 512	54 086
-D.31	less subsidies on products	−NZHC	−6 139	−6 668	−6 721	−7 575	−7 470	−6 424	−6 068	−6 027
B.1*g	**Gross Domestic Product at market prices**	**YBHA**	**654 196**	**692 987**	**733 266**	**781 726**	**830 094**	**879 102**	**928 730**	**976 533**
	Gross domestic product: Expenditure									
P.3	Final consumption expenditure									
P.41	Actual individual consumption									
P.3	Household final consumption expenditure	ABPB	406 808	426 710	448 720	482 041	512 482	546 888	582 371	616 558
P.3	Final consumption expenditure of NPISH	ABNV	14 202	15 520	16 617	18 371	19 600	21 082	22 185	23 531
P.31	Individual govt. final consumption expenditure	NNAQ	75 600	78 970	82 313	87 519	90 004	94 783	102 742	109 297
P.41	Total actual individual consumption	NQEO	496 610	521 200	547 650	587 931	622 086	662 753	707 298	749 386
P.32	Collective govt. final consumption expenditure	NQEP	58 181	59 308	60 719	61 248	60 648	61 707	66 910	72 675
P.3	Total final consumption expenditure	ABKW	554 791	580 508	608 369	649 179	682 734	724 460	774 208	822 061
P.3	Households and NPISH	NSSG	421 010	442 230	465 337	500 412	532 082	567 970	604 556	640 089
P.3	Central government	NMBJ	82 911	85 511	87 966	92 476	93 897	97 156	103 594	110 829
P.3	Local government	NMMT	50 870	52 767	55 066	56 291	56 755	59 334	66 058	71 143
P.5	Gross capital formation									
P.51	Gross fixed capital formation	NPQX	103 997	111 623	121 364	130 346	138 307	155 997	161 722	167 172
P.52	Changes in inventories	ABMP	329	3 708	4 512	1 771	4 621	5 026	6 060	5 271
P.53	Acquisitions less disposals of valuables	NPJO	−29	113	−121	−160	−27	429	229	3
P.5	Total gross capital formation	NQFM	104 297	115 444	125 755	131 957	142 901	161 452	168 011	172 446
P.6	Exports of goods and services	KTMW	165 834	183 215	207 147	229 047	237 478	233 284	242 691	269 819
-P.7	less imports of goods and services	−KTMX	−170 726	−186 180	−208 005	−228 457	−233 019	−240 094	−256 180	−287 793
B.11	External balance of goods and services	KTMY	−4 892	−2 965	−858	590	4 459	−6 810	−13 489	−17 974
de	Statistical discrepancy between expenditure components and GDP	RVFD	−	−	−	−	−	−	−	−
B.1*g	**Gross Domestic Product at market prices**	**YBHA**	**654 196**	**692 987**	**733 266**	**781 726**	**830 094**	**879 102**	**928 730**	**976 533**
	Gross domestic product: Income									
B.2g	Operating surplus, gross									
	Non-financial corporations									
	Public non-financial corporations	NRJT	6 812	7 117	8 880	8 787	7 229	7 734	7 664	7 176
	Private non-financial corporations	NRJK	113 554	130 786	141 620	157 852	169 428	172 500	176 468	182 115
	Financial corporations	NQNV	19 048	18 562	15 798	20 128	20 991	17 600	18 009	10 996
	General government	NMXV	7 520	7 926	8 500	8 813	9 003	8 999	9 262	9 542
	Households and non-profit institutions serving households	QWLS	28 220	30 213	33 658	35 480	38 111	42 232	45 134	49 172
B.2g	Total operating surplus, gross	ABNF	175 154	194 604	208 456	231 060	244 762	249 065	256 537	259 001
B.3	Mixed income	QWLT	41 589	42 898	45 288	49 407	50 559	52 077	54 942	56 931
D.1	Compensation of employees	HAEA	356 595	369 146	386 035	403 887	429 967	466 080	495 793	532 179
D.2	Taxes on production and imports	NZGX	88 127	94 034	101 266	105 936	113 226	119 355	128 527	135 358
-D.3	less subsidies	−AAXJ	−7 269	−7 695	−7 779	−8 564	−8 420	−7 475	−7 069	−6 936
di	Statistical discrepancy between income components and GDP	RVFC	−	−	−	−	−	−	−	−
B.1*g	**Gross domestic product at market prices**	**YBHA**	**654 196**	**692 987**	**733 266**	**781 726**	**830 094**	**879 102**	**928 730**	**976 533**
	GROSS NATIONAL INCOME at market prices									
B.1*g	**Gross Domestic Product at market prices**	**YBHA**	**654 196**	**692 987**	**733 266**	**781 726**	**830 094**	**879 102**	**928 730**	**976 533**
D.1	Compensation of employees									
	receipts from the rest of the world (ROW)	KTMN	595	681	887	911	1 007	840	960	1 032
	less payments to the rest of the world (ROW)	−KTMO	−560	−851	−1 183	−818	−924	−850	−759	−882
D.1	Total	KTMP	35	−170	−296	93	83	−10	201	150
	less Taxes on products paid to the ROW									
-D.21+D.31	plus Subsidies received from the ROW	−QZOZ	−4 725	−3 349	−5 220	−3 116	−2 919	−3 651	−3 438	−4 098
+D.29-D.39	Other subsidies on production	−IBJL	215	286	293	261	208	241	338	335
D.4	Property and entrepreneurial income									
	receipts from the rest of the world	HMBN	70 944	72 585	85 490	89 794	93 360	102 551	100 733	131 902
	less payments to the rest of the world	−HMBO	−73 491	−71 064	−86 036	−92 254	−93 119	−90 738	−101 977	−130 090
D.4	Total	HMBM	−2 547	1 521	−546	−2 460	241	11 813	−1 244	1 812
B.5*g	**Gross National Income at market prices**	**ABMX**	**647 174**	**691 275**	**727 497**	**776 504**	**827 707**	**887 495**	**924 587**	**974 732**

1.2 UK gross domestic product and national income

Current prices

continued

£ million

			2001	2002	2003	2004	2005	2006	2007
	GROSS DOMESTIC PRODUCT								
	Gross domestic product: Output								
B.1g	Gross value added, at basic prices								
P.1	Output of goods and services	NQAF	1 861 011	1 939 534	2 040 175	2 138 303	2 257 351	2 384 827	..
-P.2	*less* intermediate consumption	-NQAJ	-953 417	-982 440	-1 025 167	-1 069 729	-1 142 230	-1 207 595	..
B.1g	**Total Gross Value Added**	**ABML**	**907 594**	**957 094**	**1 015 008**	**1 068 574**	**1 115 121**	**1 177 232**	**1 247 721**
D.211	Value added taxes (VAT) on products	QYRC	67 097	71 059	77 335	81 550	83 415	87 753	92 000
D.212,4	Other taxes on products	NSUI	52 845	53 945	54 813	58 307	59 167	62 869	66 704
-D.31	*less* subsidies on products	-NZHC	-5 708	-6 534	-7 410	-7 836	-5 198	-5 994	-5 383
B.1*g	**Gross Domestic Product at market prices**	**YBHA**	**1 021 828**	**1 075 564**	**1 139 746**	**1 200 595**	**1 252 505**	**1 321 860**	**1 401 042**
	Gross domestic product: Expenditure								
P.3	Final consumption expenditure								
P.41	Actual individual consumption								
P.3	Household final consumption expenditure	ABPB	647 778	680 964	714 608	747 502	780 265	814 659	858 827
P.3	Final consumption expenditure of NPISH	ABNV	25 111	26 422	27 668	28 748	30 402	32 209	34 587
P.31	Individual govt. final consumption expenditure	NNAQ	118 458	130 816	143 954	148 944	160 456	173 115	183 031
P.41	Total actual individual consumption	NQEO	791 347	838 202	886 230	925 194	971 123	1 019 983	1 076 445
P.32	Collective govt. final consumption expenditure	NQEP	76 126	81 761	88 865	102 825	108 182	112 554	113 869
P.3	Total final consumption expenditure	ABKW	867 473	919 963	975 095	1 028 019	1 079 305	1 132 537	1 190 314
P.3	Households and NPISH	NSSG	672 889	707 386	742 276	776 250	810 667	846 868	893 414
P.3	Central government	NMBJ	118 778	130 348	142 658	152 563	161 800	173 905	180 546
P.3	Local government	NMMT	75 806	82 229	90 161	99 206	106 838	111 764	116 354
P.5	Gross capital formation								
P.51	Gross fixed capital formation	NPQX	171 782	180 551	186 700	200 672	211 318	227 920	249 238
P.52	Changes in inventories	ABMP	6 189	2 909	3 983	4 695	4 973	4 322	7 901
P.53	Acquisitions less disposals of valuables	NPJO	396	214	-37	-37	-377	285	374
P.5	Total gross capital formation	NQFM	178 367	183 674	190 646	205 330	215 914	232 527	257 513
P.6	Exports of goods and services	KTMW	276 866	280 536	290 677	303 392	331 028	376 384	368 337
-P.7	*less* imports of goods and services	-KTMX	-300 878	-308 609	-316 672	-336 146	-373 742	-419 588	-415 817
B.11	External balance of goods and services	KTMY	-24 012	-28 073	-25 995	-32 754	-42 714	-43 204	-47 480
de	Statistical discrepancy between expenditure components and GDP	RVFD	–	–	–	–	–	–	695
B.1*g	**Gross Domestic Product at market prices**	**YBHA**	**1 021 828**	**1 075 564**	**1 139 746**	**1 200 595**	**1 252 505**	**1 321 860**	**1 401 042**
	Gross domestic product: Income								
B.2g	Operating surplus, gross								
	Non-financial corporations								
	Public non-financial corporations	NRJT	6 879	6 586	7 200	7 038	8 928	9 872	9 514
	Private non-financial corporations	NRJK	183 157	188 444	201 091	214 851	222 175	236 916	253 355
	Financial corporations	NQNV	12 965	27 125	33 218	32 460	32 300	36 628	46 290
	General government	NMXV	9 796	10 289	10 807	11 429	12 174	12 931	14 523
	Households and non-profit institutions serving households	QWLS	53 000	55 647	60 984	65 182	68 632	71 963	79 858
B.2g	Total operating surplus, gross	ABNF	265 797	288 091	313 300	330 960	344 209	368 310	403 540
B.3	Mixed income	QWLT	61 282	64 967	68 324	72 816	74 858	78 908	83 628
D.1	Compensation of employees	HAEA	564 194	587 396	616 893	648 099	682 205	715 496	744 857
D.2	Taxes on production and imports	NZGX	137 507	143 117	150 665	158 710	162 288	171 453	180 262
-D.3	*less* subsidies	-AAXJ	-6 952	-8 007	-9 436	-9 990	-11 055	-12 307	-12 079
di	Statistical discrepancy between income components and GDP	RVFC	–	–	–	–	–	–	834
B.1*g	**Gross domestic product at market prices**	**YBHA**	**1 021 828**	**1 075 564**	**1 139 746**	**1 200 595**	**1 252 505**	**1 321 860**	**1 401 042**
	GROSS NATIONAL INCOME at market prices								
B.1*g	**Gross Domestic Product at market prices**	**YBHA**	**1 021 828**	**1 075 564**	**1 139 746**	**1 200 595**	**1 252 505**	**1 321 860**	**1 401 042**
D.1	Compensation of employees								
	receipts from the rest of the world (ROW)	KTMN	1 087	1 121	1 116	931	974	1 058	1 159
	less payments to the rest of the world (ROW)	-KTMO	-1 021	-1 054	-1 057	-1 425	-1 584	-1 803	-1 824
D.1	Total	KTMP	66	67	59	-494	-610	-745	-665
	less Taxes on products paid to the ROW								
-D.21+D.31	*plus* Subsidies received from the ROW	-QZOZ	-3 920	-2 890	-2 596	-1 234	-4 260	-4 496	-4 731
+D.29-D.39	Other subsidies on production	-IBJL	582	519	592	592	3 408	3 220	2 943
D.4	Property and entrepreneurial income								
	receipts from the rest of the world	HMBN	137 447	120 543	122 069	137 382	185 765	237 448	284 586
	less payments to the rest of the world	-HMBO	-128 088	-102 324	-104 605	-119 058	-163 283	-226 606	-275 315
D.4	Total	HMBM	9 359	18 219	17 464	18 324	22 482	10 842	9 271
B.5*g	**Gross National Income at market prices**	**ABMX**	**1 027 915**	**1 091 479**	**1 155 265**	**1 217 783**	**1 273 525**	**1 330 681**	**1 407 860**

1 These series are not available for the latest year.

1.3 UK gross domestic product
Chained volume measures (Reference year 2003)

£ million

			1993	1994	1995	1996	1997	1998	1999	2000
	GROSS DOMESTIC PRODUCT									
	Gross domestic product: expenditure approach									
P.3	Final consumption expenditure									
P.41	Actual individual consumption									
P.3	Household final consumption expenditure	**ABPF**	499 198	513 133	522 624	543 774	564 549	588 048	619 651	647 796
P.3	Final consumption expenditure of non-profit institutions serving households	**ABNU**	20 404	21 991	22 798	23 022	23 665	25 382	25 341	27 536
P.31	Individual government final consumption expenditure	**NSZK**	116 742	117 360	120 125	122 749	124 199	125 944	129 050	131 426
P.41	Total actual individual consumption	**YBIO**	633 720	650 131	663 007	687 367	710 706	738 146	773 446	806 541
P.32	Collective government final consumption expenditure	**NSZL**	74 629	75 923	75 766	74 774	72 556	73 075	77 030	80 972
P.3	Total final consumption expenditure	**ABKX**	708 002	725 702	738 452	761 911	783 208	811 259	850 491	887 499
P.5	Gross capital formation									
P.51	Gross fixed capital formation	**NPQR**	119 167	124 640	128 300	135 270	144 472	164 249	169 117	173 710
P.52	Changes in inventories	**ABMQ**	−256	4 259	3 919	1 231	3 394	4 291	5 803	4 648
P.53	Acquisitions less disposals of valuables	**NPJP**	−39	−1	−60	−75	−35	30	−	−28
P.5	Total gross capital formation	**NPQU**	118 322	128 539	132 866	136 937	148 592	169 054	175 118	178 660
	Gross domestic final expenditure	**YBIK**	823 835	852 429	869 681	897 140	930 880	980 637	1 025 828	1 066 206
P.6	Exports of goods and services	**KTMZ**	167 147	182 498	199 735	217 271	234 973	242 305	251 355	274 338
	Gross final expenditure	**ABME**	984 136	1 029 597	1 066 357	1 113 221	1 166 159	1 222 696	1 276 817	1 340 692
-P.7	*less* imports of goods and services	**−KTNB**	−163 114	−172 769	−182 331	−200 084	−219 514	−239 873	−258 861	−282 018
de	Statistical discrepancy between expenditure components and GDP	**GIXS**	−	−	−	−	−	−	−	−
B.1*g	**Gross Domestic Product at market prices**	**ABMI**	**832 910**	**868 560**	**894 988**	**920 757**	**951 208**	**985 506**	**1 019 735**	**1 059 658**
B.11	*of which* External balance of goods and services	**KTNC**	4 033	9 729	17 404	17 187	15 459	2 432	−7 506	−7 680

1.3 UK gross domestic product

Chained volume measures (Reference year 2003)

continued

£ million

			2001	2002	2003	2004	2005	2006	2007
	GROSS DOMESTIC PRODUCT								
	Gross domestic product: expenditure approach								
P.3	Final consumption expenditure								
P.41	Actual individual consumption								
P.3	Household final consumption expenditure	**ABPF**	668 482	693 124	714 608	736 857	751 288	766 378	789 163
P.3	Final consumption expenditure of non-profit								
	institutions serving households	**ABNU**	27 567	27 576	27 668	27 198	27 212	28 289	29 269
P.31	Individual government final consumption expenditure	**NSZK**	134 867	139 546	143 954	148 660	151 049	153 227	156 750
P.41	Total actual individual consumption	**YBIO**	830 840	860 237	886 230	912 715	929 549	947 894	975 182
P.32	Collective government final consumption expenditure	**NSZL**	82 620	85 437	88 865	92 012	93 801	95 549	96 450
P.3	Total final consumption expenditure	**ABKX**	913 470	945 687	975 095	1 004 727	1 023 350	1 043 443	1 071 632
P.5	Gross capital formation								
P.51	Gross fixed capital formation	**NPQR**	178 203	184 701	186 700	195 782	200 187	212 146	227 188
P.52	Changes in inventories	**ABMQ**	5 577	2 289	3 982	4 371	4 814	4 575	6 849
P.53	Acquisitions less disposals of valuables	**NPJP**	342	183	−37	−42	−354	290	535
P.5	Total gross capital formation	**NPQU**	184 462	187 374	190 646	200 111	204 647	217 011	234 572
	Gross domestic final expenditure	**YBIK**	1 098 000	1 133 077	1 165 741	1 204 838	1 227 997	1 260 454	1 306 204
P.6	Exports of goods and services	**KTMZ**	282 607	285 433	290 677	304 699	329 491	365 818	349 290
	Gross final expenditure	**ABME**	1 380 763	1 418 530	1 456 418	1 509 537	1 557 487	1 626 272	1 655 493
-P.7	*less* imports of goods and services	**−KTNB**	−295 491	−309 982	−316 672	−338 359	−362 211	−397 076	−389 724
de	Statistical discrepancy between								
	expenditure components and GDP	**GIXS**	−	−	−	−	−	−	628
B.1*g	**Gross Domestic Product at market prices**	**ABMI**	**1 085 745**	**1 108 508**	**1 139 746**	**1 171 178**	**1 195 276**	**1 229 196**	**1 266 397**
B.11	*of which* External balance of goods and services	**KTNC**	−12 884	−24 549	−25 995	−33 660	−32 720	−31 258	−40 434

1.4 Indices of value, volume, prices and costs

Indices 2003=100

			1993	1994	1995	1996	1997	1998	1999	2000
	INDICES OF VALUE AT CURRENT PRICES									
	Gross measures, before deduction of fixed capital consumption									
	at current market prices									
B.1*g	Gross domestic product at current market prices ("money GDP")	YBEU	57.4	60.8	64.3	68.6	72.8	77.1	81.5	85.7
B.5*g	Gross national income at current market prices	YBEV	56.0	59.8	63.0	67.2	71.6	76.8	80.0	84.4
B.6*g	Gross national disposable income at current market prices	YBEW	56.4	60.1	63.2	67.5	71.9	76.9	80.2	84.4
	at current basic prices									
B.1g	Gross value added at current basic prices	YBEX	57.9	61.1	64.4	68.8	72.9	77.0	81.1	85.2
	CHAINED VOLUME INDICES ("real terms")									
	Gross measures, before deduction of fixed capital consumption at market prices									
B.1*g	Gross domestic product at market prices	YBEZ	73.1	76.2	78.5	80.8	83.5	86.5	89.5	93.0
	Categories of GDP expenditure									
P.3	Final consumption expenditure by households and	YBFA	72.6	74.4	75.7	78.1	80.3	83.2	87.2	91.0
	non-profit institutions serving households	YBFB	70.0	72.1	73.4	76.3	79.2	82.6	86.9	91.0
	by general government	YBFC	82.4	83.2	84.3	84.9	84.4	85.4	88.5	91.2
P.51	Gross fixed capital formation	YBFG	63.8	66.8	68.7	72.5	77.4	88.0	90.6	93.0
	Gross domestic final expenditure	YBFH	70.7	73.1	74.6	77.0	79.9	84.1	88.0	91.5
P.6	Exports of goods and services	YBFI	57.5	62.8	68.7	74.7	80.8	83.4	86.5	94.4
	of which, goods	YBFJ	60.3	66.3	72.8	78.4	84.9	85.8	88.6	99.3
	services	YBFK	52.0	55.7	60.3	67.6	72.8	78.8	82.8	85.0
	Gross final expenditure	YBFF	67.6	70.7	73.2	76.4	80.1	84.0	87.7	92.1
P.7	Imports of goods and services	YBFL	51.5	54.6	57.6	63.2	69.3	75.7	81.7	89.1
	of which, goods	YBFM	52.8	55.1	58.5	64.1	70.4	76.4	81.5	89.1
	services	YBFN	47.1	52.6	54.3	60.1	65.8	73.7	82.6	89.0
B.5*g	Gross national income at market prices	YBFO	70.2	73.5	74.8	77.4	81.0	85.2	87.3	90.7
B.6*g	Gross national disposable income at market prices	YBFP	70.6	73.7	75.0	77.7	81.3	85.4	87.5	90.7
	Adjustment to basic prices									
D.21-D.31	Taxes *less* subsidies on products	YBFQ	68.5	72.8	77.2	79.9	82.6	84.3	86.5	89.8
B.1g	Gross value added at basic prices	CGCE	73.7	76.6	78.7	80.9	83.6	86.8	89.9	93.4
	PRICE INDICES (IMPLIED DEFLATORS)[1]									
	Categories of GDP expenditure at market prices									
P.3	Final consumption expenditure by households and	YBGA	78.4	80.0	82.4	85.2	87.2	89.3	91.0	92.6
	non-profit institutions serving households	YBFS	81.0	82.7	85.4	88.3	90.5	92.6	93.7	94.8
	by general government	YBFT	69.8	71.4	72.9	75.3	76.7	78.7	82.4	85.7
P.51	Gross fixed capital formation	YBFU	87.3	89.6	94.6	96.4	95.7	95.0	95.6	96.2
	Total domestic expenditure	YBFV	80.0	81.6	84.4	87.1	88.7	90.3	91.8	93.3
P.6	Exports of goods and services	YBFW	99.2	100.4	103.7	105.4	101.1	96.3	96.6	98.4
	of which, goods	BQNK	109.0	109.6	113.4	114.7	108.9	102.7	99.6	100.5
	services	FKNW	81.9	84.4	86.8	89.5	88.0	85.8	90.3	94.1
	Total final expenditure	YBFY	83.8	85.4	88.3	90.7	91.2	91.5	92.8	94.3
P.7	Imports of goods and services	YBFZ	104.7	107.8	114.1	114.2	106.2	100.1	99.0	102.0
	of which, goods	BQNL	107.4	111.3	118.7	118.4	109.8	102.1	101.1	104.6
	services	FHMA	94.3	95.1	97.9	99.1	93.0	92.2	92.5	94.3
B.1*g	Gross domestic product at market prices	YBGB	78.5	79.8	81.9	84.9	87.3	89.2	91.1	92.2
	HOME COSTS PER UNIT OF OUTPUT[2]									
B.1*g	Total home costs (based on expenditure components of GDP)	YBGC	77.8	79.1	81.3	84.6	86.8	88.5	89.9	90.9
D.1	Compensation of employees	YBGD	79.1	78.5	79.7	81.0	83.5	87.4	89.8	92.8
B.2g,B.3g	Gross operating surplus and mixed income	YBGE	77.7	81.7	84.7	91.0	92.7	91.3	91.2	89.0

1 Implied deflators are derived by dividing the estimates for each component at current market prices by the corresponding chained volume estimate.
2 These index numbers show how employment and operating incomes relate to the implied deflator of GDP at market prices.

1.4 Indices of value, volume, prices and costs

continued

Indices 2003=100

			2001	2002	2003	2004	2005	2006	2007
	INDICES OF VALUE AT CURRENT PRICES								
	Gross measures, before deduction of fixed capital consumption								
	at current market prices								
B.1*g	Gross domestic product at current market prices ("money GDP")	YBEU	89.7	94.4	100.0	105.3	109.9	116.0	122.9
B.5*g	Gross national income at current market prices	YBEV	89.0	94.5	100.0	105.4	110.2	115.2	121.9
B.6*g	Gross national disposable income at current market prices	YBEW	89.3	94.6	100.0	105.3	110.0	115.0	121.7
	at current basic prices								
B.1g	Gross value added at current basic prices	YBEX	89.4	94.3	100.0	105.3	109.9	116.0	122.9
	CHAINED VOLUME INDICES ("real terms")								
	Gross measures, before deduction of fixed capital consumption at market prices								
B.1*g	Gross domestic product at market prices	YBEZ	95.3	97.3	100.0	102.8	104.9	107.8	111.1
	Categories of GDP expenditure								
P.3	Final consumption expenditure	YBFA	93.7	97.0	100.0	103.0	104.9	107.0	109.9
	by households and								
	non-profit institutions serving households	YBFB	93.8	97.1	100.0	102.9	104.9	107.1	110.3
	by general government	YBFC	93.4	96.6	100.0	103.4	105.2	106.9	108.8
P.51	Gross fixed capital formation	YBFG	95.4	98.9	100.0	104.9	107.2	113.6	121.7
	Gross domestic final expenditure	YBFH	94.2	97.2	100.0	103.4	105.3	108.1	112.0
P.6	Exports of goods and services	YBFI	97.2	98.2	100.0	104.8	113.4	125.9	120.2
	of which, goods	YBFJ	101.5	100.3	100.0	101.5	111.0	125.2	110.2
	services	YBFK	89.2	94.3	100.0	110.9	117.7	127.1	138.5
	Gross final expenditure	YBFF	94.8	97.4	100.0	103.6	106.9	111.7	113.7
P.7	Imports of goods and services	YBFL	93.3	97.9	100.0	106.8	114.4	125.4	123.1
	of which, goods	YBFM	93.8	98.2	100.0	106.9	114.6	127.5	122.1
	services	YBFN	91.8	97.0	100.0	106.7	113.6	119.0	126.1
B.5*g	Gross national income at market prices	YBFO	93.6	97.0	100.0	102.9	104.4	106.3	109.8
B.6*g	Gross national disposable income at market prices	YBFP	93.9	97.1	100.0	102.8	104.2	106.1	109.6
	Adjustment to basic prices								
D.21-D.31	Taxes less subsidies on products	YBFQ	93.5	97.5	100.0	103.0	104.6	107.1	110.9
B.1g	Gross value added at basic prices	CGCE	95.5	97.2	100.0	102.7	104.9	107.9	111.1
	PRICE INDICES (IMPLIED DEFLATORS)[1]								
	Categories of GDP expenditure at market prices								
P.3	Final consumption expenditure	YBGA	95.0	97.3	100.0	102.3	105.5	108.5	111.1
	by households and								
	non-profit institutions serving households	YBFS	96.7	98.2	100.0	101.6	104.1	106.6	109.2
	by general government	YBFT	89.5	94.5	100.0	104.6	109.7	114.8	117.3
P.51	Gross fixed capital formation	YBFU	96.4	97.8	100.0	102.5	105.6	107.4	109.7
	Total domestic expenditure	YBFV	95.2	97.4	100.0	102.4	105.5	108.3	110.8
P.6	Exports of goods and services	YBFW	98.0	98.3	100.0	99.6	100.5	102.9	105.5
	of which, goods	BQNK	98.9	98.8	100.0	99.8	101.2	103.3	106.3
	services	FKNW	96.1	97.4	100.0	99.2	99.1	102.1	104.2
	Total final expenditure	YBFY	95.8	97.6	100.0	101.8	104.4	107.1	109.7
P.7	Imports of goods and services	YBFZ	101.8	99.6	100.0	99.3	103.2	105.7	106.7
	of which, goods	BQNL	103.6	100.7	100.0	99.4	103.2	105.9	107.2
	services	FHMA	96.4	96.2	100.0	99.2	103.3	105.0	105.3
B.1*g	Gross domestic product at market prices	YBGB	94.1	97.0	100.0	102.5	104.8	107.5	110.6
	HOME COSTS PER UNIT OF OUTPUT[2]								
	Total home costs (based on expenditure								
B.1*g	components of GDP)	YBGC	93.4	96.9	100.0	102.6	105.1	107.9	111.1
D.1	Compensation of employees	YBGD	96.0	97.9	100.0	102.2	105.4	107.5	108.7
B.2g,B.3g	Gross operating surplus and mixed income	YBGE	90.0	95.1	100.0	103.0	104.7	108.7	114.9

1 Implied deflators are derived by dividing the estimates for each component at current market prices by the corresponding chained volume estimate.
2 These index numbers show how employment and operating incomes relate to the implied deflator of GDP at market prices.

1.5 Population, employment and GDP per head

			1999	2000	2001	2002	2003	2004	2005	2006	2007
	POPULATION AND EMPLOYMENT (thousands)[1]										
POP	Home population[4]	**DYAY**	58 684	58 886	59 113	59 323	59 557	59 846	60 238	60 587	60 975
	Household population aged 16+										
ESE	Self-employed[2]	**MGRQ**	3 306	3 256	3 296	3 337	3 565	3 618	3 636	3 738	3 806
EEM	Employees[2]	**MGRN**	23 603	23 975	24 183	24 386	24 427	24 645	24 929	25 098	25 204
ETO	Total employment[2],[3]	**MGRZ**	27 167	27 483	27 710	27 921	28 186	28 485	28 774	29 030	29 222
EUN	Unemployed[2]	**MGSC**	1 728	1 588	1 490	1 529	1 489	1 424	1 465	1 669	1 653
	All economically active[2]	**MGSF**	28 895	29 070	29 200	29 450	29 675	29 909	30 239	30 698	30 875
	Economically inactive[2]	**MGSI**	17 043	17 124	17 302	17 337	17 411	17 538	17 632	17 570	17 793
	Total[2]	**MGSL**	45 937	46 194	46 502	46 787	47 087	47 448	47 871	48 268	48 668

			1999	2000	2001	2002	2003	2004	2005	2006	2007
	GROSS DOMESTIC PRODUCT PER HEAD £										
	At current prices										
	Gross domestic product at market prices[4]	**IHXT**	15 826	16 582	17 285	18 131	19 138	20 065	20 792	21 817	22 977
	Chained volume measures										
	Gross domestic product at market prices[4]	**IHXW**	17 377	17 995	18 368	18 686	19 138	19 573	19 843	20 289	20 769
	Gross value added at basic prices[4]	**YBGT**	15 542	16 097	16 398	16 635	17 042	17 424	17 677	18 082	18 500

1 Components may not sum to totals due to rounding.
2 These seasonally adjusted data are 4 quarter annual averages derived from quarterly Labour Force Survey, which does not include those resident in communal establishments except for those in student halls of residence and NHS accommodation.
3 Includes people on Government-supported training and employment programmes and unpaid family workers.
4 This data is consistent with the population estimates published on 22 August 2007.

1.6.0 UK summary accounts
Total economy ESA95 sector S.1

£ million

			1999	2000	2001	2002	2003	2004	2005	2006	2007
0	**GOODS AND SERVICES ACCOUNT**										
	Resources										
P.1	Output										
P.11	Market output[1]	NQAG	1 426 374	1 502 213	1 565 295	1 620 136	1 691 680	1 766 597	1 861 050	1 963 066	..
P.12	Output for own final use[1]	NQAH	65 577	69 644	76 021	80 399	88 008	91 189	97 261	103 883	..
P.13	Other non-market output[1]	NQAI	191 837	205 503	219 695	238 999	260 487	280 517	299 040	317 878	..
P.1	Total output[1]	NQAF	1 683 788	1 777 360	1 861 011	1 939 534	2 040 175	2 138 303	2 257 351	2 384 827	..
D.21	Taxes on products	NZGW	112 024	118 275	119 942	125 004	132 148	139 857	142 582	150 622	158 704
-D.31	*less* Subsidies on products	−NZHC	−6 068	−6 027	−5 708	−6 534	−7 410	−7 836	−5 198	−5 994	−5 383
P.7	Imports of goods and services	KTMX	256 180	287 793	300 878	308 609	316 672	336 146	373 742	419 588	415 817
Total	Total resources[1]	NQBM	2 045 924	2 177 401	2 276 123	2 366 613	2 481 585	2 606 470	2 768 477	2 949 043	..
	Uses										
P.2	Intermediate consumption[1]	NQAJ	861 014	913 075	953 417	982 440	1 025 167	1 069 729	1 142 230	1 207 595	..
P.3	Final consumption expenditure										
P.31	By households	ABPB	582 371	616 558	647 778	680 964	714 608	747 502	780 265	814 659	858 827
P.31	By non-profit institutions serving households	ABNV	22 185	23 531	25 111	26 422	27 668	28 748	30 402	32 209	34 587
P.3	By government										
P.31	For individual consumption	NNAQ	102 742	109 297	118 458	130 816	143 954	148 944	160 456	173 115	183 031
P.32	For collective consumption	NQEP	66 910	72 675	76 126	81 761	88 865	102 825	108 182	112 554	113 869
P.3	Total by government	NMRK	169 652	181 972	194 584	212 577	232 819	251 769	268 638	285 669	296 900
P.3	Total final consumption expenditure[2]	ABKW	774 208	822 061	867 473	919 963	975 095	1 028 019	1 079 305	1 132 537	1 190 314
P.5	Gross capital formation										
P.51	Gross fixed capital formation	NPQX	161 722	167 172	171 782	180 551	186 700	200 672	211 318	227 920	249 238
P.52	Changes in inventories	ABMP	6 060	5 271	6 189	2 909	3 983	4 695	4 973	4 322	7 901
P.53	Acquisitions less disposals of valuables	NPJO	229	3	396	214	−37	−37	−377	285	374
P.5	Total gross capital formation	NQFM	168 011	172 446	178 367	183 674	190 646	205 330	215 914	232 527	257 513
P.6	Exports of goods and services	KTMW	242 691	269 819	276 866	280 536	290 677	303 392	331 028	376 384	368 337
de	Statistical discrepancy between expenditure components and GDP	RVFD	–	–	–	–	–	–	–	–	695
Total	Total uses[1]	NQBM	2 045 924	2 177 401	2 276 123	2 366 613	2 481 585	2 606 470	2 768 477	2 949 043	..

1 These series are not available for the latest year
2 For the total economy, Total final consumption expenditure = P.4 Actual final
consumption

1.6.1 UK summary accounts
Total economy ESA95 sector S.1

£ million

			1999	2000	2001	2002	2003	2004	2005	2006
I	**PRODUCTION ACCOUNT**									
	Resources									
P.1	Output									
P.11	Market output	NQAG	1 426 374	1 502 213	1 565 295	1 620 136	1 691 680	1 766 597	1 861 050	1 963 066
P.12	Output for own final use	NQAH	65 577	69 644	76 021	80 399	88 008	91 189	97 261	103 883
P.13	Other non-market output	NQAI	191 837	205 503	219 695	238 999	260 487	280 517	299 040	317 878
P.1	Total output	NQAF	1 683 788	1 777 360	1 861 011	1 939 534	2 040 175	2 138 303	2 257 351	2 384 827
D.21	Taxes on products	NZGW	112 024	118 275	119 942	125 004	132 148	139 857	142 582	150 622
-D.31	less Subsidies on products	-NZHC	-6 068	-6 027	-5 708	-6 534	-7 410	-7 836	-5 198	-5 994
Total	Total resources	NQBP	1 789 744	1 889 608	1 975 245	2 058 004	2 164 913	2 270 324	2 394 735	2 529 455
	Uses									
P.2	Intermediate consumption	NQAJ	861 014	913 075	953 417	982 440	1 025 167	1 069 729	1 142 230	1 207 595
B.1*g	**Gross Domestic Product**	YBHA	**928 730**	**976 533**	**1 021 828**	**1 075 564**	**1 139 746**	**1 200 595**	**1 252 505**	**1 321 860**
Total	Total uses	NQBP	1 789 744	1 889 608	1 975 245	2 058 004	2 164 913	2 270 324	2 394 735	2 529 455
B.1*g	**Gross Domestic Product**	YBHA	**928 730**	**976 533**	**1 021 828**	**1 075 564**	**1 139 746**	**1 200 595**	**1 252 505**	**1 321 860**
-K.1	less Fixed capital consumption	-NQAE	-105 507	-111 251	-115 796	-121 914	-125 603	-135 184	-138 520	-147 858
B.1*n	Net domestic product	NHRK	823 223	865 282	906 032	953 650	1 014 143	1 065 411	1 113 985	1 174 002

1.6.2 UK summary accounts
Total economy ESA95 sector S.1

£ million

			1999	2000	2001	2002	2003	2004	2005	2006
II	**DISTRIBUTION AND USE OF INCOME ACCOUNTS**									
II.1	**PRIMARY DISTRIBUTION OF INCOME ACCOUNT**									
II.1.1	**GENERATION OF INCOME ACCOUNT**									
	Resources									
B.1*g	**Total resources (Gross Domestic Product)**	YBHA	928 730	976 533	1 021 828	1 075 564	1 139 746	1 200 595	1 252 505	1 321 860
	Uses									
D.1	Compensation of employees									
D.11	Wages and salaries	NQAU	431 594	462 355	490 978	508 614	527 630	549 393	574 542	600 206
D.12	Employers' social contributions	NQAV	64 199	69 824	73 216	78 782	89 263	98 706	107 663	115 290
D.1	Total	HAEA	495 793	532 179	564 194	587 396	616 893	648 099	682 205	715 496
D.2	Taxes on production and imports, paid									
D.21	Taxes on products and imports	QZPQ	112 024	118 275	119 942	125 004	132 148	139 857	142 582	150 622
D.29	Production taxes other than on products	NMYD	16 503	17 083	17 565	18 113	18 517	18 853	19 706	20 831
D.2	Total taxes on production and imports	NZGX	128 527	135 358	137 507	143 117	150 665	158 710	162 288	171 453
-D.3	less Subsidies, received									
-D.31	Subsidies on products	-NZHC	-6 068	-6 027	-5 708	-6 534	-7 410	-7 836	-5 198	-5 994
-D.39	Production subsidies other than on products	-LIUB	-1 001	-909	-1 244	-1 473	-2 026	-2 154	-5 857	-6 313
-D.3	Total subsidies on production	-AAXJ	-7 069	-6 936	-6 952	-8 007	-9 436	-9 990	-11 055	-12 307
B.2g	Operating surplus, gross	ABNF	256 537	259 001	265 797	288 091	313 300	330 960	344 209	368 310
B.3g	Mixed income, gross	QWLT	54 942	56 931	61 282	64 967	68 324	72 816	74 858	78 908
di	Statistical discrepancy between income components and GDP	RVFC	–	–	–	–	–	–	–	–
B.1*g	**Total uses (Gross Domestic Product)**	YBHA	928 730	976 533	1 021 828	1 075 564	1 139 746	1 200 595	1 252 505	1 321 860
-K.1	After deduction of fixed capital consumption:	-NQAE	-105 507	-111 251	-115 796	-121 914	-125 603	-135 184	-138 520	-147 858
B.2n	Operating surplus, net	NQAR	162 262	159 986	163 347	181 567	203 059	215 692	225 195	244 071
B.3n	Mixed income, net	QWLV	43 710	44 695	47 936	49 577	52 962	52 900	55 352	55 289

1.6.3 UK summary accounts

Total economy ESA95 sector S.1

£ million

			2000	2001	2002	2003	2004	2005	2006	2007
II.1.2	**ALLOCATION OF PRIMARY INCOME ACCOUNT**									
	Resources									
B.2g	Operating surplus, gross	ABNF	259 001	265 797	288 091	313 300	330 960	344 209	368 310	403 540
B.3g	Mixed income, gross	QWLT	56 931	61 282	64 967	68 324	72 816	74 858	78 908	83 628
D.1	Compensation of employees									
D.11	Wages and salaries	NQBI	462 505	491 044	508 681	527 689	548 899	573 932	599 461	626 566
D.12	Employers' social contributions	NQBJ	69 824	73 216	78 782	89 263	98 706	107 663	115 290	117 626
D.1	Total	NVCK	532 329	564 260	587 463	616 952	647 605	681 595	714 751	744 192
di	Statistical discrepancy between income components and GDP	RVFC	–	–	–	–	–	–	–	834
D.2	Taxes on production and imports, received									
D.21	Taxes on products									
D.211	Value added tax (VAT)	NZGF	59 985	63 522	68 251	74 595	79 761	81 416	85 586	89 681
D.212	Taxes and duties on imports excluding VAT	NMBU	–	–	–	–	–	–	–	–
D.2121	Import duties	NMXZ	–	–	–	–	–	–	–	–
D.2122	Taxes on imports excluding VAT and import duties	NMBT	–	–	–	–	–	–	–	–
D.214	Taxes on products excluding VAT and import duties	NMYB	51 956	50 745	52 001	52 858	56 137	56 906	60 540	64 292
D.21	Total taxes on products	NVCE	111 941	114 267	120 252	127 453	135 898	138 322	146 126	153 973
D.29	Other taxes on production	NMYD	17 083	17 565	18 113	18 517	18 853	19 706	20 831	21 558
D.2	Total taxes on production and imports, received	NMYE	129 024	131 832	138 365	145 970	154 751	158 028	166 957	175 531
-D.3	*less* Subsidies, paid									
-D.31	Subsidies on products	−NMYF	−3 791	−3 953	−4 672	−5 311	−5 111	−5 198	−5 994	−5 383
-D.39	Other subsidies on production	−LIUF	−574	−662	−954	−1 434	−1 562	−2 449	−3 093	−3 753
-D.3	Total subsidies	−NMRL	−4 365	−4 615	−5 626	−6 745	−6 673	−7 647	−9 087	−9 136
D.4	Property income, received									
D.41	Interest	NHQY	264 238	250 938	204 672	204 964	250 327	306 560	385 810	501 128
D.42	Distributed income of corporations	NHQZ	124 990	141 883	129 617	155 010	156 899	170 416	177 963	177 575
D.43	Reinvested earnings on direct foreign investment	NHSK	25 178	27 220	32 209	21 456	31 076	43 555	47 795	54 296
D.44	Property income attributed to insurance policy holders	QYNF	53 460	53 671	52 456	55 472	55 049	64 703	67 316	73 243
D.45	Rent	NHRP	1 540	2 170	2 155	1 823	1 445	1 492	1 493	1 510
D.4	Total property income	NHRO	469 406	475 882	421 109	438 725	494 796	586 726	680 377	807 752
Total	Total resources	NQBR	1 442 326	1 494 438	1 494 369	1 576 526	1 694 255	1 837 769	2 000 216	2 206 341
	Uses									
D.4	Property income, paid									
D.41	Interest	NHQW	278 125	262 993	218 948	218 423	264 760	327 887	408 256	529 858
D.42	Distributed income of corporations	NHQX	122 647	147 557	124 488	136 872	145 557	158 559	168 507	159 911
D.43	Reinvested earnings on direct foreign investment	NHSJ	10 788	−992	3 647	7 429	8 558	10 501	22 930	33 118
D.44	Property income attributed to insurance policy holders	NQCG	54 494	54 795	53 652	56 715	56 150	65 805	68 349	74 084
D.45	Rent	NHRN	1 540	2 170	2 155	1 823	1 445	1 492	1 493	1 510
D.4	Total property income	NHRL	467 594	466 523	402 890	421 262	476 470	564 244	669 535	798 481
B.5*g	**Gross National Income (GNI)**	ABMX	**974 732**	**1 027 915**	**1 091 479**	**1 155 265**	**1 217 783**	**1 273 525**	**1 330 681**	**1 407 860**
Total	Total uses	NQBR	1 442 326	1 494 438	1 494 369	1 576 526	1 694 255	1 837 769	2 000 216	2 206 341
-K.1	After deduction of fixed capital consumption	−NQAE	−111 251	−115 796	−121 914	−125 603	−135 184	−138 520	−147 858	−158 143
B.5*n	National income, net	NSRX	863 481	912 119	969 565	1 029 662	1 082 599	1 135 005	1 182 823	1 249 717

1.6.4 UK summary accounts
Total economy ESA95 sector S.1

£ million

			1999	2000	2001	2002	2003	2004	2005	2006	2007
II.2		**SECONDARY DISTRIBUTION OF INCOME ACCOUNT**									
		Resources									
B.5*g		**Gross National Income**	ABMX	**924 587**	**974 732**	**1 027 915**	**1 091 479**	**1 155 265**	**1 217 783**	**1 273 525**	**1 330 681**	**1 407 860**
D.5		Current taxes on income, wealth, etc.										
D.51		Taxes on income	NMZJ	129 553	140 002	147 264	142 842	144 234	154 127	172 498	192 812	199 289
D.59		Other current taxes	NVCQ	19 519	20 287	22 068	23 664	26 016	28 001	29 444	30 906	32 627
D.5		Total	NMZL	149 072	160 289	169 332	166 506	170 250	182 128	201 942	223 718	231 916
D.61		Social contributions										
D.611		Actual social contributions										
D.6111		Employers' actual social contributions	NQDA	52 529	57 288	60 296	64 805	77 571	87 675	95 732	103 551	105 298
D.6112		Employees' social contributions	NQDE	57 523	58 862	60 658	62 535	66 534	70 487	78 554	84 185	87 513
D.6113		Social contributions by self- and non-employed persons	NQDI	1 883	2 049	2 183	2 318	2 595	2 727	2 825	2 930	3 013
D.611		Total	NQCY	111 935	118 199	123 137	129 658	146 700	160 889	177 111	190 666	195 824
D.612		Imputed social contributions	NQDK	11 670	12 536	12 920	13 977	11 692	11 031	11 931	11 739	12 328
D.61		Total	NQCX	123 605	130 735	136 057	143 635	158 392	171 920	189 042	202 405	208 152
D.62		Social benefits other than social transfers in kind	QZQP	157 647	162 833	171 814	182 673	193 596	198 680	211 686	225 891	226 334
D.7		Other current transfers										
D.71		Net non-life insurance premiums	NQBY	22 894	24 550	19 553	26 620	23 000	28 148	31 711	36 531	27 745
D.72		Non-life insurance claims	NQDX	20 409	22 482	16 107	23 631	20 811	25 014	25 594	29 958	22 774
D.73		Current transfers within general government	NQDY	64 446	66 187	72 522	77 592	85 224	94 720	101 369	110 407	113 046
D.74		Current international cooperation from institutions of the EC	NQEA	3 176	2 084	4 568	3 112	3 570	3 673	3 726	3 674	3 573
D.75		Miscellaneous current transfers	QYNA	25 033	28 192	29 757	33 748	35 401	35 599	38 568	39 320	40 434
D.7		Total other current transfers	NQDU	135 958	143 495	142 507	164 703	168 006	187 154	200 968	219 890	207 572
Total		Total resources	NQBT	1 490 869	1 572 084	1 647 625	1 748 996	1 845 508	1 957 667	2 077 163	2 202 585	2 281 834
		Uses									
D.5		Current taxes on income, wealth etc.										
D.51		Taxes on income	NQCR	129 898	140 420	147 389	142 959	144 303	154 180	172 541	192 627	199 282
D.59		Other current taxes	NQCU	19 519	20 287	22 068	23 664	26 016	28 001	29 444	30 906	32 627
D.5		Total	NQCQ	149 417	160 707	169 457	166 623	170 319	182 181	201 985	223 533	231 909
D.61		Social contributions										
D.611		Actual social contributions										
D.6111		Employers' actual social contributions	NQDB	52 529	57 288	60 296	64 805	77 571	87 675	95 732	103 551	105 298
D.6112		Employees' actual social contributions	NQDF	57 434	58 807	60 599	62 458	66 490	70 451	78 540	84 129	87 487
D.6113		Social contributions by self- and non-employed persons	NQDJ	1 883	2 049	2 183	2 318	2 595	2 727	2 825	2 930	3 013
D.611		Total actual social contributions	NQCZ	111 846	118 144	123 078	129 581	146 656	160 853	177 097	190 610	195 798
D.612		Imputed social contributions	QZQQ	11 670	12 536	12 920	13 977	11 692	11 031	11 931	11 739	12 328
D.61		Total	NQBS	123 516	130 680	135 998	143 558	158 348	171 884	189 028	202 349	208 126
D.62		Social benefits other than social transfers in kind	NQDN	158 892	164 086	173 145	184 115	195 081	200 301	213 383	227 628	228 195
D.7		Other current transfers										
D.71		Net non-life insurance premiums	NQDW	20 409	22 482	16 107	23 631	20 811	25 014	25 594	29 958	22 774
D.72		Non-life insurance claims	NQBZ	22 894	24 550	19 553	26 620	23 000	28 148	31 711	36 531	27 745
D.73		Current transfers within general government	NNAF	64 446	66 187	72 522	77 592	85 224	94 720	101 369	110 407	113 046
D.74		Current international cooperation to institutions of the EC	NMDZ	1 456	2 181	2 190	2 362	2 433	3 080	3 255	3 632	3 909
D.75		Miscellaneous current transfers	NUHK	29 476	32 495	33 920	39 516	42 871	44 199	48 365	48 523	50 213
		Of which: GNP based fourth own resource	NMFH	4 632	4 379	3 858	5 335	6 772	7 549	8 732	8 521	8 323
D.7		Total other current transfers	NQDV	138 681	147 895	144 292	169 721	174 339	195 161	210 294	229 051	217 687
B.6*g		**Gross National Disposable Income**	NQCO	**920 363**	**968 716**	**1 024 733**	**1 084 979**	**1 147 422**	**1 208 138**	**1 262 473**	**1 320 024**	**1 395 917**
Total		Total uses	NQBT	1 490 869	1 572 084	1 647 625	1 748 996	1 845 508	1 957 667	2 077 163	2 202 585	2 281 834
-K.1		After deduction of fixed capital consumption	-NQAE	-105 507	-111 251	-115 796	-121 914	-125 603	-135 184	-138 520	-147 858	-158 143
B.6*n		Disposable income, net	NQCP	814 856	857 465	908 937	963 065	1 021 819	1 072 954	1 123 953	1 172 166	1 237 774

1.6.5 UK summary accounts
Total economy ESA95 sector S.1

£ million

			1999	2000	2001	2002	2003	2004	2005	2006	2007
II.3	**REDISTRIBUTION OF INCOME IN KIND ACCOUNT**										
	Resources										
B.6*g	**Gross National Disposable Income**	**NQCO**	920 363	968 716	1 024 733	1 084 979	1 147 422	1 208 138	1 262 473	1 320 024	1 395 917
D.63	Social transfers in kind										
D.631	Social benefits in kind										
D.6313	Social assistance benefits in kind	**NRNC**	–	–	–	–	–	–	–	–	–
D.632	Transfers of individual non-market goods and services	**NRNE**	124 927	132 828	143 569	157 238	171 622	177 692	190 858	205 324	217 618
D.63	Total social transfers in kind	**NRNF**	124 927	132 828	143 569	157 238	171 622	177 692	190 858	205 324	217 618
Total	Total resources	**NQCB**	1 045 290	1 101 544	1 168 302	1 242 217	1 319 043	1 385 832	1 453 331	1 525 348	1 613 535
	Uses										
D.63	Social transfers in kind										
D.631	Social benefits in kind										
D.6313	Social assistance benefits in kind	**NRNI**	–	–	–	–	–	–	–	–	–
D.632	Transfers of individual non-market goods and services	**NRNK**	124 927	132 828	143 569	157 238	171 622	177 692	190 858	205 324	217 618
D.63	Total social transfers in kind	**NRNL**	124 927	132 828	143 569	157 238	171 622	177 692	190 858	205 324	217 618
B.7g	Adjusted disposable income, gross	**NRNM**	920 363	968 716	1 024 733	1 084 979	1 147 421	1 208 140	1 262 473	1 320 024	1 395 917
Total	Total uses	**NQCB**	1 045 290	1 101 544	1 168 302	1 242 217	1 319 043	1 385 832	1 453 331	1 525 348	1 613 535

1.6.6 UK summary accounts
Total economy ESA95 sector S.1

£ million

			1999	2000	2001	2002	2003	2004	2005	2006	2007
II.4	**USE OF INCOME ACCOUNT**										
II.4.1	**USE OF DISPOSABLE INCOME ACCOUNT**										
	Resources										
B.6g	Gross National Disposable Income	NQCO	920 363	968 716	1 024 733	1 084 979	1 147 422	1 208 138	1 262 473	1 320 024	1 395 917
D.8	Adjustment for the change in net equity of households in pension funds	NVCI	14 016	14 154	16 038	17 784	21 377	29 468	32 888	31 714	41 943
Total	Total resources	NVCW	934 379	982 870	1 040 771	1 102 763	1 168 798	1 237 608	1 295 361	1 351 738	1 437 860
	Uses										
P.3	Final consumption expenditure										
P.31	Individual consumption expenditure	NQEO	707 298	749 386	791 347	838 202	886 230	925 194	971 123	1 019 983	1 076 445
P.32	Collective consumption expenditure	NQEP	66 910	72 675	76 126	81 761	88 865	102 825	108 182	112 554	113 869
P.3	Total	ABKW	774 208	822 061	867 473	919 963	975 095	1 028 019	1 079 305	1 132 537	1 190 314
D.8	Adjustment for the change in net equity of households in pension funds	NQEL	14 014	14 150	16 033	17 783	21 365	29 457	32 833	31 705	41 906
B.8g	Gross Saving	NQET	146 157	146 659	157 265	165 017	172 338	180 132	183 223	187 496	205 640
Total	Total uses	NVCW	934 379	982 870	1 040 771	1 102 763	1 168 798	1 237 608	1 295 361	1 351 738	1 437 860
-K.1	After deduction of fixed capital consumption	−NQAE	−105 507	−111 251	−115 796	−121 914	−125 603	−135 184	−138 520	−147 858	−158 143
B.8n	Saving, net	NQEJ	40 650	35 408	41 469	43 103	46 735	44 948	44 703	39 638	47 497
II.4.2	**USE OF ADJUSTED DISPOSABLE INCOME ACCOUNT**										
	Resources										
B.7g	Adjusted disposable income	NRNM	920 363	968 716	1 024 733	1 084 979	1 147 421	1 208 140	1 262 473	1 320 024	1 395 917
D.8	Adjustment for the change in net equity of households in pension funds	NVCI	14 016	14 154	16 038	17 784	21 377	29 468	32 888	31 714	41 943
Total	Total resources	NVCW	934 379	982 870	1 040 771	1 102 763	1 168 798	1 237 608	1 295 361	1 351 738	1 437 860
	Uses										
P.4	Actual final consumption										
P.41	Actual individual consumption	NQEO	707 298	749 386	791 347	838 202	886 230	925 194	971 123	1 019 983	1 076 445
P.42	Actual collective consumption	NRMZ	66 910	72 675	76 126	81 761	88 865	102 825	108 182	112 554	113 869
P.4	Total actual final consumption	NRMX	774 208	822 061	867 473	919 963	975 095	1 028 019	1 079 305	1 132 537	1 190 314
D.8	Adjustment for the change in net equity of households in pension funds	NQEL	14 014	14 150	16 033	17 783	21 365	29 457	32 833	31 705	41 906
B.8g	Gross Saving	NQET	146 157	146 659	157 265	165 017	172 338	180 132	183 223	187 496	205 640
Total	Total uses	NVCW	934 379	982 870	1 040 771	1 102 763	1 168 798	1 237 608	1 295 361	1 351 738	1 437 860

1.6.7 UK summary accounts
Total economy ESA95 sector S.1

£ million

			1999	2000	2001	2002	2003	2004	2005	2006	2007
III	ACCUMULATION ACCOUNTS										
III.1	CAPITAL ACCOUNT										
III.1.1	CHANGE IN NET WORTH DUE TO SAVING & CAPITAL TRANSFERS										
	Changes in liabilities and net worth										
B.8g	Gross Saving	NQET	146 157	146 659	157 265	165 017	172 338	180 132	183 223	187 496	205 640
D.9	Capital transfers receivable										
D.91	Capital taxes	NQEY	1 951	2 215	2 396	2 381	2 416	2 871	3 150	3 575	3 890
D.92	Investment grants	NQFB	8 935	9 667	11 645	13 679	17 614	16 898	21 076	21 443	24 508
D.99	Other capital transfers	NQFD	1 499	1 924	4 794	3 612	7 656	7 256	19 352	6 446	7 101
D.9	Total	NQEW	12 385	13 806	18 835	19 672	27 686	27 025	43 578	31 464	35 499
-D.9	*less* Capital transfers payable										
-D.91	Capital taxes	−NQCC	−1 951	−2 215	−2 396	−2 381	−2 416	−2 871	−3 150	−3 575	−3 890
-D.92	Investment grants	−NVDG	−8 774	−8 821	−11 313	−13 646	−17 335	−16 176	−19 990	−21 163	−24 056
-D.99	Other capital transfers	−NQCE	−925	−1 091	−3 711	−2 581	−6 398	−5 595	−18 677	−5 759	−4 932
-D.9	Total	−NQCF	−11 650	−12 127	−17 420	−18 608	−26 149	−24 642	−41 817	−30 497	−32 878
B.10.1g	Total change in liabilities and net worth	NQCT	146 892	148 338	158 680	166 081	173 875	182 515	184 984	188 463	208 261
	Changes in assets										
B.10.1g	Changes in net worth due to gross saving and capital transfers	NQCT	146 892	148 338	158 680	166 081	173 875	182 515	184 984	188 463	208 261
-K.1	After deduction of fixed capital consumption	−NQAE	−105 507	−111 251	−115 796	−121 914	−125 603	−135 184	−138 520	−147 858	−158 143
B.10.1n	Changes in net worth due to net saving and capital transfers	NQER	41 385	37 087	42 884	44 167	48 272	47 331	46 464	40 605	50 118
III.1.2	ACQUISITION OF NON-FINANCIAL ASSETS ACCOUNT										
	Changes in liabilities and net worth										
B.10.1n	Changes in net worth due to net saving and capital transfers	NQER	41 385	37 087	42 884	44 167	48 272	47 331	46 464	40 605	50 118
K.1	Consumption of fixed capital	NQAE	105 507	111 251	115 796	121 914	125 603	135 184	138 520	147 858	158 143
Total	Total change in liabilities and net worth	NQCT	146 892	148 338	158 680	166 081	173 875	182 515	184 984	188 463	208 261
	Changes in assets										
P.5	Gross capital formation										
P.51	Gross fixed capital formation	NPQX	161 722	167 172	171 782	180 551	186 700	200 672	211 318	227 920	249 238
P.52	Changes in inventories	ABMP	6 060	5 271	6 189	2 909	3 983	4 695	4 973	4 322	7 901
P.53	Acquisitions less disposals of valuables	NPJO	229	3	396	214	−37	−37	−377	285	374
P.5	Total	NQFM	168 011	172 446	178 367	183 674	190 646	205 330	215 914	232 527	257 513
K.2	Acquisitions less disposals of non-produced non-financial assets	NQFJ	−12	−24	98	132	71	319	258	−8	−20
de	Statistical discrepancy between expenditure components and GDP	RVFD	−	−	−	−	−	−	−	−	695
B.9	**Net lending(+) / net borrowing(-)**	NQFH	−21 107	−24 084	−19 785	−17 725	−16 842	−23 134	−31 188	−44 056	−49 927
Total	Total change in assets	NQCT	146 892	148 338	158 680	166 081	173 875	182 515	184 984	188 463	208 261

1.6.8 UK summary accounts

Total economy ESA95 sector S.1. Unconsolidated

£ million

			1999	2000	2001	2002	2003	2004	2005	2006	2007
III.2	**FINANCIAL ACCOUNT**										
F.A	**Net acquisition of financial assets**										
F.1	Monetary gold and special drawing rights (SDRs)	NQAD	−374	−956	−808	−240	−2	−37	−8	47	−50
F.2	Currency and deposits										
F.21	Currency	NYPY	5 314	583	1 020	1 680	3 123	5 544	1 075	1 949	1 129
F.22	Transferable deposits										
F.221	Deposits with UK monetary financial institutions	NYQC	29 196	146 280	164 858	129 283	227 744	252 370	307 220	450 012	293 383
F.229	Deposits with rest of the world monetary financial institutions	NYQK	27 280	187 527	122 793	53 299	190 273	212 831	367 335	278 279	508 210
F.29	Other deposits	NYQM	−1 572	4 998	−5 454	2 464	2 498	3 318	6 109	4 754	12 528
F.2	Total currency and deposits	NQAK	60 218	339 388	283 217	186 726	423 638	474 063	681 739	734 994	815 250
F.3	Securities other than shares										
F.331	Short term: money market instruments										
F.3311	Issued by UK central government	NYQQ	−814	−1 401	8 319	10 510	442	−974	−2 879	−2 499	−4 913
F.3312	Issued by UK local government	NYQY	–	–	–	–	–	–	–	–	–
F.3315	Issued by UK monetary financial institutions	NYRA	17 595	−14 324	3 756	6 639	−11 824	48	1 033	7 946	2 918
F.3316	Issued by other UK residents	NYRK	946	−1 330	−609	−1 969	2 142	−3 136	2 846	6 298	−1 883
F.3319	Issued by the rest of the world	NYRM	13 930	−2 551	11 493	−6 133	12 224	−2 634	7 377	14 543	−1 922
F.332	Medium (1 to 5 year) and long term (over 5 year) bonds										
F.3321	Issued by UK central government	NYRQ	721	−12 399	−16 547	5 190	20 277	21 602	9 228	16 118	13 629
F.3322	Issued by UK local government	NYRW	−2	−12	–	47	18	−226	213	360	−9
F.3325	Medium term bonds issued by UK MFIs[1]	NYRY	7 585	2 045	−480	2 463	11 387	11 063	15 105	14 499	20 764
F.3326	Other medium & long term bonds issued by UK residents	NYSE	36 404	67 609	48 488	24 816	37 610	32 571	34 342	44 288	36 401
F.3329	Long term bonds issued by the rest of the world	NYSG	−10 300	53 299	30 261	9 900	818	88 342	84 672	101 268	68 455
F.34	Financial derivatives	NYSI	−2 724	−1 570	−8 507	−1 433	5 136	7 682	−9 418	−7 869	18 668
F.3	Total securities other than shares	NQAL	63 341	89 366	76 174	50 030	78 230	154 338	142 519	194 952	152 108
F.4	Loans										
F.41	Short term loans										
F.411	Loans by UK monetary financial institutions, excluding loans secured on dwellings & financial leasing	NYSS	66 698	150 664	108 353	87 544	159 494	235 263	255 959	305 306	516 001
F.42	Long term loans										
F.421	Direct investment	NYTE	28 607	14 517	11 291	26 584	8 912	20 975	25 670	15 150	50 327
F.422	Loans secured on dwellings	NYTK	37 900	42 206	54 323	83 644	101 994	102 280	89 948	109 993	107 675
F.423	Finance leasing	NYTS	341	367	440	979	1 195	1 655	1 594	963	1 175
F.424	Other long-term loans by UK residents	NYTU	25 485	25 226	13 349	6 389	11 001	11 833	40 105	49 788	48 194
F.4	Total loans	NQAN	159 031	232 980	187 756	205 140	282 596	372 006	413 276	481 200	723 372
F.5	Shares and other equity										
F.51	Shares and other equity, excluding mutual funds' shares										
F.514	Quoted UK shares	NYUG	−1 249	95 761	13 796	16 127	1 284	15 523	−54 486	−8 135	−16 292
F.515	Unquoted UK shares	NYUI	5 036	21 675	8 020	2 159	8 375	11 887	8 967	19 059	4 987
F.516	Other UK equity (including direct investment in property)	NYUK	−2 052	−2 374	−2 520	−3 064	−5 504	−3 803	−3 850	−3 543	−2 171
F.517	UK shares and bonds issued by other UK residents	NSQJ	–	–	–	–	–	–	–	–	–
F.519	Shares and other equity issued by the rest of the world	NYUQ	137 968	193 618	88 797	55 592	61 972	107 366	119 152	93 054	142 395
F.52	Mutual funds' shares										
F.521	UK mutual funds' shares	NYUY	14 716	14 059	9 333	6 251	8 208	3 461	8 251	14 395	−2 054
F.529	Rest of the world mutual funds' shares	NYVA	70	63	33	−8	41	536	1 810	783	−110
F.5	Total shares and other equity	NQAP	154 489	322 802	117 459	77 057	74 376	134 970	79 844	115 613	126 755
F.6	Insurance technical reserves										
F.61	Net equity of households in life assurance and pension funds' reserves	NQAX	34 691	29 716	35 851	46 181	34 449	44 953	53 727	55 998	72 738
F.62	Prepayments of insurance premiums and reserves for outstanding claims	NQBD	−999	524	−1 596	1 446	2 058	3 546	3 244	4 828	59
F.6	Total insurance technical reserves	NQAW	33 692	30 240	34 255	47 627	36 507	48 499	56 971	60 826	72 797
F.7	Other accounts receivable	NQBK	13 324	30 506	8 875	19 944	11 064	15 224	13 662	79 913	22 313
F.A	**Total net acquisition of financial assets**	NQBL	483 721	1 044 326	706 928	586 284	906 409	1 199 063	1 388 003	1 667 545	1 912 545

1 UK monetary financial institutions

1.6.8 UK summary accounts

Total economy ESA95 sector S.1. Unconsolidated

£ million

			1999	2000	2001	2002	2003	2004	2005	2006	2007
III.2	**FINANCIAL ACCOUNT** continued										
F.L	**Net acquisition of financial liabilities**										
F.2	Currency and deposits										
F.21	Currency	NYPZ	5 422	674	966	1 712	3 174	5 631	1 125	1 899	1 166
F.22	Transferable deposits										
F.221	Deposits with UK monetary financial institutions	NYQD	35 792	345 481	286 540	218 055	399 447	540 924	586 768	783 929	981 443
F.29	Other deposits	NYQN	−879	5 526	−5 632	2 440	2 730	2 441	6 052	5 228	12 229
F.2	Total currency and deposits	NQCK	40 335	351 681	281 874	222 207	405 351	548 996	593 945	791 056	994 838
F.3	Securities other than shares										
F.331	Short term: money market instruments										
F.3311	Issued by UK central government	NYQR	−404	−1 652	8 623	10 330	2 592	999	−3 902	−1 752	−1 367
F.3312	Issued by UK local government	NYQZ	–	–	–	–	–	–	–	–	–
F.3315	Issued by UK monetary financial institutions	NYRB	31 135	23 941	22 835	25 599	−11 489	8 024	−3 488	53 189	17 860
F.3316	Issued by other UK residents	NYRL	2 729	1 370	−372	8 850	−2 181	−2 953	222	2 827	1 021
F.332	Medium (1 to 5 year) and long term (over 5 year) bonds										
F.3321	Issued by UK central government	NYRR	−4 560	−12 700	−17 219	1 555	31 474	34 219	39 917	41 013	38 951
F.3322	Issued by UK local government	NYRX	−2	−12	–	47	18	−226	213	360	−9
F.3325	Medium term bonds issued by UK MFIs[1]	NYRZ	12 081	4 750	3 575	4 238	25 258	29 810	37 843	40 534	57 261
F.3326	Other medium & long term bonds issued by UK residents	NYSF	63 484	75 893	51 333	45 132	101 297	88 872	114 344	119 616	149 680
F.34	Financial derivatives	NYSJ	−39	−67	−95	−274	−75	−175	−207	−110	−312
F.3	Total securities other than shares	NQCM	104 424	91 523	68 680	95 477	146 894	158 570	184 942	255 677	263 085
F.4	Loans										
F.41	Short term loans										
F.411	Loans by UK monetary financial institutions, excluding loans secured on dwellings & financial leasing	NYST	49 476	95 740	60 262	70 027	88 503	123 225	120 733	185 893	289 473
F.419	Loans by rest of the world monetary financial institutions	NYTB	46 782	35 217	115 728	−25 874	70 716	136 801	206 923	46 383	46 048
F.42	Long term loans										
F.421	Direct investment	NYTF	30 111	41 688	31 172	50 445	12 927	18 354	44 408	36 510	26 275
F.422	Loans secured on dwellings	NYTL	37 900	42 206	54 323	83 644	101 994	102 280	89 948	109 993	107 675
F.423	Finance leasing	NYTT	341	367	440	979	1 195	1 655	1 594	963	1 175
F.424	Other long-term loans by UK residents	NYTV	25 832	26 721	13 321	7 847	11 293	11 955	41 762	53 144	48 895
F.429	Other long-term loans by the rest of the world	NYTX	−120	−293	17	−30	124	904	94	228	−12
F.4	Total loans	NQCN	190 322	241 646	275 263	187 038	286 752	395 174	505 462	433 114	519 529
F.5	Shares and other equity										
F.51	Shares and other equity, excluding mutual funds' shares										
F.514	Quoted UK shares	NYUH	87 750	225 687	22 303	18 881	14 175	19 893	6 323	24 345	14 646
F.515	Unquoted UK shares	NYUJ	30 846	81 978	34 409	16 008	27 066	32 202	50 444	53 528	66 587
F.516	Other UK equity (including direct investment in property)	NYUL	−1 239	−745	−1 729	−2 316	−5 109	−3 180	−3 253	−3 076	187
F.517	UK shares and bonds issued by other UK residents	NSQK	–	–	–	–	–	–	–	–	–
F.52	Mutual funds' shares										
F.521	UK mutual funds' shares	NYUZ	14 719	14 102	9 338	6 259	8 212	3 489	8 300	14 445	−2 032
F.5	Total shares and other equity	NQCS	132 076	321 022	64 321	38 832	44 344	52 404	61 814	89 242	79 388
F.6	Insurance technical reserves										
F.61	Net equity of households in life assurance and pension funds' reserves	NQCD	34 689	29 712	35 846	46 180	34 437	44 942	53 672	55 989	72 701
F.62	Prepayments of insurance premiums and reserves for outstanding claims	NQDD	−1 601	1 466	−1 753	1 781	687	3 778	3 969	6 011	39
F.6	Total insurance technical reserves	NQCV	33 088	31 178	34 093	47 961	35 124	48 720	57 641	62 000	72 740
F.7	Other accounts payable	NQDG	12 981	30 408	9 893	18 974	10 497	14 763	14 780	78 331	22 795
F.L	**Total net acquisition of financial liabilities**	NQDH	513 226	1 067 458	734 124	610 489	928 962	1 218 627	1 418 584	1 709 420	1 952 375
B.9	**Net lending / borrowing**										
F.A	Total net acquisition of financial assets	NQBL	483 721	1 044 326	706 928	586 284	906 409	1 199 063	1 388 003	1 667 545	1 912 545
-F.L	*less* Total net acquisition of financial liabilities	−NQDH	−513 226	−1 067 458	−734 124	−610 489	−928 962	−1 218 627	−1 418 584	−1 709 420	−1 952 375
B.9f	Net lending (+) / net borrowing (-), from financial account	NQDL	−29 505	−23 132	−27 196	−24 205	−22 553	−19 564	−30 581	−41 875	−39 830
dB.9f	Statistical discrepancy between financial and non-financial accounts	NYVK	8 398	−952	7 411	6 480	5 711	−3 570	−607	−2 181	−10 097
B.9	**Net lending (+) / net borrowing (-), from capital account**	NQFH	**−21 107**	**−24 084**	**−19 785**	**−17 725**	**−16 842**	**−23 134**	**−31 188**	**−44 056**	**−49 927**

1 UK monetary financial institutions

1.6.9 UK summary accounts

Total economy ESA95 sector S.1. Unconsolidated

£ billion

			1999	2000	2001	2002	2003	2004	2005	2006	2007
IV.3	FINANCIAL BALANCE SHEET at end of period										
AN	Non-financial assets	CGJB	3 877.5	4 245.1	4 484.8	5 076.8	5 522.2	6 069.0	6 283.0	6 863.1	7 380.0
AF.A	Financial assets										
AF.1	Monetary gold and special drawing rights (SDRs)	NYVN	4.0	3.1	2.4	2.4	2.6	2.5	3.2	3.4	4.3
AF.2	Currency and deposits										
AF.21	Currency	NYVV	37.4	37.9	38.9	40.5	43.6	49.0	50.1	52.0	53.0
AF.22	Transferable deposits										
AF.221	Deposits with UK monetary financial institutions institutions	NYVZ	1 154.3	1 317.8	1 462.0	1 595.3	1 913.5	2 129.6	2 477.7	2 961.3	2 751.9
AF.229	Deposits with rest of the world monetary financial institutions	NYWH	870.9	1 087.2	1 185.8	1 203.3	1 399.9	1 605.5	2 055.1	2 189.5	2 760.6
AF.29	Other deposits	NYWJ	71.4	76.6	71.5	73.6	75.1	78.4	85.5	90.1	102.6
AF.2	Total currency and deposits	NYVT	2 134.0	2 519.5	2 758.2	2 912.7	3 432.0	3 862.6	4 668.4	5 292.8	5 668.2
AF.3	Securities other than shares										
AF.331	Short term: money market instruments										
AF.3311	Issued by UK central government	NYWP	4.1	2.6	11.1	21.2	22.1	21.2	18.3	15.8	10.8
AF.3312	Issued by UK local government	NYWX	–	–	–	–	–	–	–	–	–
AF.3315	Issued by UK monetary financial institutions	NYWZ	166.3	154.9	157.9	162.3	151.5	152.5	155.6	165.1	164.0
AF.3316	Issued by other UK residents	NYXJ	20.3	24.5	25.5	21.0	21.8	19.6	27.9	48.9	51.1
AF.3319	Issued by the rest of the world	NYXL	44.3	45.3	56.7	48.7	62.0	58.5	64.1	75.6	77.1
AF.332	Medium (1 to 5 year) and long term (over 5 year) bonds										
AF.3321	Issued by UK central government	NYXP	273.1	266.8	240.6	254.8	265.8	289.1	313.5	315.8	334.6
AF.3322	Issued by UK local government	NYXV	0.8	0.8	0.8	0.8	0.8	0.6	0.8	1.2	1.2
AF.3325	Medium term bonds issued by UK MFIs[1]	NYXX	33.0	36.2	35.1	37.4	53.3	63.8	80.0	91.0	118.4
AF.3326	Other medium & long term bonds issued by UK residents	NYYD	185.0	238.4	269.5	288.7	319.8	355.0	417.4	471.8	502.5
AF.3329	Long term bond issued by the rest of the world	NYYF	392.4	478.6	523.7	538.2	550.1	611.3	717.2	796.0	905.1
AF.34	Financial derivatives	NYYH	–0.4	–	0.7	0.2	–	0.2	0.6	0.7	–0.4
AF.3	Total securities other than shares	NYWL	1 118.8	1 247.9	1 321.6	1 373.4	1 447.4	1 571.8	1 795.6	1 981.9	2 164.3
AF.4	Loans										
AF.41	Short term loans										
AF.411	Loans by UK monetary financial institutions, excluding loans secured on dwellings & financial leasing	NYYT	809.4	976.8	1 074.7	1 142.5	1 283.9	1 493.7	1 761.9	1 975.9	2 538.9
AF.42	Long term loans										
AF.421	Direct investment	NYZF	133.5	142.1	157.5	176.2	175.3	205.5	222.6	229.5	279.9
AF.422	Loans secured on dwellings	NYZL	492.9	535.1	590.2	669.4	772.9	881.1	965.4	1 077.2	1 181.4
AF.423	Finance leasing	NYZT	25.1	25.8	26.2	27.2	28.3	30.2	31.8	31.5	32.7
AF.424	Other long-term loans by UK residents	NYZV	137.7	138.9	146.9	147.7	161.0	180.8	185.1	212.3	212.5
AF.4	Total loans	NYYP	1 598.6	1 818.6	1 995.5	2 162.8	2 421.4	2 791.3	3 166.8	3 526.4	4 245.3
AF.5	Shares and other equity										
AF.51	Shares and other equity, excluding mutual funds' shares										
AF.514	Quoted UK shares	NZAJ	1 162.5	1 112.5	951.2	707.4	833.6	891.8	989.9	1 065.6	1 016.2
AF.515	Unquoted UK shares	NZAL	432.3	472.0	428.6	373.3	414.8	455.8	503.8	545.9	537.2
AF.516	Other UK equity (including direct investment in property)	NZAN	84.8	83.6	89.7	97.2	105.8	116.0	131.4	123.1	120.2
AF.517	UK shares and bonds issued by other UK residents	NSRC	–	–	–	–	–	–	–	–	–
AF.519	Shares and other equity issued by the rest of the world	NZAT	836.6	1 020.8	992.2	931.3	1 049.0	1 128.8	1 348.3	1 456.3	1 651.0
AF.52	Mutual funds' shares										
AF.521	UK mutual funds' shares	NZBB	297.0	302.9	267.0	214.9	265.2	302.7	383.5	450.7	505.8
AF.529	Rest of the world mutual fund share	NZBD	2.1	1.7	1.7	1.4	1.4	1.7	4.1	6.0	3.5
AF.5	Total shares and other equity	NYZZ	2 815.3	2 993.5	2 730.4	2 325.5	2 669.8	2 896.8	3 361.0	3 647.5	3 833.9
AF.6	Insurance technical reserves										
AF.61	Net equity of households in life assurance and pension funds' reserves	NZBH	1 631.3	1 599.0	1 531.3	1 384.1	1 509.2	1 603.2	1 894.3	2 071.7	2 186.7
AF.62	Prepayments of insurance premiums and reserves for outstanding claims	NZBN	44.8	52.0	48.4	50.1	53.3	55.9	57.0	59.0	59.1
AF.6	Total insurance technical reserves	NZBF	1 676.1	1 651.0	1 579.6	1 434.2	1 562.4	1 659.1	1 951.3	2 130.7	2 245.8
AF.7	Other accounts receivable	NZBP	235.9	270.5	275.4	290.7	318.5	331.2	341.1	410.6	434.1
AF.A	Total financial assets	NZBV	9 582.6	10 504.2	10 663.1	10 501.7	11 854.1	13 115.1	15 287.3	16 993.4	18 596.0

1 UK monetary financial institutions

1.6.9 UK summary accounts

Total economy ESA95 sector S.1. Unconsolidated

continued

£ billion

			1999	2000	2001	2002	2003	2004	2005	2006	2007
IV.3	**FINANCIAL BALANCE SHEET** continued at end of period										
AF.L	**Financial liabilities**										
AF.2	Currency and deposits										
AF.21	Currency	NYVW	38.0	38.6	39.5	41.1	44.2	49.8	50.9	52.8	53.9
AF.22	Transferable deposits										
AF.221	Deposits with UK monetary financial institutions	NYWA	2 186.4	2 582.3	2 834.8	3 034.7	3 518.7	3 984.9	4 677.5	5 332.0	5 895.3
AF.29	Other deposits	NYWK	72.7	78.5	73.2	75.3	77.0	79.4	86.4	91.5	103.7
AF.2	Total currency and deposits	NYVU	2 297.1	2 699.4	2 947.5	3 151.1	3 639.9	4 114.2	4 814.8	5 476.3	6 052.9
AF.3	Securities other than shares										
AF.331	Short term: money market instruments										
AF.3311	Issued by UK central government	NYWQ	4.2	2.6	11.2	21.4	24.0	25.0	21.1	19.4	18.0
AF.3312	Issued by UK local government	NYWY	–	–	–	–	–	–	–	–	–
AF.3315	Issued by UK monetary financial institutions	NYXA	233.5	265.8	291.0	302.6	282.1	283.2	291.7	327.7	346.1
AF.3316	Issued by other UK residents	NYXK	38.1	46.2	48.1	51.6	45.6	42.1	50.1	65.2	70.2
AF.332	Medium (1 to 5 year) and long term (over 5 year) bonds										
AF.3321	Issued by UK central government	NYXQ	334.0	329.2	300.5	311.1	331.9	372.9	424.2	451.3	492.8
AF.3322	Issued by UK local government	NYXW	0.8	0.8	0.8	0.8	0.8	0.6	0.8	1.2	1.2
AF.3325	Medium term bonds issued by UK MFIs[1]	NYXY	67.7	74.6	77.6	81.0	107.0	134.7	175.4	205.8	285.3
AF.3326	Other medium & long term bonds issued by UK residents	NYYE	330.2	409.6	458.1	517.6	615.5	716.8	881.4	1 002.9	1 108.4
AF.34	Financial derivatives	NYYI	–0.4	–0.1	0.3	–	–	0.1	0.2	0.7	–0.5
AF.3	Total securities other than shares	NYWM	1 008.2	1 128.7	1 187.6	1 286.2	1 407.0	1 575.5	1 845.1	2 074.2	2 321.6
AF.4	Loans										
AF.41	Short term loans										
AF.411	Loans by UK monetary financial institutions, excluding loans secured on dwellings & financial leasing	NYYU	594.2	696.9	751.7	814.1	885.5	997.3	1 119.4	1 266.9	1 583.0
AF.419	Loans by rest of the world monetary financial institutions	NYZC	347.9	368.9	470.6	446.9	520.2	646.7	881.3	896.5	965.2
AF.42	Long term loans										
AF.421	Direct investment	NYZG	167.1	196.5	239.9	284.1	280.6	305.1	358.7	376.4	402.6
AF.422	Loans secured on dwellings	NYZM	492.9	535.1	590.2	669.4	772.9	881.1	965.4	1 077.2	1 181.4
AF.423	Finance leasing	NYZU	25.1	25.8	26.2	27.2	28.3	30.2	31.8	31.5	32.7
AF.424	Other long-term loans by UK residents	NYZW	127.5	130.3	138.1	140.4	153.8	173.4	177.8	206.2	206.1
AF.429	Other long-term loans by the rest of the world	NYZY	2.0	2.1	2.1	2.0	2.2	3.2	3.2	3.4	3.3
AF.4	Total loans	NYYQ	1 756.7	1 955.6	2 218.6	2 384.0	2 643.6	3 037.0	3 537.7	3 858.0	4 374.4
AF.5	Shares and other equity										
AF.51	Shares and other equity, excluding mutual funds' shares										
AF.514	Quoted UK shares	NZAK	1 751.1	1 754.3	1 494.3	1 126.1	1 334.0	1 441.7	1 644.5	1 804.5	1 791.9
AF.515	Unquoted UK shares	NZAM	636.8	729.4	713.9	609.8	670.2	729.1	852.5	997.7	1 088.8
AF.516	Other UK equity (including direct investment in property)	NZAO	96.4	97.1	103.9	113.1	121.7	133.8	149.8	143.2	145.0
AF.517	UK shares and bonds issued by other UK residents	NSRD	–	–	–	–	–	–	–	–	–
AF.52	Mutual funds' shares										
AF.521	UK mutual funds' shares	NZBC	298.7	304.5	268.2	215.8	266.3	303.9	385.0	452.4	507.5
AF.5	Total shares and other equity	NZAA	2 783.0	2 885.4	2 580.3	2 064.7	2 392.2	2 608.5	3 031.8	3 397.9	3 533.1
AF.6	Insurance technical reserves										
AF.61	Net equity of households in life assurance and pension funds' reserves	NZBI	1 631.5	1 599.2	1 531.5	1 384.3	1 509.4	1 603.4	1 894.5	2 071.9	2 186.9
AF.62	Prepayments of insurance premiums and reserves for outstanding claims	NZBO	58.9	62.8	59.0	62.8	63.5	67.2	71.2	77.2	77.3
AF.6	Total insurance technical reserves	NZBG	1 690.4	1 662.0	1 590.5	1 447.1	1 572.9	1 670.6	1 965.7	2 149.1	2 264.2
AF.7	Other accounts payable	NZBQ	235.4	269.3	275.1	288.6	315.7	329.3	340.3	408.6	431.4
AF.L	**Total financial liabilities**	NZBW	9 770.8	10 600.4	10 799.7	10 621.7	11 971.3	13 335.1	15 535.5	17 364.1	18 977.6
BF.90	**Net financial assets / liabilities**										
AF.A	Total financial assets	NZBV	9 582.6	10 504.2	10 663.1	10 501.7	11 854.1	13 115.1	15 287.3	16 993.4	18 596.0
-AF.L	*less* Total financial liabilities	–NZBW	–9 770.8	–10 600.4	–10 799.7	–10 621.7	–11 971.3	–13 335.1	–15 535.5	–17 364.1	–18 977.6
BF.90	**Net financial assets (+) / liabilities (-)**	NQFT	–188.2	–96.2	–136.5	–120.0	–117.2	–220.0	–248.2	–370.7	–381.6
	Net worth										
AN	Non-financial assets	CGJB	3 877.5	4 245.1	4 484.8	5 076.8	5 522.2	6 069.0	6 283.0	6 863.1	7 380.0
BF.90	Net financial assets (+) / liabilities (-)	NQFT	–188.2	–96.2	–136.5	–120.0	–117.2	–220.0	–248.2	–370.7	–381.6
B.90	**Net worth**	CGDA	3 689.3	4 148.9	4 348.2	4 956.8	5 405.0	5 849.0	6 034.9	6 492.4	6 998.4

1 UK monetary financial institutions

1.7A UK summary accounts 2004

Total economy: all sectors and the rest of the world

£ million

		RESOURCES						USES		TOTAL
		UK total economy	Non-financial corporations	Financial corporations	General government	Households & NPISH	Not sector-ised	Rest of the world	Goods & services	
		S.1	S.11	S.12	S.13	S.14+S.15	S.N	S.2		
	Current accounts									
I	**PRODUCTION / EXTERNAL**									
0	**ACCOUNT OF GOODS AND SERVICES**									
P.7	Imports of goods and services							336 146		336 146
P.6	Exports of goods and services								303 392	303 392
P.1	Output at basic prices	2 138 303	1 370 009	151 071	278 450	338 773				2 138 303
P.2	Intermediate consumption								1 069 729	1 069 729
D.21-D.31	Taxes *less* subsidies on products	132 021					132 021			132 021
II.1.1	**GENERATION OF INCOME**									
B.1g	**Gross domestic product, value added at market prices**	**1 200 595**	**654 414**	**73 655**	**143 440**	**197 065**	**132 021**			**1 200 595**
B.11	External balance of goods and services							32 754		32 754
II.1.2	**ALLOCATION OF PRIMARY INCOME**									
D.1	Compensation of employees	647 605				647 605		1 425		649 030
D.21-D.31	Taxes *less* subsidies on products	130 787			130 787			1 234		132 021
D.29-D.39	Other taxes *less* subsidies on production	16 699	15 784	1 443	–	–528		–592		16 699
B.2g	Operating surplus, gross	330 960	221 889	32 460	11 429	65 182				330 960
B.3g	Mixed income, gross	72 816				72 816				72 816
di	Statistical discrepancy between income components and GDP	–					–			–
D.4	Property income	494 796	80 467	268 416	10 768	135 145		119 058		613 854
II.2	**SECONDARY DISTRIBUTION OF INCOME**									
B.5g	National income, balance of primary incomes, gross	1 217 783	166 282	30 924	143 262	877 317	–			1 217 783
D.5	Current taxes on income, wealth etc	182 128			182 128			535		182 663
D.61	Social contributions	171 920	3 810	70 628	96 983	499		–		171 920
D.62	Social benefits other than social transfers in kind	198 680				198 680		1 621		200 301
D.7	Other current transfers	187 154	6 550	28 828	99 452	52 324		17 939		205 093
II.3	**REDISTRIBUTION OF INCOME IN KIND**									
B.6g	Disposable income, gross	1 208 138	138 491	53 057	237 253	779 339	–			1 208 138
D.63	Social transfers in kind	177 692				177 692				177 692
II.4	**USE OF INCOME**									
B.7g	Adjusted disposable income, gross	1 208 140	138 491	53 057	88 309	928 283	–			1 208 140
B.6g	Disposable income, gross	1 208 138	138 491	53 057	237 253	779 339	–			1 208 138
P.4	Actual final consumption								1 028 019	1 028 019
P.3	Final consumption expenditure								1 028 019	1 028 019
D.8	Adjustment for change in households' net equity in pension funds	29 468				29 468		–11		29 457
	Accumulation accounts									
III.1.1	**CHANGE IN NET WORTH DUE TO SAVING AND CAPITAL TRANSFERS**									
B.8g	Saving, gross	180 132	138 491	23 600	–14 516	32 557	–			180 132
B.12	Current external balance							25 200		25 200
D.9	Capital transfers receivable	27 025	5 859	328	13 636	7 202		1 026		28 051
D.9	Capital transfers payable	–24 642	–419	–328	–20 072	–3 823		–3 409		–28 051
III.1.2	**ACQUISITION ON NON-FINANCIAL ASSETS** **Changes in liabilities and net worth**									
B.10.1.g	Changes in net worth due to saving and capital transfers	182 515	143 931	23 600	–20 952	35 936	–	22 817		205 332
P.51	Gross fixed capital formation								200 672	200 672
-K.1	(Consumption of fixed capital)									
P.52	Changes in inventories								4 695	4 695
P.53	Acquisitions less disposals of valuables								–37	–37
K.2	Acquisitions less disposals of non-produced non-financial assets									
de	Statistical discrepancy between expenditure components and GDP								–	–
III.2	**FINANCIAL ACCOUNT**									
B.9	**Net lending(+) / net borrowing(-)**	–23 134	30 983	18 477	–43 061	–29 533	–	23 136		2
	Changes in liabilities									
F.2	Currency and deposits	548 996	–	546 402	2 594	–		212 877		761 873
F.3	Securities other than shares	158 570	5 451	118 064	34 992	63		93 565		252 135
F.4	Loans	395 174	90 610	157 794	8 992	137 778		132 891		528 065
F.5	Shares and other equity	52 404	14 959	37 445		–		107 902		160 306
F.6	Insurance technical reserves	48 720		48 720						48 720
F.7	Other accounts payable	14 763	2 169	8 851	–1 181	4 924		303		15 066

1.7A UK summary accounts 2004

continued

Total economy: all sectors and the rest of the world   £ million

		USES						RESOURCES		TOTAL
		UK total economy	Non-financial corporations	Financial corporations	General government	Households & NPISH	Not sector-ised	Rest of the world	Goods & services	
		S.1	S.11	S.12	S.13	S.14+S.15	S.N	S.2		
	Current accounts									
I	**PRODUCTION / EXTERNAL**									
0	**ACCOUNT OF GOODS AND SERVICES**									
P.7	Imports of goods and services								336 146	336 146
P.6	Exports of goods and services							303 392		303 392
P.1	Output at basic prices								2 138 303	2 138 303
P.2	Intermediate consumption	1 069 729	715 595	77 416	135 010	141 708				1 069 729
D.21-D.31	Taxes *less* subsidies on products								132 021	132 021
B.1g	**Gross domestic product, value added at market prices**	**1 200 595**	**654 414**	**73 655**	**143 440**	**197 065**	**132 021**			**1 200 595**
B.11	External balance of goods and services							32 754		32 754
II.1.1	**GENERATION OF INCOME**									
D.1	Compensation of employees	648 099	416 741	39 752	132 011	59 595		931		649 030
D.21-D.31	Taxes *less* subsidies on products	132 021					132 021			132 021
D.29-D.39	Other taxes *less* subsidies on production	16 699			16 699					16 699
B.2g	Operating surplus, gross	330 960	221 889	32 460	11 429	65 182				330 960
B.3g	Mixed income, gross	72 816				72 816				72 816
di	Statistical discrepancy between income components and GDP	–					–			–
II.1.2	**ALLOCATION OF PRIMARY INCOME**									
D.4	Property income	476 470	136 074	269 952	27 013	43 431		137 382		613 852
B.5g	National income, balance of primary incomes, gross	1 217 783	166 282	30 924	143 262	877 317		–		1 217 783
II.2	**SECONDARY DISTRIBUTION OF INCOME**									
D.5	Current taxes on income, wealth etc	182 181	27 368	7 221	924	146 668		482		182 663
D.61	Social contributions	171 884				171 884		36		171 920
D.62	Social benefits other than social transfers in kind	200 301	3 810	41 171	154 332	988				200 301
D.7	Other current transfers	195 161	6 973	28 931	129 316	29 941		9 932		205 093
B.6g	Disposable income, gross	1 208 138	138 491	53 057	237 253	779 339	–			1 208 138
II.3	**REDISTRIBUTION OF INCOME IN KIND**									
B.7g	Adjusted disposable income, gross	1 208 140	138 491	53 057	88 309	928 283	–			1 208 140
D.63	Social transfers in kind	177 692			148 944	28 748				177 692
II.4	**USE OF INCOME**									
B.6g	Disposable income, gross									
P.4	Actual final consumption	1 028 019			102 825	925 194				1 028 019
P.3	Final consumption expenditure	1 028 019			251 769	776 250				1 028 019
D.8	Adjustment for change in households' net equity in pension funds	29 457		29 457						29 457
B.8g	Saving, gross	180 132	138 491	23 600	–14 516	32 557	–			180 132
B.12	Current external balance							25 200		25 200
	Accumulation accounts									
III.1.1	**CHANGE IN NET WORTH DUE TO SAVING AND CAPITAL TRANSFERS**									
D.9	Capital transfers receivable									
D.9	Capital transfers payable									
B.10.1.g	Changes in net worth due to saving and capital transfers	182 515	143 931	23 600	–20 952	35 936	–	22 817		205 332
III.1.2	**ACQUISITION OF NON-FINANCIAL ASSETS**									
	Changes in assets									
P.51	Gross fixed capital formation	200 672	106 795	5 254	23 219	65 404				200 672
-K.1	(Consumption of fixed capital)	–135 184	–75 559	–5 687	–11 429	–42 509				–135 184
P.52	Changes in inventories	4 695	4 567	48	–46	126				4 695
P.53	Acquisitions less disposals of valuables	–37	–99	–173	20	215				–37
K.2	Acquisitions less disposals of non-produced non-financial assets	319	1 685	–6	–1 084	–276		–319		–
de	Statistical discrepancy between expenditure components and GDP	–					–			–
B.9	**Net lending(+) / net borrowing(-)**	**–23 134**	**30 983**	**18 477**	**–43 061**	**–29 533**	**–**	**23 136**		**2**
III.2	**FINANCIAL ACCOUNT: changes in assets**									
F.1	Monetary gold and SDRs	–37			–37			37		
F.2	Currency and deposits	474 063	69 678	335 534	–77	68 928		287 810		761 873
F.3	Securities other than shares	154 338	367	159 608	1 856	–7 493		97 797		252 135
F.4	Loans	372 006	19 291	351 815	2 504	–1 604		156 059		528 065
F.5	Shares and other equity	134 970	48 369	84 729	–3 637	5 509		25 336		160 306
F.6	Insurance technical reserves	48 499	956	102	42	47 399		221		48 720
F.7	Other accounts receivable	15 224	–591	4 315	2 276	9 224		–158		15 066
dB.9f	Statistical discrepancy between non-financial and financial transactions	–3 570	6 102	–350	–591	–8 731	–	3 572		2

1.7B UK summary accounts 2005

Total economy: all sectors and the rest of the world

£ million

		RESOURCES							USES	TOTAL
		UK total economy	Non-financial corporations	Financial corporations	General government	Households & NPISH	Not sector-ised	Rest of the world	Goods & services	
		S.1	S.11	S.12	S.13	S.14+S.15	S.N	S.2		
	Current accounts									
I 0	**PRODUCTION / EXTERNAL ACCOUNT OF GOODS AND SERVICES**									
P.7	Imports of goods and services							373 742		373 742
P.6	Exports of goods and services								331 028	331 028
P.1	Output at basic prices	2 257 351	1 441 217	158 560	299 444	358 130				2 257 351
P.2	Intermediate consumption								1 142 230	1 142 230
D.21-D.31	Taxes less subsidies on products	137 384					137 384			137 384
II.1.1	**GENERATION OF INCOME**									
B.1g	**Gross domestic product, value added at market prices**	**1 252 505**	**680 974**	**78 050**	**153 202**	**202 895**	**137 384**			**1 252 505**
B.11	External balance of goods and services							42 714		42 714
II.1.2	**ALLOCATION OF PRIMARY INCOME**									
D.1	Compensation of employees	681 595				681 595		1 584		683 179
D.21-D.31	Taxes less subsidies on products	133 124			133 124			4 260		137 384
D.29-D.39	Other taxes less subsidies on production	17 257	18 159	1 479	–	–2 381		–3 408		13 849
B.2g	Operating surplus, gross	344 209	231 103	32 300	12 174	68 632				344 209
B.3g	Mixed income, gross	74 858				74 858				74 858
di	Statistical discrepancy between income components and GDP	–						–		–
D.4	Property income	586 726	98 171	323 126	10 580	154 849		163 283		750 009
II.2	**SECONDARY DISTRIBUTION OF INCOME**									
B.5g	National income, balance of primary incomes, gross	1 273 525	176 832	20 056	143 666	932 971	–			1 273 525
D.5	Current taxes on income, wealth etc	201 942			201 942			589		202 531
D.61	Social contributions	189 042	3 535	80 256	104 745	506		–		189 042
D.62	Social benefits other than social transfers in kind	211 686				211 686		1 697		213 383
D.7	Other current transfers	200 968	7 261	32 517	106 151	55 039		22 758		223 726
II.3	**REDISTRIBUTION OF INCOME IN KIND**									
B.6g	Disposable income, gross	1 262 473	142 742	44 070	254 750	820 911	–			1 262 473
D.63	Social transfers in kind	190 858				190 858				190 858
II.4	**USE OF INCOME**									
B.7g	Adjusted disposable income, gross	1 262 473	142 742	44 070	94 294	981 367	–			1 262 473
B.6g	Disposable income, gross	1 262 473	142 742	44 070	254 750	820 911	–			1 262 473
P.4	Actual final consumption								1 079 305	1 079 305
P.3	Final consumption expenditure								1 079 305	1 079 305
D.8	Adjustment for change in households' net equity in pension funds	32 888				32 888		–55		32 833
	Accumulation accounts									
III.1.1	**CHANGE IN NET WORTH DUE TO SAVING AND CAPITAL TRANSFERS**									
B.8g	Saving, gross	183 223	142 742	11 237	–13 888	43 132	–			183 223
B.12	Current external balance							32 691		32 691
D.9	Capital transfers receivable	43 578	18 600	321	15 207	9 450		2 212		45 790
D.9	Capital transfers payable	–41 817	–1 257	–321	–36 162	–4 077		–3 973		–45 790
III.1.2	**ACQUISITION ON NON-FINANCIAL ASSETS** **Changes in liabilities and net worth**									
B.10.1.g	Changes in net worth due to saving and capital transfers	184 984	160 085	11 237	–34 843	48 505	–	30 930		215 914
P.51	Gross fixed capital formation								211 318	211 318
-K.1	(Consumption of fixed capital)									
P.52	Changes in inventories								4 973	4 973
P.53	Acquisitions less disposals of valuables								–377	–377
K.2	Acquisitions less disposals of non-produced non-financial assets									
de	Statistical discrepancy between expenditure components and GDP							–		–
III.2	**FINANCIAL ACCOUNT**									
B.9	**Net lending(+) / net borrowing(-)**	–31 188	22 285	5 036	–40 778	–17 731	–	31 188		–
	Changes in liabilities									
F.2	Currency and deposits	593 945	–	588 263	5 682	–		367 349		961 294
F.3	Securities other than shares	184 942	12 248	136 278	36 228	188		82 838		267 780
F.4	Loans	505 462	102 686	283 388	6 254	113 134		159 239		664 701
F.5	Shares and other equity	61 814	14 830	46 984		–		120 962		182 776
F.6	Insurance technical reserves	57 641		57 641						57 641
F.7	Other accounts payable	14 780	5 286	3 096	2 777	3 621		–960		13 820

1.7B UK summary accounts 2005

continued   **Total economy: all sectors and the rest of the world**   £ million

		USES						RESOURCES		TOTAL
		UK total economy	Non-financial corporations	Financial corporations	General government	Households & NPISH	Not sector-ised	Rest of the world	Goods & services	
		S.1	S.11	S.12	S.13	S.14+S.15	S.N	S.2		
	Current accounts									
I	**PRODUCTION / EXTERNAL**									
0	**ACCOUNT OF GOODS AND SERVICES**									
P.7	Imports of goods and services							373 742		373 742
P.6	Exports of goods and services							331 028		331 028
P.1	Output at basic prices								2 257 351	2 257 351
P.2	Intermediate consumption	1 142 230	760 243	80 510	146 242	155 235			1 142 230	
D.21-D.31	Taxes *less* subsidies on products								137 384	137 384
B.1g	**Gross domestic product, value added at market prices**	**1 252 505**	**680 974**	**78 050**	**153 202**	**202 895**	**137 384**			**1 252 505**
B.11	External balance of goods and services							42 714		42 714
II.1.1	**GENERATION OF INCOME**									
D.1	Compensation of employees	682 205	434 161	44 271	141 028	62 745		974		683 179
D.21-D.31	Taxes *less* subsidies on products	137 384					137 384			137 384
D.29-D.39	Other taxes *less* subsidies on production	13 849			13 849					13 849
B.2g	Operating surplus, gross	344 209	231 103	32 300	12 174	68 632				344 209
B.3g	Mixed income, gross	74 858				74 858				74 858
di	Statistical discrepancy between income components and GDP	–					–			–
II.1.2	**ALLOCATION OF PRIMARY INCOME**									
D.4	Property income	564 244	152 442	335 370	29 469	46 963		185 765		750 009
B.5g	National income, balance of primary incomes, gross	1 273 525	176 832	20 056	143 666	932 971	–			1 273 525
II.2	**SECONDARY DISTRIBUTION OF INCOME**									
D.5	Current taxes on income, wealth etc	201 985	33 602	8 739	1 022	158 622		546		202 531
D.61	Social contributions	189 028				189 028		14		189 042
D.62	Social benefits other than social transfers in kind	213 383	3 535	47 423	161 425	1 000				213 383
D.7	Other current transfers	210 294	7 749	32 597	139 307	30 641		13 432		223 726
B.6g	Disposable income, gross	1 262 473	142 742	44 070	254 750	820 911	–			1 262 473
II.3	**REDISTRIBUTION OF INCOME IN KIND**									
B.7g	Adjusted disposable income, gross	1 262 473	142 742	44 070	94 294	981 367	–			1 262 473
D.63	Social transfers in kind	190 858			160 456	30 402				190 858
II.4	**USE OF INCOME**									
B.6g	Disposable income, gross									
P.4	Actual final consumption	1 079 305			108 182	971 123				1 079 305
P.3	Final consumption expenditure	1 079 305			268 638	810 667				1 079 305
D.8	Adjustment for change in households' net equity in pension funds	32 833		32 833						32 833
B.8g	Saving, gross	183 223	142 742	11 237	–13 888	43 132	–			183 223
B.12	Current external balance							32 691		32 691
	Accumulation accounts									
III.1.1	**CHANGE IN NET WORTH DUE TO SAVING AND CAPITAL TRANSFERS**									
D.9	Capital transfers receivable									
D.9	Capital transfers payable									
B.10.1.g	Changes in net worth due to saving and capital transfers	184 984	160 085	11 237	–34 843	48 505	–	30 930		215 914
III.1.2	**ACQUISITION OF NON-FINANCIAL ASSETS**									
	Changes in assets									
P.51	Gross fixed capital formation	211 318	131 035	6 453	7 091	66 739				211 318
-K.1	(Consumption of fixed capital)	–138 520	–77 278	–5 811	–12 174	–43 257				–138 520
P.52	Changes in inventories	4 973	5 191	48	–6	–260				4 973
P.53	Acquisitions less disposals of valuables	–377	–171	–299	16	77				–377
K.2	Acquisitions less disposals of non-produced non-financial assets	258	1 745	–1	–1 166	–320		–258		–
de	Statistical discrepancy between expenditure components and GDP	–					–			–
B.9	**Net lending(+) / net borrowing(-)**	–31 188	22 285	5 036	–40 778	–17 731	–	31 188		–
III.2	**FINANCIAL ACCOUNT: changes in assets**									
F.1	Monetary gold and SDRs	–8				–8		8		
F.2	Currency and deposits	681 739	58 854	556 623	–1 257	67 519		279 555		961 294
F.3	Securities other than shares	142 519	–4 347	153 605	3 315	–10 054		125 261		267 780
F.4	Loans	413 276	37 020	368 690	5 175	2 391		251 425		664 701
F.5	Shares and other equity	79 844	68 717	43 111	–3 606	–28 378		102 932		182 776
F.6	Insurance technical reserves	56 971	965	107	44	55 855		670		57 641
F.7	Other accounts receivable	13 662	1 451	3 425	5 517	3 269		158		13 820
dB.9f	Statistical discrepancy between non-financial and financial transactions	–607	–5 325	–4 875	983	8 610	–	607		–

1.7C UK summary accounts 2006

Total economy: all sectors and the rest of the world

£ million

		RESOURCES							USES	TOTAL
		UK total economy	Non-financial corporations	Financial corporations	General government	Households & NPISH	Not sector-ised	Rest of the world	Goods & services	
		S.1	S.11	S.12	S.13	S.14+S.15	S.N	S.2		
	Current accounts									
I	**PRODUCTION / EXTERNAL**									
0	**ACCOUNT OF GOODS AND SERVICES**									
P.7	Imports of goods and services							419 588		419 588
P.6	Exports of goods and services								376 384	376 384
P.1	Output at basic prices	2 384 827	1 516 232	170 837	318 890	378 868				2 384 827
P.2	Intermediate consumption								1 207 595	1 207 595
D.21-D.31	Taxes *less* subsidies on products	144 628					144 628			144 628
II.1.1	**GENERATION OF INCOME**									
B.1g	**Gross domestic product, value added at market prices**	**1 321 860**	**714 508**	**89 529**	**160 371**	**212 824**	**144 628**			**1 321 860**
B.11	External balance of goods and services							43 204		43 204
II.1.2	**ALLOCATION OF PRIMARY INCOME**									
D.1	Compensation of employees	714 751				714 751		1 803		716 554
D.21-D.31	Taxes *less* subsidies on products	140 132			140 132			4 496		144 628
D.29-D.39	Other taxes *less* subsidies on production	17 738	19 202	1 578	–	–3 042		–3 220		14 518
B.2g	Operating surplus, gross	368 310	246 788	36 628	12 931	71 963				368 310
B.3g	Mixed income, gross	78 908				78 908				78 908
di	Statistical discrepancy between income components and GDP	–					–			–
D.4	Property income	680 377	106 500	405 561	10 901	157 415		226 606		906 983
II.2	**SECONDARY DISTRIBUTION OF INCOME**									
B.5g	National income, balance of primary incomes, gross	1 330 681	184 547	21 061	151 310	973 763	–			1 330 681
D.5	Current taxes on income, wealth etc	223 718			223 718			464		224 182
D.61	Social contributions	202 405	3 425	87 845	110 621	514		–		202 405
D.62	Social benefits other than social transfers in kind	225 891				225 891		1 737		227 628
D.7	Other current transfers	219 890	8 368	37 409	115 059	59 054		23 459		243 349
II.3	**REDISTRIBUTION OF INCOME IN KIND**									
B.6g	Disposable income, gross	1 320 024	146 890	37 211	283 480	852 443	–			1 320 024
D.63	Social transfers in kind	205 324				205 324				205 324
II.4	**USE OF INCOME**									
B.7g	Adjusted disposable income, gross	1 320 024	146 890	37 211	110 365	1 025 558	–			1 320 024
B.6g	Disposable income, gross	1 320 024	146 890	37 211	283 480	852 443	–			1 320 024
P.4	Actual final consumption								1 132 537	1 132 537
P.3	Final consumption expenditure								1 132 537	1 132 537
D.8	Adjustment for change in households' net equity in pension funds	31 714				31 714		–9		31 705
	Accumulation accounts									
III.1.1	**CHANGE IN NET WORTH DUE TO SAVING AND CAPITAL TRANSFERS**									
B.8g	Saving, gross	187 496	146 890	5 506	–2 189	37 289	–			187 496
B.12	Current external balance							45 031		45 031
D.9	Capital transfers receivable	31 464	8 122	446	14 652	8 244		2 426		33 890
D.9	Capital transfers payable	–30 497	–630	–446	–24 689	–4 732		–3 393		–33 890
III.1.2	**ACQUISITION ON NON-FINANCIAL ASSETS**									
	Changes in liabilities and net worth									
	Changes in net worth due to saving and									
B.10.1.g	capital transfers	188 463	154 382	5 506	–12 226	40 801	–	44 064		232 527
P.51	Gross fixed capital formation								227 920	227 920
-K.1	(Consumption of fixed capital)									
P.52	Changes in inventories								4 322	4 322
P.53	Acquisitions less disposals of valuables								285	285
K.2	Acquisitions less disposals of non-produced non-financial assets									
de	Statistical discrepancy between expenditure components and GDP								–	–
III.2	**FINANCIAL ACCOUNT**									
B.9	**Net lending(+) / net borrowing(-)**	–44 056	27 728	–3 275	–34 866	–33 643	–	44 056		–
	Changes in liabilities									
F.2	Currency and deposits	791 056	–	785 662	5 394	–		278 416		1 069 472
F.3	Securities other than shares	255 677	11 961	202 988	39 621	1 107		108 052		363 729
F.4	Loans	433 114	151 059	148 132	1 356	132 567		131 207		564 321
F.5	Shares and other equity	89 242	6 937	82 305		–		93 837		183 079
F.6	Insurance technical reserves	62 000		62 000						62 000
F.7	Other accounts payable	78 331	5 021	35 177	1 953	36 180		1 639		79 970

1.7C UK summary accounts 2006

continued

Total economy: all sectors and the rest of the world

£ million

		USES						RESOURCES		TOTAL
		UK total economy	Non-financial corporations	Financial corporations	General government	Households & NPISH	Not sector-ised	Rest of the world	Goods & services	
		S.1	S.11	S.12	S.13	S.14+S.15	S.N	S.2		

Current accounts

I	**PRODUCTION / EXTERNAL**									
0	**ACCOUNT OF GOODS AND SERVICES**									
P.7	Imports of goods and services								419 588	419 588
P.6	Exports of goods and services							376 384		376 384
P.1	Output at basic prices								2 384 827	2 384 827
P.2	Intermediate consumption	1 207 595	801 724	81 308	158 519	166 044			1 207 595	
D.21-D.31	Taxes less subsidies on products								144 628	144 628
B.1g	**Gross domestic product, value added at market prices**	**1 321 860**	**714 508**	**89 529**	**160 371**	**212 824**	**144 628**			**1 321 860**
B.11	External balance of goods and services							43 204		43 204
II.1.1	**GENERATION OF INCOME**									
D.1	Compensation of employees	715 496	451 611	51 323	147 440	65 122		1 058		716 554
D.21-D.31	Taxes less subsidies on products	144 628					144 628			144 628
D.29-D.39	Other taxes less subsidies on production	14 518			14 518					14 518
B.2g	Operating surplus, gross	368 310	246 788	36 628	12 931	71 963				368 310
B.3g	Mixed income, gross	78 908				78 908				78 908
di	Statistical discrepancy between income components and GDP	–					–			–
II.1.2	**ALLOCATION OF PRIMARY INCOME**									
D.4	Property income	669 535	168 741	421 128	30 392	49 274		237 448		906 983
B.5g	National income, balance of primary incomes, gross	1 330 681	184 547	21 061	151 310	973 763	–			1 330 681
II.2	**SECONDARY DISTRIBUTION OF INCOME**									
D.5	Current taxes on income, wealth etc	223 533	37 183	15 475	1 075	169 800		649		224 182
D.61	Social contributions	202 349				202 349		56		202 405
D.62	Social benefits other than social transfers in kind	227 628	3 425	56 140	167 053	1 010				227 628
D.7	Other current transfers	229 051	8 842	37 489	149 100	33 620		14 298		243 349
B.6g	Disposable income, gross	1 320 024	146 890	37 211	283 480	852 443	–			1 320 024
II.3	**REDISTRIBUTION OF INCOME IN KIND**									
B.7g	Adjusted disposable income, gross	1 320 024	146 890	37 211	110 365	1 025 558	–			1 320 024
D.63	Social transfers in kind	205 324			173 115	32 209				205 324
II.4	**USE OF INCOME**									
B.6g	Disposable income, gross									
P.4	Actual final consumption	1 132 537			112 554	1 019 983				1 132 537
P.3	Final consumption expenditure	1 132 537			285 669	846 868				1 132 537
D.8	Adjustment for change in households' net equity in pension funds	31 705		31 705						31 705
B.8g	Saving, gross	187 496	146 890	5 506	–2 189	37 289	–			187 496
B.12	Current external balance							45 031		45 031

Accumulation accounts

III.1.1	**CHANGE IN NET WORTH DUE TO SAVING AND CAPITAL TRANSFERS**									
D.9	Capital transfers receivable									
D.9	Capital transfers payable									
B.10.1.g	Changes in net worth due to saving and capital transfers	188 463	154 382	5 506	–12 226	40 801	–	44 064		232 527
III.1.2	**ACQUISITION OF NON-FINANCIAL ASSETS**									
	Changes in assets									
P.51	Gross fixed capital formation	227 920	121 173	8 650	23 667	74 430				227 920
-K.1	(Consumption of fixed capital)	–147 858	–80 360	–5 944	–12 931	–48 623				–147 858
P.52	Changes in inventories	4 322	4 142	199	–4	–15				4 322
P.53	Acquisitions less disposals of valuables	285	–42	–74	14	387				285
K.2	Acquisitions less disposals of non-produced non-financial assets	–8	1 381	6	–1 037	–358		8		–
de	Statistical discrepancy between expenditure components and GDP	–					–			–
B.9	**Net lending(+) / net borrowing(-)**	–44 056	27 728	–3 275	–34 866	–33 643	–	44 056		–
III.2	**FINANCIAL ACCOUNT: changes in assets**									
F.1	Monetary gold and SDRs	47				47		–47		
F.2	Currency and deposits	734 994	64 725	583 092	6 913	80 264		334 478		1 069 472
F.3	Securities other than shares	194 952	6 513	197 815	2 245	–11 621		168 777		363 729
F.4	Loans	481 200	52 896	426 472	4 494	–2 662		83 121		564 321
F.5	Shares and other equity	115 613	76 443	57 566	–2 541	–15 855		67 466		183 079
F.6	Insurance technical reserves	60 826	1 371	144	61	59 250		1 174		62 000
F.7	Other accounts receivable	79 913	5 254	40 887	2 897	30 875		57		79 970
dB.9f	Statistical discrepancy between non-financial and financial transactions	–2 181	–4 496	7 013	–658	–4 040	–	2 181		–

1.7D UK summary accounts 2007

Total economy: all sectors and the rest of the world

£ million

		RESOURCES							USES	TOTAL
		UK total economy	Non-financial corporations	Financial corporations	General government	Households & NPISH	Not sector-ised	Rest of the world	Goods & services	
		S.1	S.11	S.12	S.13	S.14+S.15	S.N	S.2		
	Current accounts									
I	**PRODUCTION / EXTERNAL**									
0	**ACCOUNT OF GOODS AND SERVICES**									
P.7	Imports of goods and services							415 817		415 817
P.6	Exports of goods and services								368 337	368 337
P.1	Output at basic prices	..	..	..	..	..				..
P.2	Intermediate consumption								..	..
D.21-D.31	Taxes less subsidies on products	153 321					153 321			153 321
II.1.1	**GENERATION OF INCOME**									
B.1g	**Gross domestic product, value added at market prices**	**1 401 042**	..	**101 584**	..	..154 155				**1 401 042**
B.11	External balance of goods and services							47 480		47 480
II.1.2	**ALLOCATION OF PRIMARY INCOME**									
D.1	Compensation of employees	744 192				744 192		1 824		746 016
D.21-D.31	Taxes less subsidies on products	148 590			148 590			4 731		153 321
D.29-D.39	Other taxes less subsidies on production	17 805	19 821	1 677	−	−3 693		−2 943		14 862
B.2g	Operating surplus, gross	403 540	262 869	46 290	14 523	79 858				403 540
B.3g	Mixed income, gross	83 628				83 628				83 628
di	Statistical discrepancy between income components and GDP	834					834			834
D.4	Property income	807 752	113 663	510 456	12 400	171 233		275 315		1 083 067
II.2	**SECONDARY DISTRIBUTION OF INCOME**									
B.5g	National income, balance of primary incomes, gross	1 407 860	196 639	38 843	159 086	1 012 458	834			1 407 860
D.5	Current taxes on income, wealth etc	231 916			231 916			633		232 549
D.61	Social contributions	208 152	3 508	87 934	116 192	518		−		208 152
D.62	Social benefits other than social transfers in kind	226 334				226 334		1 861		228 195
D.7	Other current transfers	207 572	6 376	28 411	117 480	55 305		22 171		229 743
II.3	**REDISTRIBUTION OF INCOME IN KIND**									
B.6g	Disposable income, gross	1 395 917	157 903	70 636	292 513	874 031	834			1 395 917
D.63	Social transfers in kind	217 618				217 618				217 618
II.4	**USE OF INCOME**									
B.7g	Adjusted disposable income, gross	1 395 917	157 903	70 636	109 482	1 057 062	834			1 395 917
B.6g	Disposable income, gross	1 395 917	157 903	70 636	292 513	874 031	834			1 395 917
P.4	Actual final consumption								1 190 314	1 190 314
P.3	Final consumption expenditure								1 190 314	1 190 314
D.8	Adjustment for change in households' net equity in pension funds	41 943				41 943		−37		41 906
	Accumulation accounts									
III.1.1	**CHANGE IN NET WORTH DUE TO SAVING AND CAPITAL TRANSFERS**									
B.8g	Saving, gross	205 640	157 903	28 730	−4 387	22 560	834			205 640
B.12	Current external balance							52 568		52 568
D.9	Capital transfers receivable	35 499	8 468	388	16 864	9 779		1 189		36 688
D.9	Capital transfers payable	−32 878	−758	−388	−26 715	−5 017		−3 810		−36 688
III.1.2	**ACQUISITION ON NON-FINANCIAL ASSETS** Changes in liabilities and net worth									
B.10.1.g	Changes in net worth due to saving and capital transfers	208 261	165 613	28 730	−14 238	27 322	834	49 947		258 208
P.51	Gross fixed capital formation								249 238	249 238
-K.1	(Consumption of fixed capital)									
P.52	Changes in inventories								7 901	7 901
P.53	Acquisitions less disposals of valuables								374	374
K.2	Acquisitions less disposals of non-produced non-financial assets									
de	Statistical discrepancy between expenditure components and GDP								695	695
III.2	**FINANCIAL ACCOUNT**									
B.9	**Net lending(+) / net borrowing(-)**	−49 927	22 626	20 724	−38 322	−55 094	139	49 927		−
	Changes in liabilities									
F.2	Currency and deposits	994 838	−	986 785	8 053	−		508 220		1 503 058
F.3	Securities other than shares	263 085	24 646	200 233	37 575	631		85 513		348 598
F.4	Loans	519 529	156 240	240 635	2 062	120 592		276 154		795 683
F.5	Shares and other equity	79 388	32 394	46 994		−		142 285		221 673
F.6	Insurance technical reserves	72 740		72 740						72 740
F.7	Other accounts payable	22 795	2 310	11 035	−1 442	10 892		−237		22 558

1.7D UK summary accounts 2007

continued

Total economy: all sectors and the rest of the world

£ million

		USES							RESOURCES	TOTAL
		UK total economy	Non-financial corporations	Financial corporations	General government	Households & NPISH	Not sector -ised	Rest of the world	Goods & services	
		S.1	S.11	S.12	S.13	S.14+S.15	S.N	S.2		
	Current accounts									
I	**PRODUCTION / EXTERNAL**									
0	**ACCOUNT OF GOODS AND SERVICES**									
P.7	Imports of goods and services								415 817	415 817
P.6	Exports of goods and services							368 337		368 337
P.1	Output at basic prices								..	..
P.2	Intermediate consumption	..	..	..	..	..				
D.21-D.31	Taxes *less* subsidies on products								153 321	153 321
B.1g	**Gross domestic product, value added at market prices**	**1 401 042**	..	**101 584**	..	..154 155				**1 401 042**
B.11	External balance of goods and services							47 480		47 480
II.1.1	**GENERATION OF INCOME**									
D.1	Compensation of employees	744 857	471 167	53 121	152 776	67 793		1 159		746 016
D.21-D.31	Taxes *less* subsidies on products	153 321					153 321			153 321
D.29-D.39	Other taxes *less* subsidies on production	14 862			14 862					14 862
B.2g	Operating surplus, gross	403 540	262 869	46 290	14 523	79 858				403 540
B.3g	Mixed income, gross	83 628				83 628				83 628
di	Statistical discrepancy between income components and GDP	834					834			834
II.1.2	**ALLOCATION OF PRIMARY INCOME**									
D.4	Property income	798 481	179 893	517 903	34 232	66 453		284 586		1 083 067
B.5g	National income, balance of primary incomes, gross	1 407 860	196 639	38 843	159 086	1 012 458	834			1 407 860
II.2	**SECONDARY DISTRIBUTION OF INCOME**									
D.5	Current taxes on income, wealth etc	231 909	38 260	10 033	1 111	182 505		640		232 549
D.61	Social contributions	208 126				208 126		26		208 152
D.62	Social benefits other than social transfers in kind	228 195	3 508	46 028	177 645	1 014				228 195
D.7	Other current transfers	217 687	6 852	28 491	153 405	28 939		12 056		229 743
B.6g	Disposable income, gross	1 395 917	157 903	70 636	292 513	874 031	834			1 395 917
II.3	**REDISTRIBUTION OF INCOME IN KIND**									
B.7g	Adjusted disposable income, gross	1 395 917	157 903	70 636	109 482	1 057 062	834			1 395 917
D.63	Social transfers in kind	217 618			183 031	34 587				217 618
II.4	**USE OF INCOME**									
B.6g	Disposable income, gross									
P.4	Actual final consumption	1 190 314			113 869	1 076 445				1 190 314
P.3	Final consumption expenditure	1 190 314			296 900	893 414				1 190 314
D.8	Adjustment for change in households' net equity in pension funds	41 906		41 906						41 906
B.8g	Saving, gross	205 640	157 903	28 730	−4 387	22 560	834			205 640
B.12	Current external balance							52 568		52 568
	Accumulation accounts									
III.1.1	**CHANGE IN NET WORTH DUE TO SAVING AND CAPITAL TRANSFERS**									
D.9	Capital transfers receivable									
D.9	Capital transfers payable									
B.10.1.g	Changes in net worth due to saving and capital transfers	208 261	165 613	28 730	−14 238	27 322	834	49 947		258 208
III.1.2	**ACQUISITION OF NON-FINANCIAL ASSETS**									
	Changes in assets									
P.51	Gross fixed capital formation	249 238	134 148	7 831	25 210	82 049				249 238
-K.1	(Consumption of fixed capital)	−158 143	−83 565	−6 099	−13 816	−54 663				−158 143
P.52	Changes in inventories	7 901	7 421	206	−20	294				7 901
P.53	Acquisitions less disposals of valuables	374	−22	−35	18	413				374
K.2	Acquisitions less disposals of non-produced non-financial assets	−20	1 440	4	−1 124	−340		20		−
de	Statistical discrepancy between expenditure components and GDP	695					695			695
B.9	**Net lending(+) / net borrowing(-)**	−49 927	22 626	20 724	−38 322	−55 094	139	49 927		−
III.2	**FINANCIAL ACCOUNT: changes in assets**									
F.1	Monetary gold and SDRs	−50			−50			50		
F.2	Currency and deposits	815 250	91 633	646 062	10 155	67 400		687 808		1 503 058
F.3	Securities other than shares	152 108	329	160 049	227	−8 497		196 490		348 598
F.4	Loans	723 372	45 212	681 234	4 484	−7 558		72 311		795 683
F.5	Shares and other equity	126 755	92 508	87 753	−6 118	−47 388		94 918		221 673
F.6	Insurance technical reserves	72 797	10	−	−	72 787		−57		72 740
F.7	Other accounts receivable	22 313	541	13 506	−1 741	10 007		245		22 558
dB.9f	Statistical discrepancy between non-financial and financial transactions	−10 097	7 983	−9 458	969	−9 730	139	10 097		−

1.7.1 UK summary accounts 2006

Total economy: all sectors and the rest of the world
£ million

		UK total economy S.1	Non-financial corporations S.11	Financial corporations S.12	Monetary financial institutions S.121+S.122	Other financial intermediaries & auxiliaries S.123+S.124	Insurance corporations & pension funds S.125
I	**PRODUCTION ACCOUNT**						
	Resources						
P.1	Output						
P.11	Market output*	1 963 066	1 501 215	167 725			
P.12	Output for own final use	103 883	15 017	3 112			
P.13	Other non-market output	317 878					
P.1	Total output	2 384 827	1 516 232	170 837			
D.21	Taxes on products	150 622					
-D.31	*less* Subsidies on products	−5 994					
Total	Total resources	2 529 455	1 516 232	170 837			
	Uses						
P.2	Intermediate consumption	1 207 595	801 724	81 308			
B.1*g	**Gross Domestic Product**	**1 321 860**	**714 508**	**89 529**	**55 003**	**16 352**	**18 174**
Total	Total uses	2 529 455	1 516 232	170 837			
B.1*g	**Gross Domestic Product**	**1 321 860**	**714 508**	**89 529**	**55 003**	**16 352**	**18 174**
-K.1	*less* Fixed capital consumption	−147 858	−80 360	−5 944			
B.1*n	Net domestic product	1 174 002	634 148	83 585			

1.7.2 UK summary accounts 2006

Total economy: all sectors and the rest of the world
£ million

		UK total economy S.1	Non-financial corporations S.11	Financial corporations S.12	Monetary financial institutions S.121+S.122	Other financial intermediaries & auxiliaries S.123+S.124	Insurance corporations & pension funds S.125
II	**DISTRIBUTION AND USE OF INCOME ACCOUNTS**						
II.1	**PRIMARY DISTRIBUTION OF INCOME ACCOUNT**						
II.1.1	**GENERATION OF INCOME ACCOUNT**						
	Resources						
B.1*g	**Total resources (Gross Domestic Product)** external balance of goods & services	1 321 860	714 508	89 529	55 003	16 352	18 174
	Uses						
D.1	Compensation of employees						
D.11	Wages and salaries	600 206	383 224	42 488	21 359	14 884	6 245
D.12	Employers' social contributions	115 290	68 387	8 835	4 440	3 095	1 300
D.1	Total	715 496	451 611	51 323	25 799	17 979	7 545
D.2	Taxes on production and imports, paid						
D.21	Taxes on products and imports	150 622					
D.29	Production taxes other than on products	20 831	19 202	1 578	586	608	384
D.2	Total taxes on production and imports	171 453	19 202	1 578	586	608	384
-D.3	*less* Subsidies, received						
-D.31	Subsidies on products	−5 994					
-D.39	Production subsidies other than on products	−6 313	−3 093	–	–	–	–
-D.3	Total subsidies on production	−12 307	−3 093	–	–	–	–
B.2g	Operating surplus, gross	368 310	246 788	36 628	28 618	−2 235	10 245
B.3g	Mixed income, gross	78 908					
di	Statistical discrepancy between income components and GDP	–					
B.1*g	**Total uses (Gross Domestic Product)**	**1 321 860**	**714 508**	**89 529**	**55 003**	**16 352**	**18 174**
-K.1	After deduction of fixed capital consumption	−147 858	−80 360	−5 944			
B.2n	Operating surplus, net	244 071	166 428	30 684			
B.3n	Mixed income, net	55 289					

1.7.1 UK summary accounts 2006

continued
Total economy: all sectors and the rest of the world

£ million

		General government	Central government	Local government	Households & NPISH	Not sector-ised	Taxes less subsidies	Rest of the world
		S.13	S.1311	S.1313	S.14+S.15	S.N		S.2
I	**PRODUCTION ACCOUNT**							
	Resources							
P.1	Output							
P.11	Market output*	33 038	9 380	23 658	261 088			
P.12	Output for own final use	183	3	180	85 571			
P.13	Other non-market output	285 669	173 905	111 764	32 209			
P.1	Total output	318 890	183 288	135 602	378 868			
D.21	Taxes on products					150 622	150 622	
-D.31	*less* Subsidies on products					−5 994	−5 994	
Total	Total resources	318 890	183 288	135 602	378 868	144 628	144 628	
	Uses							
P.2	Intermediate consumption	158 519	97 096	61 423	166 044			
B.1*g	**Gross Domestic Product**	**160 371**	**86 192**	**74 179**	**212 824**	**144 628**	144 628	
Total	Total uses	318 890	183 288	135 602	378 868	144 628	144 628	
B.1*g	**Gross Domestic Product**	**160 371**	**86 192**	**74 179**	**212 824**	**144 628**	144 628	
-K.1	*less* Fixed capital consumption	−12 931	−6 566	−6 365	−48 623			
B.1*n	Net domestic product	147 440	79 626	67 814	164 201	144 628	144 628	..

1.7.2 UK summary accounts 2006

continued
Total economy: all sectors and the rest of the world

£ million

		General government	Central government	Local government	Households & NPISH	Not sector-ised	Taxes less subsidies	Rest of the world
		S.13	S.1311	S.1313	S.14+S.15	S.N		S.2
II	**DISTRIBUTION AND USE OF INCOME ACCOUNTS**							
II.1	**PRIMARY DISTRIBUTION OF INCOME ACCOUNT**							
II.1.1	**GENERATION OF INCOME ACCOUNT**							
	Resources							
B.1*g	**Total Resources (Gross Domestic Product)**	**160 371**	**86 192**	**74 179**	**212 824**	**144 628**	144 628	
	external balance of goods & services							43 204
	Uses							
D.1	Compensation of employees							
D.11	Wages and salaries	122 159	65 724	56 435	52 335			1 058
D.12	Employers' social contributions	25 281	13 902	11 379	12 787			
D.1	Total	147 440	79 626	67 814	65 122			1 058
D.2	Taxes on production and imports, paid							
D.21	Taxes on products and imports					150 622	150 622	−
D.29	Production taxes other than on products	−	−	−	51			
D.2	Total taxes on production and imports	−	−	−	51	150 622	150 622	−
-D.3	*less* Subsidies, received							
-D.31	Subsidies on products					−5 994	−5 994	
-D.39	Production subsidies other than on products	−	−	−	−3 220			
-D.3	Total subsidies on production	−	−	−	−3 220	−5 994	−5 994	
B.2g	Operating surplus, gross	12 931	6 566	6 365	71 963			
B.3g	Mixed income, gross				78 908			
di	Statistical discrepancy between income components and GDP					−		
B.1*g	**Total uses (Gross Domestic Product)**	**160 371**	**86 192**	**74 179**	**212 824**	**144 628**	144 628	
-K.1	After deduction of fixed capital consumption	−12 931	−6 566	−6 365	−48 623			
B.2n	Operating surplus, net	−	−	−	46 959			
B.3n	Mixed income, net				55 289			

1.7.3 UK summary accounts 2006

Total economy: all sectors and the rest of the world

£ million

		UK total economy	Non-financial corporations	Financial corporations	Monetary financial institutions	Other financial intermediaries & auxiliaries	Insurance corporations & pension funds
		S.1	S.11	S.12	S.121+S.122	S.123+S.124	S.125
II.1.2	**ALLOCATION OF PRIMARY INCOME ACCOUNT**						
	Resources						
B.2g	Operating surplus, gross	368 310	246 788	36 628	28 618	−2 235	10 245
B.3g	Mixed income, gross	78 908					
D.1	Compensation of employees						
D.11	Wages and salaries	599 461					
D.12	Employers' social contributions	115 290					
D.1	Total	714 751					
di	Statistical discrepancy between income components and GDP	−					
D.2	Taxes on production and imports, received						
D.21	Taxes on products						
D.211	Value added tax (VAT)	85 586					
D.212	Taxes and duties on imports excluding VAT	−					
D.2121	Import duties	−					
D.2122	Taxes on imports excluding VAT and import duties	−					
D.214	Taxes on products excluding VAT and import duties	60 540					
D.21	Total taxes on products	146 126					
D.29	Other taxes on production	20 831					
D.2	Total taxes on production and imports, received	166 957					
-D.3	*less* Subsidies, paid						
-D.31	Subsidies on products	−5 994					
-D.39	Other subsidies on production	−3 093					
-D.3	Total subsidies	−9 087					
D.4	Property income, received						
D.41	Interest	385 810	24 562	311 433	237 356	46 212	27 865
D.42	Distributed income of corporations	177 963	44 582	82 883	13 506	42 267	27 110
D.43	Reinvested earnings on direct foreign investment	47 795	36 642	11 153	5 938	2 600	2 615
D.44	Property income attributed to insurance policy holders	67 316	590	61	15	13	33
D.45	Rent	1 493	124	31	−	−	31
D.4	Total property income	680 377	106 500	405 561	256 815	91 092	57 654
Total	Total resources	2 000 216	353 288	442 189	285 433	88 857	67 899
	Uses						
D.4	Property income, paid						
D.41	Interest	408 256	45 229	283 589	222 823	58 566	2 200
D.42	Distributed income of corporations	168 507	105 445	63 062	26 663	31 494	4 905
D.43	Reinvested earnings on direct foreign investment	22 930	16 802	6 128	1 487	3 141	1 500
D.44	Property income attributed to insurance policy holders	68 349		68 349			68 349
D.45	Rent	1 493	1 265	−	−	−	
D.4	Total property income	669 535	168 741	421 128	250 973	93 201	76 954
B.5*g	**Gross National Income (GNI)**	**1 330 681**	**184 547**	**21 061**	**34 460**	**−4 344**	**−9 055**
Total	Total uses	2 000 216	353 288	442 189	285 433	88 857	67 899
-K.1	After deduction of fixed capital consumption	−147 858	−80 360	−5 944			
B.5*n	National income, net	1 182 823	104 187	15 117			

1.7.3

continued

UK summary accounts
2006

Total economy: all sectors and the rest of the world

£ million

		General government	Central government	Local government	Households & NPISH	Not sector -ised	Rest of the world
		S.13	S.1311	S.1313	S.14+S.15	S.N	S.2
II.1.2	**ALLOCATION OF PRIMARY INCOME ACCOUNT**						
	Resources						
B.2g	Operating surplus, gross	12 931	6 566	6 365	71 963		
B.3g	Mixed income, gross				78 908		
D.1	Compensation of employees						
D.11	Wages and salaries				599 461		1 803
D.12	Employers' social contributions				115 290		
D.1	Total				714 751		1 803
di	Statistical discrepancy between income components and GDP					−	
D.2	Taxes on production and imports, received						
D.21	Taxes on products						
D.211	Value added tax (VAT)	85 586	85 586				2 167
D.212	Taxes and duties on imports excluding VAT						
D.2121	Import duties	−	−				2 329
D.2122	Taxes on imports excluding VAT and import duties	−	−				−
D.214	Taxes on products excluding VAT and import duties	60 540	60 540				−
D.21	Total taxes on products	146 126	146 126				4 496
D.29	Other taxes on production	20 831	20 629	202			
D.2	Total taxes on production and imports, received	166 957	166 755	202			4 496
-D.3	*less* Subsidies, paid						
-D.31	Subsidies on products	−5 994	−4 258	−1 736			−
-D.39	Other subsidies on production	−3 093	−1 432	−1 661			−3 220
-D.3	Total subsidies	−9 087	−5 690	−3 397			−3 220
D.4	Property income, received						
D.41	Interest	7 109	5 864	1 245	42 706		157 867
D.42	Distributed income of corporations	2 541	1 866	675	47 957		44 776
D.43	Reinvested earnings on direct foreign investment						22 930
D.44	Property income attributed to insurance policy holders	25		25	66 640		1 033
D.45	Rent	1 210	1 226	−	112		
D.4	Total property income	10 901	8 956	1 945	157 415		226 606
Total	Total resources	181 702	176 587	5 115	1 023 037	−	
	Uses						
D.4	Property income, paid						
D.41	Interest	30 392	26 738	3 654	49 046		135 421
D.42	Distributed income of corporations						54 232
D.43	Reinvested earnings on direct foreign investment						47 795
D.44	Property income attributed to insurance policy holders						
D.45	Rent				228		
D.4	Total property income	30 392	26 738	3 654	49 274		237 448
B.5*g	**Gross National Income (GNI)**	**151 310**	**149 849**	**1 461**	**973 763**	**−**	
Total	Total uses	181 702	176 587	5 115	1 023 037	−	
-K.1	After deduction of fixed capital consumption	−12 931	−6 566	−6 365	−48 623		
B.5*n	National income, net	138 379	143 283	−4 904	925 140		

1.7.4 UK summary accounts 2006

Total economy: all sectors and the rest of the world

£ million

	UK total economy S.1	Non-financial corporations S.11	Financial corporations S.12	Monetary financial institutions S.121+S.122	Other financial intermediaries & auxiliaries S.123+S.124	Insurance corporations & pension funds S.125
II.2 SECONDARY DISTRIBUTION OF INCOME ACCOUNT						
Resources						
B.5*g **Gross National Income**	**1 330 681**	**184 547**	**21 061**	**34 460**	**−4 344**	**−9 055**
D.5 Current taxes on income, wealth etc.						
D.51 Taxes on income	192 812					
D.59 Other current taxes	30 906					
D.5 Total	223 718					
D.61 Social contributions						
D.611 Actual social contributions						
D.6111 Employers' actual social contributions	103 551		47 527			47 527
D.6112 Employees' social contributions	84 185		39 807	–	–	39 807
D.6113 Social contributions by self- and non-employed persons	2 930		–	–	–	–
D.611 Total	190 666		87 334	–		87 334
D.612 Imputed social contributions	11 739	3 425	511	256	179	76
D.61 Total	202 405	3 425	87 845	256	179	87 410
D.62 Social benefits other than social transfers in kind	225 891					
D.7 Other current transfers						
D.71 Net non-life insurance premiums	36 531		36 531			36 531
D.72 Non-life insurance claims	29 958	8 368	878	219	183	476
D.73 Current transfers within general government	110 407					
D.74 Current international cooperation from institutions of the EC	3 674					
D.75 Miscellaneous current transfers	39 320	–	–	–	–	
D.7 Total, other current transfers	219 890	8 368	37 409	219	183	37 007
Total Total resources	2 202 585	196 340	146 315	34 935	−3 982	115 362
Uses						
D.5 Current taxes on income, wealth etc.						
D.51 Taxes on income	192 627	37 183	15 475	5 224	6 472	3 779
D.59 Other current taxes	30 906					
D.5 Total	223 533	37 183	15 475	5 224	6 472	3 779
D.61 Social contributions						
D.611 Actual social contributions						
D.6111 Employers' actual social contributions	103 551					
D.6112 Employees' actual social contributions	84 129					
D.6113 Social contributions by self- and non-employed persons	2 930					
D.611 Total actual social contributions	190 610					
D.612 Imputed social contributions	11 739					
D.61 Total	202 349					
D.62 Social benefits other than social transfers in kind	227 628	3 425	56 140	256	179	55 705
D.7 Other current transfers						
D.71 Net non-life insurance premiums	29 958	8 368	878	219	183	476
D.72 Non-life insurance claims	36 531		36 531			36 531
D.73 Current transfers within general government	110 407					
D.74 Current international cooperation to institutions of the EC	3 632					
D.75 Miscellaneous current transfers	48 523	474	80	56	24	–
Of which: GNP based fourth own resource	8 521					
D.7 Total other current transfers	229 051	8 842	37 489	275	207	37 007
B.6*g **Gross National Disposable Income**	**1 320 024**	**146 890**	**37 211**	**29 180**	**−10 840 g**	**18 871**
Total Total uses	2 202 585	196 340	146 315	34 935	−3 982	115 362
-K.1 After deduction of fixed capital consumption	−147 858	−80 360	−5 944			
B.6*n Disposable income, net	1 172 166	66 530	31 267			

1.7.4

UK summary accounts
2006

continued

Total economy: all sectors and the rest of the world

£ million

		General government	Central government	Local government	Households & NPISH	Not sector -ised	Rest of the world
		S.13	S.1311	S.1313	S.14+S.15	S.N	S.2
II.2	**SECONDARY DISTRIBUTION OF INCOME ACCOUNT**						
	Resources						
B.5*g	**Gross National Income**	**151 310**	**149 849**	**1 461**	**973 763**	–	
D.5	Current taxes on income, wealth etc.						
D.51	Taxes on income	192 812	192 812				464
D.59	Other current taxes	30 906	8 687	22 219			
D.5	Total	223 718	201 499	22 219			464
D.61	Social contributions						
D.611	Actual social contributions						
D.6111	Employers' actual social contributions	56 024	56 024				
D.6112	Employees' social contributions	44 378	43 581	797			–
D.6113	Social contributions by self- and non-employed persons	2 930	2 930				
D.611	Total	103 332	102 535	797			–
D.612	Imputed social contributions	7 289	4 863	2 426	514		
D.61	Total	110 621	107 398	3 223	514		–
D.62	Social benefits other than social transfers in kind				225 891		1 737
D.7	Other current transfers						
D.71	Net non-life insurance premiums						39
D.72	Non-life insurance claims	366	–	366	20 346		6 612
D.73	Current transfers within general government	110 407	–	110 407			
	Current international cooperation						3 632
D.74	from institutions of the EC	3 674	3 594	80			
D.75	Miscellaneous current transfers	612	612		38 708		13 176
	Of which: GNP based fourth own resource						8 521
D.7	Total, other current transfers	115 059	4 206	110 853	59 054		23 459
Total	Total resources	600 708	462 952	137 756	1 259 222	–	
	Uses						
D.5	Current taxes on income, wealth etc.						
D.51	Taxes on income				139 969		649
D.59	Other current taxes	1 075		1 075	29 831		
D.5	Total	1 075		1 075	169 800		649
D.61	Social contributions						
D.611	Actual social contributions						
D.6111	Employers' actual social contributions				103 551		
D.6112	Employees' actual social contributions				84 129		56
D.6113	Social contributions by self- and non-employed persons				2 930		
D.611	Total actual social contributions				190 610		56
D.612	Imputed social contributions				11 739		
D.61	Total				202 349		56
D.62	Social benefits other than social transfers in kind	167 053	147 998	19 055	1 010		1 305
D.7	Other current transfers						
D.71	Net non-life insurance premiums	366	–	366	20 346		6 612
D.72	Non-life insurance claims						39
D.73	Current transfers within general government	110 407	110 407	–			
	Current international cooperation						3 674
D.74	to institutions of the EC	3 632	3 632				
D.75	Miscellaneous current transfers	34 695	34 670	25	13 274		3 973
	Of which: GNP based fourth own resource	8 521	8 521				
D.7	Total other current transfers	149 100	148 709	391	33 620		14 298
B.6*g	**Gross National Disposable Income**	**283 480**	**166 245**	**117 235**	**852 443**	–	
Total	Total uses	600 708	462 952	137 756	1 259 222	–	
-K.1	After deduction of fixed capital consumption	–12 931	–6 566	–6 365	–48 623		
B.6*n	Disposable income, net	270 549	159 679	110 870	803 820	–	

1.7.5 UK summary accounts 2006

Total economy: all sectors and the rest of the world

£ million

		UK total economy S.1	Non-financial corporations S.11	Financial corporations S.12	Monetary financial institutions S.121+S.122	Other financial intermediaries & auxiliaries S.123+S.124	Insurance corporations & pension funds S.125
II.3	**REDISTRIBUTION OF INCOME IN KIND ACCOUNT**						
	Resources						
B.6*g	**Gross National Disposable Income**	**1 320 024**	**146 890**	**37 211**	**29 180**	**−10 840**	**18 871**
D.63	Social transfers in kind						
D.631	Social benefits in kind						
D.6313	Social assistance benefits in kind	−					
D.632	Transfers of individual non-market goods and services	205 324					
D.63	Total social transfers in kind	205 324					
Total	Total resources	1 525 348	146 890	37 211	29 180	−10 840	18 871
	Uses						
D.63	Social transfers in kind						
D.631	Social benefits in kind						
D.6313	Social assistance benefits in kind	−					
D.632	Transfers of individual non-market goods and services	205 324					
D.63	Total social transfers in kind	205 324					
B.7g	Adjusted disposable income, gross	1 320 024	146 890	37 211	29 180	−10 840	18 871
Total	Total uses	1 525 348	146 890	37 211	29 180	−10 840	18 871

1.7.5

UK summary accounts
2006

continued

Total economy: all sectors and the rest of the world

£ million

		General government	Central government	Local government	Households & NPISH	Not sector -ised	Rest of the world
		S.13	S.1311	S.1313	S.14+S.15	S.N	S.2
II.3	**REDISTRIBUTION OF INCOME IN KIND ACCOUNT**						
	Resources						
B.6*g	**Gross National Disposable Income**	**283 480**	**166 245**	**117 235**	**852 443**	–	
D.63	Social transfers in kind						
D.631	Social benefits in kind						
D.6313	Social assistance benefits in kind				–		
D.632	Transfers of individual non-market goods and services				205 324		
D.63	Total social transfers in kind				205 324		
Total	Total resources	283 480	166 245	117 235	1 057 767	–	
	Uses						
D.63	Social transfers in kind						
D.631	Social benefits in kind						
D.6313	Social assistance benefits in kind				–		
D.632	Transfers of individual non-market goods and services	173 115	98 532	74 583	32 209		
D.63	Total social transfers in kind	173 115	98 532	74 583	32 209		
B.7g	Adjusted disposable income, gross	110 365	67 713	42 652	1 025 558	–	
Total	Total uses	283 480	166 245	117 235	1 057 767	–	

1.7.6 UK summary accounts 2006

Total economy: all sectors and the rest of the world

£ million

		UK total economy S.1	Non-financial corporations S.11	Financial corporations S.12	Monetary financial institutions S.121+S.122	Other financial intermediaries & auxiliaries S.123+S.124	Insurance corporations & pension funds S.125
II.4	**USE OF INCOME ACCOUNT**						
II.4.1	**USE OF DISPOSABLE INCOME ACCOUNT**						
	Resources						
B.6g	**Gross National Disposable Income**	**1 320 024**	**146 890**	**37 211**	**29 180**	**−10 840**	**18 871**
D.8	Adjustment for the change in net equity of households in pension funds	31 714					
Total	Total resources	1 351 738	146 890	37 211	29 180	−10 840	18 871
	Uses						
P.3	Final consumption expenditure						
P.31	Individual consumption expenditure	1 019 983					
P.32	Collective consumption expenditure	112 554					
P.3	Total	1 132 537					
D.8	Adjustment for the change in net equity of households in pension funds	31 705		31 705			31 705
B.8g	**Gross Saving**	**187 496**	**146 890**	**5 506**	**29 180**	**−10 840**	**−12 834**
B.12	Current external balance						
Total	Total uses	1 351 738	146 890	37 211	29 180	−10 840	18 871
-K.1	After deduction of fixed capital consumption	−147 858	−80 360	−5 944			
B.8n	Saving, net	39 638	66 530	−438			
II.4.2	**USE OF ADJUSTED DISPOSABLE INCOME ACCOUNT**						
	Resources						
B.7g	Adjusted disposable income	1 320 024	146 890	37 211	29 180	−10 840	18 871
D.8	Adjustment for the change in net equity of households in pension funds	31 714					
Total	Total resources	1 351 738	146 890	37 211	29 180	−10 840	18 871
	Uses						
P.4	Actual final consumption						
P.41	Actual individual consumption	1 019 983					
P.42	Actual collective consumption	112 554					
P.4	Total actual final consumption	1 132 537					
D.8	Adjustment for the change in net equity of households in pension funds	31 705		31 705			
B.8g	**Gross Saving**	**187 496**	**146 890**	**5 506**	**29 180**	**−10 840**	**−12 834**
Total	Total uses	1 351 738	146 890	37 211	29 180	−10 840	18 871

1.7.6

UK summary accounts
2006

Total economy: all sectors and the rest of the world

£ million

		General government	Central government	Local government	Households & NPISH	Not sector -ised	Rest of the world
		S.13	S.1311	S.1313	S.14+S.15	S.N	S.2
II.4	**USE OF INCOME ACCOUNT**						
II.4.1	**USE OF DISPOSABLE INCOME ACCOUNT**						
	Resources						
B.6g	**Gross National Disposable Income**	**283 480**	**166 245**	**117 235**	**852 443**	–	
D.8	Adjustment for the change in net equity of households in pension funds				31 714		–9
Total	Total resources	283 480	166 245	117 235	884 157	–	
	Uses						
P.3	Final consumption expenditure						
P.31	Individual consumption expenditure	173 115	98 532	74 583	846 868		
P.32	Collective consumption expenditure	112 554	75 373	37 181			
P.3	Total	285 669	173 905	111 764	846 868		
D.8	Adjustment for the change in net equity of households in pension funds						
B.8g	**Gross Saving**	**–2 189**	**–7 660**	**5 471**	**37 289**	–	
B.12	Current external balance						45 031
Total	Total uses	283 480	166 245	117 235	884 157	–	
-K.1	After deduction of fixed capital consumption	–12 931	–6 566	–6 365	–48 623		
B.8n	Saving, net	–15 120	–14 226	–894	–11 334	–	
II.4.2	**USE OF ADJUSTED DISPOSABLE INCOME ACCOUNT**						
	Resources						
B.7g	Adjusted disposable income	110 365	67 713	42 652	1 025 558	–	
D.8	Adjustment for the change in net equity of households in pension funds				31 714		–9
Total	Total resources	110 365	67 713	42 652	1 057 272	–	
	Uses						
P.4	Actual final consumption						
P.41	Actual individual consumption				1 019 983		
P.42	Actual collective consumption	112 554	75 373	37 181			
P.4	Total actual final consumption	112 554	75 373	37 181	1 019 983		
D.8	Adjustment for the change in net equity of households in pension funds						
B.8g	**Gross Saving**	**–2 189**	**–7 660**	**5 471**	**37 289**	–	
Total	Total uses	110 365	67 713	42 652	1 057 272	–	

1.7.7 UK summary accounts 2006

Total economy: all sectors and the rest of the world

£ million

		UK total economy S.1	Non-financial corporations S.11	Financial corporations S.12	Monetary financial institutions S.121+S.122	Other financial intermediaries & auxiliaries S.123+S.124	Insurance corporations & pension funds S.125
III	**ACCUMULATION ACCOUNTS**						
III.1	**CAPITAL ACCOUNT**						
III.1.1	**CHANGE IN NET WORTH DUE TO SAVING & CAPITAL TRANSFERS**						
	Changes in liabilities and net worth						
B.8g	**Gross Saving**	**187 496**	**146 890**	**5 506**	**29 180**	**−10 840**	**−12 834**
B.12	Current external balance						
D.9	Capital transfers receivable						
D.91	Capital taxes	3 575					
D.92	Investment grants	21 443	7 673	–	–	–	–
D.99	Other capital transfers	6 446	449	446	–	–	446
D.9	Total	31 464	8 122	446	–	–	446
-D.9	*less* Capital transfers payable						
-D.91	Capital taxes	−3 575	–	–	–	–	–
-D.92	Investment grants	−21 163					
-D.99	Other capital transfers	−5 759	−630	−446	–	–	−446
-D.9	Total	−30 497	−630	−446	–	–	−446
B.10.1g	Total change in liabilities and net worth	188 463	154 382	5 506	29 180	−10 840	−12 834
	Changes in assets						
B.10.1g	Changes in net worth due to gross saving and capital transfers	188 463	154 382	5 506	29 180	−10 840	−12 834
-K.1	After deduction of fixed capital consumption	−147 858	−80 360	−5 944			
B.10.1n	Changes in net worth due to net saving and capital transfers	40 605	74 022	−438			
III.1.2	**ACQUISITION OF NON-FINANCIAL ASSETS ACCOUNT**						
	Changes in liabilities and net worth						
B.10.1n	Changes in net worth due to net saving and capital transfers	40 605	74 022	−438			
K.1	Consumption of fixed capital	147 858	80 360	5 944			
B.10.1g	Total change in liabilities and net worth	188 463	154 382	5 506	29 180	−10 840	−12 834
	Changes in assets						
P.5	Gross capital formation						
P.51	Gross fixed capital formation	227 920	121 173	8 650	4 872	1 366	2 412
P.52	Changes in inventories	4 322	4 142	199	199	–	–
P.53	Acquisitions less disposals of valuables	285	−42	−74	–	–	−74
P.5	Total	232 527	125 273	8 775	5 071	1 366	2 338
K.2	Acquisitions less disposals of non-produced non-financial assets	−8	1 381	6	–	20	−14
de	Statistical discrepancy between expenditure components and GDP	–					
B.9	**Net lending(+) / net borrowing(-)**	**−44 056**	**27 728**	**−3 275**	**24 109**	**−12 226**	**−15 158**
Total	Total change in assets	188 463	154 382	5 506	29 180	−10 840	−12 834

1.7.7

**UK summary accounts
2006**

Total economy: all sectors and the rest of the world

£ million

		General government	Central government	Local government	Households & NPISH	Not sector -ised	Rest of the world
		S.13	S.1311	S.1313	S.14+S.15	S.N	S.2
III	**ACCUMULATION ACCOUNTS**						
III.1	**CAPITAL ACCOUNT**						
III.1.1	**CHANGE IN NET WORTH DUE TO SAVING SAVING & CAPITAL TRANSFERS**						
	Changes in liabilities and net worth						
B.8g	**Gross Saving**	−2 189	−7 660	5 471	37 289	−	
B.12	Current external balance						45 031
D.9	Capital transfers receivable						
D.91	Capital taxes	3 575	3 575				
D.92	Investment grants	8 515		8 515	5 255		388
D.99	Other capital transfers	2 562	1 488	1 074	2 989		2 038
D.9	Total	14 652	5 063	9 589	8 244		2 426
-D.9	*less* Capital transfers payable						
-D.91	Capital taxes				−3 575		
-D.92	Investment grants	−21 163	−19 528	−1 635			−668
-D.99	Other capital transfers	−3 526	−2 641	−885	−1 157		−2 725
-D.9	Total	−24 689	−22 169	−2 520	−4 732		−3 393
B.10.1g	Total change in liabilities and net worth	−12 226	−24 766	12 540	40 801	−	44 064
	Changes in assets						
B.10.1g	Changes in net worth due to gross saving and capital transfers	−12 226	−24 766	12 540	40 801	−	44 064
-K.1	After deduction of fixed capital consumption	−12 931	−6 566	−6 365	−48 623		
B.10.1n	Changes in net worth due to net saving and capital transfers	−25 157	−31 332	6 175	−7 822	−	
III.1.2	**ACQUISITION OF NON-FINANCIAL ASSETS ACCOUNT**						
	Changes in liabilities and net worth						
B.10.1n	Changes in net worth due to net saving and capital transfers	−25 157	−31 332	6 175	−7 822	−	
K.1	Consumption of fixed capital	12 931	6 566	6 365	48 623		
B.10.1g	Total change in liabilities and net worth	−12 226	−24 766	12 540	40 801	−	44 064
	Changes in assets						
P.5	Gross capital formation						
P.51	Gross fixed capital formation	23 667	9 860	13 807	74 430		
P.52	Changes in inventories	−4	−4	−	−15		
P.53	Acquisitions less disposals of valuables	14	14		387		
P.5	Total	23 677	9 870	13 807	74 802		
K.2	Acquisitions less disposals of non-produced non-financial assets	−1 037	−90	−947	−358		8
de	Statistical discrepancy between expenditure components and GDP					−	
B.9	**Net lending(+) / net borrowing(-)**	**−34 866**	**−34 546**	**−320**	**−33 643**	**−**	44 056
Total	Total change in assets	−12 226	−24 766	12 540	40 801	−	44 064

1.7.8 UK summary accounts 2007

Total economy: all sectors and the rest of the world. Unconsolidated

£ million

		UK total economy S.1	Non-financial corporations S.11	Financial corporations S.12	Monetary financial institutions S.121+S.122	Other financial intermediaries & auxiliaries S.123+S.124	Insurance corporations & pension funds S.125
III.2	**FINANCIAL ACCOUNT**						
F.A	**Net acquisition of financial assets**						
F.1	Monetary gold and special drawing rights (SDRs)	−50					
F.2	Currency and deposits						
F.21	Currency	1 129	293	−1 413	−1 413	−	
F.22	Transferable deposits						
F.221	Deposits with UK monetary financial institutions	293 383	18 488	221 698	96 409	107 882	17 407
F.229	Deposits with rest of the world monetary financial institutions	508 210	72 738	423 529	375 379	36 409	11 741
F.29	Other deposits	12 528	114	2 248	−11	2 259	−
F.2	Total currency and deposits	815 250	91 633	646 062	470 364	146 550	29 148
F.3	Securities other than shares						
F.331	Short term: money market instruments						
F.3311	Issued by UK central government	−4 913	408	−5 270	−6 513	1 258	−15
F.3312	Issued by UK local authorities	−	−	−	−	−	
F.3315	Issued by UK monetary financial institutions	2 918	3 020	2 200	−8 676	6 913	3 963
F.3316	Issued by other UK residents	−1 883	1 659	−3 072	−3 768	183	513
F.3319	Issued by the rest of the world	−1 922	−9 820	5 773	8 534	−3 618	857
F.332	Medium (1 to 5 year) and long term (over 5 year) bonds						
F.3321	Issued by UK central government	13 629	492	22 317	2 302	24 174	−4 159
F.3322	Issued by UK local authorities	−9	−	−29		−	−29
F.3325	Medium term bonds issued by UK MFIs[1]	20 764	658	20 106	1 091	4 802	14 213
F.3326	Other medium & long term bonds issued by UK residents	36 401	3 733	32 952	27 954	3 788	1 210
F.3329	Long term bonds issued by the rest of the world	68 455	169	66 071	43 738	−14 561	36 894
F.34	Financial derivatives	18 668	10	19 001	19 001		
F.3	Total securities other than shares	152 108	329	160 049	83 663	22 939	53 447
F.4	Loans						
F.41	Short term loans						
F.411	Loans by UK monetary financial institutions, excluding loans secured on dwellings & financial leasing	516 001		516 001	516 001		
F.419	Loans by rest of the world monetary financial institutions						
F.42	Long term loans						
F.421	Direct investment	50 327	47 098	3 229	−	2 569	660
F.422	Loans secured on dwellings	107 675	−	107 252	26 718	80 549	−15
F.423	Finance leasing	1 175	559	616	−6	622	
F.424	Other long term loans	48 194	−2 445	54 136	−168	58 363	−4 059
F.429	Other long term loans by the rest of the world						
F.4	Total loans	723 372	45 212	681 234	542 545	142 103	−3 414
F.5	Shares and other equity						
F.51	Shares and other equity, excluding mutual funds' shares						
F.514	Quoted UK shares	−16 292	11 794	10 266	3 635	34 819	−28 188
F.515	Unquoted UK shares	4 987	11 311	9 916	10 308	−55	−337
F.516	Other UK equity (including direct investment in property)	−2 171					
F.517	UK shares and bonds issued by other UK residents	−	−	−	−	−	−
F.519	Shares and other equity issued by the rest of the world	142 395	69 396	68 894	20 620	36 379	11 895
F.52	Mutual funds' shares						
F.521	UK mutual funds' shares	−2 054	7	−1 323	22	42	−1 387
F.529	Rest of the world mutual funds' shares	−110					
F.5	Total shares and other equity	126 755	92 508	87 753	34 585	71 185	−18 017
F.6	Insurance technical reserves						
F.61	Net equity of households in life assurance and pension funds' reserves	72 738					
F.62	Prepayments of insurance premiums and reserves for outstanding claims	59	10	−	−	−1	1
F.6	Total insurance technical reserves	72 797	10	−	−	−1	1
F.7	Other accounts receivable	22 313	541	13 506	−37	645	12 898
F.A	**Total net acquisition of financial assets**	1 912 545	230 233	1 588 604	1 131 120	383 421	74 063

1 UK monetary financial institutions

1.7.8 UK summary accounts 2007

continued

Total economy: all sectors and the rest of the world. Unconsolidated

£ million

		General government	Central government	Local government	Households & NPISH	Rest of the world
		S.13	S.1311	S.1313	S.14+S.15	S.2
III.2	**FINANCIAL ACCOUNT**					
F.A	**Net acquisition of financial assets**					
F.1	Monetary gold and special drawing rights (SDRs)	−50	−50			50
F.2	Currency and deposits					
F.21	Currency				2 249	47
F.22	Transferable deposits					
F.221	Deposits with UK monetary financial institutions	6 363	2 024	4 339	46 834	688 060
F.229	Deposits with rest of the world monetary financial institutions	−550	−550		12 493	
F.29	Other deposits	4 342	3 761	581	5 824	−299
F.2	Total currency and deposits	10 155	5 235	4 920	67 400	687 808
F.3	Securities other than shares					
F.331	Short term: money market instruments					
F.3311	Issued by UK central government	−51		−51	−	3 546
F.3312	Issued by UK local authorities	−			−	
F.3315	Issued by UK monetary financial institutions	−2 991	−2 038	−953	689	14 942
F.3316	Issued by other UK residents	−472	−1 142	670	2	2 904
F.3319	Issued by the rest of the world	2 125	2 125			
F.332	Medium (1 to 5 year) and long term (over 5 year) bonds					
F.3321	Issued by UK central government	−126		−126	−9 054	25 322
F.3322	Issued by UK local authorities				20	−
F.3325	Medium term bonds issued by UK MFIs[1]					36 497
F.3326	Other medium & long term bonds issued by UK residents	−42	−42	−	−242	113 279
F.3329	Long term bonds issued by the rest of the world	2 127	2 127		88	
F.34	Financial derivatives	−343	−343		−	
F.3	Total securities other than shares	227	687	−460	−8 497	196 490
F.4	Loans					
F.41	Short term loans					
F.411	Loans by UK monetary financial institutions, excluding loans secured on dwellings & financial leasing					
F.419	Loans by rest of the world monetary financial institutions					46 048
F.42	Long term loans					
F.421	Direct investment					26 275
F.422	Loans secured on dwellings	423	−	423		
F.423	Finance leasing					
F.424	Other long-term loans by UK residents	4 061	4 360	−299	−7 558	
F.429	Other long-term loans by the rest of the world					−12
F.4	Total loans	4 484	4 360	124	−7 558	72 311
F.5	Shares and other equity					
F.51	Shares and other equity, excluding mutual funds' shares					
F.514	Quoted UK shares	−2 484	−2 316	−168	−35 868	30 938
F.515	Unquoted UK shares	−2 188	−2 060	−128	−14 052	61 600
F.516	Other UK equity (including direct investment in property)	−2 171	−76	−2 095	−	2 358
F.517	UK shares and bonds issued by other UK residents	−	−	−		−
F.519	Shares and other equity issued by the rest of the world	725	725		3 380	
F.52	Mutual funds' shares					
F.521	UK mutual funds' shares				−738	22
F.529	Rest of the world mutual funds' shares				−110	
F.5	Total shares and other equity	−6 118	−3 727	−2 391	−47 388	94 918
F.6	Insurance technical reserves					
F.61	Net equity of households in life assurance and pension funds' reserves				72 738	−37
F.62	Prepayments of insurance premiums and reserves for outstanding claims	−		−	49	−20
F.6	Total insurance technical reserves	−		−	72 787	−57
F.7	Other accounts receivable	−1 741	−1 684	−57	10 007	245
F.A	**Total net acquisition of financial assets**	6 957	4 821	2 136	86 751	1 051 765

1 UK monetary financial institutions

1.7.8 UK summary accounts 2007

continued

Total economy: all sectors and the rest of the world. Unconsolidated

£ million

		UK total economy	Non-financial corporations	Financial corporations	Monetary financial institutions	Other financial intermediaries & auxiliaries	Insurance corporations & pension funds
		S.1	S.11	S.12	S.121+S.122	S.123+S.124	S.125
III.2	**FINANCIAL ACCOUNT** continued						
F.L	**Net acquisition of financial liabilities**						
F.2	Currency and deposits						
F.21	Currency	1 166		1 043	1 043		
F.22	Transferable deposits						
F.221	Deposits with UK monetary financial institutions	981 443		981 443	981 443		
F.229	Deposits with rest of the world monetary financial institutions						
F.29	Other deposits	12 229	–	4 299		4 299	
F.2	Total currency and deposits	994 838	–	986 785	982 486	4 299	
F.3	Securities other than shares						
F.331	Short term: money market instruments						
F.3311	Issued by UK central government	−1 367					
F.3312	Issued by UK local authorities	–					
F.3315	Issued by UK monetary financial institutions	17 860		17 860	17 860		
F.3316	Issued by other UK residents	1 021	677	−287		−287	
F.3319	Issued by the rest of the world						
F.332	Medium (1 to 5 year) and long term (over 5 year) bonds						
F.3321	Issued by UK central government	38 951					
F.3322	Issued by UK local authorities	−9					
F.3325	Medium term bonds issued by UK MFIs[1]	57 261		57 261	57 261		
F.3326	Other medium & long term bonds issued by UK residents	149 680	23 969	125 711	−12 681	137 678	714
F.3329	Long term bonds issued by the rest of the world						
F.34	Financial derivatives	−312	–	−312	−312		
F.3	Total securities other than shares	263 085	24 646	200 233	62 128	137 391	714
F.4	Loans						
F.41	Short term loans						
	Loans by UK monetary financial institutions,						
F.411	excluding loans secured on dwellings & financial leasing	289 473	80 518	197 788		202 011	−4 223
F.419	Loans by rest of the world monetary financial institutions	46 048	−7 105	52 943		52 111	832
F.42	Long term loans						
F.421	Direct investment	26 275	21 163	5 112	−56	6 288	−1 120
F.422	Loans secured on dwellings	107 675	3 830				
F.423	Finance leasing	1 175	546	187	108	79	
F.424	Other long-term loans by UK residents	48 895	57 294	−15 421		−6 053	−9 368
F.429	Other long-term loans by the rest of the world	−12	−6	26		26	
F.4	Total loans	519 529	156 240	240 635	52	254 462	−13 879
F.5	Shares and other equity						
F.51	Shares and other equity, excluding mutual funds' shares						
F.514	Quoted UK shares	14 646	5 392	9 254	6 263	2 058	933
F.515	Unquoted UK shares	66 587	26 815	39 772	3 248	35 937	587
F.516	Other UK equity (including direct investment in property)	187	187	–	–	–	
F.517	UK shares and bonds issued by other UK residents	–	–	–	–	–	
F.519	Shares and other equity issued by the rest of the world						
F.52	Mutual funds' shares						
F.521	UK mutual funds' shares	−2 032		−2 032		−2 032	
F.529	Rest of the world mutual funds' shares						
F.5	Total shares and other equity	79 388	32 394	46 994	9 511	35 963	1 520
F.6	Insurance technical reserves						
	Net equity of households in life assurance and						
F.61	pension funds' reserves	72 701		72 701			72 701
	Prepayments of insurance premiums and reserves for						
F.62	outstanding claims	39		39			39
F.6	Total insurance technical reserves	72 740		72 740			72 740
F.7	Other accounts payable	22 795	2 310	11 035	1 694	−1 029	10 370
F.L	**Total net acquisition of financial liabilities**	1 952 375	215 590	1 558 422	1 055 871	431 086	71 465
B.9	**Net lending / borrowing**						
F.A	Total net acquisition of financial assets	1 912 545	230 233	1 588 604	1 131 120	383 421	74 063
-F.L	*less* Total net acquisition of financial liabilities	−1 952 375	−215 590	−1 558 422	−1 055 871	−431 086	−71 465
B.9f	Net lending (+) / net borrowing (-), from financial account	−39 830	14 643	30 182	75 249	−47 665	2 598
dB.9f	Statistical discrepancy between financial & non-financial accounts	−10 097	7 983	−9 458	−32 718	34 325	−11 065
B.9	**Net lending (+) / net borrowing (-), from capital account**	**−49 927**	**22 626**	**20 724**	**42 531**	**−13 340**	**−8 467**

1.7.8 UK summary accounts 2007

continued

Total economy: all sectors and the rest of the world. Unconsolidated

£ million

		General government	Central government	Local government	Households & NPISH	Not sector -ised	Rest of the world
		S.13	S.1311	S.1313	S.14+S.15	S.N	S.2
III.2	**FINANCIAL ACCOUNT** continued						
F.L	**Net acquisition of financial liabilities**						
F.2	Currency and deposits						
F.21	Currency	123	123				10
F.22	Transferable deposits						
F.221	Deposits with UK monetary financial institutions						
F.229	Deposits with rest of the world monetary financial institutions						508 210
F.29	Other deposits	7 930	7 930				
F.2	Total currency and deposits	8 053	8 053				508 220
F.3	Securities other than shares						
F.331	Short term: money market instruments						
F.3311	Issued by UK central government	−1 367	−1 367				
F.3312	Issued by UK local authorities	−		−			
F.3315	Issued by UK monetary financial institutions						
F.3316	Issued by other UK residents				631		
F.3319	Issued by the rest of the world						−1 922
F.332	Medium (1 to 5 year) and long term (over 5 year) bonds						
F.3321	Issued by UK central government	38 951	38 951				
F.3322	Issued by UK local authorities	−9		−9			
F.3325	Medium term bonds issued by UK MFIs[1]						
F.3326	Other medium & long term bonds issued by UK residents				−		
F.3329	Long term bonds issued by the rest of the world						68 455
F.34	Financial derivatives				−		18 980
F.3	Total securities other than shares	37 575	37 584	−9	631		85 513
F.4	Loans						
F.41	Short term loans						
	Loans by UK monetary financial institutions,						
F.411	excluding loans secured on dwellings & financial leasing	386	−1 068	1 454	10 781		226 528
F.419	Loans by rest of the world monetary financial institutions	−	−	−	210		
F.42	Long term loans						
F.421	Direct investment						50 327
F.422	Loans secured on dwellings				103 845		
F.423	Finance leasing	442	442	−			−
F.424	Other long-term loans by UK residents	1 266	−6	1 272	5 756		−701
F.429	Other long-term loans by the rest of the world	−32	−3	−29			
F.4	Total loans	2 062	−635	2 697	120 592		276 154
F.5	Shares and other equity						
F.51	Shares and other equity, excluding mutual funds' shares						
F.514	Quoted UK shares						
F.515	Unquoted UK shares						
F.516	Other UK equity (including direct investment in property)						
F.517	UK shares and bonds issued by other UK residents						
F.519	Shares and other equity issued by the rest of the world						142 395
F.52	Mutual funds' shares						
F.521	UK mutual funds' shares						
F.529	Rest of the world mutual funds' shares						−110
F.5	Total shares and other equity						142 285
F.6	Insurance technical reserves						
F.61	Net equity of households in life assurance and pension funds' reserves						
F.62	Prepayments of insurance premiums and reserves for outstanding claims						
F.6	Total insurance technical reserves						
F.7	Other accounts payable	−1 442	−1 658	216	10 892		−237
F.L	**Total net acquisition of financial liabilities**	46 248	43 344	2 904	132 115		1 011 935
B.9	**Net lending / borrowing**						
F.A	Total net acquisition of financial assets	6 957	4 821	2 136	86 751		1 051 765
-F.L	*less* Total net acquisition of financial liabilities	−46 248	−43 344	−2 904	−132 115		−1 011 935
B.9f	Net lending (+) / net borrowing (-), from financial account	−39 291	−38 523	−768	−45 364		39 830
dB.9f	Statistical discrepancy between financial & non-financial accounts	969	961	8	−9 730	139	10 097
B.9	**Net lending (+) / net borrowing (-), from capital account**	**−38 322**	**−37 562**	**−760**	**−55 094**	**139**	**49 927**

1.7.9 UK summary accounts 2007

Total economy: all sectors and the rest of the world. Unconsolidated

£ billion

		UK total economy	Non-financial corporations	Financial corporations	Monetary financial institutions	Other financial intermediaries & auxiliaries	Insurance corporations & pension funds
		S.1	S.11	S.12	S.121+S.122	S.123+S.124	S.125
IV.3	**FINANCIAL BALANCE SHEET** at end of period						
AF.A	**Financial assets**						
AF.1	Monetary gold and special drawing rights (SDRs)	4.3					
AF.2	Currency and deposits						
AF.21	Currency	53.0	4.8	8.7	8.6	0.1	
AF.22	Transferable deposits						
AF.221	Deposits with UK monetary financial institutions	2 751.9	274.3	1 533.1	842.6	605.6	84.9
AF.229	Deposits with rest of the world monetary financial institutions	2 760.6	355.2	2 329.5	1 714.1	569.4	46.0
AF.29	Other deposits	102.6	9.6	3.8	–	3.7	–
AF.2	Total currency and deposits	5 668.2	643.9	3 875.0	2 565.3	1 178.8	130.9
AF.3	Securities other than shares						
AF.331	Short term: money market instruments						
AF.3311	Issued by UK central government	10.8	0.4	10.3	5.6	4.1	0.6
AF.3312	Issued by UK local authorities	–	–	–	–	–	
AF.3315	Issued by UK monetary financial institutions	164.0	9.3	148.2	88.7	26.4	33.1
AF.3316	Issued by other UK residents	51.1	43.7	5.7	1.3	1.0	3.4
AF.3319	Issued by the rest of the world	77.1	6.4	65.2	53.8	7.6	3.8
AF.332	Medium (1 to 5 year) and long term (over 5 year) bonds						
AF.3321	Issued by UK central government	334.6	1.2	329.4	−5.5	92.5	242.4
AF.3322	Issued by UK local authorities	1.2	–	0.5			0.5
AF.3325	Medium term bonds issued by UK MFIs[1]	118.4	2.5	115.9	25.2	23.2	67.5
AF.3326	Other medium & long term bonds issued by UK residents	502.5	5.2	491.2	209.4	99.5	182.4
AF.3329	Long term bonds issued by the rest of the world	905.1	11.6	867.7	555.2	53.0	259.5
AF.34	Financial derivatives	−0.4		–	–		
AF.3	Total securities other than shares	2 164.3	80.3	2 034.1	933.6	307.2	793.2
AF.4	Loans						
AF.41	Short term loans						
AF.411	Loans by UK monetary financial institutions, excluding loans secured on dwellings & financial leasing	2 538.9		2 538.9	2 538.9		
AF.419	Loans by rest of the world monetary financial institutions						
AF.42	Long term loans						
AF.421	Direct investment	279.9	254.3	25.5	–	19.8	5.7
AF.422	Loans secured on dwellings	1 181.4	–	1 179.3	829.7	348.8	0.8
AF.423	Finance leasing	32.7	4.9	27.7	2.6	25.1	
AF.424	Other long term loans	212.5	10.5	116.5	3.3	14.6	98.6
AF.429	Other long term loans by the rest of the world						
AF.4	Total loans	4 245.3	269.7	3 887.9	3 374.6	408.4	105.0
AF.5	Shares and other equity						
AF.51	Shares and other equity, excluding mutual funds' shares						
AF.514	Quoted UK shares	1 016.2	26.0	802.1	26.2	316.9	459.0
AF.515	Unquoted UK shares	537.2	63.3	312.9	123.2	186.4	3.3
AF.516	Other UK equity (including direct investment in property)	120.2					
AF.517	UK shares and bonds issued by other UK residents	–	–	–	–	–	
AF.519	Shares and other equity issued by the rest of the world	1 651.0	671.4	887.4	190.4	–	417.9
AF.52	Mutual funds' shares						
AF.521	UK mutual funds' shares	505.8	0.6	288.6	1.7	4.5	282.4
AF.529	Rest of the world mutual funds' shares	3.5					
AF.5	Total shares and other equity	3 833.9	761.3	2 291.0	341.4	786.9	1 162.6
AF.6	Insurance technical reserves						
AF.61	Net equity of households in life assurance and pension funds' reserves	2 186.7					
AF.62	Prepayments of insurance premiums and reserves for outstanding claims	59.1	17.6	1.9		0.9	1.0
AF.6	Total insurance technical reserves	2 245.8	17.6	1.9		0.9	1.0
AF.7	Other accounts receivable	434.1	126.9	112.7	–	15.2	97.4
AF.A	**Total financial assets**	18 596.0	1 899.7	12 202.5	7 214.9	2 697.4	2 290.2

1 UK monetary financial institutions

1.7.9

UK summary accounts
2007

continued

Total economy: all sectors and the rest of the world. Unconsolidated

£ billion

		General government	Central government	Local government	Households & NPISH	Rest of the world
		S.13	S.1311	S.1313	S.14+S.15	S.2
IV.3	**FINANCIAL BALANCE SHEET** at end of period					
AF.A	**Financial assets**					
AF.1	Monetary gold and special drawing rights (SDRs)	4.3	4.3			
AF.2	Currency and deposits					
AF.21	Currency				39.6	1.6
AF.22	Transferable deposits					
AF.221	Deposits with UK monetary financial institutions	41.0	9.8	31.2	903.5	3 143.4
AF.229	Deposits with rest of the world monetary financial institutions	1.0	1.0		74.9	
AF.29	Other deposits	4.6	3.8	0.8	84.8	1.1
AF.2	Total currency and deposits	46.6	14.6	32.0	1 102.7	3 146.1
AF.3	Securities other than shares					
AF.331	Short term: money market instruments					
AF.3311	Issued by UK central government	0.1		0.1	–	7.2
AF.3312	Issued by UK local authorities	–			–	
AF.3315	Issued by UK monetary financial institutions	2.3	0.8	1.6	4.2	182.0
AF.3316	Issued by other UK residents	1.3	0.1	1.3	0.4	19.1
AF.3319	Issued by the rest of the world	5.5	5.5			
AF.332	Medium (1 to 5 year) and long term (over 5 year) bonds					
AF.3321	Issued by UK central government	0.1		0.1	3.9	158.2
AF.3322	Issued by UK local authorities	–	–		0.7	–
AF.3325	Medium term bonds issued by UK MFIs[1]					167.0
AF.3326	Other medium & long term bonds issued by UK residents	0.5	0.3	0.2	5.5	605.9
AF.3329	Long term bonds issued by the rest of the world	18.2	18.2		7.6	
AF.34	Financial derivatives	–0.4	–0.4		–	
AF.3	Total securities other than shares	27.6	24.4	3.2	22.3	1 139.4
AF.4	Loans					
AF.41	Short term loans					
AF.411	Loans by UK monetary financial institutions, excluding loans secured on dwellings & financial leasing					
AF.419	Loans by rest of the world monetary financial institutions					965.2
AF.42	Long term loans					
AF.421	Direct investment					402.6
AF.422	Loans secured on dwellings	2.1	0.1	2.0		
AF.423	Finance leasing					
AF.424	Other long-term loans by UK residents	82.1	81.9	0.3	3.4	
AF.429	Other long-term loans by the rest of the world					3.3
AF.4	Total loans	84.2	82.0	2.3	3.4	1 371.2
AF.5	Shares and other equity					
AF.51	Shares and other equity, excluding mutual funds' shares					
AF.514	Quoted UK shares	1.8	0.6	1.2	186.2	775.7
AF.515	Unquoted UK shares	–0.9	–1.3	0.4	162.0	551.6
AF.516	Other UK equity (including direct investment in property)	118.8	7.4	111.4	1.4	24.8
AF.517	UK shares and bonds issued by other UK residents	–	–	–		–
AF.519	Shares and other equity issued by the rest of the world	10.3	10.3		82.0	
AF.52	Mutual funds' shares					
AF.521	UK mutual funds' shares				216.6	1.7
AF.529	Rest of the world mutual funds' shares				3.5	
AF.5	Total shares and other equity	130.0	17.0	113.0	651.6	1 353.7
AF.6	Insurance technical reserves					
AF.61	Net equity of households in life assurance and pension funds' reserves				2 186.7	0.2
AF.62	Prepayments of insurance premiums and reserves for outstanding claims	0.8		0.8	38.9	18.2
AF.6	Total insurance technical reserves	0.8		0.8	2 225.6	18.4
AF.7	Other accounts receivable	54.4	53.1	1.3	140.2	2.2
AF.A	**Total financial assets**	348.0	195.4	152.5	4 145.8	7 031.0

1 UK monetary financial institutions

1.7.9 UK summary accounts 2007

continued

Total economy: all sectors and the rest of the world. Unconsolidated £ billion

		UK total economy S.1	Non-financial corporations S.11	Financial corporations S.12	Monetary financial institutions S.121+S.122	Other financial intermediaries & auxiliaries S.123+S.124	Insurance corporations & pension funds S.125
IV.3	**FINANCIAL BALANCE SHEET** continued at end of period						
AF.L	**Financial liabilities**						
AF.2	Currency and deposits						
AF.21	Currency	53.9		50.0	50.0		
AF.22	Transferable deposits						
AF.221	Deposits with UK monetary financial institutions	5 895.3		5 895.3	5 895.3		
AF.229	Deposits with rest of the world monetary financial institutions						
AF.29	Other deposits	103.7	–	5.9		5.9	
AF.2	Total currency and deposits	6 052.9	–	5 951.3	5 945.4	5.9	
AF.3	Securities other than shares						
AF.331	Short term: money market instruments						
AF.3311	Issued by UK central government	18.0					
AF.3312	Issued by UK local authorities	–					
AF.3315	Issued by UK monetary financial institutions	346.1		346.1	346.1		
AF.3316	Issued by other UK residents	70.2	22.2	46.8		46.8	
AF.3319	Issued by the rest of the world						
AF.332	Medium (1 to 5 year) and long term (over 5 year) bonds						
AF.3321	Issued by UK central government	492.8					
AF.3322	Issued by UK local authorities	1.2					
AF.3325	Medium term bonds issued by UK MFIs[1]	285.3		285.3	285.3		
AF.3326	Other medium & long term bonds issued by UK residents	1 108.4	351.6	753.6	112.9	639.2	1.5
AF.3329	Long term bonds issued by the rest of the world						
AF.34	Financial derivatives	–0.5		–0.5	–0.5		
AF.3	Total securities other than shares	2 321.6	373.8	1 431.4	743.9	686.0	1.5
AF.4	Loans						
AF.41	Short term loans						
AF.411	Loans by UK monetary financial institutions, excluding loans secured on dwellings & financial leasing	1 583.0	477.6	879.2	–	870.5	8.7
AF.419	Loans by rest of the world monetary financial institutions	965.2	224.5	709.9		673.5	36.4
AF.42	Long term loans						
AF.421	Direct investment	402.6	346.3	56.3	1.3	45.1	9.9
AF.422	Loans secured on dwellings	1 181.4	34.8				
AF.423	Finance leasing	32.7	24.2	3.9	2.1	1.8	
AF.424	Other long-term loans by UK residents	206.1	102.4	20.3	–	19.8	0.5
AF.429	Other long-term loans by the rest of the world	3.3	0.8	0.5		0.5	
AF.4	Total loans	4 374.4	1 210.7	1 670.1	3.3	1 611.3	55.5
AF.5	Shares and other equity						
AF.51	Shares and other equity, excluding mutual funds' shares						
AF.514	Quoted UK shares	1 791.9	1 366.2	425.7	5.0	353.4	67.3
AF.515	Unquoted UK shares	1 088.8	693.2	395.6	133.3	243.1	19.2
AF.516	Other UK equity (including direct investment in property)	145.0	145.0	–	–	–	–
AF.517	UK shares and bonds issued by other UK residents	–	–	–	–	–	–
AF.519	Shares and other equity issued by the rest of the world						
AF.52	Mutual funds' shares						
AF.521	UK mutual funds' shares	507.5		507.5		507.5	
AF.529	Rest of the world mutual funds' shares						
AF.5	Total shares and other equity	3 533.1	2 204.4	1 328.8	138.3	1 103.9	86.5
AF.6	Insurance technical reserves						
AF.61	Net equity of households in life assurance and pension funds' reserves	2 186.9		2 186.9			2 186.9
AF.62	Prepayments of insurance premiums and reserves for outstanding claims	77.3		77.3			77.3
AF.6	Total insurance technical reserves	2 264.2		2 264.2			2 264.2
AF.7	Other accounts payable	431.4	155.1	95.3	7.6	2.5	85.1
AF.L	**Total financial liabilities**	18 977.6	3 944.1	12 740.9	6 838.5	3 409.7	2 492.7
BF.90	**Net financial assets / liabilities**						
AF.A	Total financial assets	18 596.0	1 899.7	12 202.5	7 214.9	2 697.4	2 290.2
-AF.L	*less* Total financial liabilities	–18 977.6	–3 944.1	–12 740.9	–6 838.5	–3 409.7	–2 492.7
BF.90	**Net financial assets (+) / liabilities (-)**	–381.6	–2 044.3	–538.4	376.4	–712.3	–202.5

1 UK monetary financial institutions

1.7.9

UK summary accounts
2007

Total economy: all sectors and the rest of the world. Unconsolidated

£ billion

		General government	Central government	Local government	Households & NPISH	Rest of the world
		S.13	S.1311	S.1313	S.14+S.15	S.2
IV.3	**FINANCIAL BALANCE SHEET** continued at end of period					
AF.L	**Financial liabilities**					
AF.2	Currency and deposits					
AF.21	Currency	3.9	3.9			0.8
AF.22	Transferable deposits					
AF.221	Deposits with UK monetary financial institutions					
AF.229	Deposits with rest of the world monetary financial institutions					2 760.6
AF.29	Other deposits	97.8	97.8			
AF.2	Total currency and deposits	101.6	101.6			2 761.4
AF.3	Securities other than shares					
AF.331	Short term: money market instruments					
AF.3311	Issued by UK central government	18.0	18.0			
AF.3312	Issued by UK local authorities	–		–		
AF.3315	Issued by UK monetary financial institutions					
AF.3316	Issued by other UK residents				1.2	
AF.3319	Issued by the rest of the world					77.1
AF.332	Medium (1 to 5 year) and long term (over 5 year) bonds					
AF.3321	Issued by UK central government	492.8	492.8			
AF.3322	Issued by UK local authorities	1.2		1.2		
AF.3325	Medium term bonds issued by UK MFIs[1]					
AF.3326	Other medium & long term bonds issued by UK residents			–	3.2	
AF.3329	Long term bonds issued by the rest of the world					905.1
AF.34	Financial derivatives				–	0.1
AF.3	Total securities other than shares	512.0	510.8	1.2	4.4	982.2
AF.4	Loans					
AF.41	Short term loans					
AF.411	Loans by UK monetary financial institutions, excluding loans secured on dwellings & financial leasing	34.7	24.4	10.3	191.5	955.9
AF.419	Loans by rest of the world monetary financial institutions	–	–	–	30.8	
AF.42	Long term loans					
AF.421	Direct investment					279.9
AF.422	Loans secured on dwellings				1 146.6	
AF.423	Finance leasing	4.5	4.5	0.1		–
AF.424	Other long-term loans by UK residents	51.1	–	51.1	32.3	6.3
AF.429	Other long-term loans by the rest of the world	2.1	–	2.1		
AF.4	Total loans	92.4	28.9	63.5	1 401.2	1 242.1
AF.5	Shares and other equity					
AF.51	Shares and other equity, excluding mutual funds' shares					
AF.514	Quoted UK shares					
AF.515	Unquoted UK shares					
AF.516	Other UK equity (including direct investment in property)					
AF.517	UK shares and bonds issued by other UK residents					
AF.519	Shares and other equity issued by the rest of the world					1 651.0
AF.52	Mutual funds' shares					
AF.521	UK mutual funds' shares					
AF.529	Rest of the world mutual funds' shares					3.5
AF.5	Total shares and other equity					1 654.5
AF.6	Insurance technical reserves					
AF.61	Net equity of households in life assurance and pension funds' reserves					
AF.62	Prepayments of insurance premiums and reserves for outstanding claims					
AF.6	Total insurance technical reserves					
AF.7	Other accounts payable	47.8	37.0	10.8	133.2	4.9
AF.L	**Total financial liabilities**	753.8	678.3	75.5	1 538.8	6 645.1
BF.90	**Net financial assets / liabilities**					
AF.A	Total financial assets	348.0	195.4	152.5	4 145.8	7 031.0
-AF.L	*less* Total financial liabilities	−753.8	−678.3	−75.5	−1 538.8	−6 645.1
BF.90	**Net financial assets (+) / liabilities (-)**	−405.9	−482.9	77.0	2 607.0	385.9

1 UK monetary financial institutions

1.8A FISIM impact on UK gross domestic product and national income
Current prices

£ million

			2001	2002	2003	2004	2005	2006	2007
	IMPACT OF FISIM ON GROSS DOMESTIC PRODUCT								
	Gross domestic product: Output								
P.1	Output of services								
	Financial intermediaries	D8NH	34 535	35 595	38 051	39 100	43 124	48 634	48 385
	Non-Market	D8N9	472	567	603	591	349	283	142
-P.2	Intermediate comsumption								
	Non-financial corporations	−G7VJ	−7 918	−7 175	−7 919	−8 904	−11 035	−13 445	−15 092
	Financial corporations	−D8OO	−1 164	−948	−882	−593	55	−237	1 626
	General Government	−C5PR	−81	−113	−120	−142	−66	−31	58
	Households and NPISH	−IV8A	−7 313	−8 155	−8 232	−7 820	−9 914	−10 930	−8 157
B.1*g	**Gross Domestic Product at market prices**	C95M	18 531	19 771	21 501	22 232	22 513	24 274	26 962
	Gross domestic product: Expenditure								
P.3	Total Final consumption expenditure								
	Households and NPISH	IV8B	15 673	16 856	17 931	19 769	21 302	23 149	24 222
	General Government	C5PR	81	113	120	142	66	31	−58
P.6	Exports of services	C6FD	3 726	4 025	5 280	4 943	4 967	5 500	7 995
-P.7	*less* imports of services	−C6F7	−949	−1 223	−1 830	−2 622	−3 822	−4 406	−5 197
B.1*g	**Gross Domestic Product at market prices**	C95M	18 531	19 771	21 501	22 232	22 513	24 274	26 962
	Gross domestic product: Income								
B.2g	Operating surplus, gross								
	Non-financial corporations	IV8H	−7 918	−7 175	−7 919	−8 904	−11 035	−13 445	−15 092
	Financial corporations	IV8I	33 371	34 647	37 169	38 507	43 179	48 397	50 011
	Households	IV8J	−6 922	−7 701	−7 749	−7 371	−9 631	−10 678	−7 957
B.1*g	**Gross Domestic Product at current prices**	C95M	18 531	19 771	21 501	22 232	22 513	24 274	26 962
	IMPACT OF FISIM ON GROSS NATIONAL INCOME								
B.1*g	Gross domestic product at market prices	C95M	18 531	19 771	21 501	22 232	22 513	24 274	26 962
D.4	Property and entreprenurial income								
	receipts from the rest of the world	IV8E	−1 009	−1 138	−1 166	−524	259	391	−84
	less payments to the rest of the world (ROW)	−IV8F	−1 768	−1 664	−2 284	−1 797	−1 404	−1 485	−2 714
B.5*g	**Gross National Income at market prices**	IV8G	15 754	16 969	18 051	19 911	21 368	23 180	24 164

1.8B FISIM impact on UK gross domestic product and national income
Chained volume measures (Reference year 2003)

£ million

			2001	2002	2003	2004	2005	2006	2007
	IMPACT OF FISIM ON GROSS DOMESTIC PRODUCT								
	Gross domestic product: Expenditure								
P.3	Total Final consumption expenditure								
	Households and NPISH	IV8D	15 607	16 755	17 931	19 194	20 428	20 876	21 419
	General Government	C5Q9	97	100	120	147	165	186	208
P.6	Exports of services	C6FM	4 889	4 781	5 280	5 753	6 587	7 449	8 352
-P.7	*less* imports of services	−C6FL	−1 013	−1 262	−1 830	−2 558	−3 645	−4 095	−4 707
B.1*g	**Gross Domestic Product at market prices**	DZ4H	19 509	20 392	21 501	22 536	23 535	24 416	25 272

The industrial analyses

Part 2

Chapter 2

The industrial analyses at a glance from Table 2.1

Gross value added at basic prices by industry

An analysis of the eleven broad industrial sectors shows that in 2006, the financial intermediation and other business services sector provided the largest contribution (31.0 per cent) to gross valued added at current basic prices, at £364.7 billion out of a total of £1,177.2 billion. The distribution and hotels sector contributed 14.4 per cent, the manufacturing sector accounted for 13.0 per cent and the education, health and social work sector 12.8 per cent.

Breakdown of gross value added at basic prices by industry for 2006

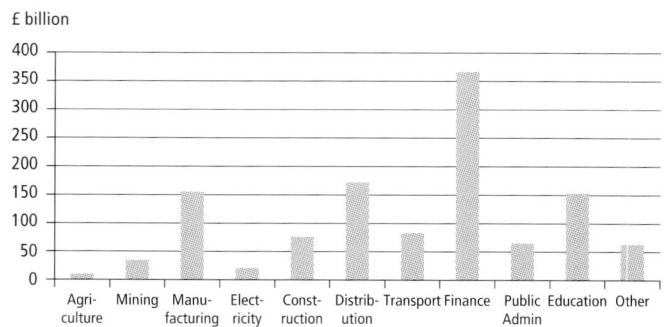

Final demand

In 2006, just under half (46.8 per cent) of all goods and services entering into final demand were purchased by consumers, 21.6 per cent were exported, and 16.4 per cent consumed by government, both central and local. Gross capital formation by all sectors of the economy amounted to 13.4 per cent of the total.

Composition of final demand for 2006

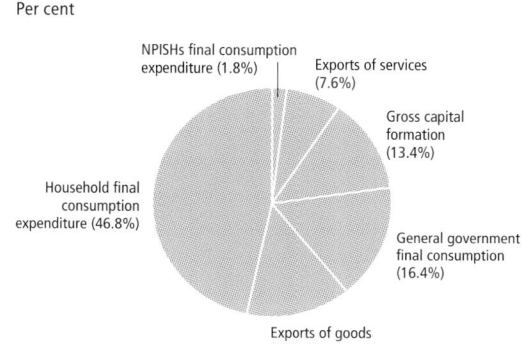

Compensation of employees by industry

The financial intermediation and other business services sector showed the highest level of compensation of employees in 2006 at £168.9 billion. After the financial sector, the second largest industry in terms of its contribution to total compensation of employees was the education, health and social work sector at £131.7 billion. The manufacturing industries' provided the largest contribution to the level of compensation of employees for years up to and including 2000. Thereafter, the financial services sector became the largest contributor.

Compensation of employees by industry 2006

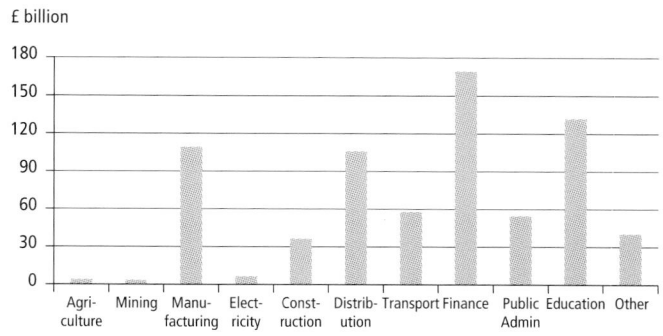

Explanation of industrial analyses

Input-Output Supply and Use Tables

The annual estimates prepared for the *Blue Book* incorporate the results of annual inquiries which become available in the first part of the year, although estimates for the latest year are still based largely on quarterly information. As new data are collected it is likely that revisions will be necessary. The process of reassessing these estimates involves the preparation of Supply and Use Tables. This approach amalgamates all the available information on inputs, outputs, gross value added, income and expenditure. Similarly the production of the consolidated sector and financial accounts requires the preparation of 'top-to-bottom' sector and sub-sector accounts to identify discrepancies in the estimates relating to each sector. The thorough and detailed nature of this estimation process require a large amount of time and resource and so estimates for earlier years are not normally revisited unless there are strong reasons for doing so.

GDP and the balancing of the annual accounts

As discussed in Part 1, there are three different approaches to the estimation of current price GDP in the UK: the income approach, the expenditure approach and the production approach. In theory the three different approaches should produce the same result. However, the different approaches are based on different surveys and administrative data sources and each produces estimates which, like all statistical estimates, are subject to errors and omissions. A definitive GDP estimate can only emerge after a process of balancing and adjustment. ONS believes that the most reliable 'definitive' estimate of the current price level of GDP is that derived using the annual Supply and Use Tables framework. Thus, for the years when Supply and Use Tables are available, GDP is set at the level derived from that year's balance. For periods subsequent to the latest Supply and Use Tables, the level of GDP is carried forward using movements in income, expenditure and production totals.

The Supply and Use framework

The accounting framework shown in Figure 1 in the Introduction is mainly concerned with the composition and value of goods and services entering into final demand (for example, purchases by consumers) and the outputs and incomes generated in the production process. It does not display the inter-industry transactions which link these activities.

The UK Supply and Use Tables, however, do include these intermediate transactions which form inputs into these processes, thus providing an extra dimension. The analyses are constructed to show a balanced and complete picture of the flows of products in the economy and illustrate the relationships between producers and consumers of goods and services. On an annual basis, Supply and Use Tables are used to achieve consistency in the economic accounts' aggregates by linking the components of value added, inputs, outputs and final demand. As the income, production and expenditure measures of GDP can all be calculated from the Supply and Use Tables, a single estimate of GDP can be derived by balancing the supply and demand for goods and services and reconciling them with the corresponding value added estimates. For the years 1989 to 2006, the balancing process has been used to set the level of current price GDP and has disposed of the need for statistical discrepancies in the form of a GDP expenditure adjustment and a GDP income adjustment.

Industrial analyses

The process, which produces Supply and Use Tables annually, has been speeded up considerably over the last few years and can now produce the first balance for a year around eighteen months after the end of that year. These full Supply and Use Tables, consistent with the National Accounts *Blue Book*, are published as a separate web-only publication at the same time as the *Blue Book*. The latest annual Supply and Use tables[1] cover the periods 2004 to 2006, with summary information provided in the *Blue Book* itself.

Some background on the structure of the Supply and Use Tables

The Supply and Use Tables are based on a framework which incorporates estimates of industry inputs, outputs and value added. The tables consist of two matrices: the *Supply* matrix and the *Use* matrix, each of which breaks down and balances 108 different industries and 123 products at purchasers' prices. The following paragraphs summarise the methodology. For more detail see Akers and Clifton-Fearnside (2008).[2]

Supply table

At a very aggregate level the *Supply* table can be represented as follows:

	Output by industry	Imports of goods and services	Dis-tributors' trading margins	Taxes *less* subsidies on products
Output by product				

The main part of the Supply table shows estimates of domestic industries' output (total sales adjusted for changes in inventories of work in progress and finished goods) compiled at basic prices. Basic prices value the goods leaving the factory gate but exclude any taxes on products and include any subsidies on products. However, for the balancing process, the estimates of supply of products are required at purchasers' prices, that is, those actually paid by the purchasers to take delivery of the goods, excluding any deductible VAT. To convert the estimates of domestic output valued at basic prices to the total supply of products valued at purchasers' prices requires the addition of:

- the value of imports of goods and services

- distributors' trading margins

- taxes on products (for example, VAT, excise duties, air passenger tax, insurance premium tax etc)

less

- subsidies on products (for example, agricultural and transport subsidies)

Use table

The Use table reveals the input structure of each industry in terms of combined domestic and imported goods and services.

It also shows the product composition of final demand and, for each industry, the intermediate purchases adjusted for changes in inventories of materials and fuels. Consumption of products is represented in the rows of the balance while purchases by industries, and final demands, are represented in the columns. At a very aggregate level the Use table can be considered in three parts as shown below.

The body of the matrix, which represents consumption of products, is at purchasers' prices and so already includes the product-specific taxes and subsidies separately added in the Supply table.

The Supply-Use balance is effectively achieved when:

For industries:

Inputs (from the *Use* table)

equals

Outputs (from the *Supply* table)

For products:

Supply (from the *Supply* table)

equals

Demand (from the *Use* table)

That is, when the data from the income, expenditure and production approaches used to fill the matrices all produce the same estimate of current price GDP at market prices. GDP at current market prices can be derived from the balances by taking the estimate of total gross value added at basic prices (from the Use table) and adding taxes on products and deducting subsidies on products (from the Supply table).

The BB08 balancing process

The supply and use tables produced this year will appear little different to those of the past, in terms of level of detail and coverage. What is being published this year provides the foundation for future improvements. What is fundamentally different this year is the process used to balance the supply and use tables. Previously balancing supply and use tables has been achieved by means of a dedicated central team. Their role was to maintain the system to bring together all the data sources necessary to populate the supply and use framework and

Industry consumption/final demand table

	Industry consumption	Final demands
Products consumed	Shows consumption by each industry to produce their own output (that is, intermediate consumption)	Shows final demand categories (for example, households' expenditure) and the values of products going to these categories
Primary inputs	Shows the gross value added components of each industry, taxes *less* subsidies on production other than product specific taxes and subsidies, compensation of employees and gross operating surplus.	

produce a balance. A detailed description of the methods and process used previously can be found in Mahajan (2006).[3]

For this year's *Blue Book* we have used a more decentralised approach to balancing. The sources of data used to populate the supply and use framework have not changed significantly although the computing systems used to marshal together the data and represent the supply and use framework are new. These new systems are an output from the ONS programme for the modernisation of its statistical systems and processes. The process of balancing is, however, somewhat different to what has been done in the past. Balancing no longer relies on a separate team allocated specifically to balancing the supply and use tables. Those involved in balancing are the compilers of the basic data that form the input to the process. These individuals bring with them an understanding of the data that is being used to populate the supply and use framework. If we considered the supply and use framework as a column (industry) and row (product) matrix the confrontation of the data can be viewed as a process of separate column, row and column confrontations of the data.

The process used to produce and balance the national accounts in the past has relied on the knowledge and experience of a small group of people. The new process aims to open up the process and make it more transparent. In this way we aim to place less reliance on specific individuals, thus ensuring our ability to balance in the longer term is more secure. Also, by including more individuals in the balancing process we hope to benefit from the wider experience those involved bring to the process.

The first interrogation of data takes place before the supply and use framework is populated. It consists of an examination of the columns in the framework being reviewed for plausibility independently of each other. For example, estimates of household consumption expenditure, by product, are produced and analysed to ensure the overall picture of household spending and its breakdown by product presents a credible story in their own right. Similarly, for those components with an industry dimension, such as output, the initial stage scrutinises these data to ensure the story for industries look plausible. This first stage of confrontation is carried out by the compilers of the original data.

The second stage is a confrontation within the framework of the rows (products) in the supply and use framework. This challenges the data in each row with the aim of achieving a balance across the row to ensure that the accounting relationship that the supply of a product is equal to the demand for that product. This process identifies areas of inconsistency between the various sources which can then be investigated. Data within the row are then subsequently adjusted to achieve a balance. This adjustment process reviews

the quality of the data used to populate the individual cells within a row and makes use of this information to adjust the original data.

The third stage of the balancing process is to interrogate the columns. Unlike the confrontation within the column, carried out during the first stage this time it is carried out in the context of the supply and use framework. Whilst the second stage of balancing results in a balance of the rows it does not result in satisfying the accounting relationship for the columns. This needs to ensure that for each industry the inputs to the process of production equal its outputs. This third stage of balancing has the objective of confirming that this column identity is satisfied.

Once stage three is complete there is a strong potential that the row identities balanced during stage two of the process will have subsequently been broken. The process of repeating stages two and three continues until both the row and column identities are satisfied or a balance can not be achieved. This iterative process of row and column balancing effectively homes in on a position of balance by way of narrowing the degree of imbalance remaining in the supply and use framework after each balancing cycle. Whilst the description above may seem to indicate a fairly mechanistic balancing approach a significant amount of knowledge of the methods and quality of the basis data are used as part of the process. Alongside this the evolving balance is reviewed at each stage to see how the economic story is developing and make sure that story is credible.

Current price analysis (Tables 2.1, 2.2 and 2.3)

The analyses of gross value added and other variables by industry shown in Part 2 reflect estimates based on the Standard Industrial Classification (SIC(2003)). Tables 2.1, 2.2 and 2.3 are based on current price data reconciled through the I-O process for 1992 to 2006. The aggregate figures for the latest year, 2007, as shown in Tables 2.2 and 2.3, are based on data reconciled through the National Accounts balancing process. This process is explained in chapter 11 of *Concepts, Sources and Methods*.[5] The industry detail for the year 2007 is based on current price output estimates from a variety of sources, both within ONS and in other government departments. These estimates will be revised when the first I-O Supply and Use Tables for 2007 become available.

Estimates of total output and gross value added are valued at basic prices, the method recommended by ESA95. Thus the only taxes included in the price will be taxes paid as part of the production process (such as business rates and vehicle excise duty), and not any taxes specifically levied on the production of a unit of output (such as VAT). Any subsidies on products received will also be included in the valuation of output.

Chained volume indices (2003=100) analyses (Table 2.4)

Table 2.4 shows chained volume estimates of gross value added at basic prices by industry. The basic methodology for these estimates can be found in the Government Statistical Service methodological publications *Gross Domestic Product: Output approach*.[6,7] A more detailed explanation is in *Concepts, Sources and Methods*.[5]

The output approach provides the lead indicator of economic change in the short-term. However in the longer-term, it is required to follow the annual path indicated by the expenditure measure of real GDP (usually within 0.2 per cent of the average annual gross value added growth). To achieve this, balancing adjustments are sometimes applied to the output based gross value added estimates.

An examination of the chained volume gross value added and expenditure measures of GDP shows what are considered to be excessive differences in growth for a number of recent years.

During the five years of 1995 to 1999 the output-based estimate increased more than the expenditure measure.

The output-based estimate grew more slowly than the expenditure measure in the years of 2000 2002 and 2003[4].

In the years 2001, 2004, 2005 and 2006 output growth was greater than expenditure.

The largest the difference in growth between the output and expenditure GVA measure was 0.6 percent, which occurred over the 1998 year.

To reduce these discrepancies, a number of balancing adjustments have been made to the chained volume gross value added annual growth rates.

Assigning adjustments: improvements for the 2008 *Blue Book*

For this year's *Blue Book*, balancing adjustments have been applied on the same basis as for the 2006 *Blue Book*. For technical and other reasons, the adjustments are not at present made to the non-service industries for any years.

Apportioning between industries

Under the revisions policy in the 2005 *Blue Book*, revisions were only permitted for the predominantly 'government' components between 1996 and 2000. Consequently all adjustments to annual growth rates in these years were achieved via the following industries: public administration and defence; compulsory social security (section L), education (section M) and health and social work (section N). In some cases this restriction led to an inappropriate allocation across the components of gross value added.

The revisions policy for the 2006 *Blue Book* permits revisions to all components . The revision policy for the 2008 *Blue Book* permits revisions to all components for all years as a result of the allocation of FISIM. This has enabled a more appropriate allocation of the adjustments across industries.

Applying the adjustments

ONS has developed an automatic function for assigning the annual adjustments to gross value added. This is designed to be as faithful as possible to the quarterly paths whilst adjusting the overall annual growth rate of a group of series. The 2006 *Blue Book* is the first time that all adjustments to all industries have been assigned using this system. Details of the new adjustments are given below. Using the automatic function produces some differences in the adjustments within the groupings shown. These differences are generally no greater than 0.2 per cent.

For 1995:

A downward adjustment of 0.6 per cent has been applied to:

- distribution, hotels and restaurants; (sections G and H)

A downward adjustment of 0.7 per cent has been applied to:

- transport storage and communication (section I)

A downward adjustment of 0.7 per cent has been applied to:

- Business Services and Finance (section J and K)

A downward adjustment of 0.3 per cent has been applied to:

- government and other services (sections L to P)

The total effect of these adjustments is to reduce the 1994/1995 growth rate by 0.3 per cent.

For 1996:

A downward adjustment of 0.6 per cent has been applied to:

- distribution, hotels and restaurants; (sections G and H)

A downward adjustment of 0.9 per cent has been applied to:

- transport storage and communication (section I)

A downward adjustment of 0.6 per cent has been applied to:

- Business Services and Finance (section J and K)

A downward adjustment of 0.6 per cent has been applied to:

- government and other services (sections L to P)

The total effect of these adjustments is to reduce the 1995/1996 growth rate by 0.4 per cent.

For 1997:

A downward adjustment of 0.4 per cent has been applied to:

- distribution, hotels and restaurants; (sections G and H)

A downward adjustment of 0.6 per cent has been applied to:

- transport storage and communication (section I)

A downward adjustment of 0.5 per cent has been applied to:

- Business Services and Finance (section J and K)

A downward adjustment of 0.5 per cent has been applied to:

- government and other services (sections L to P)

The total effect of these adjustments is to reduce the 1996/1997 growth rate by 0.3 per cent.

1998:

A downward adjustment of 0.7 per cent has been applied to:

- distribution, hotels and restaurants; (sections G and H)

A downward adjustment of 0.4 per cent has been applied to:

- transport storage and communication (section I)

A downward adjustment of 0.6 per cent has been applied to:

- Business Services and Finance (section J and K)

A downward adjustment of 1.3 per cent has been applied to:

- government and other services (sections L to P)

The total effect of these adjustments is to reduce the 1997/1998 growth rate by 0.6 per cent.

1999:

A downward adjustment of 0.2 per cent has been applied to:

- distribution, hotels and restaurants; (sections G and H)

An upward adjustment of 0.1 per cent has been applied to:

- transport storage and communication (section I)

A downward adjustment of 0.3 per cent has been applied to:

- Business Services and Finance (section J and K)

A downward adjustment of 0.3 per cent has been applied to:

- government and other services (sections L to P)

The total effect of these adjustments is to reduce the 1998/1999 growth rate by 0.1 per cent.

2000:

An upward adjustment of 0.1 per cent has been applied to:

- distribution, hotels and restaurants; (sections G and H)

An upward adjustment of 0.2 per cent has been applied to:

- transport storage and communication (section I)

A downward adjustment of less than 0.1 per cent has been applied to:

- Business Services and Finance (section J and K)

A downward adjustment of less than 0.1 per cent has been applied to:

- government and other services (sections L to P)

The total effect of these adjustments is to increase the 1999/2000 growth rate by less than 0.1 per cent.

For 2001:

A downward adjustment of 0.1 per cent has been applied to:

- distribution, hotels and restaurants; (sections G and H)

An downward adjustment of 0.2 per cent has been applied to:

- transport storage and communication (section I)

An upward adjustment of less than 0.1 per cent has been applied to:

- Business Services and Finance (section J and K)

A downward adjustment of less than 0.1 per cent has been applied to:

- government and other services (sections L to P)

The total effect of these adjustments is to decrease the 2000/2001 growth rate by less than 0.1 per cent.

For 2002:

An upward adjustment of 0.4 per cent has been applied to:

- distribution, hotels and restaurants; (sections G and H)

An upward adjustment of 0.3 per cent has been applied to:

- transport storage and communication (section I)

An upward adjustment of 0.2 per cent has been applied to:

- Business Services and Finance (section J and K)

An upward adjustment of 0.3 per cent has been applied to:

- government and other services (sections L to P)

The total effect of these adjustments is to increase the 2001/2002 growth rate by 0.2 per cent.

For 2003:

A downward adjustment of 0.6 per cent has been applied to:

- distribution, hotels and restaurants; (sections G and H)

A downward adjustment of 1.0 per cent has been applied to:

- transport storage and communication (section I)

An upward adjustment of 0.3 per cent has been applied to:

■ Business Services and Finance (section J and K)

An upward adjustment of 0.5 per cent has been applied to:

■ government and other services (sections L to P)

The total effect of these adjustments is to increase the 2002/2003 growth rate by less than 0.1 per cent.

For 2004:

A downward adjustment of 0.5 per cent has been applied to:

■ distribution, hotels and restaurants; (sections G and H)

A downward adjustment of 0.4 per cent has been applied to:

■ transport storage and communication (section I)

A downward adjustment of 0.5 per cent has been applied to:

■ Business Services and Finance (section J and K)

A downward adjustment of 0.8 per cent has been applied to:

■ government and other services (sections L to P)

The total effect of these adjustments is to decrease the 2003/2004 growth rate by 0.4 per cent.

For 2005:

A downward adjustment of 0.5 per cent has been applied to:

■ distribution, hotels and restaurants; (sections G and H)

A downward adjustment of 0.5 per cent has been applied to:

■ transport storage and communication (section I)

A downward adjustment of 0.5 per cent has been applied to:

■ Business Services and Finance (section J and K)

A downward adjustment of 0.7 per cent has been applied to:

■ government and other services (sections L to P)

The total effect of these adjustments is to decrease the 2004/2005 growth rate by 0.4 per cent.

For 2006:

A downward adjustment of 0.3 per cent has been applied to:

■ distribution, hotels and restaurants; (sections G and H)

A downward adjustment of 0.3 per cent has been applied to:

■ transport storage and communication (section I)

A downward adjustment of 0.3 per cent has been applied to:

■ Business Services and Finance (section J and K)

A downward adjustment of 0.2 per cent has been applied to:

■ government and other services (sections L to P)

The total effect of these adjustments is to decrease the 2005/2006 growth rate by 0.2 per cent.

Employment analyses (Table 2.5)

Table 2.5 breaks down employment data into six broad industry groupings. Employee jobs, the main component of the employment figures, uses an industry breakdown which is consistent with most other parts of the National Accounts. This is because employee figures are obtained from surveys of businesses whose details are stored on National Statistics' Business Register. This is the same register which is used for all other business surveys collecting economic data.

The estimates of self-employment jobs come from the Labour Force Survey. This is a household survey which codes respondents according to their own view of the industry in which they work. Because of this, the industrial coding of the self employment jobs may not be consistent with the industrial codes for employees. Note that the data do not include UK armed forces or government supported trainees, which are the other components of the Workforce Jobs series.

References:

1 Office for National Statistics (2008) Supply-Use Tables 2008: www.statistics.gov.uk/about/methodology_by_theme/inputoutput/latestdata.asp

2 Akers R and Clifton-Fearnside A (2008) forthcoming.

3 Mahajan S (2006) Compilation and Use of Input-Output Supply and Use Tables in the UK National Accounts *Economic Trends* No. 634.

4 Office for National Statistics (1998) *National Accounts Concepts, Sources and Methods*, 1998 edition. The Stationery Office: London.

5 Humphries S (2006) Revisions planned for the 2006 annual Blue Book, Pink Book and Input-Output analyses. *Economic Trends* No. 629, pp 20–23: www.statistics.gov.uk/cci/article.asp?ID=1476

6 Government Statistical Service (1998) *Gross Domestic Product: Output methodological guide.*

7 Government Statistical Service (1998) *Gross Domestic Product: Output approach (Gross Valued Added).* GSS Methodology Series No 15.

8 Office for National Statistics (2000) Review of Short-Term Output Indicators: National Statistics. *Quality Review Series Report* No. 1.

2.1 Supply and Use Tables for the United Kingdom, 2004

Supply Table

£ million

2004	Domestic output of products at basic prices	SUPPLY OF PRODUCTS				
		Imports		Distributors' trading margins	Taxes *less* subsidies on products	Total supply of products at purchasers' prices
		Goods	Services			
PRODUCTS[1]						
Agriculture, forestry & fishing [1-3]	21 216	6 142	375	3 858	-2 186	29 405
Mining & quarrying [4-7]	32 418	14 517	483	1 660	504	49 582
Manufacturing [8-84]	378 195	228 154	14 862	211 845	78 793	911 849
Electricity, gas & water supply [85-87]	49 093	327	55	-	1 993	51 468
Construction [88]	170 705	-	203	-	11 980	182 888
Distribution & hotels [89-92]	322 862	-	13 564	-217 363	14 063	133 126
Transport & communication [93-99]	167 696	-	18 557	-	2 783	189 036
Finance & business services [100-114]	562 881	228	29 567	-	15 506	608 182
Public administration & defence [115]	115 066	-	32	-	-	115 098
Education, health & social work [116-118]	225 688	-	1 943	-	2 148	229 779
Other services [119-123]	92 483	2 406	4 731	-	6 437	106 057
Total	2 138 303	251 774	84 372	-	132 021	2 606 470
of which:						
Market output	1 766 597					
Output for own final use	91 189					
Other non-market output	280 517					

Use Table at Purchasers' prices

2004	INTERMEDIATE CONSUMPTION BY INDUSTRY GROUP[1 2]										
	1	2	3	4	5	6	7	8	9	10	11
	Agriculture	Mining & quarrying	Manufac-turing	Electricity, gas & water supply	Construc-tion	Distribution & hotels	Transport & communi-cation	Finance & business services	Public adminis-tration & defence	Education, health & social work	Other services
PRODUCTS[1]											
Agriculture, forestry & fishing [1-3]	2 131	1	9 859	5	215	1 680	42	12	8	211	29
Mining & quarrying [4-7]	6	3 332	16 027	11 736	2 612	151	105	8	6	7	21
Manufacturing [8-84]	5 948	2 188	179 511	3 559	26 910	43 664	20 582	12 239	21 056	27 295	6 500
Electricity, gas & water supply [85-87]	428	500	8 528	14 949	276	2 146	927	1 608	1 162	1 706	603
Construction [88]	243	851	1 127	752	50 423	1 945	1 923	12 154	4 631	1 206	867
Distribution & hotels [89-92]	684	123	1 119	170	1 558	6 938	3 155	5 513	1 631	1 983	682
Transport & communication [93-99]	424	1 267	13 940	496	1 202	31 835	35 071	25 684	4 757	5 896	2 664
Finance & business services [100-114]	2 082	2 891	31 091	3 273	20 760	53 442	25 907	137 995	18 620	18 887	17 427
Public administration & defence [115]	12	20	517	35	338	214	1 323	5 351	266	75	66
Education, health & social work [116-118]	187	32	1 097	154	170	916	1 171	4 847	4 272	29 420	907
Other services [119-123]	228	90	3 027	184	161	1 848	1 754	3 554	3 264	3 427	15 024
Total consumption	12 373	11 295	265 843	35 313	104 625	144 779	91 960	208 965	59 673	90 113	44 790
Taxes *less* subsidies on production	-446	187	2 451	1 275	651	7 655	1 087	2 737	-	152	950
Compensation of employees	3 454	3 105	104 260	4 873	31 147	99 529	53 793	146 628	47 599	119 073	34 638
Gross operating surplus	7 592	19 268	40 550	10 524	32 157	51 517	24 948	172 725	7 794	17 006	19 695
Gross value added at basic prices	10 600	22 560	147 261	16 672	63 955	158 701	79 828	322 090	55 393	136 231	55 283
Output at basic prices	22 973	33 855	413 104	51 985	168 580	303 480	171 788	531 055	115 066	226 344	100 073

2.1 Supply and Use Tables for the United Kingdom, 2004

continued

Gross value added at basic prices

£ billion

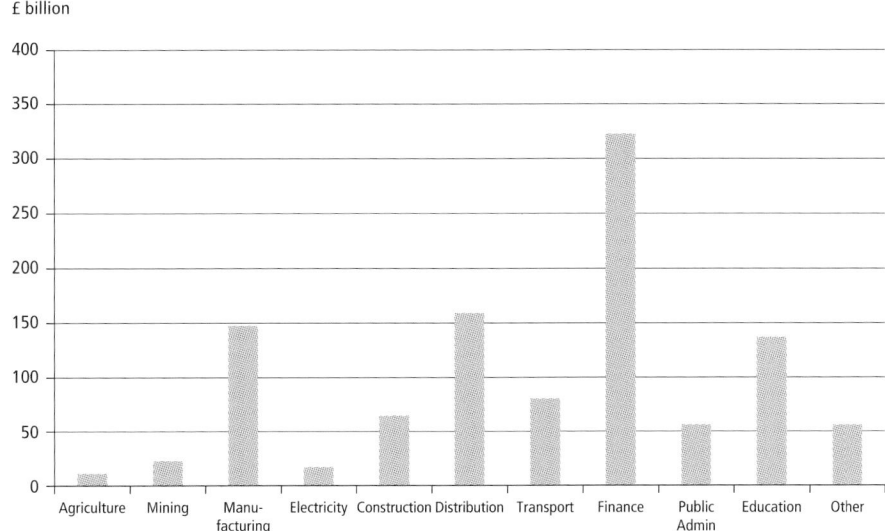

Components of final demand

Per cent

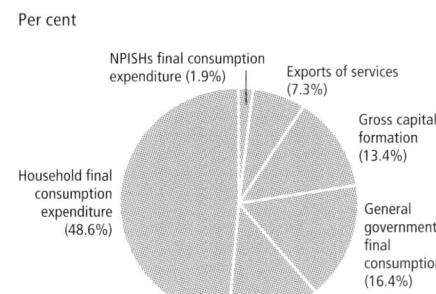

NPISHs final consumption expenditure (1.9%)

Exports of services (7.3%)

Gross capital formation (13.4%)

Household final consumption expenditure (48.6%)

General government final consumption (16.4%)

Exports of goods (12.4%)

£ million

2004	Total intermediate consumption	FINAL CONSUMPTION EXPENDITURE			GROSS CAPITAL FORMATION			EXPORTS		TOTAL
		Households	NPISHs	GGFC	GFCF	Valuables	Changes in inventories	Goods	Services	
PRODUCTS¹										
Agriculture, forestry & fishing [1-3]	14 193	12 300	-	-	757	-	486	1 559	110	29 405
Mining & quarrying [4-7]	34 011	326	-	-	387	-	11	14 658	189	49 582
Manufacturing [8-84]	349 452	322 214	-	-	61 691	- 402	2 428	171 204	5 262	911 849
Electricity, gas & water supply [85-87]	32 833	18 413	-	-	-	-	4	155	63	51 468
Construction [88]	76 122	6 126	-	-	99 062	-	1 265	-	313	182 888
Distribution & hotels [89-92]	23 556	101 294	-	-	-	365	- 16	-	7 927	133 126
Transport & communication [93-99]	123 236	45 032	-	-	1 128	-	3	-	19 637	189 036
Finance & business services [100-114]	332 375	167 583	1 009	-	33 562	-	433	354	72 866	608 182
Public administration & defence [115]	8 217	3 076	-	100 993	1 768	-	-	-	1 044	115 098
Education, health & social work [116-118]	43 173	24 570	21 597	138 603	-	-	21	-	1 815	229 779
Other services [119-123]	32 561	46 568	6 142	2 173	2 317	-	60	2 944	3 292	106 057
Total consumption	1 069 729	747 502	28 748	251 769	200 769	-37	4 695	190 874	112 518	2 606 470
Taxes *less* subsidies on production	16 699									
Compensation of employees	648 099									
Gross operating surplus	403 776									
Gross value added at basic prices	1 068 574									
Output at basic prices	2 138 303									

Notes for information

(1) Some of the industry/product group headings have been truncated.
(2) Purchases of products by industry and by final consumption categories are valued at purchasers' prices.

NPISHs represents Non-Profit Institutions Serving Households.
GGFC represents General Government Final Consumption.
GFCF represents Gross Fixed Capital Formation.

Gross value added at basic prices *plus* taxes *less* subsidies on products gives GDP at market prices.
Gross operating surplus includes gross mixed income.
Changes in inventories includes materials and fuels, work-in-progress and finished goods.
Valuables include both 'transfer costs' and 'acquisitions *less* disposals'.

2.1 Supply and Use Tables for the United Kingdom, 2005

Supply Table

£ million

2005	Domestic output of products at basic prices	SUPPLY OF PRODUCTS		Distributors' trading margins	Taxes *less* subsidies on products	Total supply of products at purchasers' prices
		Imports				
		Goods	Services			
PRODUCTS[1]						
Agriculture, forestry & fishing [1-3]	18 349	6 748	407	3 845	653	30 002
Mining & quarrying [4-7]	39 197	19 883	480	1 680	510	61 750
Manufacturing [8-84]	393 201	250 258	15 558	216 942	80 286	956 245
Electricity, gas & water supply [85-87]	59 149	421	54	-	2 079	61 703
Construction [88]	178 514	-	636	-	12 168	191 318
Distribution & hotels [89-92]	333 574	-	13 986	-222 467	14 384	139 477
Transport & communication [93-99]	177 848	-	20 453	-	2 777	201 078
Finance & business services [100-114]	592 278	326	35 033	-	15 790	643 427
Public administration & defence [115]	123 193	-	44	-	-	123 237
Education, health & social work [116-118]	243 083	-	2 001	-	2 183	247 267
Other services [119-123]	98 965	2 561	4 893	-	6 554	112 973
Total	2 257 351	280 197	93 545	-	137 384	2 768 477
of which:						
Market output	1 861 050					
Output for own final use	97 261					
Other non-market output	299 040					

Use Table at Purchasers' prices

2005	INTERMEDIATE CONSUMPTION BY INDUSTRY GROUP[1][2]										
	1 Agriculture	2 Mining & quarrying	3 Manufac-turing	4 Electricity, gas & water supply	5 Construc-tion	6 Distribution & hotels	7 Transport & communi-cation	8 Finance & business services	9 Public adminis-tration & defence	10 Education, health & social work	11 Other services
PRODUCTS[1]											
Agriculture, forestry & fishing [1-3]	2 315	1	10 226	6	230	1 677	42	12	-	221	32
Mining & quarrying [4-7]	6	4 301	19 940	16 214	2 996	158	121	10	-	6	24
Manufacturing [8-84]	5 947	2 461	187 493	3 756	27 718	45 384	22 926	12 447	21 866	29 617	6 920
Electricity, gas & water supply [85-87]	457	771	9 675	19 865	326	2 514	1 116	1 800	1 228	2 140	717
Construction [88]	243	748	1 094	792	50 979	1 583	1 816	12 303	4 811	998	841
Distribution & hotels [89-92]	684	127	1 155	173	1 813	7 826	3 502	6 045	1 762	2 167	760
Transport & communication [93-99]	422	1 345	14 175	583	1 233	32 921	39 543	27 724	4 997	5 745	2 792
Finance & business services [100-114]	2 127	3 230	31 609	3 944	21 945	55 379	27 368	145 396	20 039	21 974	18 023
Public administration & defence [115]	12	22	550	38	383	247	1 859	6 777	266	90	77
Education, health & social work [116-118]	186	36	1 135	203	168	909	1 241	5 156	4 627	32 429	942
Other services [119-123]	221	110	3 015	216	169	1 953	1 868	3 842	3 501	3 696	15 868
Total consumption	12 620	13 152	280 067	45 790	107 960	150 551	101 402	221 512	63 097	99 083	46 996
Taxes *less* subsidies on production	-3 252	241	2 384	1 248	624	8 386	1 165	1 917	-	180	956
Compensation of employees	3 653	3 330	106 616	5 049	33 409	102 301	54 942	156 326	51 799	125 913	38 867
Gross operating surplus	7 021	24 098	39 591	10 370	33 986	52 234	24 403	180 448	8 297	18 590	20 029
Gross value added at basic prices	7 422	27 669	148 591	16 667	68 019	162 921	80 510	338 691	60 096	144 683	59 852
Output at basic prices	20 042	40 821	428 658	62 457	175 979	313 472	181 912	560 203	123 193	243 766	106 848

2.1 Supply and Use Tables for the United Kingdom, 2005

continued

Gross value added at basic prices

£ billion

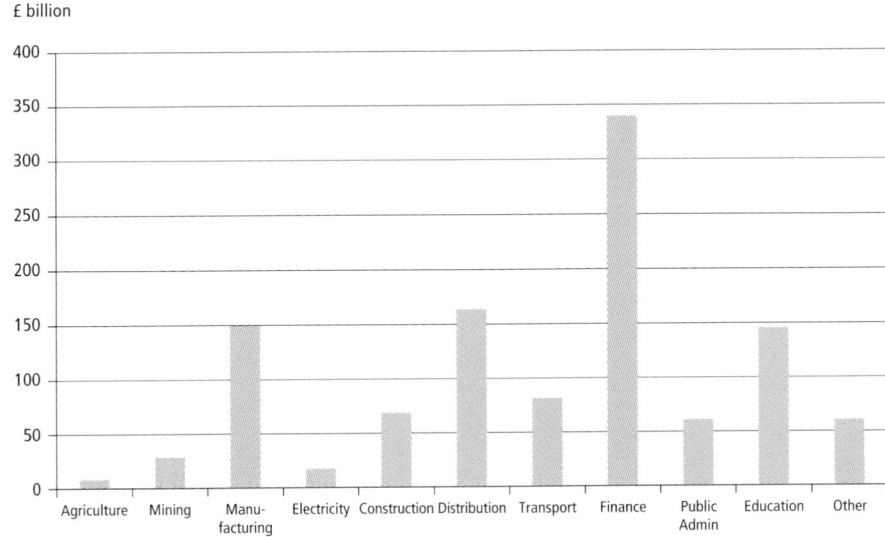

Components of final demand

Per cent

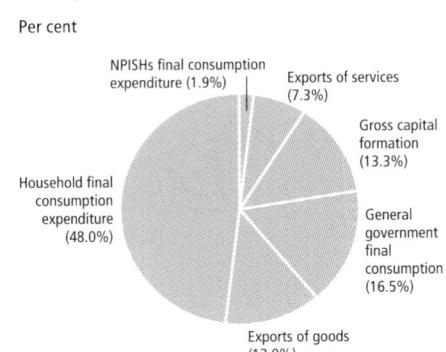

£ million

2005	Total intermediate consumption	FINAL CONSUMPTION EXPENDITURE			GROSS CAPITAL FORMATION			EXPORTS		TOTAL
		Households	NPISHs	GGFC	GFCF	Valuables	Changes in inventories	Goods	Services	

PRODUCTS[1]

Agriculture, forestry & fishing [1-3]	14 762	13 004	-	-	780	-	- 266	1 600	122	30 002
Mining & quarrying [4-7]	43 776	360	-	-	391	-	340	16 722	161	61 750
Manufacturing [8-84]	366 535	330 042	-	-	62 680	- 762	3 082	188 994	5 674	956 245
Electricity, gas & water supply [85-87]	40 609	20 926	-	-	-	-	- 4	102	70	61 703
Construction [88]	76 208	6 306	-	-	107 082	-	1 082	-	640	191 318
Distribution & hotels [89-92]	26 014	104 142	-	-	-	385	-	-	8 936	139 477
Transport & communication [93-99]	131 480	47 107	-	-	1 213	-	1	-	21 277	201 078
Finance & business services [100-114]	351 034	179 010	1 199	-	34 670	-	853	613	76 048	643 427
Public administration & defence [115]	10 321	3 626	-	106 191	2 036	-	-	-	1 063	123 237
Education, health & social work [116-118]	47 032	26 133	22 614	149 527	-	-	1	-	1 960	247 267
Other services [119-123]	34 459	49 609	6 589	12 920	2 466	-	-116	3 577	3 469	112 973

Total consumption	1 142 230	747 502	28 748	251 769	200 769	-37	4 695	190 874	112 518	2 606 470

Taxes *less* subsidies on production	13 849
Compensation of employees	682 205
Gross operating surplus	419 067
Gross value added at basic prices	1 115 121
Output at basic prices	2 257 351

Notes for information

(1) Some of the industry/product group headings have been truncated.
(2) Purchases of products by industry and by final consumption categories are valued at purchasers' prices.

NPISHs represents Non-Profit Institutions Serving Households.
GGFC represents General Government Final Consumption.
GFCF represents Gross Fixed Capital Formation.

Gross value added at basic prices *plus* taxes *less* subsidies on products gives GDP at market prices.
Gross operating surplus includes gross mixed income.
Changes in inventories includes materials and fuels, work-in-progress and finished goods.
Valuables include both 'transfer costs' and 'acquisitions *less* disposals'.

2.1 Supply and Use Tables for the United Kingdom, 2006

Supply Table

£ million

2006	Domestic output of products at basic prices	Imports		Distributors' trading margins	Taxes *less* subsidies on products	Total supply of products at purchasers' prices
		Goods	Services			
		SUPPLY OF PRODUCTS				

PRODUCTS[1]

Agriculture, forestry & fishing [1-3]	19 172	7 173	421	3 909	632	31 307
Mining & quarrying [4-7]	45 351	24 218	543	1 760	545	72 417
Manufacturing [8-84]	412 610	284 924	16 168	224 165	84 881	1 022 748
Electricity, gas & water supply [85-87]	69 567	399	63	-	2 148	72 177
Construction [88]	189 007	-	692	-	12 948	202 647
Distribution & hotels [89-92]	345 519	-	14 425	-229 834	15 134	145 244
Transport & communication [93-99]	183 218	-	20 534	-	2 399	206 151
Finance & business services [100-114]	628 641	298	39 799	-	16 682	685 420
Public administration & defence [115]	129 377	-	61	-	-	129 438
Education, health & social work [116-118]	259 119	-	1 979	-	2 318	263 416
Other services [119-123]	103 246	2 935	4 956	-	6 941	118 078
Total	2 384 827	319 947	99 641	-	144 628	2 949 043

of which:

Market output	1 963 066
Output for own final use	103 883
Other non-market output	317 878

Use Table at Purchasers' prices

2006	INTERMEDIATE CONSUMPTION BY INDUSTRY GROUP[1][2]										
	1	2	3	4	5	6	7	8	9	10	11
	Agriculture	Mining & quarrying	Manufac- turing	Electricity, gas & water supply	Construc- tion	Distribution & hotels	Transport & communi- cation	Finance & business services	Public adminis- tration & defence	Education, health & social work	Other services

PRODUCTS[1]

Agriculture, forestry & fishing [1-3]	2 495	1	10 520	6	240	1 678	42	12	2	223	34
Mining & quarrying [4-7]	10	5 172	23 743	19 802	3 271	169	124	12	-	9	28
Manufacturing [8-84]	6 206	2 530	196 391	4 068	29 694	46 955	25 508	13 661	23 472	32 899	7 635
Electricity, gas & water supply [85-87]	423	779	9 928	24 061	344	2 675	1 151	1 906	1 321	2 453	838
Construction [88]	243	872	1 128	839	51 437	1 451	1 880	12 433	4 954	1 076	869
Distribution & hotels [89-92]	693	146	1 201	193	2 172	8 781	4 097	6 713	1 826	2 589	890
Transport & communication [93-99]	440	1 431	14 733	611	1 273	33 905	40 256	5 173	5 967	2 885
Finance & business services [100-114]	2 145	3 504	32 454	4 213	23 087	57 006	28 224	150 358	21 096	24 046	19 215
Public administration & defence [115]	12	25	540	41	439	283	2 019	7 037	292	109	94
Education, health & social work [116-118]	188	40	1 160	218	166	894	1 257	5 490	4 825	35 038	979
Other services [119-123]	233	117	3 194	233	183	2 048	2 012	4 114	3 383	4 089	16 607
Total consumption	13 088	14 617	294 992	54 285	112 306	155 845	106 570	230 976	66 344	108 498	50 074
Taxes *less* subsidies on production	-3088	284	2 464	1 256	678	8 747	1 058	1 893	-	201	1 025
Compensation of employees	3 551	3 122	108 830	6 142	36 031	105 609	57 303	168 893	54 246	131 680	40 089
Gross operating surplus	7 402	28 796	41 861	11 472	37 284	55 480	22 666	193 869	8 787	19 347	20 254
Gross value added at basic prices	7 865	32 202	153 155	18 870	73 993	169 836	81 027	364 655	63 033	151 228	61 368
Output at basic prices	20 953	46 819	448 147	73 155	186 299	325 681	187 597	595 631	129 377	259 726	111 442

2.1 Supply and Use Tables for the United Kingdom, 2006

continued

Gross value added at basic prices

£ billion

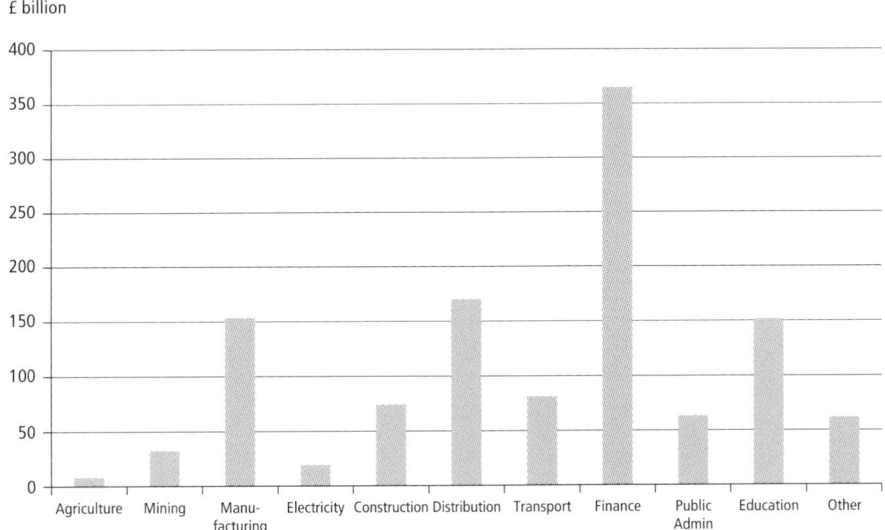

Components of final demand

Per cent

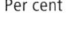
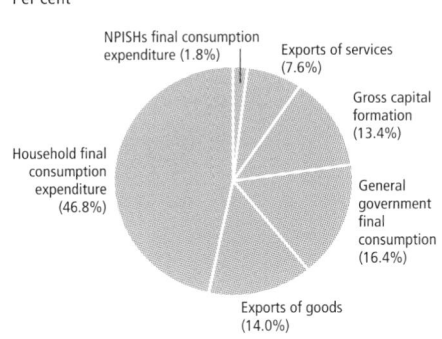

£ million

2006	Total intermediate consumption	FINAL CONSUMPTION EXPENDITURE			GROSS CAPITAL FORMATION			EXPORTS		TOTAL
		Households	NPISHs	GGFC	GFCF	Valuables	Changes in inventories	Goods	Services	
PRODUCTS[1]										
Agriculture, forestry & fishing [1-3]	15 253	13 629	-	-	890	-	- 251	1 650	136	31 307
Mining & quarrying [4-7]	52 340	398	-	-	504	-	102	18 895	178	72 417
Manufacturing [8-84]	389 019	340 277	-	-	64 540	- 110	3 649	219 198	6 175	1 022 748
Electricity, gas & water supply [85-87]	45 879	26 086	-	-	-	-	32	104	76	72 177
Construction [88]	77 182	7 022	-	-	117 398	-	214	-	831	202 647
Distribution & hotels [89-92]	29 301	106 235	-	-	-	395	- 23	-	9 336	145 244
Transport & communication [93-99]	135 914	49 194	-	-	1 241	-	-	-	19 802	206 151
Finance & business services [100-114]	365 348	189 552	1 267	-	38 727	-	699	452	89 375	685 420
Public administration & defence [115]	10 891	3 729	-	111 716	2 012	-	-	-	1 090	129 438
Education, health & social work [116-118]	50 255	27 034	23 765	160 302	-	-	24	-	2 036	263 416
Other services [119-123]	36 213	51 503	7 177	13 651	2 608	-	-124	3 336	3 714	118 078
Total consumption	1 207 595	814 659	32 209	285 669	227 920	285	4 322	243 635	132 749	2 949 043
Taxes *less* subsidies on production	14 518									
Compensation of employees	715 496									
Gross operating surplus	447 218									
Gross value added at basic prices	1 177 232									
Output at basic prices	2 384 827									

Notes for information

(1) Some of the industry/product group headings have been truncated.
(2) Purchases of products by industry and by final consumption categories are valued at purchasers' prices.

NPISHs represents Non-Profit Institutions Serving Households.
GGFC represents General Government Final Consumption.
GFCF represents Gross Fixed Capital Formation.

Gross value added at basic prices *plus* taxes *less* subsidies on products gives GDP at market prices.
Gross operating surplus includes gross mixed income.
Changes in inventories includes materials and fuels, work-in-progress and finished goods.
Valuables include both 'transfer costs' and 'acquisitions *less* disposals'.

2.2 Output and capital formation: by industry[1,2]
Gross value added at current basic prices

£ million

			1999	2000	2001	2002	2003	2004	2005	2006
	Agriculture, hunting, forestry and fishing									
P.1	Output									
D.1	Compensation of employees	CFHE	3 249	3 243	3 245	3 225	3 286	3 454	3 653	3 551
D.29-D.39	Taxes *less* subsidies on production other than those on products	EWTZ	−155	−169	−429	−348	−397	−446	−3 252	−3 088
B.2g/B.3g	Operating surplus/Mixed income, gross	ESMU	5 928	5 458	5 517	6 130	6 917	7 592	7 021	7 402
B.1g	Gross value added at basic prices	QTOP	9 022	8 532	8 333	9 007	9 806	10 600	7 422	7 865
P.2	Intermediate consumption at purchasers' prices	EWSI	12 349	11 955	11 335	11 374	11 782	12 373	12 620	13 088
P.1	Total output at basic prices	EWSJ	21 371	20 487	19 668	20 381	21 588	22 973	20 042	20 953
P.5	Gross capital formation	EWSK	1 960	1 874	2 083	2 675	2 879	2 664	2 751	3 001
	Mining and quarrying									
P.1	Output									
D.1	Compensation of employees	CFHF	2 808	3 003	2 945	2 856	2 834	3 105	3 330	3 122
D.29-D.39	Taxes *less* subsidies on production other than those on products	EWUA	161	171	222	143	123	187	241	284
B.2g/B.3g	Operating surplus/Mixed income, gross	ESMQ	13 976	21 391	19 953	18 919	18 485	19 268	24 098	28 796
B.1g	Gross value added at basic prices	QTOT	16 945	24 565	23 120	21 918	21 442	22 560	27 669	32 202
P.2	Intermediate consumption at purchasers' prices	EWSM	9 199	10 096	10 340	9 749	10 219	11 295	13 152	14 617
P.1	Total output at basic prices	EWSN	26 144	34 661	33 460	31 667	31 661	33 855	40 821	46 819
P.5	Gross capital formation	EWSO	4 830	3 384	4 568	5 201	4 621	4 344	4 241	4 735
	Manufacturing[3]									
P.1	Output									
D.1	Compensation of employees	CFHG	102 707	104 735	104 381	104 091	103 802	104 260	106 616	108 830
D.29-D.39	Taxes *less* subsidies on production other than those on products	EWUB	2 578	2 573	2 642	2 690	2 588	2 451	2 384	2 464
B.2g/B.g	Operating surplus/Mixed income, gross	ESMT	45 872	42 701	42 200	39 527	38 455	40 550	39 591	41 861
B.1g	Gross value added at basic prices	QTPI	151 157	150 009	149 223	146 308	144 845	147 261	148 591	153 155
P.2	Intermediate consumption at purchasers' prices	EWSQ	254 175	264 591	262 690	259 319	259 646	265 843	280 067	294 992
P.1	Total output at basic prices	EWSR	405 332	414 600	411 913	405 627	404 491	413 104	428 658	448 147
P.5	Gross capital formation	EWSS	19 596	20 735	17 805	14 084	13 726	13 604	15 839	15 756

1 The contribution of each industry to the gross domestic product before providing for consumption of fixed capital. The industrial composition in this table is consistent with the Input-Output Supply and Use Tables in Table 2.1, which show data from 2004-2006
2 Components may not sum to totals due to rounding.
3 Further detail is given in Table 2.3.

2.2 Output and capital formation: by industry[1,2]
Gross value added at current basic prices

continued

£ million

			1999	2000	2001	2002	2003	2004	2005	2006
	Electricity, gas and water supply									
P.1	Output									
D.1	Compensation of employees	CFHI	4 742	4 522	4 497	4 606	4 762	4 873	5 049	6 142
D.29-D.39	Taxes *less* subsidies on production other than those on products	EWUC	1 257	1 289	1 277	1 214	1 233	1 275	1 248	1 256
B.2g/B.3g	Operating surplus/Mixed income, gross	ESMV	9 704	9 987	9 886	10 232	10 410	10 524	10 370	11 472
B.1g	Gross value added at basic prices	QTPJ	15 703	15 798	15 660	16 052	16 405	16 672	16 667	18 870
P.2	Intermediate consumption at purchasers' prices	EWSU	30 814	33 420	32 872	31 940	32 676	35 313	45 790	54 285
P.1	Total output at basic prices	EWSV	46 517	49 218	48 532	47 992	49 081	51 985	62 457	73 155
P.5	Gross capital formation	EWSW	5 955	5 855	5 943	5 204	5 288	3 067	4 834	5 930
	Construction									
P.1	Output									
D.1	Compensation of employees	CFHU	21 445	24 196	25 714	27 472	29 302	31 147	33 409	36 031
D.29-D.39	Taxes *less* subsidies on production other than those on products	EWUD	611	638	512	533	565	651	624	678
B.2g/B.3g	Operating surplus/Mixed income, gross	ESMW	20 180	20 792	24 300	26 679	29 655	32 157	33 986	37 284
B.1g	Gross value added at basic prices	QTPL	42 236	45 626	50 526	54 684	59 522	63 955	68 019	73 993
P.2	Intermediate consumption at purchasers' prices	EWSY	74 456	77 454	82 918	90 607	98 422	104 625	107 960	112 306
P.1	Total output at basic prices	EWSZ	116 692	123 080	133 444	145 291	157 944	168 580	175 979	186 299
P.5	Gross capital formation	EWTA	2 896	1 556	3 803	3 783	4 234	3 960	4 507	2 342
	Distribution, hotels and catering									
P.1	Output									
D.1	Compensation of employees	CFIK	76 079	82 205	88 158	91 802	96 364	99 529	102 301	105 609
D.29-D.39	Taxes *less* subsidies on production other than those on products	EWUE	6 125	6 712	7 250	7 330	7 515	7 655	8 386	8 747
B.2g/B.3g	Operating surplus/Mixed income, gross	ESMX	41 451	40 097	41 769	43 284	46 761	51 517	52 234	55 480
B.1g	Gross value added at basic prices	EWTB	123 655	129 014	137 177	142 416	150 640	158 701	162 921	169 836
P.2	Intermediate consumption at purchasers' prices	EWTC	120 360	126 268	133 316	137 498	143 798	144 779	150 551	155 845
P.1	Total output at basic prices	EWTD	244 015	255 282	270 493	279 914	294 438	303 480	313 472	325 681
P.5	Gross capital formation	EWTE	20 622	20 399	20 542	20 628	19 449	26 863	24 292	26 391

See footnotes on first page of this table.

2.2 Output and capital formation: by industry[1,2]
Gross value added at current basic prices

continued

£ million

			1999	2000	2001	2002	2003	2004	2005	2006
	Transport, storage and communication									
P.1	Output									
D.1	Compensation of employees	CFIM	42 591	45 160	48 434	50 638	51 796	53 793	54 942	57 303
D.29-D.39	Taxes less subsidies on production other than those on products	EWUF	1 365	1 396	1 195	1 495	1 341	1 087	1 165	1 058
B.2g/B.3g	Operating surplus/Mixed income, gross	ESMY	21 005	22 645	20 873	20 931	23 450	24 948	24 403	22 666
B.1g	Gross value added at basic prices	QTPQ	64 961	69 201	70 502	73 064	76 587	79 828	80 510	81 027
P.2	Intermediate consumption at purchasers' prices	EWTG	70 398	75 822	79 429	81 370	87 198	91 960	101 402	106 570
P.1	Total output at basic prices	EWTH	135 359	145 023	149 931	154 434	163 785	171 788	181 912	187 597
P.5	Gross capital formation	EWTI	22 395	26 581	26 016	24 937	23 633	25 901	22 532	24 938
	Business services and finance									
P.1	Output									
D.1	Compensation of employees	CFIP	100 042	112 699	123 101	127 913	136 240	146 628	156 326	168 893
D.29-D.39	Taxes less subsidies on production other than those on products	EWUG	2 692	2 585	2 690	2 495	2 411	2 737	1 917	1 893
B.2g/B.3g	Operating surplus/Mixed income, gross	ESMZ	119 139	118 065	126 451	147 807	165 083	172 725	180 448	193 869
B.1g	Gross value added at basic prices	EWTJ	221 873	233 349	252 242	278 215	303 734	322 090	338 691	364 655
P.2	Intermediate consumption at purchasers' prices	EWTK	162 997	176 902	194 053	198 288	205 417	208 965	221 512	230 976
P.1	Total output at basic prices	EWTL	384 870	410 251	446 295	476 503	509 151	531 055	560 203	595 631
P.5	Gross capital formation	EWTM	31 186	31 763	32 908	32 958	34 249	22 953	30 201	30 728
	Public administration and defence									
P.1	Output									
D.1	Compensation of employees	CFIV	34 635	36 327	38 450	40 608	44 035	47 599	51 799	54 246
D.29-D.39	Taxes less subsidies on production other than those on products	EWUH	–	–	–	–	–	–	–	–
B.2g	Operating surplus, gross	EWUW	6 274	6 385	6 575	6 920	7 267	7 794	8 297	8 787
B.1g	Gross value added at basic prices	QTPV	40 909	42 712	45 025	47 528	51 302	55 393	60 096	63 033
P.2	Intermediate consumption at purchasers' prices	EWTO	35 938	40 953	43 236	48 394	52 942	59 673	63 097	66 344
P.1	Total output at basic prices	EWTP	76 847	83 665	88 261	95 922	104 244	115 066	123 193	129 377
P.5	Gross capital formation	EWTQ	6 448	6 071	6 987	8 490	11 141	13 269	12 070	12 014

See footnotes on first page of this table.

2.2 Output and capital formation: by industry[1,2]
Gross value added at current basic prices

continued   £ million

			1999	2000	2001	2002	2003	2004	2005	2006
	Education, health and social work									
P.1	Output									
D.1	Compensation of employees	CFIW	83 574	89 797	96 724	103 787	112 124	119 073	125 913	131 680
D.29-D.39	Taxes *less* subsidies on production other than those on products	EWUI	144	162	130	190	152	152	180	201
B.2g/B.3g	Operating surplus/Mixed income, gross	EWSF	12 773	13 434	14 370	15 614	16 645	17 006	18 590	19 347
B.1g	Gross value added at basic prices	EWTR	96 491	103 393	111 224	119 591	128 921	136 231	144 683	151 228
P.2	Intermediate consumption at purchasers' prices	EWTS	57 491	61 007	66 240	73 261	80 745	90 113	99 083	108 498
P.1	Total output at basic prices	EWTT	153 982	164 400	177 464	192 852	209 666	226 344	243 766	259 726
P.5	Gross capital formation	EWTU	7 026	6 891	8 119	8 630	9 447	10 667	11 961	13 294
	Other services									
P.1	Output									
D.1	Compensation of employees	CFIX	23 921	26 292	28 545	30 398	32 348	34 638	38 867	40 089
D.29-D.39	Taxes *less* subsidies on production other than those on products	EWUJ	724	817	832	898	960	950	956	1 025
B.2g/B.3g	Operating surplus/Mixed income, gross	EWSG	15 177	14 977	15 184	17 016	18 496	19 695	20 029	20 254
B.1g	Gross value added at basic prices	QTPY	39 822	42 086	44 561	48 312	51 804	55 283	59 852	61 368
P.2	Intermediate consumption at purchasers' prices	EWTW	32 837	34 607	36 988	40 640	42 322	44 790	46 996	50 074
P.1	Total output at basic prices	EWTX	72 659	76 693	81 549	88 952	94 126	100 073	106 848	111 442
P.5	Gross capital formation	EWTY	11 364	10 737	9 244	9 735	11 000	16 324	18 648	18 216
	Not allocated to industries									
P.5	Gross capital formation[4]	EWUV	33 733	36 600	40 348	47 350	50 979	61 714	64 038	75 182
	All industries									
P.1	Output									
D.1	Compensation of employees	HAEA	495 793	532 179	564 194	587 396	616 893	648 099	682 205	715 496
D.29-D.39	Taxes *less* subsidies on production other than those on products	QZPC	15 502	16 174	16 321	16 640	16 491	16 699	13 849	14 518
B.2g	Operating surplus, gross	ABNF	256 537	259 001	265 797	288 091	313 300	330 960	344 209	368 310
B.3g	Mixed income, gross	QWLT	54 942	56 931	61 282	64 967	68 324	72 816	74 858	78 908
di	Statistical discrepancy between income and GDP	RVFC	–	–	–	–	–	–	–	–
B.1g	Gross value added at basic prices	ABML	822 774	864 285	907 594	957 094	1 015 008	1 068 574	1 115 121	1 177 232
P.2	Intermediate consumption at purchasers' prices	NQAJ	861 014	913 075	953 417	982 440	1 025 167	1 069 729	1 142 230	1 207 595
P.1	Total output at basic prices	NQAF	1 683 788	1 777 360	1 861 011	1 939 534	2 040 175	2 138 303	2 257 351	2 384 827
P.5	Gross capital formation									
P.51	Gross fixed capital formation	NPQX	161 722	167 172	171 782	180 551	186 700	200 672	211 318	227 920
P.52	Changes in inventories	ABMP	6 060	5 271	6 189	2 909	3 983	4 695	4 973	4 322
P.53	Acquisitions less disposals of valuables	NPJO	229	3	396	214	–37	–37	–377	285
P.5	Total gross capital formation	NQFM	168 011	172 446	178 367	183 674	190 646	205 330	215 914	232 527

See footnotes on first page of this table.

4 Includes investment in dwellings, transfer costs of land and existing buildings, and valuables.

2.3 Gross value added at current basic prices: by industry[1,2]

£ million

			1999	2000	2001	2002	2003	2004	2005	2006	2007
A,B	**Agriculture, hunting, forestry and fishing**	**QTOP**	9 022	8 532	8 333	9 007	9 806	10 600	7 422	7 865	8 910
C,D,E	**Production**										
C	Mining and quarrying										
CA	Mining and quarrying of energy producing materials										
C10	Mining of coal	QTOQ	639	607	545	538	472	398	323	314	309
C11	Extraction of mineral oil and natural gas	QTOR	14 606	22 174	20 825	19 911	19 451	20 321	25 265	29 776	29 831
CB	Other mining and quarrying	QTOS	1 700	1 784	1 750	1 469	1 519	1 841	2 081	2 112	2 291
C	Total mining and quarrying	QTOT	16 945	24 565	23 120	21 918	21 442	22 560	27 669	32 202	32 431
D	Manufacturing										
DA	Food; beverages and tobacco	QTOU	19 953	19 963	20 655	20 834	21 408	21 979	21 826	22 143	22 996
DB	Textiles and textile products	QTOV	6 220	5 813	5 343	4 818	4 282	4 240	3 977	3 944	3 887
DC	Leather and leather products	QTOW	803	747	645	590	462	474	424	418	429
DD	Wood and wood products	QTOX	2 204	2 294	2 332	2 479	2 655	2 790	3 052	3 200	3 603
DE	Pulp, paper and paper products; publishing and printing	QTOY	19 558	20 187	20 129	20 008	19 780	19 378	19 315	19 246	19 530
DF	Coke, petroleum products and nuclear fuel	QTOZ	2 533	2 336	2 488	2 435	2 377	2 439	2 529	2 506	2 636
DG	Chemicals, chemical products and man-made fibres	QTPA	15 165	15 040	16 077	16 083	16 149	17 321	17 246	18 847	18 874
DH	Rubber and plastic products	QTPB	7 708	7 609	7 656	7 569	7 516	7 380	7 563	7 928	7 929
DI	Other non-metal mineral products	QTPC	4 908	4 965	5 033	5 296	5 417	5 528	5 193	5 469	5 718
DJ	Basic metals and fabricated metal products	QTPD	16 580	15 903	15 525	14 897	14 774	15 678	16 402	16 400	17 312
DK	Machinery and equipment not elsewhere classified	QTPE	12 726	12 346	12 256	12 085	12 146	12 381	12 525	13 901	14 876
DL	Electrical and optical equipment	QTPF	20 331	20 337	18 347	16 468	15 545	15 661	16 117	15 908	15 730
DM	Transport equipment	QTPG	16 113	15 987	16 091	16 178	15 903	15 652	15 932	16 305	16 805
DN	Manufacturing not elsewhere classified	QTPH	6 354	6 477	6 643	6 567	6 429	6 361	6 491	6 938	7 403
D	Total manufacturing	QTPI	151 157	150 009	149 223	146 308	144 845	147 261	148 591	153 155	157 728
E	Electricity, gas and water supply	QTPJ	15 703	15 798	15 660	16 052	16 405	16 672	16 667	18 870	18 696
C,D,E	Total production	QTPK	183 803	190 367	188 000	184 277	182 690	186 494	192 928	204 225	208 855
F	**Construction**	QTPL	42 236	45 626	50 526	54 684	59 522	63 955	68 019	73 993	79 623
G-Q	**Service industries**										
G	Wholesale and retail trade (including motor trade); repair of motor vehicles, personal and household goods	QTPM	99 510	103 409	110 250	113 778	120 520	127 411	130 952	136 071	142 402
H	Hotels and restaurants	QTPN	24 145	25 605	26 927	28 638	30 120	31 290	31 969	33 765	36 645
I	Transport, storage and communication										
	Transport and storage	QTPO	40 973	42 476	43 184	44 501	47 022	49 576	50 203	50 491	53 434
	Communication	QTPP	23 990	26 726	27 317	28 562	29 566	30 253	30 307	30 537	31 892
I	Total	QTPQ	64 961	69 201	70 502	73 064	76 587	79 828	80 510	81 027	85 326
J	Financial intermediation	QTPR	48 546	44 990	48 202	63 368	71 530	75 042	79 356	91 011	95 398
K	Real estate, renting and business activities										
	Letting of dwellings including imputed rent of owner occupiers	QTPS	53 502	57 261	61 352	64 249	69 298	76 166	80 155	84 809	90 065
	Other real estate, renting and business activities	QTPT	119 825	131 098	142 688	150 598	162 906	170 882	179 180	188 835	212 540
K	Total	QTPU	173 327	188 359	204 040	214 847	232 204	247 048	259 335	273 644	302 605
L	Public administration and defence (PAD)	QTPV	40 909	42 712	45 025	47 528	51 302	55 393	60 096	63 033	64 012
M	Education	QTPW	44 914	48 111	51 675	55 099	58 328	61 814	66 186	69 345	73 105
N	Health and social work	QTPX	51 577	55 282	59 549	64 492	70 593	74 417	78 497	81 883	86 689
O,P,Q	Other social and personal services, private households with employees and extra-territorial organisations	QTPY	39 822	42 086	44 561	48 312	51 804	55 283	59 852	61 368	64 151
G-Q	Total service industries	QTPZ	587 715	619 756	660 729	709 122	762 988	807 529	846 753	891 148	950 333
B.1g	**All industries**	ABML	822 774	864 285	907 594	957 094	1 015 008	1 068 574	1 115 121	1 177 232	1 247 721

1 Components may not sum to totals as a result of rounding.
2 Because of differences in the annual and monthly production inquiries, estimates of current price output and gross value added by industry derived from the current price Input-Output Supply and Use Tables are not consistent with the equivalent measures of chained volume measures growth given in 2.4. These differences do not affect GDP totals.

2.4 Gross value added at basic prices: by industry[1,2,3]
Chained volume indices

Indices 2003=100

		Weight per 1000[1]		1999	2000	2001	2002	2003	2004	2005	2006	2007
		2003										
A,B	**Agriculture, hunting, forestry and fishing**	9.7	**GDQA**	100.9	100.1	91.1	101.7	100.0	99.8	105.1	107.9	107.0
C,D,E	**Production**											
C	Mining and quarrying											
CA	Mining and quarrying of energy producing materials											
C10	Mining of coal	0.5	**CKZP**	132.7	112.5	112.9	105.9	100.0	85.9	67.2	64.4	57.6
C11	Extraction of mineral oil and natural gas	19.2	**CKZO**	117.4	113.5	107.1	105.8	100.0	91.5	82.4	75.1	73.2
CB	Other mining and quarrying	1.5	**CKZQ**	83.9	86.4	81.5	98.8	100.0	102.1	112.6	119.2	127.1
C	Total mining and quarrying	21.1	**CKYX**	114.6	111.0	104.9	105.3	100.0	92.1	84.2	78.0	76.7
D	Manufacturing											
DA	Food; beverages and tobacco	21.1	**CKZA**	98.4	98.4	98.9	101.7	100.0	102.0	103.6	102.9	102.3
DB	Textiles and textile products	4.2	**CKZB**	125.0	122.1	105.7	99.6	100.0	91.2	90.0	89.9	88.0
DC	Leather and leather products	0.5	**CKZC**	154.0	139.0	128.2	116.5	100.0	73.6	67.0	70.2	71.7
DD	Wood and wood products	2.6	**CKZD**	95.6	98.0	97.9	98.6	100.0	105.3	101.2	98.8	103.0
DE	Pulp, paper and paper products; publishing and printing	19.5	**CKZE**	101.5	102.0	101.6	101.8	100.0	99.0	95.0	94.3	94.2
DF	Coke, petroleum products and nuclear fuel	2.3	**CKZF**	106.9	113.0	106.9	109.2	100.0	107.8	111.0	105.4	109.3
DG	Chemicals, chemical products and man-made fibres	15.9	**CKZG**	89.6	93.3	98.4	99.2	100.0	103.6	106.5	110.0	109.0
DH	Rubber and plastic products	7.4	**CKZH**	106.8	106.2	103.2	99.1	100.0	98.3	97.2	101.3	100.8
DI	Other non-metallic mineral products	5.3	**CKZI**	93.6	96.0	96.8	95.8	100.0	106.2	106.2	109.1	109.4
DJ	Basic metals and fabricated metal products	14.6	**CKZJ**	101.1	103.0	100.2	101.3	100.0	102.7	103.6	105.1	106.1
DK	Machinery and equipment not elsewhere classified	12.0	**CKZK**	102.7	102.4	104.4	98.8	100.0	105.9	109.3	116.1	121.3
DL	Electrical and optical equipment	15.3	**CKZL**	111.5	127.0	119.6	103.9	100.0	102.2	98.0	98.3	99.3
DM	Transport equipment	15.7	**CKZM**	102.9	99.9	98.4	95.4	100.0	105.3	105.2	111.3	111.1
DN	Manufacturing not elsewhere classified	6.3	**CKZN**	101.0	100.5	98.9	100.1	100.0	100.2	100.7	101.7	104.5
D	Total manufacturing	142.7	**CKYY**	101.6	103.9	102.5	100.3	100.0	102.2	102.0	103.8	104.5
E	Electricity, gas and water supply	16.2	**CKYZ**	92.1	95.0	97.7	98.3	100.0	101.0	100.7	100.1	101.3
C,D,E	Total production	180.0	**CKYW**	102.1	103.9	102.3	100.7	100.0	100.9	99.8	100.5	100.9
F	**Construction**	58.6	**GDQB**	88.8	89.5	91.6	95.2	100.0	103.4	104.5	105.5	108.6
G-Q	**Service industries**											
G	Wholesale and retail trade (including motor trade); repair of motor vehicles, personal and household goods	118.7	**GDQC**	86.6	89.0	91.5	96.6	100.0	104.1	105.2	108.0	111.8
H	Hotels and restaurants	29.7	**GDQD**	91.8	92.2	94.5	97.2	100.0	101.7	103.9	109.4	112.0
I	Transport, storage and communication											
	Transport and storage	46.3	**GDQF**	98.4	100.8	99.9	101.3	100.0	104.5	108.8	111.7	115.3
	Communication	29.1	**GDQG**	68.1	84.3	94.4	93.4	100.0	102.5	107.6	109.8	113.1
I	Total	75.5	**GDQH**	85.0	93.8	97.6	98.0	100.0	103.7	108.3	111.0	114.5
J	Financial intermediation	70.5	**GDQI**	80.4	85.4	89.4	93.4	100.0	104.2	109.2	117.4	126.8
K	Real estate, renting and business activities											
	Letting of dwellings, including imputed rent of owner occupiers	68.3	**GDQL**	95.2	96.5	97.4	98.3	100.0	100.4	101.1	102.6	103.2
	Other real estate, renting and business activities	160.5	**GDQK**	82.0	89.6	95.2	95.5	100.0	106.6	113.5	121.4	129.8
K	Total	228.8	**GDQM**	85.7	91.6	95.9	96.3	100.0	104.7	109.8	115.8	121.9
L	Public administration and defence (PAD)	50.5	**GDQO**	91.0	91.2	92.5	95.1	100.0	101.1	101.6	101.9	102.0
M	Education	57.5	**GDQP**	95.2	96.0	97.1	99.1	100.0	99.4	99.8	99.3	98.8
N	Health and social work	69.5	**GDQQ**	86.1	89.0	92.4	96.2	100.0	103.7	106.1	108.7	112.4
O,P,Q	Other social and personal services, private households with employees and extra-territorial organisations	51.0	**GDQR**	90.4	93.5	97.0	99.2	100.0	99.3	100.5	102.2	102.3
G-Q	Total service industries	751.7	**GDQS**	86.9	91.1	94.3	96.6	100.0	103.2	106.3	110.2	114.3
B.1g	**All industries**	1 000.0	**CGCE**	89.9	93.4	95.5	97.2	100.0	102.7	104.9	107.9	111.1

1 The weights shown are in proportion to total gross value added (GVA) in 2003 and are used to combine the industry output indices to calculate the totals. For 2003 and earlier, totals are calculated using the equivalent weights for the previous year (e.g. totals for 2003 use 2002 weights). Weights may not sum to totals due to rounding.

2 As GVA is expressed in index number form, it is inappropriate to show as a statistical adjustment any divergence from the other measures of GDP. Such an adjustment does, however, exist implicitly.

3 See footnote 2 to Table 2.3.

2.5 Employment: by industry

Thousands

			1999	2000	2001	2002	2003	2004	2005	2006	2007
A,B	**Agriculture, hunting & forestry; fishing**										
	Self-employment jobs	YEKN	210	203	203	185	194	197	206	207	204
	Employee jobs	YEKO	320	323	280	257	230	226	240	228	240
	Total employed	YEKP	530	527	483	442	424	422	446	435	444
C-E	**Production industries, including energy**										
	Self-employment jobs	YEKQ	296	278	262	281	277	289	258	285	278
	Employee jobs	YEKR	4 292	4 185	4 036	3 816	3 611	3 434	3 276	3 144	3 092
	Total employed	YEKS	4 588	4 463	4 298	4 097	3 887	3 723	3 534	3 429	3 371
F	**Construction**										
	Self-employment jobs	YEKT	705	678	706	755	808	852	870	849	930
	Employee jobs	YEKU	1 144	1 217	1 206	1 186	1 181	1 207	1 239	1 306	1 296
	Total employed	YEKV	1 849	1 895	1 912	1 942	1 989	2 059	2 109	2 154	2 227
G-I	**Wholesale & retail trade (including motor trade); repair of motor vehicles, personal & household goods; hotels and restaurants; transport, storage & communication**										
	Self-emloyment jobs	YEKW	914	869	881	889	891	893	853	869	879
	Employee jobs	YEKX	7 467	7 614	7 791	7 883	7 935	8 000	8 069	7 991	7 997
	Total employed	YEKY	8 381	8 484	8 672	8 772	8 827	8 893	8 922	8 860	8 876
J-K	**Financial intermediation; real estate, renting & business activities**										
	Self-employment jobs	YEKZ	694	691	721	695	798	803	828	807	850
	Employee jobs	YELA	4 648	4 819	5 027	5 071	5 104	5 205	5 402	5 595	5 725
	Total employed	YELB	5 342	5 510	5 748	5 765	5 901	6 008	6 230	6 403	6 575
L-Q	**Other service activities** Public administration & defence, education, health and social work, other community, social & personal services, private households with employees										
	Self-employment jobs	YEJW	892	883	854	890	939	946	947	1 050	1 057
	Employee jobs	YEJX	7 554	7 825	7 945	8 161	8 388	8 601	8 812	8 917	8 927
	Total employed	YEJY	8 446	8 708	8 799	9 051	9 327	9 548	9 759	9 967	9 984
A-Q	**All industries**										
ESE	Self-employment jobs	BCAG	3 714	3 606	3 629	3 696	3 908	3 982	3 966	4 072	4 204
EEM	Employee jobs	IK6H	25 425	25 983	26 285	26 374	26 449	26 673	27 038	27 181	27 278
ETO	Total employed	YEJZ	29 140	29 589	29 914	30 070	30 357	30 655	31 004	31 253	31 482

1 Data sources are: Labour Force Survey for self-employed; employer surveys for employees. Figures as at June of each year.

The sector accounts

Part 3

The sector accounts at a glance

Net lending/borrowing

Net borrowing by general government increased in 2007 to £38.3 billion compared to net borrowing of £34.9 billion in 2006. The net borrowing figures reflect continued high government expenditure growth with lower revenues. Non-financial corporations sector was a net lender with £22.6 billion in 2007 and a net lender of £27.7 billion in 2006. This was driven by increased gross capital formation. Households and NPISH sector was a net borrower with £55.1 billion in 2007 compared to £33.6 billion in 2006. Financial corporations became net lenders in 2007 at £20.7 billion, from net borrowing of £3.3 billion in 2006. This reflects the large rise in gross trading profits, reduced payments of taxes on income and increased net interest receipts.

Net lending/borrowing, 2007

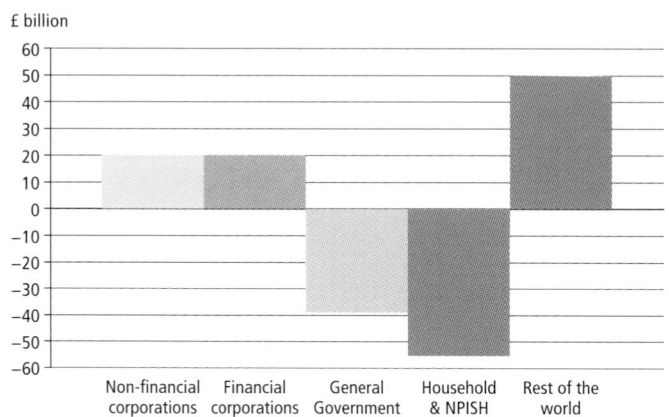

£ billion

Net financial transactions

Net financial transactions by general government showed a deficit of £39.3 billion in 2007 and a £34.2 billion deficit in 2006. The deficit has reflects the net issuance of gilts by central government. The Non-financial corporations show a surplus of £14.6 billion in 2007 down compared to a £32.2 billion surplus in 2006, following increased foreign currency loans with UK banks in 2007. Households showed a deficit of £45.4 billion in 2007 compared to a deficit of £29.6 billion in 2006. This was mainly driven by decreases acquisitions of assets.

In 2007 financial corporations showed surplus of £30.2 billion, following on from a deficit of £10.3 billion in 2006, reflecting their increased acquisition of short term loans.

Financial transactions by sector

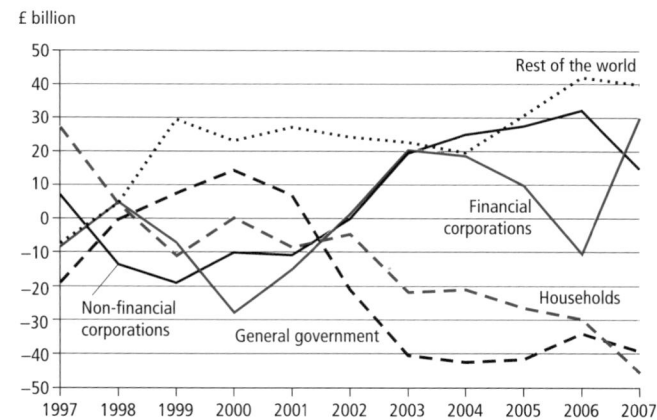

£ billion

Gross trading profits of private non-financial corporations

Gross trading profit is the largest component of private non-financial corporations' gross operating surplus. Profits rose by 7.4 per cent between 2006 and 2007 compared with profits of 6.6 per cent between 2005 and 2006.

Gross trading profits of private non-financial corporations

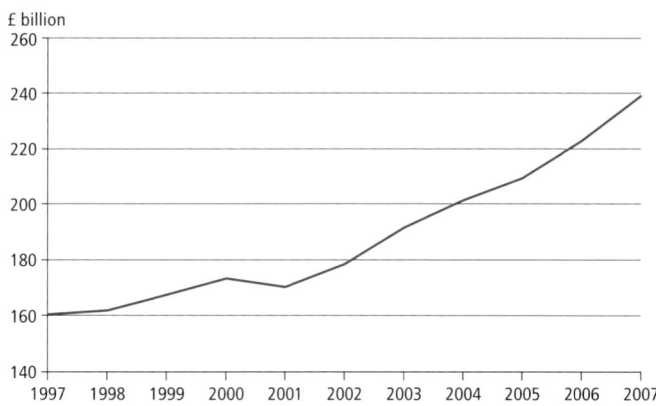

Real household disposable income

Real household disposable income (RHDI) is the amount of money in real terms the household sector has available for spending after taxes and other deductions. Between 2006 and 2007 RHDI increased by 0.1 per cent compared with an increase of 1.5 per cent between 2005 and 2006.

Annual changes in real household disposable income

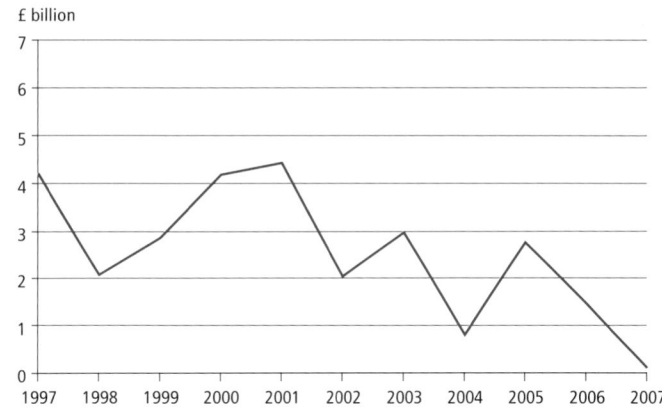

Household saving ratio

The household saving ratio reflects household gross savings as a percentage of their total available resources (the amount available to spend or save). Household resources rose by 3.6 per cent between 2006 and 2007. Household and NPISH final consumption expenditure rose by 5.5 per cent in the same period. As a consequence the household saving ratio fell from 4.2 per cent in 2006 to 2.5 per cent in 2007.

Household saving ratio

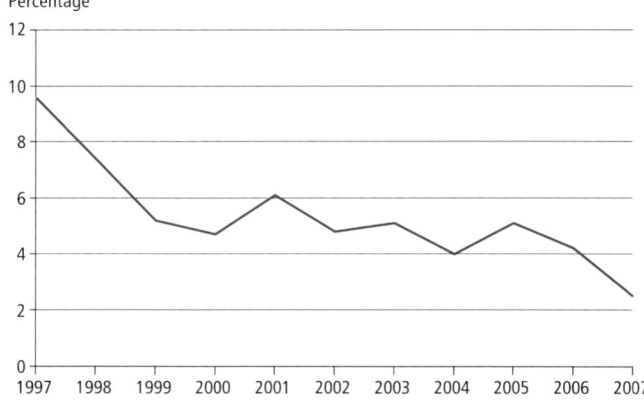

C The sector accounts: Key economic indicators

£ million

			1999	2000	2001	2002	2003	2004	2005	2006	2007
	Net lending/borrowing by:										
B.9	Non-financial corporations	**EABO**	−9 937	−4 614	−6 366	10 549	22 971	30 983	22 285	27 728	22 626
B.9	Financial corporations	**NHCQ**	−15 742	−26 988	−22 123	4 386	13 451	18 477	5 036	−3 275	20 724
B.9	General government	**NNBK**	8 623	13 954	7 660	−20 183	−41 173	−43 061	−40 778	−34 866	−38 322
B.9	Households and NPISH's	**NSSZ**	−4 051	−6 436	1 044	−12 477	−12 091	−29 533	−17 731	−33 643	−55 094
B.9	Rest of the world	**NHRB**	21 107	24 084	19 784	17 725	16 841	23 136	31 188	44 056	49 927
	Private non-financial corporations										
	Gross trading profits										
	Continental shelf profits	**CAGJ**	13 365	20 627	18 961	18 328	17 882	18 564	23 424	27 611	25 034
	Others	**CAGK**	154 082	152 682	151 364	160 068	173 584	182 976	185 873	195 399	214 415
	Rental of buildings	**FCBW**	10 821	11 747	12 394	12 904	13 891	16 097	16 936	17 350	18 011
	less Holding gains of inventories	**−DLQZ**	−1 800	−2 941	438	−2 856	−4 266	−2 786	−4 058	−3 444	−4 105
B.2g	Gross operating surplus	**NRJK**	176 468	182 115	183 157	188 444	201 091	214 851	222 175	236 916	253 355
	Households and NPISH										
B.6g	Household gross disposable income	**QWND**	623 737	657 288	700 094	725 267	760 916	779 339	820 911	852 443	874 031
	Implied deflator of household and NPISH individual consumption expenditure index (2003=100)[1]	**YBFS**	93.7	94.8	96.7	98.2	100.0	101.6	104.1	106.6	109.2
	Real household disposable income:										
	Chained volume measures (Reference year 2003)	**RVGK**	665 374	693 322	724 114	738 900	760 916	767 096	788 338	799 898	800 676
	Index (2003=100)	**OSXR**	87.4	91.1	95.2	97.1	100.0	100.8	103.6	105.1	105.2
B.8g	Gross saving	**NSSH**	33 197	31 353	43 243	35 665	40 017	32 557	43 132	37 289	22 560
	Households total resources	**NSSJ**	740 495	780 739	834 590	873 867	926 247	957 751	1 014 255	1 057 272	1 099 005
	Saving ratio, per cent	**RVGL**	5.2	4.7	6.0	4.8	5.1	4.0	5.1	4.2	2.5

1 Rounded to one decimal place

The sector accounts

The sector accounts show the relationships between different sectors of the economy and different types of transactions. They summarise the transactions of particular groups of institutions in the economy, showing how income is distributed and redistributed, and how savings are used to add wealth through investment in physical or financial assets. This section introduces the tables in Chapters 3 to 7 which deal with individual areas and subdivisions of the accounts. This introduction to the sector accounts has been divided into the following areas:

- The framework of the accounts

- The institutional sectors

- The types of transactions

- The sequence of accounts

- The statistical adjustment items

- Balance sheets

The framework of the accounts

The framework of national accounts detailed in Part 1 highlights the five main kinds of accounts; goods and services, production, distribution and use of income, capital, and financial. The production account records the activity of producing goods and services. The distribution and use of income accounts record how incomes are generated by production, distributed to institutional units with claims on the value added created by production, redistributed among institutional units, and eventually used by households, government units or non-profit institutions serving households for purposes of final consumption or saving. The capital account records the flows of non-financial assets acquired and disposed. The financial account shows how the net lending or borrowing on the capital account is financed by transactions in financial instruments.

The distribution and use of income accounts can be elaborated to form a consistent set of sector accounts. This is done in two dimensions, by sectors and types of transaction. A third dimension, related to capital and financial transactions is that of asset and liability levels, the national and sector balance sheets. The sectors and types of transaction are described below.

The institutional sectors

The system identifies two kinds of institutions: consuming units (mostly households); and production units (mainly corporations and non-profit institutions or government). Units can own goods and assets, incur liabilities and engage in economic activities and transactions with other units in their own right. All units within the country are put in one of the sectors. Also, the rest of the world is treated as a sector in respect of its dealings with the United Kingdom.

Non-financial corporations are those which exist to produce goods and non-financial services. They are, in the UK, mainly public limited companies, private companies and partnerships. They are mostly owned privately, but there are some public corporations, which are shown separately.

Financial corporations are those engaged primarily in financial activities, and are subdivided into monetary financial institutions, other financial intermediaries and financial auxiliaries, and insurance corporations and pension funds.

General government comprises central government and local government.

The Household sector contains all the resident people of the United Kingdom as receivers of income and consumers of products. It includes individuals such as prisoners as well as conventional family units. It also contains one person businesses where household and business accounts cannot be separated. This sector currently includes non-profit institutions serving households, which include productive units such as charities and universities.

The Rest of the world sector comprises those units that are not in the United Kingdom. The accounts for the rest of the world only record transactions between units in the rest of the world and units in the UK, and are equivalent to the balance of payments.

The tables in Chapters 3 to 7 are based on the sector classification detailed above. More detailed definitions of these sectors are given in the appropriate chapters of the *UK National Accounts Concepts, Sources and Methods* and, in full detail, in the Business Monitor MA23 *Sector classification for the national accounts* available from the ONS website.

The types of transactions

The other dimension is that of the types of transactions. These are divided into three types.

Transactions in products are related to goods and services, and include output, intermediate and final consumption, gross capital formation and exports and imports.

Distributive transactions transfer income or wealth between units of the economy, and include property income, taxes and subsidies, social contributions and benefits, and other current or capital transfers.

Financial transactions differ from distributive transactions in that they relate to transactions in financial claims by one unit on another, whereas distributive transactions are unrequited. The main categories in the classification of financial instruments are monetary gold and special drawing rights, currency and deposits, securities other than shares, loans, shares and other equity, insurance and pension funds reserves and other accounts receivable/payable.

The sequence of accounts

The transactions can be grouped broadly according to purpose in the production, distribution and use of income, capital or financial accounts. These are described briefly below:

Production account

The production account displays the transactions involved in the generation of income by the production of goods and services. This account is produced for the UK total economy (Table 1.6.1) and for the first four sectors (Tables 3.1.1, 4.1.1 etc.); the rest of the world does not have a production account. For each of the four sectors, the balancing item gross value added is shown as output less intermediate consumption. Gross value added at basic prices for each sector differs from gross domestic product for the UK total economy in that taxes less subsidies on products are not taken into the production accounts by sector but they are included within resources for the UK total economy. The sum of gross value added and taxes less subsidies on products for the UK economy is GDP at market prices.

Distribution and use of income account

The distribution and use of income accounts exist for all the main institutional sectors. To obtain the disposable income and savings of each sector we need to take account of transfers in and out of the sector. The accounts are not consolidated, so that in the whole economy account, transfers such as social contributions and benefits appear in both uses and resources.

These accounts describe the distribution and redistribution of income and its use in the form of final consumption. The distribution and use of income are analysed in four stages, each of which is presented as a separate account:

- The generation of income account

- The allocation of primary income account

- The secondary distribution of income account

- The use of disposable income account

Generation of income account

This is the first of the distribution and use of income accounts. It shows the sectors, sub-sectors and industries which are the source, rather than the destination, of income. It shows the derivation of the 'profit' arising from production, called the operating surplus (or mixed income in the case of unincorporated businesses in the households sector). The industry dimension is shown in Part 2, Table 2.1.

This account analyses the degree to which value added covers the compensation of employees (their wages and salaries, etc.) and other taxes less subsidies on production. So it gives a figure for the operating surplus: the surplus (or deficit) on production activities before distributions such as interest, rent and income tax charges have been considered. Hence the operating surplus is the income which units obtain from their own use of the production facilities.

Note that taxes on production and imports are shown as a use by producing sectors in this account but not as a resource of government. This is because they do not relate to productive activity by government, and cannot therefore contribute to its operating surplus. They become a resource of government in the allocation of primary income account which follows.

Allocation of primary income account

This account shows the resident units and institutional sectors as recipients rather than producers of primary income. It demonstrates the extent to which operating surpluses are distributed (for example by dividends) to the owners of the enterprises. Also recorded in this account is the property income received by an owner of a financial asset in return for providing funds to, or putting a tangible non-produced asset at the disposal of, another unit. The receipt by government of taxes on production less subsidies is shown in resources.

The resources side of the allocation of primary income accounts includes the components of the income approach to measurement of gross domestic product and this is the starting point for the quarterly sector accounts. The accounts also include property income recorded as both resources for receipts and uses for payments.

The balance of this account is the gross balance of primary income (B.5g) for each sector, and if the gross balance of primary income is aggregated across all sectors of the UK economy the result is gross national income.

Secondary distribution of income account

This account describes how the balance of primary income for each institutional sector is allocated by redistribution; through transfers such as taxes on income, social contributions and benefits and other current transfers. It excludes social transfers in kind.

The balancing item of this account is gross disposable income (B.6g) which reflects current transactions and explicitly excludes capital transfers, real holding gains and losses, and the consequences of events such as natural disasters.

Use of disposable income account

This account illustrates how disposable income is split between final consumption expenditure and saving. In the system for recording economic accounts, only the government and the households and NPISH sectors have final consumption. In addition, for households and pension funds, there is an adjustment item in the account which reflects the way that transactions between households and pension funds are recorded. (This adjustment is D.8: Adjustment for the changes in the net equity of households in pension funds reserves.)

The balancing item for this account, and thus for this whole group of distribution and use of income accounts, is gross saving (B.8g).

Thus it is only in the case of non-financial corporations (public and private), that undistributed income and saving are equivalent.

Capital account

The capital account is presented in two parts.

The first part shows that saving (B.8g) – the balance between national disposable income and final consumption expenditure from the production and distribution and use of income accounts – is reduced or increased by the balance of capital transfers (D.9) to provide an amount available for financing investment (in both non-financial and financial assets).

Then in the second part, total investment in non-financial assets is the sum of gross fixed capital formation (P.51), changes in inventories (P.52), acquisitions less disposals of valuables (P.53) and acquisitions less disposals of non-financial non-produced assets (K.2). The balance on the capital account is known as net lending or borrowing. Conceptually this net lending or borrowing for all the domestic sectors represents net lending or borrowing to the rest of the world sector.

Thus, if investment is lower than the amount available for investment, the balance will be positive and is regarded as lending (if negative the balance is borrowing). Where the capital accounts relate to the individual institutional sectors, the net lending/borrowing of a particular sector represents the amounts available for lending or borrowing to other sectors. The value of net lending/borrowing is the same irrespective of whether the accounts are shown before or after deduction of fixed capital consumption (K.1), provided a consistent approach is adopted throughout.

Financial account

The financial account elaborates the acquisition and disposal of financial assets and liabilities. Examples of financial assets include: bank deposits (which are assets of the depositors and liabilities of the banks), unit trust units (assets of the holders and liabilities of unit trusts) and Treasury Bills (assets of the holders and a liability of central government). The balance of all transactions in the financial account is net lending or borrowing.

The statistical adjustment items

Although in theory the net lending/borrowing from the financial account and the net lending/borrowing from the capital account for each sector should be equal, in practice they are not. This is because of the (sometimes substantial) errors and omissions in the accounts. The difference between the two balances is known as the statistical adjustment item.

Part of the balancing process for the economic accounts statistics for years before the latest one shown (that is, for years t–1 and earlier) involves assessing and modifying the component variables so that the estimates of net lending/borrowing made from the income and capital accounts, and from the financial accounts, are the same at the level of the whole economy, and reasonably close to each other at the sector level.

The sectoral statistical adjustment items are shown in Table D below. They provide a measure of the reliability of the accounts.

Table D: Sector statistical adjustment

										£ million
		1999	2000	2001	2002	2003	2004	2005	2006	2007
Households sector	**NZDV**	6 859	–6 875	9 348	–7 976	9 557	–8 731	8 610	–4 040	–9 730
Private non-financial corporations	**NYPM**	9 106	5 130	5 276	11 139	3 018	5 134	–5 303	–4 575	8 936
Financial corporations	**NYOX**	–8 772	684	–7 296	2 860	–6 933	–350	–4 875	7 013	–9 458
Public corporations	**NYPI**	7	431	–704	–423	607	968	–22	79	–953
Central government	**NZDW**	526	510	76	819	111	365	370	–679	961
Local government	**NYPC**	672	–832	711	61	–649	–956	613	21	8
Rest of the world	**NYPO**	–8 398	951	–7 410	–6 479	–5 712	3 572	607	2 181	10 097
Total[1]	**–RVFE**	–	–	–	–	–	–	–	–	–139

1 Equals, but opposite in sign to, the residual error observed between GDP measured by the income approach and GDP measured by the expenditure approach

Balance sheets

A financial balance sheet for each sector has been compiled using the same financial instrument classification as that used for financial transactions. The changes in the end period levels in the financial balance sheets do not equal the financial transactions because of holding gains or losses and reclassifications of units between sectors. Non-financial balance sheets for the ESA95 sectors are now included.

Further information

In addition to the articles and publications mentioned in Part 1, further information relating to the sector accounts and in particular the financial accounts can be found in the following articles and publications:

Office for National Statistics (2007) *Financial Statistics: Explanatory Handbook* 2008 edition, Palgrave Macmillan, Basingstoke.

Office for National Statistics *Financial Statistics*, monthly publication, Palgrave Macmillan, Basingstoke.

Turnbull P (Central Statistical Office) (1993) 'The UK Sector Accounts' *Economic Trends*, No. 479, HMSO.

Bank of England (2002) *Bank of England Statistical Abstract*, Bank of England.

Articles relating to the Public Sector Finances

Golland J, Savage D, Pike T and Pike S (1999) 'Monthly Statistics on Public Sector Finances. A Methodological Guide', GSS Methodology Series no. 12, Office for National Statistics.

Golland J, Louth N, Hill C (1998) 'New Format For Public Finances' *Economic Trends*, No. 535, The Stationery Office.

Articles relating to monetary aggregates (M0, M4)

Bank of England (1994) 'The Determination of M0 and M4' *Bank of England Quarterly Bulletin* February 1994, pages 46–50.

Bank of England (1993) 'Divisia measures of money' *Bank of England Quarterly Bulletin*, May 1993.

Chapter 3

Non-financial corporations

3.1.1 Non-financial corporations
ESA95 sector S.11

£ million

			1999	2000	2001	2002	2003	2004	2005	2006
I	**PRODUCTION ACCOUNT**									
	Resources									
P.1	Output									
P.11	Market output	**FAIN**	1 114 874	1 177 211	1 213 638	1 243 635	1 294 414	1 356 823	1 427 239	1 501 215
P.12	Output for own final use	**FAIO**	8 714	9 448	10 293	10 727	12 129	13 186	13 978	15 017
P.1	Total resources	**FAFA**	1 123 588	1 186 659	1 223 931	1 254 362	1 306 543	1 370 009	1 441 217	1 516 232
	Uses									
P.2	Intermediate consumption	**FAIQ**	592 568	625 800	642 548	655 448	680 238	715 595	760 243	801 724
B.1g	**Gross Value Added**	**FAIS**	**531 020**	**560 859**	**581 383**	**598 914**	**626 305**	**654 414**	**680 974**	**714 508**
Total	Total uses	**FAFA**	1 123 588	1 186 659	1 223 931	1 254 362	1 306 543	1 370 009	1 441 217	1 516 232
B.1g	**Gross Value Added**	**FAIS**	**531 020**	**560 859**	**581 383**	**598 914**	**626 305**	**654 414**	**680 974**	**714 508**
-K.1	*less* Consumption of fixed capital	**-DBGF**	−63 897	−66 420	−68 362	−70 547	−72 598	−75 559	−77 278	−80 360
B.1n	Value added, net	**FAIT**	467 123	494 439	513 021	528 367	553 707	578 855	603 696	634 148

3.1.2 Non-financial corporations
ESA95 sector S.11

£ million

			1999	2000	2001	2002	2003	2004	2005	2006
II	**DISTRIBUTION AND USE OF INCOME ACCOUNTS**									
II.1	**PRIMARY DISTRIBUTION OF INCOME ACCOUNT**									
II.1.1	**GENERATION OF INCOME ACCOUNT** before deduction of fixed capital consumption									
	Resources									
B.1g	**Total resources (Gross Value Added)**	**FAIS**	**531 020**	**560 859**	**581 383**	**598 914**	**626 305**	**654 414**	**680 974**	**714 508**
	Uses									
D.1	Compensation of employees									
D.11	Wages and salaries	**FAKT**	293 542	313 703	330 912	340 164	347 038	356 952	371 557	383 224
D.12	Employers' social contributions	**FAKU**	39 117	42 631	44 927	47 995	55 373	59 789	62 604	68 387
D.1	Total	**FCFV**	332 659	356 334	375 839	388 159	402 411	416 741	434 161	451 611
D.2	Taxes on production and imports, paid									
D.29	Production taxes other than on products	**EACJ**	14 892	15 808	16 170	16 679	17 037	17 346	18 159	19 202
-D.3	*less* Subsidies, received									
-D.39	Production subsidies other than on products	**-JQJV**	−663	−574	−662	−954	−1 434	−1 562	−2 449	−3 093
B.2g	Operating surplus, gross	**NQBE**	184 132	189 291	190 036	195 030	208 291	221 889	231 103	246 788
B.1g	**Total uses (Gross Value Added)**	**FAIS**	**531 020**	**560 859**	**581 383**	**598 914**	**626 305**	**654 414**	**680 974**	**714 508**
-K.1	After deduction of fixed capital consumption	**-DBGF**	−63 897	−66 420	−68 362	−70 547	−72 598	−75 559	−77 278	−80 360
B.2n	Operating surplus, net	**FAIR**	120 235	122 871	121 674	124 483	135 693	146 330	153 825	166 428

3.1.3 Non-financial corporations
ESA95 sector S.11

£ million

			1999	2000	2001	2002	2003	2004	2005	2006	2007
II.1.2	**ALLOCATION OF PRIMARY INCOME ACCOUNT** before deduction of fixed capital consumption										
	Resources										
B.2g	Operating surplus, gross	NQBE	184 132	189 291	190 036	195 030	208 291	221 889	231 103	246 788	262 869
D.4	Property income, received										
D.41	Interest	EABC	11 716	14 598	13 177	9 330	9 727	14 145	17 389	24 562	29 783
D.42	Distributed income of corporations	EABD	21 527	26 544	37 478	30 550	50 263	42 964	46 724	44 582	38 538
D.43	Reinvested earnings on direct foreign investment	WEYD	16 214	20 118	22 997	26 931	12 559	22 868	33 354	36 642	44 790
D.44	Attributed property income of insurance policy-holders	FAOF	338	290	333	300	401	368	582	590	428
D.45	Rent	FAOG	117	117	117	118	120	122	122	124	124
D.4	Total	FAKY	49 912	61 667	74 102	67 229	73 070	80 467	98 171	106 500	113 663
Total	Total resources	FBXJ	234 044	250 958	264 138	262 259	281 361	302 356	329 274	353 288	376 532
	Uses										
D.4	Property income, paid										
D.41	Interest	EABG	24 802	30 405	30 661	29 045	29 592	34 937	39 338	45 229	56 552
D.42	Distributed income of corporations	NVCS	86 427	84 187	103 635	87 281	93 735	93 591	106 853	105 445	98 383
D.43	Reinvested earnings on direct foreign investment	HDVB	2 776	7 348	1 699	1 614	3 955	6 325	4 983	16 802	23 676
D.45	Rent	FBXO	565	1 325	1 955	1 939	1 603	1 221	1 268	1 265	1 282
D.4	Total	FBXK	114 570	123 265	137 950	119 879	128 885	136 074	152 442	168 741	179 893
B.5g	**Balance of primary incomes, gross**	NQBG	**119 474**	**127 693**	**126 188**	**142 380**	**152 476**	**166 282**	**176 832**	**184 547**	**196 639**
Total	Total uses	FBXJ	234 044	250 958	264 138	262 259	281 361	302 356	329 274	353 288	376 532
-K.1	After deduction of fixed capital consumption	–DBGF	–63 897	–66 420	–68 362	–70 547	–72 598	–75 559	–77 278	–80 360	–83 565
B.5n	Balance of primary incomes, net	FBXQ	55 577	61 273	57 826	71 833	79 878	90 723	99 554	104 187	113 074

3.1.4 Non-financial corporations
ESA95 sector S.11

£ million

			1999	2000	2001	2002	2003	2004	2005	2006	2007
II.2	**SECONDARY DISTRIBUTION OF INCOME ACCOUNT**										
	Resources										
B.5g	**Balance of primary incomes, gross**	NQBG	**119 474**	**127 693**	**126 188**	**142 380**	**152 476**	**166 282**	**176 832**	**184 547**	**196 639**
D.61	Social contributions										
D.612	Imputed social contributions	NSTJ	3 845	4 175	4 357	4 575	4 229	3 810	3 535	3 425	3 508
D.7	Current transfers other than taxes, social contributions and benefits										
D.72	Non-life insurance claims	FCBP	3 719	5 762	3 714	5 396	6 000	6 522	7 261	8 368	6 376
D.75	Miscellaneous current transfers	CY8C	109	85	122	147	124	28	–	–	–
D.7	Total	NRJB	3 828	5 847	3 836	5 543	6 124	6 550	7 261	8 368	6 376
Total	Total resources	FCBR	127 147	137 715	134 381	152 498	162 829	176 642	187 628	196 340	206 523
	Uses										
D.5	Current taxes on income, wealth etc.										
D.51	Taxes on income	FCBS	22 948	24 497	23 177	24 038	23 702	27 368	33 602	37 183	38 260
D.62	Social benefits other than social transfers in kind	NSTJ	3 845	4 175	4 357	4 575	4 229	3 810	3 535	3 425	3 508
D.7	Current transfers other than taxes, social contributions and benefits										
D.71	Net non-life insurance premiums	FCBY	3 719	5 762	3 714	5 396	6 000	6 522	7 261	8 368	6 376
D.75	Miscellaneous current transfers	CY8B	709	553	506	480	462	451	488	474	476
D.7	Total, other current transfers	FCBX	4 428	6 315	4 220	5 876	6 462	6 973	7 749	8 842	6 852
B.6g	**Gross Disposable Income**	NRJD	**95 926**	**102 728**	**102 627**	**118 009**	**128 436**	**138 491**	**142 742**	**146 890**	**157 903**
Total	Total uses	FCBR	127 147	137 715	134 381	152 498	162 829	176 642	187 628	196 340	206 523
-K.1	After deduction of fixed capital consumption	–DBGF	–63 897	–66 420	–68 362	–70 547	–72 598	–75 559	–77 278	–80 360	–83 565
B.6n	Disposable income, net	FCCF	32 029	36 308	34 265	47 462	55 838	62 932	65 464	66 530	74 338

3.1.6 Non-financial corporations
ESA95 sector S.11

£ million

			1999	2000	2001	2002	2003	2004	2005	2006	2007
II.4.1	**USE OF DISPOSABLE INCOME ACCOUNT**										
	Resources										
B.6g	**Total resources (Gross Disposable Income)**	**NRJD**	95 926	102 728	102 627	118 009	128 436	138 491	142 742	146 890	157 903
	Uses										
B.8g	**Total uses (Gross Saving)**	**NRJD**	95 926	102 728	102 627	118 009	128 436	138 491	142 742	146 890	157 903
-K.1	After deduction of fixed capital consumption	**–DBGF**	–63 897	–66 420	–68 362	–70 547	–72 598	–75 559	–77 278	–80 360	–83 565
B.8n	Saving, net	**FCCF**	32 029	36 308	34 265	47 462	55 838	62 932	65 464	66 530	74 338

3.1.7 Non-financial corporations
ESA95 sector S.11

£ million

			1999	2000	2001	2002	2003	2004	2005	2006	2007
III	**ACCUMULATION ACCOUNTS**										
III.1	**CAPITAL ACCOUNT**										
III.1.1	**CHANGE IN NET WORTH DUE TO SAVING AND CAPITAL TRANSFERS**										
	Changes in liabilities and net worth										
B.8g	**Gross Saving**	**NRJD**	95 926	102 728	102 627	118 009	128 436	138 491	142 742	146 890	157 903
D.9	Capital transfers receivable										
D.92	Investment grants	**FCCO**	2 992	2 835	3 845	3 895	5 563	5 723	6 799	7 673	8 291
D.99	Other capital transfers	**LNZN**	150	142	915	184	148	136	11 801	449	177
D.9	Total	**FCCQ**	3 142	2 977	4 760	4 079	5 711	5 859	18 600	8 122	8 468
-D.9	*less* Capital transfers payable										
-D.91	Capital taxes	**–QYKB**	–	–	–	–	–	–	–	–	–
-D.99	Other capital transfers	**–JRWI**	–216	–290	–285	–492	–575	–419	–1 257	–630	–758
-D.9	Total	**–JRWJ**	–216	–290	–285	–492	–575	–419	–1 257	–630	–758
B.10.1g	Total change in liabilities and net worth	**FCCY**	98 852	105 415	107 102	121 596	133 572	143 931	160 085	154 382	165 613
	Changes in assets										
B.10.1g	Changes in net worth due to gross saving and capital transfers	**FCCY**	98 852	105 415	107 102	121 596	133 572	143 931	160 085	154 382	165 613
-K.1	After deduction of fixed capital consumption	**–DBGF**	–63 897	–66 420	–68 362	–70 547	–72 598	–75 559	–77 278	–80 360	–83 565
B.10.1n	Changes in net worth due to net saving and capital transfers	**FCCV**	34 955	38 995	38 740	51 049	60 974	68 372	82 807	74 022	82 048
III.1.2	**ACQUISITION OF NON-FINANCIAL ASSETS ACCOUNT**										
	Changes in liabilities and net worth										
B.10.1n	Changes in net worth due to net saving and capital transfers	**FCCV**	34 955	38 995	38 740	51 049	60 974	68 372	82 807	74 022	82 048
K.1	Consumption of fixed capital	**DBGF**	63 897	66 420	68 362	70 547	72 598	75 559	77 278	80 360	83 565
B.10.1g	Total change in liabilities and net worth	**FCCY**	98 852	105 415	107 102	121 596	133 572	143 931	160 085	154 382	165 613
	Changes in assets										
P.5	Gross capital formation										
P.51	Gross fixed capital formation	**DBGP**	101 701	103 951	106 310	107 012	105 712	106 795	131 035	121 173	134 148
P.52	Changes in inventories	**DBGM**	6 054	5 289	5 950	2 647	3 745	4 567	5 191	4 142	7 421
P.53	Acquisitions less disposals of valuables	**NPOV**	–17	–75	–	–43	–97	–99	–171	–42	–22
P.5	Total gross capital formation	**FCCZ**	107 738	109 165	112 260	109 616	109 360	111 263	136 055	125 273	141 547
K.2	Acquisitions less disposals of non-produced non-financial assets	**FCFY**	1 051	864	1 208	1 431	1 241	1 685	1 745	1 381	1 440
B.9	**Net lending(+) / net borrowing(-)**	**EABO**	**–9 937**	**–4 614**	**–6 366**	**10 549**	**22 971**	**30 983**	**22 285**	**27 728**	**22 626**
Total	Total change in assets	**FCCY**	98 852	105 415	107 102	121 596	133 572	143 931	160 085	154 382	165 613

3.1.8 Non-financial corporations
ESA95 sector S.11 Unconsolidated

£ million

			1999	2000	2001	2002	2003	2004	2005	2006	2007
III.2	**FINANCIAL ACCOUNT**										
F.A	**Net acquisition of financial assets**										
F.2	Currency and deposits										
F.21	Currency	**NGIJ**	378	308	277	10	338	−47	182	272	293
F.22	Transferable deposits										
F.2211	Sterling deposits with UK banks	**NGIM**	7 490	11 123	10 083	8 921	10 781	12 041	19 951	24 013	14 893
F.2212	Foreign currency deposits with UK banks	**NGIN**	2 446	3 567	1 335	−274	3 840	2 559	2 640	2 653	3 383
F.2213	Sterling deposits with building societies	**NGIO**	156	−134	301	−77	245	−313	−64	299	212
F.229	Deposits with rest of the world monetary financial institutions	**NGIP**	4 105	7 804	21 011	9 947	38 367	54 984	35 482	36 770	72 738
F.29	Other deposits	**NGIQ**	−695	−251	−566	1 109	−398	454	663	718	114
F.2	Total currency and deposits	**NGII**	13 880	22 417	32 441	19 636	53 173	69 678	58 854	64 725	91 633
F.3	Securities other than shares										
F.331	Short term: money market instruments										
F.3311	Issued by UK central government	**NGIT**	144	−78	−100	–	2	−4	1	–	408
F.3312	Issued by UK local government	**NGIX**	–	–	–	–	–	–	–	–	–
F.3315	Issued by UK monetary financial institutions	**NGIY**	−2 003	−81	234	230	622	77	−787	1 612	3 020
F.3316	Issued by other UK residents	**NGJD**	−175	−2 797	136	−2 108	821	−387	−1 604	4 402	1 659
F.3319	Issued by the rest of the world	**NGJE**	722	1 110	1 912	1 110	3 798	615	1 078	4 758	−9 820
F.332	Medium (1 to 5 year) and long term (over 5 year) bonds										
F.3321	Issued by UK central government	**NGJG**	−453	230	−579	148	−335	33	−902	−2 001	492
F.3322	Issued by UK local government	**NGJJ**	–	–	–	–	–	–	–	–	–
F.3325	Medium term bonds issued by UK MFIs[1]	**NGJK**	54	−237	−333	42	167	−23	395	466	658
F.3326	Other medium & long term bonds issued by UK residents	**NGJN**	−1 347	1 141	1 784	559	−685	−389	−3 421	−537	3 733
F.3329	Long term bonds issued by the rest of the world	**NGJO**	−934	1 792	1 759	−601	2 213	437	892	−2 186	169
F.34	Financial derivatives	**NGJP**	3	−92	−8	10	9	8	1	−1	10
F.3	Total securities other than shares	**NGIR**	−3 989	988	4 805	−610	6 612	367	−4 347	6 513	329
F.4	Loans										
F.42	Long term loans										
F.421	Direct investment	**NGKB**	28 144	13 030	8 935	21 891	9 678	17 775	22 347	13 762	47 098
F.422	Loans secured on dwellings	**NGKE**	−1	−1	–	–	–	–	–	–	–
F.423	Finance leasing	**NGKI**	607	658	118	221	471	946	1 043	297	559
F.424	Other long-term loans by UK residents	**NGKJ**	−118	13 617	4 656	−27	−4 863	570	13 630	38 837	−2 445
F.4	Total loans	**NGJT**	28 632	27 304	13 709	22 085	5 286	19 291	37 020	52 896	45 212
F.5	Shares and other equity										
F.51	Shares and other equity, excluding mutual funds' shares										
F.514	Quoted UK shares	**NGKQ**	20 143	84 735	6 636	13 999	4 944	12 620	11 641	17 786	11 794
F.515	Unquoted UK shares	**NGKR**	6 973	8 213	13 285	7 557	9 425	9 279	16 002	9 915	11 311
F.517	UK shares and bonds issued by other UK residents	**NSQC**	–	–	–	–	–	–	–	–	–
F.519	Shares and other equity issued by the rest of the world	**NGKV**	112 093	166 680	36 002	49 469	19 394	26 461	41 057	48 725	69 396
F.52	Mutual funds' shares										
F.521	UK mutual funds' shares	**NGKZ**	1	14	2	3	1	9	17	17	7
F.5	Total shares and other equity	**NGKL**	139 210	259 642	55 925	71 028	33 764	48 369	68 717	76 443	92 508
F.6	Insurance technical reserves										
F.62	Prepayments of insurance premiums and reserves for outstanding claims	**NGLE**	−291	344	−370	363	170	956	965	1 371	10
F.7	Other accounts receivable	**NGLF**	−2 324	25 027	−2 282	2 881	918	−591	1 451	5 254	541
F.A	**Total net acquisition of financial assets**	**NRGP**	175 118	335 722	104 228	115 383	99 923	138 070	162 660	207 202	230 233

1 UK monetary financial institutions

3.1.8 Non-financial corporations
ESA95 sector S.11 Unconsolidated

continued

£ million

			1999	2000	2001	2002	2003	2004	2005	2006	2007
III.2	**FINANCIAL ACCOUNT** continued										
F.L	**Net acquisition of financial liabilities**										
F.2	Currency and deposits										
F.29	Other deposits	–A4VS	28	29	30	18	–	–	–	–	–
F.2	Total currency and deposits	–A4VR	28	29	30	18	–	–	–	–	–
F.3	Securities other than shares										
F.331	Short term: money market instruments										
F.3316	Issued by UK residents other than government or monetary financial institutions	NGMH	2 716	1 331	–426	8 543	–1 541	–3 071	–172	698	677
F.332	Medium (1 to 5 year) and long term (over 5 year) bonds										
F.3326	Other medium & long term bonds issued by UK residents or monetary financial institutions	NGMR	39 378	40 595	15 478	15 330	19 426	8 550	12 420	11 263	23 969
F.34	Financial derivatives	CY7W	–42	–110	–184	–204	–138	–28	–	–	–
F.3	Total securities other than shares	NGLV	42 052	41 816	14 868	23 669	17 747	5 451	12 248	11 961	24 646
F.4	Loans										
F.41	Short term loans										
F.411	Loans by UK monetary financial institutions, excluding loans secured on dwellings & financial leasing	NGMZ	15 886	25 081	17 921	20 861	7 140	20 484	46 281	55 238	80 518
F.419	Loans by rest of the world monetary financial institutions	NGND	–7 653	–15 253	30 731	5 103	32 248	52 584	–2 962	51 781	–7 105
F.42	Long term loans										
F.421	Direct investment	NGNF	27 029	40 792	17 919	43 802	10 162	15 667	49 740	34 726	21 163
F.422	Secured on dwellings	G9JS	–	–	–	–	–	–	2 591	3 812	3 830
F.423	Finance leasing	NGNM	101	62	–52	291	389	988	944	468	546
F.424	Other long-term loans by UK residents	NGNN	2 040	–1 309	4 260	490	4 611	604	6 099	5 046	57 294
F.429	Other long-term loans by the rest of the world	NGNO	–	–	–	–	–	283	–7	–12	–6
F.4	Total loans	NGMX	37 403	49 373	70 779	70 547	54 550	90 610	102 686	151 059	156 240
F.5	Shares and other equity										
F.51	Shares and other equity, excluding mutual funds' shares										
F.514	Quoted UK shares	NGNU	85 600	209 418	9 234	16 508	–748	7 286	–4 608	–3 730	5 392
F.515	Unquoted UK shares	NGNV	22 070	45 259	18 551	4 834	11 348	10 845	22 691	13 743	26 815
F.516	Other UK equity (including direct investment in property)	NGNW	–1 239	–745	–1 772	–2 348	–5 100	–3 172	–3 253	–3 076	187
F.517	UK shares and bonds issued by other UK residents	NSQD	–	–	–	–	–	–	–	–	–
F.5	Total shares and other equity	NGNP	106 431	253 932	26 013	18 994	5 500	14 959	14 830	6 937	32 394
F.7	Other accounts payable	NGOJ	8 254	747	3 476	2 322	2 780	2 169	5 286	5 021	2 310
F.L	**Total net acquisition of financial liabilities**	NRGR	194 168	345 897	115 166	115 550	80 577	113 189	135 050	174 978	215 590
B.9	**Net lending / borrowing**										
F.A	Total net acquisition of financial assets	NRGP	175 118	335 722	104 228	115 383	99 923	138 070	162 660	207 202	230 233
-F.L	*less* Total net acquisition of financial liabilities	–NRGR	–194 168	–345 897	–115 166	–115 550	–80 577	–113 189	–135 050	–174 978	–215 590
B.9f	Net lending (+) / net borrowing (-), from financial account	NYNT	–19 050	–10 175	–10 938	–167	19 346	24 881	27 610	32 224	14 643
dB.9f	Statistical discrepancy	NYPF	9 113	5 561	4 572	10 716	3 625	6 102	–5 325	–4 496	7 983
B.9	**Net lending (+) / net borrowing (-), from capital account**	EABO	**–9 937**	**–4 614**	**–6 366**	**10 549**	**22 971**	**30 983**	**22 285**	**27 728**	**22 626**

3.1.9 Non-financial corporations
ESA95 sector S.11 Unconsolidated

£ billion

			1999	2000	2001	2002	2003	2004	2005	2006	2007
IV.3	**FINANCIAL BALANCE SHEET** at end of period										
AN	**Non-financial assets**	CGES	1 240.8	1 255.6	1 265.7	1 314.5	1 356.2	1 429.5	1 438.6	1 541.0	1 560.9
AF.A	**Financial assets**										
AF.2	Currency and deposits										
AF.21	Currency	NNZG	3.3	3.6	3.8	3.8	4.1	4.1	4.3	4.5	4.8
AF.22	Transferable deposits										
AF.221	Deposits with UK monetary financial institutions	NNZI	143.4	159.3	172.0	177.9	191.4	205.4	230.1	253.6	274.3
AF.229	Deposits with rest of the world monetary financial institutions	NNZM	46.7	57.5	66.5	65.1	121.1	194.3	255.4	286.9	355.2
AF.29	Other deposits	NNZN	8.2	8.2	7.6	8.0	6.7	7.2	8.7	9.4	9.6
AF.2	Total currency and deposits	NNZF	201.7	228.6	249.9	254.8	323.4	411.0	498.4	554.5	643.9
AF.3	Securities other than shares										
AF.331	Short term: money market instruments										
AF.3311	Issued by UK central government	NNZQ	0.2	0.1	–	–	–	–	–	0.1	0.4
AF.3312	Issued by UK local government	NNZU	–	–	–	–	–	–	–	–	–
AF.3315	Issued by UK monetary financial institutions	NNZV	5.2	5.8	6.0	5.0	5.4	5.8	5.2	7.1	9.3
AF.3316	Issued by other UK residents	NOLO	13.6	16.4	18.6	13.9	13.8	14.2	18.3	37.6	43.7
AF.3319	Issued by the rest of the world	NOLP	1.9	3.0	4.9	6.0	9.8	10.4	11.4	16.2	6.4
AF.332	Medium (1 to 5 year) and long term (over 5 year) bonds										
AF.3321	Issued by UK central government	NOLR	3.8	4.0	3.4	3.5	3.2	3.6	2.7	0.7	1.2
AF.3322	Issued by UK local government	NOLU	–	–	–	–	–	–	–	–	–
AF.3325	Medium term bonds issued by UK MFIs[1]	NOLV	0.3	0.2	0.2	0.3	0.9	1.0	1.5	1.9	2.5
AF.3326	Other medium & long term bonds issued by UK residents	NOLY	1.9	2.5	4.1	6.1	5.2	5.1	1.4	1.5	5.2
AF.3329	Long term bonds issued by the rest of the world	NOLZ	7.2	28.4	28.8	29.3	30.0	12.8	14.6	10.3	11.6
AF.3	Total securities other than shares	NNZO	34.0	60.5	66.0	64.1	68.2	52.7	55.1	75.4	80.3
AF.4	Loans										
AF.42	Long term loans										
AF.421	Direct investment	NOMM	129.3	134.1	146.3	163.3	159.1	180.3	193.7	207.2	254.3
AF.422	Loans secured on dwellings	NOMP	–	–	–	–	–	–	–	–	–
AF.423	Finance leasing	NOMT	1.8	2.4	2.5	2.7	3.2	4.4	5.4	4.4	4.9
AF.424	Other long-term loans by UK residents	NOMU	12.9	12.0	12.3	12.3	12.3	12.2	11.9	10.7	10.5
AF.4	Total loans	NOME	144.0	148.5	161.1	178.3	174.5	196.8	211.0	222.3	269.7
AF.5	Shares and other equity										
AF.51	Shares and other equity, excluding mutual funds' shares										
AF.514	Quoted UK shares	NONB	39.2	26.6	15.0	8.9	9.6	9.0	19.3	32.9	26.0
AF.515	Unquoted UK shares	NONC	64.7	63.9	52.7	39.9	46.6	50.3	57.4	61.2	63.3
AF.517	UK shares and bonds issued by other UK residents	NSQW	–	–	–	–	–	–	–	–	–
AF.519	Shares and other equity issued by the rest of the world	NONG	340.7	507.4	495.2	522.3	565.7	550.8	593.3	603.2	671.4
AF.52	Mutual funds' shares										
AF.521	UK mutual funds' shares	NONK	0.6	0.5	0.4	0.3	0.3	0.4	0.5	0.6	0.6
AF.5	Total shares and other equity	NOMW	445.2	598.5	563.3	571.4	622.3	610.5	670.4	697.9	761.3
AF.6	Insurance technical reserves										
AF.62	Prepayments of insurance premiums and reserves for outstanding claims	NONP	10.7	14.7	12.5	12.8	15.7	17.0	17.3	17.6	17.6
AF.7	Other accounts receivable	NONQ	93.0	117.7	116.5	116.8	119.9	122.3	123.1	126.8	126.9
AF.A	**Total financial assets**	NNZB	928.6	1 168.5	1 169.2	1 198.1	1 324.0	1 410.3	1 575.4	1 694.5	1 899.7

1 UK monetary financial institutions

3.1.9 Non-financial corporations
ESA95 sector S.11 Unconsolidated

continued

£ billion

			1999	2000	2001	2002	2003	2004	2005	2006	2007
IV.3	**FINANCIAL BALANCE SHEET** continued at end of period										
AF.L	**Financial liabilities**										
	Currency and deposits										
AF.29	Other deposits	**NOOF**	0.4	0.4	0.4	–	–	–	–	–	–
AF.2	Total currency and deposits	**NONX**	0.4	0.4	0.4	–	–	–	–	–	–
AF.3	Securities other than shares										
AF.331	Short term: money market instruments										
AF.3316	Issued by UK residents other than government or monetary financial institutions	**NOOS**	22.5	24.7	24.6	30.4	26.0	21.8	23.8	21.7	22.2
AF.332	Medium (1 to 5 year) and long term (over 5 year) bonds										
AF.3326	Other medium & long term bonds issued by UK residents or monetary financial institutions	**NOPC**	156.5	198.8	210.3	233.1	255.4	260.4	308.4	342.7	351.6
AF.3	Total securities other than shares	**NOOG**	179.0	223.5	234.9	263.4	281.4	282.3	332.2	364.3	373.8
AF.4	Loans										
AF.41	Short term loans										
AF.411	Loans by UK monetary financial institutions, excluding loans secured on dwellings & financial leasing	**NOPK**	221.7	249.4	266.8	285.5	286.1	299.0	346.6	397.6	477.6
AF.419	Loans by rest of the world monetary financial institutions	**NOPO**	56.9	42.0	63.9	69.1	106.8	158.5	166.0	228.8	224.5
AF.42	Long term loans										
AF.421	Direct investment	**NOPQ**	150.9	180.9	209.3	249.9	241.6	250.6	308.4	325.2	346.3
AF.422	Loans secured on dwellings	**G9JO**	–	–	–	–	–	–	27.1	30.9	34.8
AF.423	Finance leasing	**NOPX**	21.5	21.8	21.7	22.0	22.3	23.6	24.5	23.7	24.2
AF.424	Other long-term loans by UK residents	**NOPY**	48.8	50.4	55.4	56.0	71.3	83.7	77.3	95.6	102.4
AF.429	Other long-term loans by the rest of the world	**NOPZ**	0.4	0.4	0.3	0.4	0.4	0.8	0.8	0.8	0.8
AF.4	Total loans	**NOPI**	500.2	544.9	617.4	682.9	728.5	816.2	950.7	1 102.5	1 210.7
AF.5	Shares and other equity										
AF.51	Shares and other equity, excluding mutual funds' shares										
AF.514	Quoted UK shares	**NOQF**	1 394.4	1 375.5	1 134.7	857.8	1 002.0	1 080.2	1 235.4	1 318.7	1 366.2
AF.515	Unquoted UK shares	**NOQG**	462.5	490.1	455.6	353.0	393.2	423.6	514.1	608.8	693.2
AF.516	Other UK equity (including direct investment in property)	**NOQH**	96.4	97.1	103.9	113.1	121.7	133.8	149.8	143.2	145.0
AF.517	UK shares and bonds issued by other UK residents	**NSQX**	–	–	–	–	–	–	–	–	–
AF.5	Total shares and other equity	**NOQA**	1 953.3	1 962.8	1 694.2	1 323.9	1 517.0	1 637.6	1 899.2	2 070.8	2 204.4
AF.7	Other accounts payable	**NOQU**	137.5	141.5	143.1	143.0	145.4	149.0	153.7	156.0	155.1
AF.L	**Total financial liabilities**	**NONT**	2 770.4	2 873.1	2 689.9	2 413.3	2 672.2	2 885.0	3 335.8	3 693.7	3 944.1
BF.90	**Net financial assets / liabilities**										
AF.A	Total financial assets	**NNZB**	928.6	1 168.5	1 169.2	1 198.1	1 324.0	1 410.3	1 575.4	1 694.5	1 899.7
-AF.L	*less* Total financial liabilities	**−NONT**	−2 770.4	−2 873.1	−2 689.9	−2 413.3	−2 672.2	−2 885.0	−3 335.8	−3 693.7	−3 944.1
BF.90	**Net financial assets (+) / liabilities (-)**	**NYOM**	−1 841.7	−1 704.6	−1 520.8	−1 215.1	−1 348.2	−1 474.6	−1 760.4	−1 999.2	−2 044.3
	Net worth										
AN	Non-financial assets	**CGES**	1 240.8	1 255.6	1 265.7	1 314.5	1 356.2	1 429.5	1 438.6	1 541.0	1 560.9
BF.90	Net financial assets(+)/ liabilities(-)	**NYOM**	−1 841.7	−1 704.6	−1 520.8	−1 215.1	−1 348.2	−1 474.6	−1 760.4	−1 999.2	−2 044.3
B.90	**Net worth**	**CGRV**	−600.9	−449.0	−255.0	99.4	7.9	−45.1	−321.9	−458.2	−483.4

3.2.1 Public non-financial corporations[1]
ESA95 sector S.11001

£ million

			1999	2000	2001	2002	2003	2004	2005	2006
I		**PRODUCTION ACCOUNT**								
		Resources								
P.1		Output								
P.11		Market output	FCZI	29 921	30 991	31 389	34 093	37 479	42 002	43 593	43 548
P.12		Output for own final use	GIRZ	189	183	164	224	205	97	57	10
P.1		Total resources	FCZG	30 110	31 174	31 553	34 317	37 684	42 099	43 650	43 558
		Uses								
P.2		Intermediate consumption	QZLQ	11 957	12 946	13 304	15 620	18 314	21 630	21 633	22 646
B.1g		**Gross Value Added**	FACW	**18 153**	**18 228**	**18 249**	**18 697**	**19 370**	**20 469**	**22 017**	**20 912**
Total		Total uses	FCZG	30 110	31 174	31 553	34 317	37 684	42 099	43 650	43 558
B.1g		**Gross Value Added**	FACW	**18 153**	**18 228**	**18 249**	**18 697**	**19 370**	**20 469**	**22 017**	**20 912**
-K.1		*less* Consumption of fixed capital	-NSRM	-3 394	-3 470	-3 604	-3 900	-4 068	-4 077	-4 288	-4 464
B.1n		Value added, net	FACX	14 759	14 758	14 645	14 797	15 302	16 392	17 729	16 448

1 Public financial corporations are also included to avoid disclosure of commercial information

3.2.2 Public non-financial corporations[1]
ESA95 sector S.11001

£ million

			1999	2000	2001	2002	2003	2004	2005	2006
II		**DISTRIBUTION AND USE OF INCOME ACCOUNTS**								
II.1		**PRIMARY DISTRIBUTION OF INCOME ACCOUNT**								
II.1.1		**GENERATION OF INCOME ACCOUNT** before deduction of fixed capital consumption								
		Resources								
B.1g		**Total resources (Gross Value Added)**	FACW	18 153	18 228	18 249	18 697	19 370	20 469	22 017	20 912
		Uses								
D.1		Compensation of employees								
D.11		Wages and salaries	FAIZ	9 296	9 689	9 949	10 523	10 513	11 910	12 281	10 965
D.12		Employers' social contributions	FAOH	1 639	1 710	1 758	1 859	1 855	1 905	2 089	1 942
D.1		Total	FDDI	10 935	11 399	11 707	12 382	12 368	13 815	14 370	12 907
D.2		Taxes on production and imports, paid								
D.29		Production taxes other than on products	FAOK	109	103	95	95	95	86	86	85
-D.3		*less* Subsidies, received								
-D.39		Production subsidies other than on products	-ARDD	-555	-450	-432	-366	-293	-470	-1 367	-1 952
B.2g		Operating surplus, gross	NRJT	7 664	7 176	6 879	6 586	7 200	7 038	8 928	9 872
B.1g		**Total uses (Gross Value Added)**	FACW	18 153	18 228	18 249	18 697	19 370	20 469	22 017	20 912
-K.1		After deduction of fixed capital consumption	-NSRM	-3 394	-3 470	-3 604	-3 900	-4 068	-4 077	-4 288	-4 464
B.2n		Operating surplus, net	FAOO	4 270	3 706	3 275	2 686	3 132	2 961	4 640	5 408

1 Public financial corporations are also included to avoid disclosure of commercial information

3.2.3 Public non-financial corporations[1]
ESA95 sector S.11001

£ million

			1999	2000	2001	2002	2003	2004	2005	2006	2007
II.1.2	**ALLOCATION OF PRIMARY INCOME ACCOUNT** before deduction of fixed capital consumption											
	Resources											
B.2g	Operating surplus, gross	NRJT	7 664	7 176	6 879	6 586	7 200	7 038	8 928	9 872	9 514
D.4	Property income, received											
D.41	Interest	CPBV	847	898	932	813	771	1 264	1 799	921	787
D.42	Distributed income of corporations	FACT	41	44	63	59	79	62	41	38	54
D.43	Property income reinvested earnings on foreign investments	WUHM	–	–	47	38	67	155	155	216	36
D.44	Property income attributed to insurance policy-holders	FAOT	–	–	–	–	–	–	–	–	–
D.4	Total	FAOP	888	942	1 042	910	917	1 481	1 995	1 175	877
Total	Total resources	FAOU	8 552	8 118	7 921	7 496	8 117	8 519	10 923	11 047	10 391
	Uses											
D.4	Property income, paid											
D.41	Interest	XAQZ	826	304	587	649	722	1 317	1 246	1 329	1 384
D.42	Distributed income of corporations	ZOYB	3 592	3 488	2 627	1 729	1 443	866	807	696	593
D.45	Rent	FAOZ	–	–	–	–	–	–	–	–	–
D.4	Total	FAOV	4 418	3 792	3 214	2 378	2 165	2 183	2 053	2 025	1 977
B.5g	**Balance of primary incomes, gross**	NRJX	4 134	4 326	4 707	5 118	5 952	6 336	8 870	9 022	8 414
Total	Total uses	FAOU	8 552	8 118	7 921	7 496	8 117	8 519	10 923	11 047	10 391
-K.1	After deduction of fixed capital consumption	–NSRM	–3 394	–3 470	–3 604	–3 900	–4 068	–4 077	–4 288	–4 464	–4 647
B.5n	Balance of primary incomes, net	FARX	740	856	1 103	1 218	1 884	2 259	4 582	4 558	3 767

1 Public financial corporations are also included to avoid disclosure of commercial information

3.2.4 Public non-financial corporations[1]
ESA95 sector S.11001

£ million

			1999	2000	2001	2002	2003	2004	2005	2006	2007
II.2	**SECONDARY DISTRIBUTION OF INCOME ACCOUNT**											
	Resources											
B.5g	**Balance of primary incomes, gross**	NRJX	4 134	4 326	4 707	5 118	5 952	6 336	8 870	9 022	8 414
D.61	Social contributions											
D.612	Imputed social contributions	EWRS	121	108	128	138	131	131	132	135	137
D.7	Current transfers other than taxes, social contributions and benefits											
D.72	Net non-life insurance claims	FDDF	–	–	–	–	–	–	–	–	–
D.75	Miscellaneous current transfers	CY89	109	85	122	147	124	28	–	–	–
D.7	Total	FDEK	109	85	122	147	124	28	–	–	–
Total	Total resources	FDDH	4 364	4 519	4 957	5 403	6 207	6 495	9 002	9 157	8 551
	Uses											
D.5	Current taxes on income, wealth etc.											
D.51	Taxes on income	FCCS	340	218	90	61	94	75	141	372	225
D.62	Social benefits other than social transfers in kind	EWRS	121	108	128	138	131	131	132	135	137
D.7	Current transfers other than taxes, social contributions and benefits											
D.71	Net non-life insurance premiums	FDDM	–	–	–	–	–	–	–	–	–
D.75	Miscellaneous Current Transfers	CY87	140	140	95	58	28	5	–	–	–
D.7	Total	FDDL	140	140	95	58	28	5	–	–	–
B.6g	**Gross Disposable Income**	NRKD	3 763	4 053	4 644	5 146	5 954	6 284	8 729	8 650	8 189
Total	Total uses	FDDH	4 364	4 519	4 957	5 403	6 207	6 495	9 002	9 157	8 551
-K.1	After deduction of fixed capital consumption	–NSRM	–3 394	–3 470	–3 604	–3 900	–4 068	–4 077	–4 288	–4 464	–4 647
B.6n	Disposable income, net	FDDP	369	583	1 040	1 246	1 886	2 207	4 441	4 186	3 542

1 Public financial corporations are also included to avoid disclosure of commercial information

3.2.6 Public non-financial corporations
ESA95 sector S.11001

£ million

			1999	2000	2001	2002	2003	2004	2005	2006	2007
II.4.1	**USE OF DISPOSABLE INCOME ACCOUNT**										
	Resources										
B.6g	**Total resources (Gross Disposable Income)**	**NRKD**	**3 763**	**4 053**	**4 644**	**5 146**	**5 954**	**6 284**	**8 729**	**8 650**	**8 189**
	Uses										
B.8g	**Total uses (Gross Saving)**	**NRKD**	**3 763**	**4 053**	**4 644**	**5 146**	**5 954**	**6 284**	**8 729**	**8 650**	**8 189**
-K.1	After deduction of fixed capital consumption	**−NSRM**	−3 394	−3 470	−3 604	−3 900	−4 068	−4 077	−4 288	−4 464	−4 647
B.8n	Saving, net	**FDDP**	369	583	1 040	1 246	1 886	2 207	4 441	4 186	3 542

3.2.7 Public non-financial corporations[1]
ESA95 sector S.11001

£ million

			1999	2000	2001	2002	2003	2004	2005	2006	2007
III	ACCUMULATION ACCOUNTS										
III.1	CAPITAL ACCOUNT										
III.1.1	CHANGE IN NET WORTH DUE TO SAVING AND CAPITAL TRANSFERS										
	Changes in liabilities and net worth										
B.8g	**Gross Saving**	NRKD	3 763	4 053	4 644	5 146	5 954	6 284	8 729	8 650	8 189
D.9	Capital transfers receivable										
D.92	Investment grants	FDBV	1 583	1 329	797	764	504	794	1 658	1 566	477
D.99	Other capital transfers	NZGD	41	24	42	91	42	42	11 682	333	66
D.9	Total	FDBU	1 624	1 353	839	855	546	836	13 340	1 899	543
-D.9	*less* Capital transfers payable										
-D.99	Other capital transfers	−ZMLL	–	–	–	–	–	–	−801	−122	−187
B.10.1g	Total change in liabilities and net worth	FDEG	5 387	5 406	5 483	6 001	6 500	7 120	21 268	10 427	8 545
	Changes in assets										
B.10.1g	Changes in net worth due to gross saving and capital transfers	FDEG	5 387	5 406	5 483	6 001	6 500	7 120	21 268	10 427	8 545
-K.1	After deduction of fixed capital consumption	−NSRM	−3 394	−3 470	−3 604	−3 900	−4 068	−4 077	−4 288	−4 464	−4 647
B.10.1n	Changes in net worth due to net saving and capital transfers	FDED	1 993	1 936	1 879	2 101	2 432	3 043	16 980	5 963	3 898
III.1.2	ACQUISITION OF NON-FINANCIAL ASSETS ACCOUNT										
	Changes in liabilities and net worth										
B.10.1n	Changes in net worth due to net saving and capital transfers	FDED	1 993	1 936	1 879	2 101	2 432	3 043	16 980	5 963	3 898
K.1	Consumption of fixed capital	NSRM	3 394	3 470	3 604	3 900	4 068	4 077	4 288	4 464	4 647
B.10.1g	Total change in liabilities and net worth	FDEG	5 387	5 406	5 483	6 001	6 500	7 120	21 268	10 427	8 545
	Changes in assets										
P.5	Gross capital formation										
P.51	Gross fixed capital formation	FCCJ	2 712	2 354	3 183	3 830	1 857	1 260	20 576	5 440	6 191
P.52	Changes in inventories	DHHL	−120	−223	9	−30	11	1 738	−186	−40	−160
P.5	Total	FDEH	2 592	2 131	3 192	3 800	1 868	2 998	20 390	5 400	6 031
K.2	Acquisitions less disposals of non-produced non-financial assets	FDEJ	−2	13	70	176	282	346	428	512	484
B.9g	**Net lending (+) / net borrowing (-)**	CPCM	**2 797**	**3 262**	**2 221**	**2 025**	**4 350**	**3 776**	**450**	**4 515**	**2 030**
Total	Total change in assets	FDEG	5 387	5 406	5 483	6 001	6 500	7 120	21 268	10 427	8 545

1 Public financial corporations are also included to avoid disclosure of commercial information

3.2.8 Public non-financial corporations
ESA95 sector S.11001 Unconsolidated

£ million

			1999	2000	2001	2002	2003	2004	2005	2006	2007
III.2	FINANCIAL ACCOUNT										
F.A	**Net acquisition of financial assets**										
F.2	Currency and deposits										
F.21	Currency	NCXV	125	116	90	−143	141	−295	−16	23	55
F.22	Transferable deposits										
F.2211	Sterling deposits with UK banks	NCXY	8	581	748	63	−334	−296	−423	1 358	−766
F.2212	Foreign currency deposits with UK banks	NCXZ	1	68	−1	−42	29	−3	33	1 201	−1 191
F.2213	Sterling deposits with building societies	NCYA	−10	−92	102	−73	−28	−2	34	−65	−32
F.229	Deposits with rest of the world monetary financial institutions	NCYB	–	–	–	−30	3	−3	–	–	–
F.29	Other deposits	NCYC	−466	−128	−842	477	−626	592	534	345	80
F.2	Total currency and deposits	NCXU	−342	545	97	252	−815	−7	162	2 862	−1 854
F.3	Securities other than shares										
F.331	Short term: money market instruments										
F.3311	Issued by UK central government	NCYF	140	−50	−90	–	–	–	–	–	400
F.3315	Issued by UK monetary financial institutions	NCYK	–	–	–	–	–	–	–	–	–
F.3316	Issued by other UK residents	NCYP	−191	–	–	223	104	−943	240	324	−209
F.332	Medium (1 to 5 year) and long term (over 5 year) bonds										
F.3321	Issued by UK central government	NCYS	362	−183	−411	−67	−196	75	−789	−1 972	217
F.3326	Other medium & long term bonds issued by UK residents	NCYZ	–	–	–	–	–	–	–	–	–
F.3329	Long term bonds issued by the rest of the world	NCZA	–	–	–	–	–	–	–	–	–
F.34	Financial derivatives	NSUH	3	−92	−8	10	9	8	1	−1	10
F.3	Total securities other than shares	NCYD	314	−325	−509	166	−83	−860	−548	−1 649	418
F.4	Loans										
F.42	Long term loans										
F.421	Direct investment loans	CFZI	–	–	115	120	−10	2	–	−346	–
F.422	Loans secured on dwellings	NCZQ	−1	−1	–	–	–	–	–	–	–
F.424	Other long-term loans by UK residents	NCZV	90	−171	−90	−489	−380	−421	−1 769	−2 909	−648
F.4	Total loans	NCZF	89	−172	25	−369	−390	−419	−1 769	−3 255	−648
F.5	Shares and other equity										
F.51	Shares and other equity, excluding mutual funds' shares										
F.514	Quoted UK shares	NEBC	30	16	13	23	24	24	−243	–	–
F.515	Unquoted UK shares	NEBD	–	–	269	510	−2	−2	–	−1 248	–
F.517	UK shares and bonds issued by other UK residents	NSPN	–	–	–	–	–	–	–	–	–
F.519	Shares and other equity issued by the rest of the world	NEBH	290	570	97	158	−151	−64	14	−1 761	36
F.5	Total shares and other equity	NCZX	320	586	379	691	−129	−42	−229	−3 009	36
F.6	Insurance technical reserves										
F.62	Prepayments of insurance premiums and reserves for outstanding claims	NEBQ	–	–	–	–	–	–	–	–	–
F.7	Other accounts receivable	NEBR	−481	−302	−19	328	899	1 929	1 993	3 472	1 423
F.A	**Total net acquisition of financial assets**	NCXQ	−100	332	−27	1 068	−518	601	−391	−1 579	−625

3.2.8 Public non-financial corporations
ESA95 sector S.11001 Unconsolidated

continued

£ million

			1999	2000	2001	2002	2003	2004	2005	2006	2007
III.2	**FINANCIAL ACCOUNT** continued										
F.L	**Net acquisition of financial liabilities**										
F.2	Currency & deposits										
F.29	Other deposits	**WUGZ**	28	29	30	18	–	–	–	–	–
	Total currency & deposits	**–A4FK**	28	29	30	18	–	–	–	–	–
F.3	Securities other than shares										
F.332	Medium (1 to 5 year) and long term (over 5 year) bonds										
F.3326	Other medium & long term bonds issued by UK residents or monetary financial institutions	**NEOF**	–	160	–32	–1 541	–	–	856	–620	–42
F.345	Financial derivatitives issued by UK residents	**CY7U**	–42	–110	–184	–204	–138	–28	–	–	–
F.3	Total securities other than shares	**NENJ**	–42	50	–216	–1 745	–138	–28	856	–620	–42
F.4	Loans										
F.41	Short term loans										
F.411	Loans by UK monetary financial institutions, excluding loans secured on dwellings & financial leasing	**NEON**	–57	83	–153	321	–112	332	–276	12	194
F.42	Long term loans										
F.421	Direct investment	**–CFZJ**	–	–	–	–	–	–	–	–108	–
F.423	Finance leasing	**NEPA**	44	226	–111	–56	–41	472	536	–7	117
F.424	Other long-term loans by UK residents	**NEPB**	–687	–863	–290	3 019	1 661	454	–158	–187	41
F.429	Other long-term loans by the rest of the world	**NEPC**	–	–	–	–	–	283	–7	–12	–6
F.4	Total loans	**NEOL**	–700	–554	–554	3 284	1 508	1 541	95	–302	346
F.5	Shares and other equity										
F.51	Shares and other equity, excluding mutual funds' shares										
F.515	Unquoted UK shares	**NEPJ**	–	–	–	–	–	29	–495	42	–2 060
F.516	Other UK equity (including direct investment in property)	**NEPK**	–2 072	–2 350	–2 551	–3 096	–5 495	–3 795	–3 850	–3 543	–2 171
F.517	UK shares and bonds issued by other UK residents	**NSPO**	–	–	–	–	–	–	–	–	–
F.5	Total shares and other equity	**NEPD**	–2 072	–2 350	–2 551	–3 096	–5 495	–3 766	–4 345	–3 501	–4 231
F.7	Other accounts payable	**NEPX**	–104	326	339	159	–136	46	2 531	–1 592	319
F.L	**Total net acquisition of financial liabilities**	**NEBU**	–2 890	–2 499	–2 952	–1 380	–4 261	–2 207	–863	–6 015	–3 608
B.9	**Net lending / borrowing**										
F.A	Total net acquisition of financial assets	**NCXQ**	–100	332	–27	1 068	–518	601	–391	–1 579	–625
-F.L	*less* Total net acquisition of financial liabilities	**–NEBU**	2 890	2 499	2 952	1 380	4 261	2 207	863	6 015	3 608
B.9f	Net lending (+) / net borrowing (-), from financial account	**NZEC**	2 790	2 831	2 925	2 448	3 743	2 808	472	4 436	2 983
dB.9f	Statistical discrepancy	**NYPI**	7	431	–704	–423	607	968	–22	79	–953
B.9g	**Net lending (+) / net borrowing (-), from capital account**	**CPCM**	**2 797**	**3 262**	**2 221**	**2 025**	**4 350**	**3 776**	**450**	**4 515**	**2 030**

3.2.9 Public non-financial corporations
ESA95 sector S.11001

£ billion

			1999	2000	2001	2002	2003	2004	2005	2006	2007
IV.3	**FINANCIAL BALANCE SHEET** at end of period										
AN	**Non-financial assets**	CGGN	126.6	125.8	137.2	158.1	160.3	173.4	185.6	177.6	183.0
AF.A	**Financial assets**										
AF.2	Currency and deposits										
AF.21	Currency	NKDS	0.9	1.0	0.9	0.8	0.9	0.6	0.6	0.6	0.7
AF.22	Transferable deposits										
AF.221	Deposits with UK monetary financial institutions	NKDU	3.5	4.4	6.1	6.0	4.6	4.9	4.5	6.8	4.3
AF.229	Deposits with rest of the world monetary financial institutions	NKDY	–	–	–	–	–	–	–	–	–
AF.29	Other deposits	NKDZ	3.4	3.5	2.8	3.1	1.5	2.1	3.5	3.9	3.9
AF.2	Total currency and deposits	NKDR	7.8	8.9	9.8	10.0	7.0	7.7	8.7	11.3	8.9
AF.3	Securities other than shares										
AF.331	Short term: money market instruments										
AF.3311	Issued by UK central government	NKEC	0.1	0.1	–	–	–	–	–	–	0.4
AF.3315	Issued by UK monetary financial institutions	NKEH	0.4	0.4	0.4	0.4	0.4	0.4	0.4	0.4	0.4
AF.3316	Issued by other UK residents	NKEM	0.1	0.1	0.1	0.2	0.3	1.2	1.4	1.7	1.5
AF.332	Medium (1 to 5 year) and long term (over 5 year) bonds										
AF.3321	Issued by UK central government	NKEP	3.7	3.5	3.1	3.1	2.9	3.3	2.5	0.5	0.7
AF.3322	Issued by UK local government	NKES	–	–	–	–	–	–	–	–	–
AF.3326	Other medium & long term bonds issued by UK residents	NKEW	–	–	–	–	–	–	–	–	–
AF.3	Total securities other than shares	NKEA	4.4	4.1	3.6	3.7	3.6	4.9	4.3	2.6	3.0
AF.4	Loans										
AF.42	Long term loans										
AF.421	Direct investment loans	ZYBN	–	–	0.1	0.5	0.4	0.3	0.3	–	–
AF.422	Loans secured on dwellings	NKFN	–	–	–	–	–	–	–	–	–
AF.424	Other long-term loans by UK residents	NKFS	4.9	4.1	4.2	3.9	4.0	4.0	3.7	3.3	2.9
AF.4	Total loans	NKFC	4.9	4.1	4.3	4.4	4.5	4.3	4.0	3.3	2.9
AF.5	Shares and other equity										
AF.51	Shares and other equity, excluding mutual funds' shares										
AF.514	Quoted UK shares	NKFZ	0.2	0.2	0.2	0.2	0.2	0.2	–	–	–
AF.515	Unquoted UK shares	NKGA	0.3	0.3	0.3	0.3	0.3	0.3	0.3	0.3	0.3
AF.517	UK shares and bonds issued by other UK residents	NSOL	–	–	–	–	–	–	–	–	–
AF.519	Shares and other equity issued by the rest of the world	NKGE	1.2	1.8	0.8	1.0	1.1	1.6	0.5	0.5	0.3
AF.5	Total shares and other equity	NKFU	1.7	2.3	1.3	1.5	1.6	2.1	0.8	0.8	0.7
AF.6	Insurance technical reserves										
AF.62	Prepayments of insurance premiums and reserves for outstanding claims	NKGN	–	–	–	–	–	–	–	–	–
AF.7	Other accounts receivable	NKGO	4.9	5.4	5.6	6.4	7.5	9.5	11.4	16.1	17.3
AF.A	**Total financial assets**	NKFB	23.7	24.8	24.6	26.0	24.3	28.4	29.2	34.2	32.8

3.2.9 Public non-financial corporations
ESA95 sector S.11001 Unconsolidated

continued

£ billion

			1999	2000	2001	2002	2003	2004	2005	2006	2007
IV.3	**FINANCIAL BALANCE SHEET** continued at end of period										
AF.L	**Financial liabilities**										
AF.2 AF.29	Currency & deposits Other deposits	**NKHD**	0.4	0.4	0.4	–	–	–	–	–	–
AF.2	Total currency & deposits	**NKGV**	0.4	0.4	0.4	–	–	–	–	–	–
AF.3 AF.332 AF.3326	Securities other than shares Medium (1 to 5 year) and long term (over 5 year) bonds Other medium & long term bonds issued by UK residents or monetary financial institutions	**NKIA**	1.1	0.4	0.4	0.9	1.3	5.8	7.0	6.3	8.5
AF.3	Total securities other than shares	**NKHE**	1.1	0.4	0.4	0.9	1.3	5.8	7.0	6.3	8.5
AF.4 AF.41 AF.411	Loans Short term loans Loans by UK monetary financial institutions, excluding loans secured on dwellings & financial leasing	**NKII**	0.3	0.4	0.2	0.6	0.5	0.5	0.5	0.6	0.7
AF.419	Loans by rest of the world monetary financial institutions	**ZMEW**	–	–	–	–	–	–	–	–	–
AF.42 AF.421	Long term loans Direct investment	**ZYBO**	–	–	–	–	–	–		0.2	0.2
AF.423	Finance leasing	**NKIV**	0.4	0.6	0.5	0.4	0.4	1.1	1.6	0.3	0.4
AF.424	Other long-term loans by UK residents	**NKIW**	4.4	3.2	2.4	11.3	3.3	4.4	4.2	4.1	4.1
AF.429	Other long-term loans by the rest of the world	**NKIX**	–	–	–	–	–	0.4	0.4	0.4	0.4
AF.4	Total loans	**NKIG**	5.2	4.2	3.0	12.3	4.1	6.4	6.8	5.6	5.9
AF.5 AF.51 AF.514	Shares and other equity Shares and other equity, excluding mutual funds' shares Quoted UK shares	**C308**	–	–	–	–	–		3.0	3.2	5.6
AF.515	Unquoted UK shares	**NKJE**	0.5	0.5	0.8	0.8	0.8	1.5	0.9	0.8	−1.2
AF.516	Other UK equity	**H406**	83.3	82.3	88.4	95.8	104.4	114.6	130.0	121.7	118.8
AF.517	UK shares and bonds issued by other UK residents	**NSOM**	–	–	–	–	–	–	–	–	–
AF.5	Total shares and other equity	**NKIY**	83.8	82.7	89.2	96.6	105.3	116.1	133.9	125.7	123.2
AF.7	Other accounts payable	**NKJS**	10.2	12.8	13.1	13.7	13.8	14.7	16.6	15.3	15.2
AF.L	**Total financial liabilities**	**NKIF**	100.7	100.6	106.1	123.6	124.4	142.9	164.3	152.9	152.8
BF.90	**Net financial assets / liabilities**										
AF.A -AF.L	Total financial assets *less* Total financial liabilities	**NKFB** **−NKIF**	23.7 −100.7	24.8 −100.6	24.6 −106.1	26.0 −123.6	24.3 −124.4	28.4 −142.9	29.2 −164.3	34.2 −152.9	32.8 −152.8
BF.90	**Net financial assets (+) / liabilities (-)**	**NYOP**	−77.1	−75.8	−81.5	−97.6	−100.2	−114.4	−135.1	−118.7	−120.0
	Net worth										
AN BF.90	Non-financial assets Net financial assets (+) / liabilities (-)	**CGGN** **NYOP**	126.6 −77.1	125.8 −75.8	137.2 −81.5	158.1 −97.6	160.3 −100.2	173.4 −114.4	185.6 −135.1	177.6 −118.7	183.0 −120.0
B.90	**Net worth**	**CGRW**	49.5	50.0	55.7	60.5	60.1	58.9	50.6	58.9	63.0

3.3.1 Private non-financial corporations

ESA95 sectors S.11002 National controlled and S.11003 Foreign controlled

£ million

			1999	2000	2001	2002	2003	2004	2005	2006
I	**PRODUCTION ACCOUNT**									
	Resources									
P.1	Output									
P.11	Market output	**FBXS**	1 084 953	1 146 220	1 182 249	1 209 542	1 256 935	1 314 821	1 383 646	1 457 667
P.12	Output for own final use	**FDCG**	8 525	9 265	10 129	10 503	11 924	13 089	13 921	15 007
P.1	Total resources	**FBXR**	1 093 478	1 155 485	1 192 378	1 220 045	1 268 859	1 327 910	1 397 567	1 472 674
	Uses									
P.2	Intermediate consumption	**FARP**	580 611	612 854	629 244	639 828	661 924	693 965	738 610	779 078
B.1g	**Gross Value Added**	**FARR**	**512 867**	**542 631**	**563 134**	**580 217**	**606 935**	**633 945**	**658 957**	**693 596**
Total	Total uses	**FBXR**	1 093 478	1 155 485	1 192 378	1 220 045	1 268 859	1 327 910	1 397 567	1 472 674
B.1g	**Gross Value Added**	**FARR**	**512 867**	**542 631**	**563 134**	**580 217**	**606 935**	**633 945**	**658 957**	**693 596**
-K.1	*less* Consumption of fixed capital	**−NSRK**	−60 503	−62 950	−64 758	−66 647	−68 530	−71 482	−72 990	−75 896
B.1n	Value added, net	**FARS**	452 364	479 681	498 376	513 570	538 405	562 463	585 967	617 700

3.3.2 Private non-financial corporations

ESA95 sectors S.11002 National controlled and S.11003 Foreign controlled

£ million

			1999	2000	2001	2002	2003	2004	2005	2006
II	**DISTRIBUTION AND USE OF INCOME ACCOUNTS**									
II.1	**PRIMARY DISTRIBUTION OF INCOME ACCOUNT**									
II.1.1	**GENERATION OF INCOME ACCOUNT**									
	before deduction of fixed capital consumption									
	Resources									
B.1g	**Total resources (Gross Value Added)**	**FARR**	512 867	542 631	563 134	580 217	606 935	633 945	658 957	693 596
	Uses									
D.1	Compensation of employees									
D.11	Wages and salaries	**FAAX**	284 246	304 014	320 963	329 641	336 525	345 042	359 276	372 259
D.12	Employers' social contributions	**FABH**	37 478	40 921	43 169	46 136	53 518	57 884	60 515	66 445
D.1	Total	**FBDA**	321 724	344 935	364 132	375 777	390 043	402 926	419 791	438 704
D.2	Taxes on production and imports, paid									
D.29	Production taxes other than on products	**FACQ**	14 783	15 705	16 075	16 584	16 942	17 260	18 073	19 117
-D.39	Production subsidies other than on products	**−JQJW**	−108	−124	−230	−588	−1 141	−1 092	−1 082	−1 141
B.2g	Operating surplus, gross	**NRJK**	176 468	182 115	183 157	188 444	201 091	214 851	222 175	236 916
B.1g	**Total uses (Gross Value Added)**	**FARR**	**512 867**	**542 631**	**563 134**	**580 217**	**606 935**	**633 945**	**658 957**	**693 596**
-K.1	After deduction of fixed capital consumption	**−NSRK**	−60 503	−62 950	−64 758	−66 647	−68 530	−71 482	−72 990	−75 896
B.2n	Operating surplus, net	**FACU**	115 965	119 165	118 399	121 797	132 561	143 369	149 185	161 020

3.3.3 Private non-financial corporations

ESA95 sectors S.11002 National controlled and S.11003 Foreign controlled

£ million

			1999	2000	2001	2002	2003	2004	2005	2006	2007
II.1.2	**ALLOCATION OF PRIMARY INCOME ACCOUNT** before deduction of fixed capital consumption										
	Resources										
B.2g	Operating surplus, gross[1]	NRJK	176 468	182 115	183 157	188 444	201 091	214 851	222 175	236 916	253 355
D.4	Property income, received										
D.41	Interest	DSZR	10 869	13 700	12 245	8 517	8 956	12 881	15 590	23 641	28 996
D.42	Distributed income of corporations	DSZS	21 486	26 500	37 415	30 491	50 184	42 902	46 683	44 544	38 484
D.43	Reinvested earnings on direct foreign investment	HDVR	16 214	20 118	22 950	26 893	12 492	22 713	33 199	36 426	44 754
D.44	Property income attributed to insurance policy-holders	FCFP	338	290	333	300	401	368	582	590	428
D.45	Rent	FAOL	117	117	117	118	120	122	122	124	124
D.4	Total	FACV	49 024	60 725	73 060	66 319	72 153	78 986	96 176	105 325	112 786
Total	Total resources	FCFQ	225 492	242 840	256 217	254 763	273 244	293 837	318 351	342 241	366 141
	Uses										
D.4	Property income, paid										
D.41	Interest	DSZV	23 976	30 101	30 074	28 396	28 870	33 620	38 092	43 900	55 168
D.42	Distributed income of corporations	NVDC	82 835	80 699	101 008	85 552	92 292	92 725	106 046	104 749	97 790
	Of which: Dividend payments	NETZ	61 088	55 846	77 516	61 580	71 096	72 689	82 890	83 356	81 400
D.43	Reinvested earnings on direct foreign investment	HDVB	2 776	7 348	1 699	1 614	3 955	6 325	4 983	16 802	23 676
D.45	Rent	FCFU	565	1 325	1 955	1 939	1 603	1 221	1 268	1 265	1 282
D.4	Total	FCFR	110 152	119 473	134 736	117 501	126 720	133 891	150 389	166 716	177 916
B.5g	**Balance of primary incomes, gross**	NRJM	**115 340**	**123 367**	**121 481**	**137 262**	**146 524**	**159 946**	**167 962**	**175 525**	**188 225**
Total	Total uses	FCFQ	225 492	242 840	256 217	254 763	273 244	293 837	318 351	342 241	366 141
-K.1	After deduction of fixed capital consumption	-NSRK	-60 503	-62 950	-64 758	-66 647	-68 530	-71 482	-72 990	-75 896	-78 918
B.5n	Balance of primary incomes, net	FCFW	54 837	60 417	56 723	70 615	77 994	88 464	94 972	99 629	109 307

1 Companies gross trading profits and rental of buildings less holding gains of inventories, details of which are shown at Table C: The Sector Accounts Key Economic Indicators.

3.3.4 Private non-financial corporations

ESA95 sectors S.11002 National controlled and S.11003 Foreign controlled

£ million

			1999	2000	2001	2002	2003	2004	2005	2006	2007
II.2	**SECONDARY DISTRIBUTION OF INCOME ACCOUNT**										
	Resources										
B.5g	**Balance of primary incomes, gross**	NRJM	**115 340**	**123 367**	**121 481**	**137 262**	**146 524**	**159 946**	**167 962**	**175 525**	**188 225**
D.61	Social contributions										
D.612	Imputed social contributions	EWRT	3 724	4 067	4 229	4 437	4 098	3 679	3 403	3 290	3 371
D.7	Current transfers other than taxes, social contributions and benefits										
D.72	Net non-life insurance claims	FDBA	3 719	5 762	3 714	5 396	6 000	6 522	7 261	8 368	6 376
Total	Total resources	FDBC	122 783	133 196	129 424	147 095	156 622	170 147	178 626	187 183	197 972
	Uses										
D.5	Current taxes on income, wealth etc.										
D.51	Taxes on income	FCCP	22 608	24 279	23 087	23 977	23 608	27 293	33 461	36 811	38 035
D.62	Social benefits other than social transfers in kind	EWRT	3 724	4 067	4 229	4 437	4 098	3 679	3 403	3 290	3 371
D.7	Current transfers other than taxes, social contributions and benefits										
D.71	Net non-life insurance premiums	FDBH	3 719	5 762	3 714	5 396	6 000	6 522	7 261	8 368	6 376
D.75	Miscellaneous current transfers	FDBI	569	413	411	422	434	446	488	474	476
D.7	Total	FCCN	4 288	6 175	4 125	5 818	6 434	6 968	7 749	8 842	6 852
B.6g	**Gross Disposable Income**	NRJQ	**92 163**	**98 675**	**97 983**	**112 863**	**122 482**	**132 207**	**134 013**	**138 240**	**149 714**
Total	Total uses	FDBC	122 783	133 196	129 424	147 095	156 622	170 147	178 626	187 183	197 972
-K.1	After deduction of fixed capital consumption	-NSRK	-60 503	-62 950	-64 758	-66 647	-68 530	-71 482	-72 990	-75 896	-78 918
B.6n	Disposable income, net	FDBK	31 660	35 725	33 225	46 216	53 952	60 725	61 023	62 344	70 796

3.3.6 Private non-financial corporations
ESA95 sectors S.11002 National controlled and S.11003 Foreign controlled

£ million

			1999	2000	2001	2002	2003	2004	2005	2006	2007
II.4.1	**USE OF DISPOSABLE INCOME ACCOUNT**										
	Resources										
B.6g	**Total resources (Gross Disposable Income)**	NRJQ	92 163	98 675	97 983	112 863	122 482	132 207	134 013	138 240	149 714
	Uses										
B.8g	**Total uses (Gross Saving)**	NRJQ	92 163	98 675	97 983	112 863	122 482	132 207	134 013	138 240	149 714
-K.1	After deduction of fixed capital consumption	−NSRK	−60 503	−62 950	−64 758	−66 647	−68 530	−71 482	−72 990	−75 896	−78 918
B.8n	Saving, net	FDBK	31 660	35 725	33 225	46 216	53 952	60 725	61 023	62 344	70 796

3.3.7 Private non-financial corporations

ESA95 sectors S.11002 National controlled and S.11003 Foreign controlled

£ million

			1999	2000	2001	2002	2003	2004	2005	2006	2007
III	**ACCUMULATION ACCOUNTS**										
III.1	**CAPITAL ACCOUNT**										
III.1.1	**CHANGE IN NET WORTH DUE TO SAVING AND CAPITAL TRANSFERS**										
	Changes in liabilities and net worth										
B.8g	**Gross Saving**	**NRJQ**	**92 163**	**98 675**	**97 983**	**112 863**	**122 482**	**132 207**	**134 013**	**138 240**	**149 714**
D.9	Capital transfers receivable										
D.92	Investment grants	**AIBR**	1 409	1 506	3 048	3 131	5 059	4 929	5 141	6 107	7 814
D.99	Other capital transfers	**LNZM**	109	118	873	93	106	94	119	116	111
-D.9	*less* Capital transfers payable										
-D.91	Capital taxes	**-QYKB**	–	–	–	–	–	–	–	–	–
-D.99	Other capital transfers	**-CISB**	–216	–290	–285	–492	–575	–419	–456	–508	–571
-D.9	Total	**-FCFX**	–216	–290	–285	–492	–575	–419	–456	–508	–571
B.10.1g	Total change in liabilities and net worth	**NRMG**	93 465	100 009	101 619	115 595	127 072	136 811	138 817	143 955	157 068
	Changes in assets										
B.10.1g	Changes in net worth due to gross saving and capital transfers	**NRMG**	93 465	100 009	101 619	115 595	127 072	136 811	138 817	143 955	157 068
-K.1	After deduction of fixed capital consumption	**-NSRK**	–60 503	–62 950	–64 758	–66 647	–68 530	–71 482	–72 990	–75 896	–78 918
B.10.1n	Changes in net worth due to net saving and capital transfers	**FDCH**	32 962	37 059	36 861	48 948	58 542	65 329	65 827	68 059	78 150
III.1.2	**ACQUISITION OF NON-FINANCIAL ASSETS ACCOUNT**										
	Changes in liabilities and net worth										
B.10.1n	Changes in net worth due to net saving and capital transfers	**FDCH**	32 962	37 059	36 861	48 948	58 542	65 329	65 827	68 059	78 150
K.1	Consumption of fixed capital	**NSRK**	60 503	62 950	64 758	66 647	68 530	71 482	72 990	75 896	78 918
B.10.1g	Total change in liabilities and net worth	**NRMG**	93 465	100 009	101 619	115 595	127 072	136 811	138 817	143 955	157 068
	Changes in assets										
P.5	Gross capital formation										
P.51	Gross fixed capital formation	**FDBM**	98 989	101 597	103 127	103 182	103 855	105 535	110 459	115 733	127 957
P.52	Changes in inventories	**DLQX**	6 174	5 512	5 941	2 677	3 734	2 829	5 377	4 182	7 581
P.53	Acquisitions less disposals of valuables	**NPOV**	–17	–75	–	–43	–97	–99	–171	–42	–22
P.5	Total	**FDCL**	105 146	107 034	109 068	105 816	107 492	108 265	115 665	119 873	135 516
K.2	Acquisitions less disposals of non-produced non-financial assets	**FDCN**	1 053	851	1 138	1 255	959	1 339	1 317	869	956
B.9	**Net lending (+) / net borrowing (-)**	**DTAL**	**–12 734**	**–7 876**	**–8 587**	**8 524**	**18 621**	**27 207**	**21 835**	**23 213**	**20 596**
Total	Total change in assets	**NRMG**	93 465	100 009	101 619	115 595	127 072	136 811	138 817	143 955	157 068

3.3.8 Private non-financial corporations

ESA95 sectors S.11002 National controlled and S.11003 Foreign controlled. Unconsolidated

£ million

			1999	2000	2001	2002	2003	2004	2005	2006	2007
III.2	**FINANCIAL ACCOUNT**										
F.A	**Net acquisition of financial assets**										
F.2	Currency and deposits										
F.21	Currency	NEQF	253	192	187	153	197	248	198	249	238
F.22	Transferable deposits										
F.2211	Sterling deposits with UK banks	NEQI	7 482	10 542	9 335	8 858	11 115	12 337	20 374	22 655	15 659
F.2212	Foreign currency deposits with UK banks	NEQJ	2 445	3 499	1 336	−232	3 811	2 562	2 607	1 452	4 574
F.2213	Sterling deposits with building societies	NEQK	166	−42	199	−4	273	−311	−98	364	244
F.229	Deposits with rest of the world monetary financial institutions	NEQL	4 105	7 804	21 011	9 977	38 364	54 987	35 482	36 770	72 738
F.29	Other deposits	NEQM	−229	−123	276	632	228	−138	129	373	34
F.2	Total currency and deposits	NEQE	14 222	21 872	32 344	19 384	53 988	69 685	58 692	61 863	93 487
F.3	Securities other than shares										
F.331	Short term: money market instruments										
F.3311	Issued by UK central government	NEQP	4	−28	−10	–	2	−4	1	–	8
F.3315	Issued by UK monetary financial institutions	NEQU	−2 003	−81	234	230	622	77	−787	1 612	3 020
F.3316	Issued by other UK residents	NEQZ	16	−2 797	136	−2 331	717	556	−1 844	4 078	1 868
F.3319	Issued by the rest of the world	NERA	722	1 110	1 912	1 110	3 798	615	1 078	4 758	−9 820
F.332	Medium (1 to 5 year) and long term (over 5 year) bonds										
F.3321	Issued by UK central government	NERC	−815	413	−168	215	−139	−42	−113	−29	275
F.3325	Medium term bonds issued by UK MFIs[1]	NERG	54	−237	−333	42	167	−23	395	466	658
F.3326	Other medium & long term bonds issued by UK residents	NERJ	−1 347	1 141	1 784	559	−685	−389	−3 421	−537	3 733
F.3329	Long term bonds issued by the rest of the world	NERK	−934	1 792	1 759	−601	2 213	437	892	−2 186	169
F.3	Total securities other than shares	NEQN	−4 303	1 313	5 314	−776	6 695	1 227	−3 799	8 162	−89
F.4	Loans										
F.42	Long term loans										
F.4211	Outward direct investment	NERY	15 371	11 607	9 656	16 366	10 155	13 053	13 713	2 224	42 518
F.4212	Inward direct investment	NERZ	12 773	1 423	−836	5 405	−467	4 720	8 634	11 884	4 580
F.423	Finance leasing	F8Y9	607	658	118	221	471	946	1 043	297	559
F.424	Other long-term loans by UK residents	NESF	−208	13 788	4 746	462	−4 483	991	15 399	41 746	−1 797
F.4	Total loans	NERP	28 543	27 476	13 684	22 454	5 676	19 710	38 789	56 151	45 860
F.5	Shares and other equity										
F.51	Shares and other equity, excluding mutual funds' shares										
F.514	Quoted UK shares	NESM	20 113	84 719	6 623	13 976	4 920	12 596	11 884	17 786	11 794
F.515	Unquoted UK shares	NESN	6 973	8 213	13 016	7 047	9 427	9 281	16 002	11 163	11 311
F.517	UK shares and bonds issued by other UK residents	NSPP	–	–	–	–	–	–	–	–	–
F.519	Shares and other equity issued by the rest of the world	NESR	111 803	166 110	35 905	49 311	19 545	26 525	41 043	50 486	69 360
F.52	Mutual funds' shares										
F.521	UK mutual funds' shares	NESV	1	14	2	3	1	9	17	17	7
F.5	Total shares and other equity	NESH	138 890	259 056	55 546	70 337	33 893	48 411	68 946	79 452	92 472
F.6	Insurance technical reserves										
F.62	Prepayments of insurance premiums and reserves for outstanding claims	NETA	−291	344	−370	363	170	956	965	1 371	10
F.7	Other accounts receivable	NETB	−1 843	25 329	−2 263	2 553	19	−2 520	−542	1 782	−882
F.A	**Total net acquisition of financial assets**	NEQA	175 218	335 390	104 255	114 315	100 441	137 469	163 051	208 781	230 858

1 UK monetary financial institutions

3.3.8 Private non-financial corporations

ESA95 sectors S.11002 National controlled and S.11003 Foreign controlled. Unconsolidated

continued

£ million

			1999	2000	2001	2002	2003	2004	2005	2006	2007
III.2	**FINANCIAL ACCOUNT** continued										
F.L	**Net acquisition of financial liabilities**										
F.3	Securities other than shares										
F.331	Short term: money market instruments										
F.3316	Issued by UK residents other than government or monetary financial institutions	NEUD	2 716	1 331	−426	8 543	−1 541	−3 071	−172	698	677
F.332	Medium (1 to 5 year) and long term (over 5 year) bonds										
F.3326	Other medium & long term bonds issued by UK residents or monetary financial institutions	NEUN	39 378	40 435	15 510	16 871	19 426	8 550	11 564	11 883	24 011
F.3	Total securities other than shares	NETR	42 094	41 766	15 084	25 414	17 885	5 479	11 392	12 581	24 688
F.4	Loans										
F.41	Short term loans										
F.411	Loans by UK monetary financial institutions,										
F.4111	Sterling loans by UK banks	NEUW	7 985	21 404	15 218	22 428	11 577	18 894	36 461	48 253	57 119
F.4112	Foreign currency loans by UK banks	NEUX	6 411	1 940	984	−3 818	−5 556	630	9 171	3 984	21 668
F.4113	Sterling loans by building societies	NEUY	1 547	1 654	1 872	1 930	1 231	628	925	2 989	1 537
F.419	Loans by rest of the world monetary financial institutions	ZMFI	7 653	15 253	−30 731	−5 103	−32 248	−52 584	2 962	−51 781	7 105
F.42	Long term loans										
F.4211	Outward direct investment	NEVC	9 978	30 178	13 746	38 989	12 030	9 173	27 467	25 377	25 328
F.4212	Inward direct investment	NEVD	17 051	10 614	4 173	4 813	−1 868	6 494	22 273	9 457	−4 165
F.423	Finance leasing	NEVI	57	−164	59	347	430	516	408	475	429
F.424	Other long-term loans by UK residents	NEVJ	2 727	−446	4 550	−2 529	2 950	150	6 257	5 233	57 253
F.429	Other long-term loans by the rest of the world	NEVK	–	–	–	–	–	–	–	–	–
F.4	Total loans	NEUT	38 103	49 927	71 333	67 263	53 042	89 069	102 591	151 361	155 894
F.5	Shares and other equity										
F.51	Shares and other equity, excluding mutual funds' shares										
F.514	Quoted UK shares	NEVQ	85 600	209 418	9 234	16 508	−748	7 286	−4 608	−3 730	5 392
F.515	Unquoted UK shares	NEVR	22 070	45 259	18 551	4 834	11 348	10 816	23 186	13 701	28 875
F.516	Other UK equity (including direct investment in property)	NEVS	833	1 605	779	748	395	623	597	467	2 358
F.517	UK shares and bonds issued by other UK residents	NSPQ	–	–	–	–	–	–	–	–	–
F.5	Total shares and other equity	NEVL	108 503	256 282	28 564	22 090	10 995	18 725	19 175	10 438	36 625
F.7	Other accounts payable	NEWF	8 358	421	3 137	2 163	2 916	2 123	2 755	6 613	1 991
F.L	**Total net acquisition of financial liabilities**	NETE	197 058	348 396	118 118	116 930	84 838	115 396	135 913	180 993	219 198
B.9	**Net lending / borrowing**										
F.A	Total net acquisition of financial assets	NEQA	175 218	335 390	104 255	114 315	100 441	137 469	163 051	208 781	230 858
-F.L	*less* Total net acquisition of financial liabilities	-NETE	−197 058	−348 396	−118 118	−116 930	−84 838	−115 396	−135 913	−180 993	−219 198
B.9f	Net lending (+) / net borrowing (-), from financial account	NYOA	−21 840	−13 006	−13 863	−2 615	15 603	22 073	27 138	27 788	11 660
dB.9f	Statistical discrepancy	NYPM	9 106	5 130	5 276	11 139	3 018	5 134	−5 303	−4 575	8 936
B.9	**Net lending (+) / net borrowing (-), from capital account**	DTAL	−12 734	−7 876	−8 587	8 524	18 621	27 207	21 835	23 213	20 596

3.3.9 Private non-financial corporations

ESA95 sectors S.11002 National controlled and S.11003 Foreign controlled. Unconsolidated

£ billion

			1999	2000	2001	2002	2003	2004	2005	2006	2007
IV.3	**FINANCIAL BALANCE SHEET** at end of period										
AN	**Non-financial assets**	TMPL	1 114.2	1 129.8	1 128.6	1 156.4	1 195.9	1 256.2	1 253.0	1 363.3	1 377.9
AF.A	**Financial assets**										
AF.2	Currency and deposits										
AF.21	Currency	NKKA	2.4	2.7	2.8	3.0	3.2	3.4	3.6	3.9	4.1
AF.22	Transferable deposits										
AF.2211	Sterling deposits with UK banks	NKKD	117.8	128.6	136.8	145.7	157.7	170.0	191.3	213.4	230.9
AF.2212	Foreign currency deposits with UK banks	NKKE	19.5	24.1	24.6	23.7	26.4	28.0	31.9	30.7	36.2
AF.2213	Sterling deposits with building societies	NKKF	2.5	2.2	4.4	2.4	2.7	2.4	2.3	2.7	2.9
AF.229	Deposits with rest of the world monetary financial institutions	NKKG	46.7	57.5	66.5	65.1	121.1	194.3	255.4	286.9	355.2
AF.29	Other deposits	NKKH	4.8	4.6	4.9	4.9	5.1	5.1	5.2	5.6	5.6
AF.2	Total currency and deposits	NKJZ	193.9	219.7	240.1	244.8	316.3	403.3	489.8	543.2	634.9
AF.3	Securities other than shares										
AF.331	Short term: money market instruments										
AF.3311	Issued by UK central government	NKKK	–	–	–	–	–	–	–	–	–
AF.3315	Issued by UK monetary financial institutions	NKKP	4.8	5.4	5.6	4.6	5.0	5.4	4.8	6.7	8.9
AF.3316	Issued by other UK residents	NKKU	13.5	16.3	18.5	13.7	13.5	13.0	16.9	35.9	42.2
AF.3319	Issued by the rest of the world	NKKV	1.9	3.0	4.9	6.0	9.8	10.4	11.4	16.2	6.4
AF.332	Medium (1 to 5 year) and long term (over 5 year) bonds										
AF.3321	Issued by UK central government	NKKX	0.1	0.5	0.3	0.5	0.3	0.3	0.2	0.2	0.5
AF.3322	Issued by UK local government	NKLA	–	–	–	–	–	–	–	–	–
AF.3325	Medium term bonds issued by UK MFIs[1]	NKLB	0.3	0.2	0.2	0.3	0.9	1.0	1.5	1.9	2.5
AF.3326	Other medium & long term bonds issued by UK residents	NKLE	1.8	2.5	4.1	6.1	5.2	5.1	1.4	1.5	5.2
AF.3329	Long term bonds issued by the rest of the world	NKLF	7.2	28.4	28.8	29.3	30.0	12.8	14.6	10.3	11.6
AF.3	Total securities other than shares	NKKI	29.7	56.4	62.3	60.4	64.6	47.8	50.8	72.7	77.3
AF.4	Loans										
AF.42	Long term loans										
AF.4211	Outward direct investment	NKXH	78.2	85.9	97.5	110.5	110.7	124.5	125.9	130.5	173.0
AF.4212	Inward direct investment	NKXI	51.1	48.2	48.7	52.2	48.0	55.5	67.4	76.7	81.3
AF.423	Finance leasing	F8YG	1.8	2.4	2.5	2.7	3.2	4.4	5.4	4.4	4.9
AF.424	Other long-term loans by UK residents	NKXO	8.0	7.9	8.1	8.4	8.2	8.2	8.2	7.4	7.6
AF.4	Total loans	NKWY	139.0	144.5	156.8	173.9	170.1	192.5	207.0	219.0	266.8
AF.5	Shares and other equity										
AF.51	Shares and other equity, excluding mutual funds' shares										
AF.514	Quoted UK shares	NKXV	39.0	26.4	14.8	8.7	9.4	8.8	19.3	32.9	26.0
AF.515	Unquoted UK shares	NKXW	64.4	63.5	52.4	39.6	46.3	50.0	57.1	60.9	63.0
AF.517	UK shares and bonds issued by other UK residents	NSON	–	–	–	–	–	–	–	–	–
AF.519	Shares and other equity issued by the rest of the world	NKYA	339.4	505.6	494.4	521.3	564.6	549.2	592.8	602.7	671.1
AF.52	Mutual funds' shares										
AF.521	UK mutual funds' shares	NKYE	0.6	0.5	0.4	0.3	0.3	0.4	0.5	0.6	0.6
AF.5	Total shares and other equity	NKXQ	443.4	596.1	562.0	569.9	620.7	608.3	669.6	697.1	760.6
AF.6	Insurance technical reserves										
AF.62	Prepayments of insurance premiums and reserves for outstanding claims	NKYJ	10.7	14.7	12.5	12.8	15.7	17.0	17.3	17.6	17.6
AF.7	Other accounts receivable	NKYK	88.2	112.3	110.9	110.4	112.3	112.9	111.7	110.7	109.7
AF.A	**Total financial assets**	NKWX	904.9	1 143.7	1 144.5	1 172.1	1 299.7	1 381.9	1 546.1	1 660.3	1 867.0

1 UK monetary financial institutions

3.3.9 Private non-financial corporations

ESA95 sectors S.11002 National controlled and S.11003 Foreign controlled. Unconsolidated

continued

£ billion

			1999	2000	2001	2002	2003	2004	2005	2006	2007
IV.3		**FINANCIAL BALANCE SHEET** continued at end of period									
AF.L		**Financial liabilities**									
AF.3		Securities other than shares									
AF.331		Short term: money market instruments									
AF.3316		Issued by UK residents other than government or monetary financial institutions	**NKZM**	22.5	24.7	24.6	30.4	26.0	21.8	23.8	21.7	22.2
AF.332		Medium (1 to 5 year) and long term (over 5 year) bonds									
AF.3326		Other medium & long term bonds issued by UK residents or monetary financial institutions	**NKZW**	155.4	198.4	209.9	232.2	254.1	254.7	301.5	336.4	343.1
AF.3		Total securities other than shares	**NKZA**	177.9	223.1	234.5	262.5	280.2	276.5	325.2	358.1	365.4
AF.4		Loans									
AF.41		Short term loans									
AF.4111		Sterling deposits with UK banks	**NLBF**	175.9	198.1	213.1	235.1	242.2	256.0	291.8	339.1	393.6
AF.4112		Foreign currency deposits with UK banks	**NLBG**	41.4	45.2	45.9	40.3	32.7	31.8	42.4	43.1	66.9
AF.4113		Sterling deposits with building societies loans secured on dwellings & financial leasing	**NLBH**	4.1	5.7	7.6	9.5	10.7	10.7	11.8	14.8	16.3
AF.419		Loans by rest of the world monetary financial institutions	**ZMEV**	56.9	42.0	63.9	69.1	106.8	158.5	166.0	228.8	224.5
AF.42		Long term loans									
AF.4211		Outward direct investment	**NLBL**	56.8	80.6	94.0	125.0	124.2	125.6	159.2	164.9	190.2
AF.4212		Inward direct investment	**NLBM**	94.2	100.4	115.3	124.9	117.4	125.0	149.3	160.1	155.9
AF.422		Secured on dwellings	**G9JM**	–	–	–	–	–	–	27.1	30.9	34.8
AF.423		Finance leasing	**NLBR**	21.0	21.1	21.2	21.5	22.0	22.5	22.9	23.4	23.8
AF.424		Other long-term loans by UK residents	**NLBS**	44.3	47.2	53.1	44.7	68.0	79.2	73.1	91.5	98.3
AF.429		Other long-term loans by the rest of the world	**NLBT**	0.4	0.4	0.3	0.4	0.4	0.4	0.4	0.4	0.4
AF.4		Total loans	**NLBC**	495.0	540.7	614.4	670.6	724.4	809.8	943.9	1 097.0	1 204.8
AF.5		Shares and other equity									
AF.51		Shares and other equity, excluding mutual funds' shares									
AF.514		Quoted UK shares	**NLBZ**	1 394.4	1 375.5	1 134.7	857.8	1 002.0	1 080.2	1 232.3	1 315.5	1 360.5
AF.515		Unquoted UK shares	**NLCA**	462.0	489.7	454.8	352.2	392.4	422.1	513.2	608.0	694.5
AF.516		Other UK equity (including direct investment in property)	**NLCB**	13.1	14.9	15.5	17.3	17.3	19.2	19.7	21.6	26.2
AF.517		UK shares and bonds issued by other UK residents	**NSOO**	–	–	–	–	–	–	–	–	–
AF.5		Total shares and other equity	**NLBU**	1 869.5	1 880.1	1 605.1	1 227.3	1 411.7	1 521.5	1 765.3	1 945.1	2 081.2
AF.7		Other accounts payable	**NLCO**	127.3	128.7	129.9	129.3	131.5	134.3	137.1	140.6	139.9
AF.L		**Total financial liabilities**	**NLBB**	2 669.6	2 772.6	2 583.8	2 289.7	2 547.8	2 742.1	3 171.5	3 540.8	3 791.3
BF.90		**Net financial assets / liabilities**									
AF.A		Total financial assets	**NKWX**	904.9	1 143.7	1 144.5	1 172.1	1 299.7	1 381.9	1 546.1	1 660.3	1 867.0
-AF.L		*less* Total financial liabilities	**–NLBB**	–2 669.6	–2 772.6	–2 583.8	–2 289.7	–2 547.8	–2 742.1	–3 171.5	–3 540.8	–3 791.3
BF.90		**Net financial assets (+) / liabilities (-)**	**NYOT**	–1 764.7	–1 628.8	–1 439.3	–1 117.6	–1 248.1	–1 360.2	–1 625.4	–1 880.4	–1 924.3
		Net worth									
AN		Non-financial assets	**TMPL**	1 114.2	1 129.8	1 128.6	1 156.4	1 195.9	1 256.2	1 253.0	1 363.3	1 377.9
BF.90		Net financial assets(+)/liabilities(-)	**NYOT**	–1 764.7	–1 628.8	–1 439.3	–1 117.6	–1 248.1	–1 360.2	–1 625.4	–1 880.4	–1 924.3
BF.90		**Net worth**	**TMPN**	–650.4	–499.0	–310.7	38.8	–52.2	–104.0	–372.4	–517.1	–546.4

Chapter 4
Financial corporations

4.1.1 Financial corporations
ESA95 sector S.12

£ million

			1999	2000	2001	2002	2003	2004	2005	2006
I	**PRODUCTION ACCOUNT**									
	Resources									
P.1	Output									
P.11	Market output*	NHCV	112 070	114 331	124 496	136 124	143 840	148 308	155 661	167 725
P.12	Output for own final use	NHCW	1 766	2 008	2 106	2 388	2 559	2 763	2 899	3 112
P.1	Total resources	NHCT	113 836	116 339	126 602	138 512	146 399	151 071	158 560	170 837
	Uses									
P.2	Intermediate consumption	NHCX	66 238	72 636	79 493	76 884	76 785	77 416	80 510	81 308
B.1g	**Gross Value Added**	NHDB	**47 598**	**43 703**	**47 109**	**61 628**	**69 614**	**73 655**	**78 050**	**89 529**
Total	Total uses	NHCT	113 836	116 339	126 602	138 512	146 399	151 071	158 560	170 837
B.1g	**Gross Value Added**	NHDB	**47 598**	**43 703**	**47 109**	**61 628**	**69 614**	**73 655**	**78 050**	**89 529**
-K.1	*less* Consumption of fixed capital	−NHCE	−4 372	−4 771	−4 730	−5 035	−5 295	−5 687	−5 811	−5 944
B.1n	Value added, net of fixed capital consumption	NHDC	43 226	38 932	42 379	56 593	64 319	67 968	72 239	83 585

4.1.2 Financial corporations
ESA95 sector S.12

£ million

			1999	2000	2001	2002	2003	2004	2005	2006
II	**DISTRIBUTION AND USE OF INCOME ACCOUNTS**									
II.1	**PRIMARY DISTRIBUTION OF INCOME ACCOUNT**									
II.1.1	**GENERATION OF INCOME ACCOUNT**									
	Resources									
B.1g	**Total resources (Gross Value Added)**	NHDB	47 598	43 703	47 109	61 628	69 614	73 655	78 050	89 529
	Uses									
D.1	Compensation of employees									
D.11	Wages and salaries	NHCC	24 782	27 752	28 908	29 060	30 178	32 132	35 251	42 488
D.12	Employers' social contributions	NHCD	3 268	3 736	3 888	4 067	4 799	7 620	9 020	8 835
D.1	Total	NHCR	28 050	31 488	32 796	33 127	34 977	39 752	44 271	51 323
D.2	Taxes on production and imports, paid									
D.29	Production taxes other than on products	NHCS	1 539	1 219	1 348	1 376	1 419	1 443	1 479	1 578
-D.3	*less* Subsidies, received									
-D.39	Production subsidies other than on products	−NHCA	–	–	–	–	–	–	–	–
B.2g	Operating surplus, gross	NQNV	18 009	10 996	12 965	27 125	33 218	32 460	32 300	36 628
B.1g	**Total uses (Gross Value Added)**	NHDB	**47 598**	**43 703**	**47 109**	**61 628**	**69 614**	**73 655**	**78 050**	**89 529**
-K.1	After deduction of fixed capital consumption	−NHCE	−4 372	−4 771	−4 730	−5 035	−5 295	−5 687	−5 811	−5 944
B.2n	Operating surplus, net	NHDA	13 637	6 225	8 235	22 090	27 923	26 773	26 489	30 684

4.1.3 Financial corporations
ESA95 sector S.12

£ million

			1999	2000	2001	2002	2003	2004	2005	2006	2007
II.1.2	**ALLOCATION OF PRIMARY INCOME ACCOUNT**										
	Resources										
B.2g	Operating surplus, gross	NQNV	18 009	10 996	12 965	27 125	33 218	32 460	32 300	36 628	46 290
D.4	Property income, received										
D.41	Interest	NHCK	161 557	206 749	198 445	162 001	160 855	194 828	242 706	311 433	409 731
D.42	Distributed income of corporations	NHCL	41 509	49 211	49 801	51 990	56 472	65 310	70 122	82 883	91 141
D.43	Reinvested earnings on direct foreign investment	NHEM	5 178	5 060	4 223	5 278	8 897	8 208	10 201	11 153	9 506
D.44	Attributed property income of insurance policy-holders	NHDG	53	35	37	34	44	39	66	61	46
D.45	Rent	NHDH	29	29	29	30	30	31	31	31	32
D.4	Total	NHDF	208 326	261 084	252 535	219 333	226 298	268 416	323 126	405 561	510 456
Total	Total resources	NQNW	226 335	272 080	265 500	246 458	259 516	300 876	355 426	442 189	556 746
	Uses										
D.4	Property income, paid										
D.41	Interest	NHCM	136 518	180 167	170 669	133 981	129 917	159 603	212 341	283 589	372 849
D.42	Distributed income of corporations	NHCN	29 189	38 460	43 922	37 207	43 137	51 966	51 706	63 062	61 528
D.43	Reinvested earnings on direct foreign investment	NHEO	1 831	3 440	−2 691	2 033	3 474	2 233	5 518	6 128	9 442
D.44	Attributed property income of insurance policy-holders	NQCG	54 903	54 494	54 795	53 652	56 715	56 150	65 805	68 349	74 084
D.45	Rent	NHDK	−	−	−	−	−	−	−	−	−
D.4	Total	NHDI	222 441	276 561	266 695	226 873	233 243	269 952	335 370	421 128	517 903
B.5g	**Balance of primary incomes, gross**	NQNY	**3 894**	**−4 481**	**−1 195**	**19 585**	**26 273**	**30 924**	**20 056**	**21 061**	**38 843**
Total	Total uses	NQNW	226 335	272 080	265 500	246 458	259 516	300 876	355 426	442 189	556 746
-K.1	After deduction of fixed capital consumption	−NHCE	−4 372	−4 771	−4 730	−5 035	−5 295	−5 687	−5 811	−5 944	−6 099
B.5n	Balance of primary incomes, net	NHDL	−478	−9 252	−5 925	14 550	20 978	25 237	14 245	15 117	32 744

4.1.4 Financial corporations
ESA95 sector S.12

£ million

			1999	2000	2001	2002	2003	2004	2005	2006	2007
II.2	**SECONDARY DISTRIBUTION OF INCOME ACCOUNT**										
	Resources										
B.5g	**Balance of primary incomes, gross**	NQNY	**3 894**	**−4 481**	**−1 195**	**19 585**	**26 273**	**30 924**	**20 056**	**21 061**	**38 843**
D.61	Social contributions										
D.611	Actual social contributions										
D.6111	Employers' actual social contributions	NQOB	19 128	20 891	21 836	26 025	32 504	38 473	42 963	47 527	45 995
D.6112	Employees' social contributions	NQOC	30 878	31 569	31 933	32 967	32 158	31 652	36 786	39 807	41 425
D.6113	Social contributions by self-employed persons	NQOD	−	−	−	−	−	−	−	−	−
D.611	Total	NQOA	50 006	52 460	53 769	58 992	64 662	70 125	79 749	87 334	87 420
D.612	Imputed social contributions	NHDR	448	490	484	524	502	503	507	511	514
D.61	Total	NQNZ	50 454	52 950	54 253	59 516	65 164	70 628	80 256	87 845	87 934
D.7	Other current transfers										
D.71	Net non-life insurance premiums	NQOF	22 894	24 550	19 553	26 620	23 000	28 148	31 711	36 531	27 745
D.72	Non-life insurance claims	NHDN	479	614	405	588	645	675	806	878	666
D.75	Miscellaneous current transfers	NQOG	140	140	95	58	28	5	−	−	−
D.7	Total	NQOE	23 513	25 304	20 053	27 266	23 673	28 828	32 517	37 409	28 411
Total	Total resources	NQOH	77 861	73 773	73 111	106 367	115 110	130 380	132 829	146 315	155 188
	Uses										
D.5	Current taxes on income and wealth										
D.51	Taxes on income	NHDO	10 422	10 624	12 324	6 750	7 514	7 221	8 739	15 475	10 033
D.62	Social benefits other than social transfers in kind	NHDQ	36 440	38 800	38 220	41 733	43 799	41 171	47 423	56 140	46 028
D.7	Other current transfers										
D.71	Net non-life insurance premiums	NHDU	479	614	405	588	645	675	806	878	666
D.72	Non-life insurance claims	NQOI	22 894	24 550	19 553	26 620	23 000	28 148	31 711	36 531	27 745
D.75	Miscellaneous current transfers	NHEK	184	164	202	227	204	108	80	80	80
D.7	Total	NHDT	23 557	25 328	20 160	27 435	23 849	28 931	32 597	37 489	28 491
B.6g	**Gross Disposable Income**	NQOJ	**7 442**	**−979**	**2 407**	**30 449**	**39 948**	**53 057**	**44 070**	**37 211**	**70 636**
Total	Total uses	NQOH	77 861	73 773	73 111	106 367	115 110	130 380	132 829	146 315	155 188
-K.1	After deduction of fixed capital consumption	−NHCE	−4 372	−4 771	−4 730	−5 035	−5 295	−5 687	−5 811	−5 944	−6 099
B.6n	Disposable income, net	NHDV	3 070	−5 750	−2 323	25 414	34 653	47 370	38 259	31 267	64 537

4.1.6 Financial corporations
ESA95 sector S.12

£ million

			1999	2000	2001	2002	2003	2004	2005	2006	2007
II.4.1	**USE OF DISPOSABLE INCOME ACCOUNT**										
	Resources										
B.6g	**Total resources (Gross Disposable Income)**	**NQOJ**	**7 442**	**−979**	**2 407**	**30 449**	**39 948**	**53 057**	**44 070**	**37 211**	**70 636**
	Uses										
D.8	Adjustment for the change in net equity of households in pension funds	**NQOK**	14 014	14 150	16 033	17 783	21 365	29 457	32 833	31 705	41 906
B.8g	**Gross Saving**	**NQOL**	**−6 572**	**−15 129**	**−13 626**	**12 666**	**18 583**	**23 600**	**11 237**	**5 506**	**28 730**
B.6g	**Total uses (Gross Disposable Income)**	**NQOJ**	**7 442**	**−979**	**2 407**	**30 449**	**39 948**	**53 057**	**44 070**	**37 211**	**70 636**
-K.1	After deduction of fixed capital consumption	**−NHCE**	−4 372	−4 771	−4 730	−5 035	−5 295	−5 687	−5 811	−5 944	−6 099
B.8n	Saving, net	**NQOM**	−10 944	−19 900	−18 356	7 631	13 288	17 913	5 426	−438	22 631

4.1.7 Financial corporations
ESA95 sector S.12

£ million

			1999	2000	2001	2002	2003	2004	2005	2006	2007
III	**ACCUMULATION ACCOUNTS**										
III.1	**CAPITAL ACCOUNT**										
III.1.1	**CHANGE IN NET WORTH DUE TO SAVING & CAPITAL TRANSFERS**										
	Changes in liabilities and net worth										
B.8g	**Gross Saving**	**NQOL**	−6 572	−15 129	−13 626	12 666	18 583	23 600	11 237	5 506	28 730
D.9	Capital transfers receivable										
D.92	Investment grants	**NHEA**	–	–	–	–	–	–	–	–	–
D.99	Other capital transfers	**NHEB**	–	–	412	412	391	328	321	446	388
D.9	Total	**NHDZ**	–	–	412	412	391	328	321	446	388
-D.9	*less* Capital transfers payable										
-D.91	Capital taxes	**−NHBW**	–	–	–	–	–	–	–	–	–
-D.99	Other capital transfers	**−NHCB**	–	–	−412	−412	−391	−328	−321	−446	−388
-D.9	Total	**−NHEC**	–	–	−412	−412	−391	−328	−321	−446	−388
B.10.1g	Total change in liabilities and net worth	**NQON**	−6 572	−15 129	−13 626	12 666	18 583	23 600	11 237	5 506	28 730
	Changes in assets										
B.10.1g	Changes in net worth due to gross saving and capital transfers	**NQON**	−6 572	−15 129	−13 626	12 666	18 583	23 600	11 237	5 506	28 730
-K.1	After deduction of fixed capital consumption	**−NHCE**	−4 372	−4 771	−4 730	−5 035	−5 295	−5 687	−5 811	−5 944	−6 099
B.10.1n	Changes in net worth due to net saving and capital transfers	**NHEF**	−10 944	−19 900	−18 356	7 631	13 288	17 913	5 426	−438	22 631
III.1.2	**ACQUISITION OF NON-FINANCIAL ASSETS ACCOUNT**										
	Changes in liabilities and net worth										
B.10.1n	Changes in net worth due to net saving and capital transfers	**NHEF**	−10 944	−19 900	−18 356	7 631	13 288	17 913	5 426	−438	22 631
K.1	Consumption of fixed capital	**NHCE**	4 372	4 771	4 730	5 035	5 295	5 687	5 811	5 944	6 099
Total	Total change in liabilities and net worth	**NQON**	−6 572	−15 129	−13 626	12 666	18 583	23 600	11 237	5 506	28 730
	Changes in assets										
P.5	Gross capital formation										
P.51	Gross fixed capital formation	**NHCJ**	9 188	11 976	8 482	8 323	5 253	5 254	6 453	8 650	7 831
P.52	Changes in inventories	**NHCI**	47	55	58	67	48	48	48	199	206
P.53	Acquisitions less disposals of valuables	**NPQI**	−28	−127	–	−74	−166	−173	−299	−74	−35
P.5	Total	**NHEG**	9 207	11 904	8 540	8 316	5 135	5 129	6 202	8 775	8 002
K.2	Acquisitions less disposals of non-produced non-financial assets	**NHEI**	−37	−45	−43	−36	−3	−6	−1	6	4
B.9	**Net lending(+) / net borrowing(-)**	**NHCQ**	**−15 742**	**−26 988**	**−22 123**	**4 386**	**13 451**	**18 477**	**5 036**	**−3 275**	**20 724**
Total	Total change in assets	**NQON**	−6 572	−15 129	−13 626	12 666	18 583	23 600	11 237	5 506	28 730

4.1.8 Financial corporations
ESA95 sector S.12. Unconsolidated

£ million

			1999	2000	2001	2002	2003	2004	2005	2006	2007
III.2	**FINANCIAL ACCOUNT**										
F.A	**Net acquisition of financial assets**										
F.2	Currency and deposits										
F.21	Currency	NFCV	2 717	−1 419	−1 279	165	903	3 071	−1 104	−168	−1 413
F.22	Transferable deposits										
F.221	Deposits with UK monetary financial institutions	NFCX	−8 451	85 402	120 733	78 123	159 371	179 797	226 659	349 726	221 698
F.229	Deposits with rest of the world monetary financial institutions	NFDB	18 355	178 818	97 198	41 276	147 457	151 279	329 676	235 617	423 529
F.29	Other deposits	NFDC	−10	2 685	−1 570	1 263	−1 064	1 387	1 392	−2 083	2 248
F.2	Total currency and deposits	NFCU	12 611	265 486	215 082	120 827	306 667	335 534	556 623	583 092	646 062
F.3	Securities other than shares										
F.331	Short term: money market instruments										
F.3311	Issued by UK central government	NFDF	−1 145	−1 112	8 306	10 651	478	−911	−2 894	−2 481	−5 270
F.3312	Issued by UK local government	NFDJ	–	–	–	–	–	–	–	–	–
F.3315	Issued by UK monetary financial institutions	NFDK	18 323	−15 675	2 871	7 138	−12 219	−692	2 496	3 945	2 200
F.3316	Issued by other UK residents	NFDP	1 155	1 408	−1 112	−603	2 386	−2 759	4 252	−21	−3 072
F.3319	Issued by the rest of the world	NFDQ	13 545	−3 905	9 308	−5 667	9 413	−3 355	4 834	8 422	5 773
F.332	Medium (1 to 5 year) and long term (over 5 year) bonds										
F.3321	Issued by UK central government	NFDS	6 300	−22 198	−17 976	4 364	16 765	29 441	19 828	31 695	22 317
F.3322	Issued by UK local government	NFDV	−36	60	−47	59	14	−92	139	230	−29
F.3325	Medium term bonds issued by UK MFIs[1]	NFDW	7 531	2 282	−147	2 421	11 220	11 086	14 710	14 033	20 106
F.3326	Other medium & long term bonds issued by UK residents	NFDZ	38 102	66 289	46 077	24 061	38 256	32 777	36 474	45 221	32 952
F.3329	Long term bonds issued by the rest of the world	NFEA	−5 881	45 833	30 252	8 133	−1 093	86 266	83 322	104 220	66 071
F.34	Financial derivatives	NFEB	−2 727	−1 663	−8 601	−1 205	5 263	7 847	−9 556	−7 449	19 001
F.3	Total securities other than shares	NFDD	75 167	71 319	68 931	49 352	70 483	159 608	153 605	197 815	160 049
F.4	Loans										
F.41	Short term loans										
F.411	Loans by UK monetary financial institutions, excluding loans secured on dwellings & financial leasing	NFEH	66 698	150 664	108 353	87 544	159 494	235 263	255 959	305 306	516 001
F.42	Long term loans										
F.421	Direct investment	NFEN	463	1 487	2 356	4 693	−766	3 200	3 323	1 388	3 229
F.422	Loans secured on dwellings	NFEQ	37 795	42 196	54 226	83 438	101 808	102 306	89 696	109 653	107 252
F.423	Finance leasing	NFEU	−266	−291	322	758	724	709	551	666	616
F.424	Other long term loans	NFEV	18 995	7 687	1 433	4 798	11 320	10 337	19 161	9 459	54 136
F.4	Total loans	NFEF	123 685	201 743	166 690	181 231	272 580	351 815	368 690	426 472	681 234
F.5	Shares and other equity										
F.51	Shares and other equity, excluding mutual funds' shares										
F.514	Quoted UK shares	NFFC	4 747	24 505	27 562	−13 763	−1 726	529	−42 246	−13 330	10 266
F.515	Unquoted UK shares	NFFD	−1 906	22 451	1 211	−208	747	7 520	5 163	19 399	9 916
F.517	UK shares and bonds issued by other UK residents	NSPS	–	–	–	–	–	–	–	–	–
F.519	Shares and other equity issued by the rest of the world	NFFH	24 451	26 872	50 913	5 074	38 706	76 289	68 350	41 726	68 894
F.52	Mutual funds' shares										
F.521	UK mutual funds' shares	NFFL	5 629	7 261	1 914	3 370	901	391	11 844	9 771	−1 323
F.5	Total shares and other equity	NFEX	32 921	81 089	81 600	−5 527	38 628	84 729	43 111	57 566	87 753
F.6	Insurance technical reserves										
F.62	Prepayments of insurance premiums and reserves for outstanding claims	NFFQ	−46	36	−41	42	20	102	107	144	–
F.7	Other accounts receivable	NFFR	3 215	−2 457	9 050	15 697	8 439	4 315	3 425	40 887	13 506
F.A	**Total net acquisition of financial assets**	NFCQ	247 553	617 216	541 312	361 622	696 817	936 103	1 125 561	1 305 976	1 588 604

1 UK monetary financial institutions

4.1.8 Financial corporations
ESA95 sector S.12. Unconsolidated

continued

£ million

			1999	2000	2001	2002	2003	2004	2005	2006	2007
III.2	FINANCIAL ACCOUNT continued										
F.L	**Net acquisition of financial liabilities**										
F.2	Currency and deposits										
F.21	Currency	NFFZ	5 231	448	738	1 532	2 958	5 460	945	1 745	1 043
F.22	Transferable deposits										
F.221	Deposits with UK monetary financial institutions	NFGB	35 792	345 481	286 540	218 055	399 447	540 924	586 768	783 929	981 443
F.29	Other deposits	NFGG	–	2 919	−2 578	476	−536	18	550	−12	4 299
F.2	Total currency and deposits	NFFY	41 023	348 848	284 700	220 063	401 869	546 402	588 263	785 662	986 785
F.3	Securities other than shares										
F.331	Short term: money market instruments										
F.3315	Issued by UK monetary financial institutions	NFGO	31 135	23 941	22 835	25 599	−11 489	8 024	−3 488	53 189	17 860
F.3316	Issued by other non-government UK residents	NFGT	31	−16	–	267	−567	122	237	1 422	−287
F.332	Medium (1 to 5 year) and long term (over 5 year) bonds										
F.3325	Medium term bonds issued by UK MFIs[1]	NFHA	12 081	4 750	3 575	4 238	25 258	29 810	37 843	40 534	57 261
F.3326	Other medium & long term bonds issued by UK residents	NFHD	24 106	35 298	35 807	29 802	81 671	80 255	101 893	107 953	125 711
F.34	Financial derivatives	NFHF	3	43	89	−70	63	−147	−207	−110	−312
F.3	Total securities other than shares	NFGH	67 356	64 016	62 306	59 836	94 936	118 064	136 278	202 988	200 233
F.4	Loans										
F.41	Short term loans										
F.411	Loans by UK monetary financial institutions, excluding loans secured on dwellings & financial leasing	NFHL	15 801	54 851	31 533	26 966	62 182	71 721	53 905	116 602	197 788
F.419	Loans by rest of the world monetary financial institutions	NFHP	55 329	52 224	81 231	−32 273	34 636	77 456	209 800	−12 499	52 943
F.42	Long term loans										
F.421	Direct investment	NFHR	3 082	896	13 253	6 643	2 765	2 687	−5 332	1 784	5 112
F.423	Finance leasing	NFHY	−323	−127	263	411	294	193	143	191	187
F.424	Other long-term loans by UK residents	NFHZ	8 818	18 319	9 197	3 474	5 558	5 727	24 843	42 054	−15 421
F.429	Other long-term loans by the rest of the world	NFIA	46	−30	6	−21	−42	10	29	–	26
F.4	Total loans	NFHJ	82 753	126 133	135 483	5 200	105 393	157 794	283 388	148 132	240 635
F.5	Shares and other equity										
F.51	Shares and other equity, excluding mutual funds' shares										
F.514	Quoted UK shares	NFIG	2 150	16 269	13 069	2 373	14 923	12 607	10 931	28 075	9 254
F.515	Unquoted UK shares	NFIH	8 776	36 719	15 858	11 174	15 718	21 357	27 753	39 785	39 772
F.516	Other UK equity (including direct investment in property)	NFII	–	–	43	32	−9	−8	–	–	–
F.517	UK shares and bonds issued by other UK residents	NSPT	–	–	–	–	–	–	–	–	–
F.52	Mutual funds' shares										
F.521	UK mutual funds' shares	NFIP	14 719	14 102	9 338	6 259	8 212	3 489	8 300	14 445	−2 032
F.5	Total shares and other equity	NFIB	25 645	67 090	38 308	19 838	38 844	37 445	46 984	82 305	46 994
F.6	Insurance technical reserves										
F.61	Net equity of households in life assurance and pension funds' reserves	NFIR	34 689	29 712	35 846	46 180	34 437	44 942	53 672	55 989	72 701
F.62	Prepayments of insurance premiums and reserves for outstanding claims	NFIU	−1 601	1 466	−1 753	1 781	687	3 778	3 969	6 011	39
F.6	Total insurance technical reserves	NPWS	33 088	31 178	34 093	47 961	35 124	48 720	57 641	62 000	72 740
F.7	Other accounts payable	NFIV	4 658	7 623	1 249	7 198	267	8 851	3 096	35 177	11 035
F.L	**Total net acquisition of financial liabilities**	NFFU	254 523	644 888	556 139	360 096	676 433	917 276	1 115 650	1 316 264	1 558 422
B.9	**Net lending / borrowing**										
F.A	Total net acquisition of financial assets	NFCQ	247 553	617 216	541 312	361 622	696 817	936 103	1 125 561	1 305 976	1 588 604
-F.L	*less* Total net acquisition of financial liabilities	−NFFU	−254 523	−644 888	−556 139	−360 096	−676 433	−917 276	−1 115 650	−1 316 264	−1 558 422
B.9f	Net lending (+) / net borrowing (-), from financial account	NYNL	−6 970	−27 672	−14 827	1 526	20 384	18 827	9 911	−10 288	30 182
dB.9f	Statistical discrepancy	NYOX	−8 772	684	−7 296	2 860	−6 933	−350	−4 875	7 013	−9 458
B.9	**Net lending (+) / net borrowing (-), from capital account**	NHCQ	−15 742	−26 988	−22 123	4 386	13 451	18 477	5 036	−3 275	20 724

1 UK monetary financial institutions

4.1.9 Financial corporations
ESA95 sector S.12. Unconsolidated

£ billion

			1999	2000	2001	2002	2003	2004	2005	2006	2007
IV.3	**FINANCIAL BALANCE SHEET** at end of period										
AN	**Non-financial assets**	**CGDB**	114.0	118.0	121.4	122.0	128.5	136.9	141.9	145.8	145.8
AF.A	**Financial assets**										
AF.2	Currency and deposits										
AF.21	Currency	**NLJE**	9.9	8.5	7.2	7.4	8.3	11.3	10.2	10.1	8.7
AF.22	Transferable deposits										
AF.221	Deposits with UK monetary financial institutions	**NLJG**	509.7	606.4	705.5	790.9	1 041.7	1 184.3	1 450.2	1 837.2	1 533.1
AF.229	Deposits with rest of the world monetary financial institutions	**NLJK**	789.0	994.7	1 081.2	1 099.7	1 233.1	1 357.0	1 740.0	1 838.1	2 329.5
AF.29	Other deposits	**NLJL**	0.1	2.8	1.2	1.9	0.8	2.2	3.6	1.5	3.8
AF.2	Total currency and deposits	**NLJD**	1 308.7	1 612.3	1 795.0	1 899.8	2 283.9	2 554.8	3 204.1	3 686.8	3 875.0
AF.3	Securities other than shares										
AF.331	Short term: money market instruments										
AF.3311	Issued by UK central government	**NLJO**	3.5	2.2	10.7	21.0	21.9	21.1	18.2	15.7	10.3
AF.3312	Issued by UK local government	**NLJS**	–	–	–	–	–	–	–	–	–
AF.3315	Issued by UK monetary financial institutions	**NLJT**	155.6	141.4	145.2	151.1	140.0	139.8	144.1	149.6	148.2
AF.3316	Issued by other UK residents	**NLJY**	6.3	7.4	6.0	5.3	7.3	4.8	8.9	8.7	5.7
AF.3319	Issued by the rest of the world	**NLJZ**	40.6	40.0	49.1	41.6	52.1	47.8	50.9	56.3	65.2
AF.332	Medium (1 to 5 year) and long term (over 5 year) bonds										
AF.3321	Issued by UK central government	**NLKB**	229.6	231.6	197.8	210.5	227.3	254.3	273.1	296.9	329.4
AF.3322	Issued by UK local government	**NLKE**	0.6	0.5	0.6	0.5	0.5	0.4	0.4	0.5	0.5
AF.3325	Medium term bonds issued by UK MFIs[1]	**NLKF**	32.6	36.0	34.9	37.1	52.4	62.8	78.5	89.0	115.9
AF.3326	Other medium & long term bonds issued by UK residents	**NLKI**	179.0	231.7	261.0	278.0	309.9	345.0	409.8	464.4	491.2
AF.3329	Long term bonds issued by the rest of the world	**NLKJ**	370.6	426.0	472.9	484.4	496.2	573.8	677.4	762.9	867.7
AF.34	Financial derivatives	**NLKK**	–	–	–	–	–	–	–	–	–
AF.3	Total securities other than shares	**NLJM**	1 018.4	1 116.8	1 178.2	1 229.6	1 307.6	1 449.7	1 661.4	1 844.1	2 034.1
AF.4	Loans										
AF.41	Short term loans										
AF.411	Loans by UK monetary financial institutions, excluding loans secured on dwellings & financial leasing	**NLKQ**	809.4	976.8	1 074.7	1 142.5	1 283.9	1 493.7	1 761.9	1 975.9	2 538.9
AF.42	Long term loans										
AF.421	Direct investment	**NLKW**	4.2	7.9	11.2	12.8	16.2	25.3	28.9	22.3	25.5
AF.422	Loans secured on dwellings	**NLKZ**	492.2	534.4	589.5	668.5	771.8	880.0	964.1	1 075.5	1 179.3
AF.423	Finance leasing	**NLLD**	23.3	23.4	23.7	24.5	25.2	25.9	26.4	27.1	27.7
AF.424	Other long term loans	**NLLE**	55.4	54.1	58.6	60.0	75.0	91.9	91.8	115.8	116.5
AF.4	Total loans	**NLKO**	1 384.6	1 596.7	1 757.7	1 908.2	2 172.1	2 516.8	2 873.1	3 216.7	3 887.9
AF.5	Shares and other equity										
AF.51	Shares and other equity, excluding mutual funds' shares										
AF.514	Quoted UK shares	**NLLL**	840.4	795.0	706.0	532.9	625.9	678.0	752.6	805.9	802.1
AF.515	Unquoted UK shares	**NLLM**	103.4	165.1	194.6	209.5	231.8	263.9	280.6	332.1	312.9
AF.517	UK shares and bonds issued by other UK residents	**NSQL**	–	–	–	–	–	–	–	–	–
AF.519	Shares and other equity issued by the rest of the world	**NLLQ**	464.6	481.3	464.8	376.4	441.7	526.5	682.2	770.4	887.4
AF.52	Mutual funds' shares										
AF.521	UK mutual funds' shares	**NLLU**	145.6	150.5	130.5	106.3	146.0	164.1	243.3	286.0	288.6
AF.5	Total shares and other equity	**NLLG**	1 554.0	1 591.9	1 495.9	1 225.1	1 445.3	1 632.5	1 958.6	2 194.5	2 291.0
AF.6	Insurance technical reserves										
AF.62	Prepayments of insurance premiums and reserves for outstanding claims	**NLLZ**	1.7	1.6	1.4	1.4	1.7	1.8	1.9	1.9	1.9
AF.7	Other accounts receivable	**NLMA**	25.8	27.9	29.8	47.6	63.2	62.4	63.5	98.9	112.7
AF.A	**Total financial assets**	**NLIZ**	5 293.2	5 947.2	6 258.0	6 311.8	7 273.8	8 218.0	9 762.6	11 042.8	12 202.5

1 UK monetary financial institutions

4.1.9 Financial corporations
ESA95 sector S.12. Unconsolidated

continued

£ billion

			1999	2000	2001	2002	2003	2004	2005	2006	2007
IV.3	**FINANCIAL BALANCE SHEET** continued										
	at end of period										
AF.L	**Financial liabilities**										
AF.2	Currency and deposits										
AF.21	Currency	NLMI	35.1	35.6	36.3	37.9	40.8	46.3	47.2	49.0	50.0
AF.22	Transferable deposits										
AF.221	Deposits with UK monetary financial institutions	NLMK	2 186.4	2 582.3	2 834.8	3 034.7	3 518.7	3 984.9	4 677.5	5 332.0	5 895.3
AF.29	Other deposits	NLMP	–	2.9	0.3	0.8	0.3	0.3	1.8	1.6	5.9
AF.2	Total currency and deposits	NLMH	2 221.6	2 620.8	2 871.5	3 073.3	3 559.8	4 031.5	4 726.5	5 382.6	5 951.3
AF.3	Securities other than shares										
AF.331	Short term: money market instruments										
AF.3315	Issued by UK monetary financial institutions	NLMX	233.5	265.8	291.0	302.6	282.1	283.2	291.7	327.7	346.1
AF.3316	Issued by other non-government UK residents	NLNC	15.6	21.4	23.3	21.1	19.4	20.2	26.2	42.8	46.8
AF.332	Medium (1 to 5 year) and long term (over 5 year) bonds										
AF.3325	Medium term bonds issued by UK MFIs[1]	NLNJ	67.7	74.6	77.6	81.0	107.0	134.7	175.4	205.8	285.3
AF.3326	Other medium & long term bonds issued by UK residents	NLNM	170.9	208.0	245.0	281.7	357.1	453.3	569.9	657.1	753.6
AF.34	Financial derivatives	NLNO	–0.4	–0.1	0.3	–	–	0.1	0.2	0.7	–0.5
AF.3	Total securities other than shares	NLMQ	487.4	569.8	637.3	686.4	765.7	891.5	1 063.5	1 234.1	1 431.4
AF.4	Loans										
AF.41	Short term loans										
AF.411	Loans by UK monetary financial institutions, excluding loans secured on dwellings & financial leasing	NLNU	247.1	303.8	332.3	357.2	421.9	496.0	557.8	649.6	879.2
AF.419	Loans by rest of the world monetary financial institutions	NLNY	283.9	321.6	398.9	368.8	399.7	467.7	693.5	637.5	709.9
AF.42	Long term loans										
AF.421	Direct investment	NLOA	16.2	15.6	30.6	34.1	39.0	54.5	50.3	51.2	56.3
AF.423	Finance leasing	NLOH	2.3	2.2	2.5	2.9	3.2	3.4	3.5	3.7	3.9
AF.424	Other long-term loans by UK residents	NLOI	14.0	13.8	14.4	15.1	16.2	20.2	26.7	31.4	20.3
AF.429	Other long-term loans by the rest of the world	NLOJ	0.5	0.5	0.5	0.5	0.5	0.5	0.5	0.5	0.5
AF.4	Total loans	NLNS	564.0	657.4	779.1	778.5	880.5	1 042.3	1 332.3	1 373.8	1 670.1
AF.5	Shares and other equity										
AF.51	Shares and other equity, excluding mutual funds' shares										
AF.514	Quoted UK shares	NLOP	356.7	378.8	359.6	268.3	332.0	361.5	409.2	485.7	425.7
AF.515	Unquoted UK shares	NLOQ	174.3	239.3	258.3	256.7	277.0	305.5	338.4	388.9	395.6
AF.517	UK shares and bonds issued by other UK residents	NSQM	–	–	–	–	–	–	–	–	–
AF.52	Mutual funds' shares										
AF.521	UK mutual funds' shares	NLOY	298.7	304.5	268.2	215.8	266.3	303.9	385.0	452.4	507.5
AF.5	Total shares and other equity	NLOK	829.8	922.6	886.1	740.8	875.2	971.0	1 132.6	1 327.1	1 328.8
AF.6	Insurance technical reserves										
AF.61	Net equity of households in life assurance and pension funds' reserves	NLPA	1 631.5	1 599.2	1 531.5	1 384.3	1 509.4	1 603.4	1 894.5	2 071.9	2 186.9
AF.62	Prepayments of insurance premiums and reserves for outstanding claims	NLPD	58.9	62.8	59.0	62.8	63.5	67.2	71.2	77.2	77.3
AF.6	Total insurance technical reserves	NPYI	1 690.4	1 662.0	1 590.5	1 447.1	1 572.9	1 670.6	1 965.7	2 149.1	2 264.2
AF.7	Other accounts payable	NLPE	22.8	28.6	31.6	33.8	41.9	49.5	52.3	82.6	95.3
AF.L	**Total financial liabilities**	NLMD	5 816.0	6 461.2	6 796.0	6 760.0	7 696.0	8 656.4	10 272.9	11 549.4	12 740.9
BF.90	**Net financial assets / liabilities**										
AF.A	Total financial assets	NLIZ	5 293.2	5 947.2	6 258.0	6 311.8	7 273.8	8 218.0	9 762.6	11 042.8	12 202.5
-AF.L	*less* Total financial liabilities	–NLMD	–5 816.0	–6 461.2	–6 796.0	–6 760.0	–7 696.0	–8 656.4	–10 272.9	–11 549.4	–12 740.9
BF.90	**Net financial assets (+) / liabilities (-)**	NYOE	–522.7	–514.0	–538.0	–448.2	–422.2	–438.4	–510.3	–506.5	–538.4
	Net worth										
AN	Non-financial assets	CGDB	114.0	118.0	121.4	122.0	128.5	136.9	141.9	145.8	145.8
BF.90	Net financial assets (+) / liabilities (-)	NYOE	–522.7	–514.0	–538.0	–448.2	–422.2	–438.4	–510.3	–506.5	–538.4
BF.90	**Net worth**	CGRU	–408.7	–396.0	–416.6	–326.2	–293.7	–301.5	–368.4	–360.8	–392.6

1 UK monetary financial institutions

4.2.2 Monetary financial institutions

ESA95 sectors S.121 Central bank & S.122 Other monetary financial institutions

£ million

			1999	2000	2001	2002	2003	2004	2005	2006
II	DISTRIBUTION AND USE OF INCOME ACCOUNTS									
II.1	PRIMARY DISTRIBUTION OF INCOME ACCOUNT									
II.1.1	GENERATION OF INCOME ACCOUNT before deduction of fixed capital consumption									
	Resources									
B.1g	Total resources (Gross Value Added)	NHJN	24 962	26 418	28 669	31 310	36 262	41 862	45 321	55 003
	Uses									
D.1	Compensation of employees									
D.11	Wages and salaries	NHDJ	10 995	12 629	13 036	12 750	13 821	15 270	17 117	21 359
D.12	Employers' social contributions	NHDM	1 255	1 447	1 519	1 576	1 755	3 623	4 373	4 440
D.1	Total	NHFL	12 250	14 076	14 555	14 326	15 576	18 893	21 490	25 799
D.2	Taxes on production and imports, paid									
D.29	Production taxes other than on products	NHJE	832	480	496	512	522	526	551	586
-D.3	*less* Subsidies, received									
-D.39	Production subsidies other than on products	-NHET	–	–	–	–	–	–	–	–
B.2g	Operating surplus, gross	NHBX	11 880	11 862	13 618	16 472	20 164	22 443	23 280	28 618
B.1g	**Total uses (Gross Value Added)**	NHJN	24 962	26 418	28 669	31 310	36 262	41 862	45 321	55 003

4.2.3 Monetary financial institutions
ESA95 sectors S.121 Central bank & S.122 Other monetary financial institutions

£ million

			1999	2000	2001	2002	2003	2004	2005	2006	2007
II.1.2	**ALLOCATION OF PRIMARY INCOME ACCOUNT**										
	Resources										
B.2g	Operating surplus, gross	NHBX	11 880	11 862	13 618	16 472	20 164	22 443	23 280	28 618	31 409
D.4	Property income, received										
D.41	Interest	NHFE	120 736	158 317	150 468	120 356	117 236	141 795	180 587	237 356	314 426
D.42	Distributed income of corporations	NHFF	4 630	7 599	7 257	6 660	8 076	10 862	10 447	13 506	13 267
D.43	Reinvested earnings on direct foreign investment	NHKY	1 439	1 669	2 423	2 411	3 321	4 130	4 927	5 938	3 686
D.44	Property income attributed to insurance policy-holders	NHJS	14	8	9	8	11	9	17	15	12
D.45	Rent	NHJT	–	–	–	–	–	–	–	–	–
D.4	Total	NHJR	126 819	167 593	160 157	129 435	128 644	156 796	195 978	256 815	331 391
Total	Total resources	NRKH	138 699	179 455	173 775	145 907	148 808	179 239	219 258	285 433	362 800
	Uses										
D.4	Property income, paid										
D.41	Interest	NHFG	112 836	146 802	137 037	105 415	102 070	124 717	165 501	222 823	291 033
D.42	Distributed income of corporations	NHFH	12 917	18 580	14 126	13 399	18 384	23 385	21 426	26 663	17 676
D.43	Reinvested earnings on direct foreign investment	NHLB	986	1 911	997	1 215	1 948	499	2 692	1 487	2 432
D.45	Rent	NHJW	–	–	–	–	–	–	–	–	–
D.4	Total	NHJU	126 739	167 293	152 160	120 029	122 402	148 601	189 619	250 973	311 141
B.5g	**Balance of primary incomes, gross**	NRKI	**11 960**	**12 162**	**21 615**	**25 878**	**26 406**	**30 638**	**29 639**	**34 460**	**51 659**
Total	Total uses	NRKH	138 699	179 455	173 775	145 907	148 808	179 239	219 258	285 433	362 800

4.2.4 Monetary financial institutions
ESA95 sectors S.121 Central bank & S.122 Other monetary financial institutions

£ million

			1999	2000	2001	2002	2003	2004	2005	2006	2007
II.2	**SECONDARY DISTRIBUTION OF INCOME ACCOUNT**										
	Resources										
B.5g	**Balance of primary incomes, gross**	NRKI	11 960	12 162	21 615	25 878	26 406	30 638	29 639	34 460	51 659
D.61	Social contributions										
D.612	Imputed social contributions	NHKD	195	219	215	227	224	238	245	256	262
D.7	Other current transfers										
D.72	Non-life insurance claims	NHJZ	160	146	105	134	160	168	210	219	166
D.75	Miscellaneous current transfers	CY8D	140	140	95	58	28	5	–	–	–
D.7	Total	NRKN	300	286	200	192	188	173	210	219	166
Total	Total resources	NRKP	12 455	12 667	22 030	26 297	26 818	31 049	30 094	34 935	52 087
	Uses										
D.5	Current taxes on income, wealth etc.										
D.51	Taxes on income	NHKA	4 436	4 151	4 601	4 054	4 131	3 378	3 924	5 224	3 331
D.62	Social benefits other than social transfers in kind	NHKC	195	219	215	227	224	238	245	256	262
D.7	Other current transfers										
D.71	Net non-life insurance premiums	NHKG	160	146	105	134	160	168	210	219	166
D.75	Miscellaneous current transfers	NHKW	161	140	178	203	180	84	56	56	56
D.7	Total	NHKF	321	286	283	337	340	252	266	275	222
B.6g	**Gross Disposable Income**	NRKQ	7 503	8 011	16 931	21 679	22 123	27 181	25 659	29 180	48 272
Total	Total uses	NRKP	12 455	12 667	22 030	26 297	26 818	31 049	30 094	34 935	52 087

4.2.6 Monetary financial institutions
ESA95 sectors S.121 Central bank & S.122 Other monetary financial institutions

£ million

			1999	2000	2001	2002	2003	2004	2005	2006	2007
II.4.1	**USE OF DISPOSABLE INCOME ACCOUNT**										
	Resources										
B.6g	**Total resources (Gross Disposable Income)**	NRKQ	7 503	8 011	16 931	21 679	22 123	27 181	25 659	29 180	48 272
	Uses										
B.8g	**Total uses (Gross Saving)**	NRKT	7 503	8 011	16 931	21 679	22 123	27 181	25 659	29 180	48 272

4.2.7 Monetary financial institutions

ESA95 sectors S.121 Central bank & S.122 Other monetary financial institutions

£ million

			1999	2000	2001	2002	2003	2004	2005	2006	2007
III	**ACCUMULATION ACCOUNTS**										
III.1	**CAPITAL ACCOUNT**										
III.1.1	**CHANGE IN NET WORTH DUE TO SAVING & CAPITAL TRANSFERS ACCOUNT**										
	Changes in liabilities and net worth										
B.8g	**Gross Saving**	**NRKT**	7 503	8 011	16 931	21 679	22 123	27 181	25 659	29 180	48 272
D.9	Capital transfers receivable										
D.92	Investment grants	**NHKM**	–	–	–	–	–	–	–	–	–
D.99	Other capital transfers	**NHKN**	–	–	–	–	–	–	–	–	–
D.9	Total	**NHKL**	–	–	–	–	–	–	–	–	–
-D.9	*less* Capital transfers payable										
-D.91	Capital taxes	**–NHEQ**	–	–	–	–	–	–	–	–	–
-D.99	Other capital transfers	**–NHEV**	–	–	–	–	–	–	–	–	–
-D.9	Total	**–NHKP**	–	–	–	–	–	–	–	–	–
B.10.1g	Total change in liabilities and net worth	**NRMH**	7 503	8 011	16 931	21 679	22 123	27 181	25 659	29 180	48 272
	Changes in assets										
B.10.1g	Changes in net worth due to saving and capital transfers before deduction of fixed capital consumption	**NRMH**	7 503	8 011	16 931	21 679	22 123	27 181	25 659	29 180	48 272
III.1.2	**ACQUISITION OF NON-FINANCIAL ASSETS ACCOUNT**										
B.10.1g	**Total changes in liabilities and net worth due to saving & capital transfers**	**NRMH**	7 503	8 011	16 931	21 679	22 123	27 181	25 659	29 180	48 272
	Changes in assets										
P.5	Gross capital formation										
P.51	Gross fixed capital formation	**NHFD**	3 553	3 961	4 127	5 008	4 555	4 169	4 967	4 872	5 535
P.52	Changes in inventories	**NHFC**	47	55	58	67	48	48	48	199	206
P.53	Acquisitions less disposals of valuables	**NHKT**	–	–	–	–	–	–	–	–	–
P.5	Total	**NHKS**	3 600	4 016	4 185	5 075	4 603	4 217	5 015	5 071	5 741
K.2	Acquisitions less disposals of non-produced non-financial assets	**NHKU**	–	–	–	–	–	–	–	–	–
B.9	**Net lending (+) / net borrowing (-)**	**NHFK**	3 903	3 995	12 746	16 604	17 520	22 964	20 644	24 109	42 531
B.10.1g	Total change in assets	**NRMH**	7 503	8 011	16 931	21 679	22 123	27 181	25 659	29 180	48 272

4.2.8 Monetary financial institutions

ESA95 sectors S.121 Central bank & S.122 Other monetary financial institutions. Unconsolidated

£ million

			1999	2000	2001	2002	2003	2004	2005	2006	2007
III.2	**FINANCIAL ACCOUNT**										
F.A	**Net acquisition of financial assets**										
F.2	Currency and deposits										
F.21	Currency	NGCB	2 717	−1 419	−1 279	165	903	3 071	−1 104	−168	−1 413
F.22	Transferable deposits										
F.221	Deposits with UK MFIs[1]	NGCD	1 908	39 751	83 188	75 820	128 363	131 420	129 309	231 826	96 409
F.229	Deposits with rest of the world monetary financial institutions	NGCH	−29 477	130 066	36 702	52 742	87 727	105 775	157 467	178 001	375 379
F.29	Other deposits	NGCI	−10	−6	−3	−2	−1	−6	–	–	−11
F.2	Total currency and deposits	NGCA	−24 862	168 392	118 608	128 725	216 992	240 260	285 672	409 659	470 364
F.3	Securities other than shares										
F.331	Short term: money market instruments										
F.3311	Issued by UK central government	NGCL	35	−1 222	6 859	10 798	−1 655	−2 362	−304	−3 746	−6 513
F.3312	Issued by UK local government	NGCP	–	–	–	–	–	–	–	–	–
F.3315	Issued by UK MFIs[1]	NGCQ	10 743	−19 114	6 124	330	−14 166	1 810	3 728	3 114	−8 676
F.3316	Issued by other UK residents	NGCV	63	847	−536	−225	2 139	−1 166	909	2 239	−3 768
F.3319	Issued by the rest of the world	NGCW	9 723	345	7 374	−3 982	7 432	−4 622	2 142	5 058	8 534
F.332	Medium (1 to 5 year) and long term (over 5 year) bonds										
F.3321	Issued by UK central government	NGCY	−6 471	−6 951	−4 799	−4 805	−5 030	5 121	−1 309	−4 582	2 302
F.3322	Issued by UK local government	NGDB	–	–	–	–	–	–	–	–	–
F.3325	Medium term bonds issued by UK MFIs[1]	NGDC	5 071	3 976	−1 282	−860	2 590	2 525	1 640	−58	1 091
F.3326	Other medium & long term bonds issued by UK residents	NGDF	6 867	18 579	9 204	−1 748	8 423	12 291	26 009	45 050	27 954
F.3329	Long term bonds issued by the rest of the world	NGDG	11 842	36 532	39 224	3 768	−14 511	58 779	62 415	100 963	43 738
F.34	Financial derivatives	NGDH	−2 727	−1 663	−8 601	−1 205	5 263	7 847	−9 556	−7 449	19 001
F.3	Total securities other than shares	NGCJ	35 146	31 329	53 567	2 071	−9 515	80 223	85 674	140 589	83 663
F.4	Loans										
F.41	Short term loans										
F.411	Loans by UK MFIs[1], excluding loans secured on dwellings & financial leasing	NGDN	66 698	150 664	108 353	87 544	159 494	235 263	255 959	305 306	516 001
F.42	Long term loans										
F.421	Direct investment	NGDT	–	–	–	−52	−4	–	–	–	–
F.422	Loans secured on dwellings	NGDW	32 143	28 420	37 927	59 962	66 529	60 004	46 301	46 430	26 718
F.423	Finance leasing	NGEA	37	−40	1	8	−21	−13	−14	−4	−6
F.424	Other long term loans	NGEB	−355	−1 476	187	−1 017	113	231	−106	−478	−168
F.4	Total loans	NGDL	98 523	177 568	146 468	146 445	226 111	295 485	302 140	351 254	542 545
F.5	Shares and other equity										
F.51	Shares and other equity, excluding mutual funds' shares										
F.514	Quoted UK shares	NGEI	1 477	3 395	558	−10 446	6 243	1 505	8 198	6 084	3 635
F.515	Unquoted UK shares	NGEJ	1 943	8 931	2 693	347	2 564	8 434	4 208	21 099	10 308
F.517	UK shares and bonds issued by other UK residents	NSQA	–	–	–	–	–	–	–	–	–
F.519	Shares and other equity issued by the rest of the world	NGEN	1 405	10 513	2 237	−9 268	22 544	46 981	46 341	34 106	20 620
F.52	Mutual funds' shares										
F.521	UK mutual funds' shares	NGER	3	43	5	8	4	28	49	50	22
F.5	Total shares and other equity	NGED	4 828	22 882	5 493	−19 359	31 355	56 948	58 796	61 339	34 585
F.7	Other accounts receivable	NGEX	−85	37	−29	−180	−143	−99	16	−73	−37
F.A	**Total net acquisition of financial assets**	NGBW	113 550	400 208	324 107	257 702	464 800	672 817	732 298	962 768	1 131 120

1 UK monetary financial institutions

4.2.8 Monetary financial institutions

ESA95 sectors S.121 Central bank & S.122 Other monetary financial institutions. Unconsolidated

continued   £ million

			1999	2000	2001	2002	2003	2004	2005	2006	2007
III.2	**FINANCIAL ACCOUNT** continued										
F.L	**Net acquisition of financial liabilities**										
F.2	Currency and deposits										
F.21	Currency	NGFF	5 231	448	738	1 532	2 958	5 460	945	1 745	1 043
F.22	Transferable deposits										
F.221	Deposits with UK MFIs[1]	NGFH	35 792	345 481	286 540	218 055	399 447	540 924	586 768	783 929	981 443
F.2	Total currency and deposits	NGFE	41 023	345 929	287 278	219 587	402 405	546 384	587 713	785 674	982 486
F.3	Securities other than shares										
F.331	Short term: money market instruments										
F.3315	Issued by UK MFIs[1]	NGFU	31 135	23 941	22 835	25 599	−11 489	8 024	−3 488	53 189	17 860
F.332	Medium (1 to 5 year) and long term (over 5 year) bonds										
F.3325	Medium term bonds issued by UK MFIs[1]	NGGG	12 081	4 750	3 575	4 238	25 258	29 810	37 843	40 534	57 261
F.3326	Other medium & long term bonds issued by UK residents	NGGJ	5 818	11 006	10 068	8 801	26 069	7 934	16 894	−9 678	−12 681
F.34	Financial derivatives	NGGL	3	43	89	−70	63	−147	−207	−110	−312
F.3	Total securities other than shares	NGFN	49 037	39 740	36 567	38 568	39 901	45 621	51 042	83 935	62 128
F.4	Loans										
F.42	Long term loans										
F.421	Direct investment	NGGX	9	223	165	−92	171	137	27	−7	−56
F.423	Finance leasing	NGHE	−168	−61	135	275	190	98	72	110	108
F.4	Total loans	NGGP	−159	162	300	183	361	235	99	103	52
F.5	Shares and other equity										
F.51	Shares and other equity, excluding mutual funds' shares										
F.514	Quoted UK shares	NGHM	−519	2 410	2 723	2 041	2 979	3 183	3 266	2 881	6 263
F.515	Unquoted UK shares	NGHN	1 111	10 862	3 568	1 756	2 755	1 292	3 508	2 303	3 248
F.516	Other UK equity (including direct investment in property)	NGHO	–	–	43	32	−9	−8	–	–	–
F.517	UK shares and bonds issued by other UK residents	NSQB	–	–	–	–	–	–	–	–	–
F.5	Total shares and other equity	NGHH	592	13 272	6 334	3 829	5 725	4 467	6 774	5 184	9 511
F.7	Other accounts payable	NGIB	−283	1 449	−2 376	−571	221	1 004	974	653	1 694
F.L	**Total net acquisition of financial liabilities**	NGFA	90 210	400 552	328 103	261 596	448 613	597 711	646 602	875 549	1 055 871
B.9	**Net lending / borrowing**										
F.A	Total net acquisition of financial assets	NGBW	113 550	400 208	324 107	257 702	464 800	672 817	732 298	962 768	1 131 120
−F.L	*less* Total net acquisition of financial liabilities	−NGFA	−90 210	−400 552	−328 103	−261 596	−448 613	−597 711	−646 602	−875 549	−1 055 871
B.9f	Net lending (+) / net borrowing (-), from financial account	NYNS	23 340	−344	−3 996	−3 894	16 187	75 106	85 696	87 219	75 249
dB.9f	Statistical discrepancy	NYPE	−19 437	4 339	16 742	20 498	1 333	−52 142	−65 052	−63 110	−32 718
B.9	**Net lending (+) / net borrowing (-), from capital account**	NHFK	**3 903**	**3 995**	**12 746**	**16 604**	**17 520**	**22 964**	**20 644**	**24 109**	**42 531**

1 UK monetary financial institutions

4.2.9 Monetary financial institutions

ESA95 sectors S.121 Central bank & S.122 Other monetary financial institutions. Unconsolidated

£ billion

			1999	2000	2001	2002	2003	2004	2005	2006	2007
IV.3	**FINANCIAL BALANCE SHEET** at end of period										
AF.A	**Financial assets**										
AF.2	Currency and deposits										
AF.21	Currency	NNSY	9.9	8.4	7.1	7.3	8.2	11.3	10.2	10.0	8.6
AF.22	Transferable deposits										
AF.221	Deposits with UK MFIs[1]	NNTA	308.1	355.6	417.1	509.1	736.4	835.6	1 004.7	1 285.7	842.6
AF.229	Deposits with rest of the world monetary financial institutions	NNTE	624.6	775.6	805.3	843.0	921.4	1 006.9	1 199.2	1 286.0	1 714.1
AF.29	Other deposits	NNTF	0.1	0.1	–	–	–	–	–	–	–
AF.2	Total currency and deposits	NNSX	942.6	1 139.7	1 229.6	1 359.5	1 666.1	1 853.8	2 214.1	2 581.7	2 565.3
AF.3	Securities other than shares										
AF.331	Short term: money market instruments										
AF.3311	Issued by UK central government	NNTI	2.8	1.6	8.5	19.3	18.4	16.1	15.8	12.1	5.6
AF.3312	Issued by UK local government	NNTM	–	–	–	–	–	–	–	–	–
AF.3315	Issued by UK MFIs[1]	NNTN	114.5	97.0	103.6	102.5	89.8	90.9	96.1	98.4	88.7
AF.3316	Issued by other UK residents	NNTS	0.7	1.9	1.4	1.1	3.2	1.9	2.9	5.0	1.3
AF.3319	Issued by the rest of the world	NNTT	31.7	34.9	42.1	34.6	42.8	37.2	39.8	42.8	53.8
AF.332	Medium (1 to 5 year) and long term (over 5 year) bonds										
AF.3321	Issued by UK central government	NNTV	15.8	8.6	3.7	–1.0	–6.3	–1.4	–2.8	–7.7	–5.5
AF.3322	Issued by UK local government	NNTY	–	–	–	–	–	–	–	–	–
AF.3325	Medium term bonds issued by UK MFIs[1]	NNTZ	16.6	20.7	18.8	18.5	21.1	23.4	25.2	24.5	25.2
AF.3326	Other medium & long term bonds issued by UK residents	NNUC	61.5	71.2	71.8	50.9	65.9	90.0	133.6	189.4	209.4
AF.3329	Long term bonds issued by the rest of the world	NNUD	243.1	288.7	323.4	336.3	327.3	359.7	413.7	479.3	555.2
AF.34	Financial derivatives	NNUE									
AF.3	Total securities other than shares	NNTG	486.9	524.6	573.3	562.2	562.2	618.0	724.4	843.8	933.6
AF.4	Loans										
AF.41	Short term loans										
AF.411	Loans by UK MFIs[1], excluding loans secured on dwellings & financial leasing	NNUK	809.4	976.8	1 074.7	1 142.5	1 283.9	1 493.7	1 761.9	1 975.9	2 538.9
AF.42	Long term loans										
AF.421	Direct investment	NNUQ	–	–	0.3	–	–	–	–	–	–
AF.422	Loans secured on dwellings	NNUT	458.5	493.3	532.1	591.2	653.4	708.4	749.0	795.5	829.7
AF.423	Finance leasing	NNUX	2.7	2.7	2.7	2.7	2.7	2.6	2.6	2.6	2.6
AF.424	Other long term loans	NNUY	6.0	4.8	5.1	3.8	3.7	4.2	4.3	3.4	3.3
AF.4	Total loans	NNUI	1 276.7	1 477.7	1 614.9	1 740.2	1 943.6	2 208.9	2 517.8	2 777.5	3 374.6
AF.5	Shares and other equity										
AF.51	Shares and other equity, excluding mutual funds' shares										
AF.514	Quoted UK shares	NNVF	9.8	13.2	13.8	3.3	9.6	8.6	16.6	22.7	26.2
AF.515	Unquoted UK shares	NNVG	38.3	60.4	66.1	70.7	89.4	108.8	113.8	153.0	123.2
AF.517	UK shares and bonds issued by other UK residents	NSQU	–	–	–	–	–	–	–	–	–
AF.519	Shares and other equity issued by the rest of the world	NNVK	21.1	38.0	35.9	26.4	44.2	87.4	129.1	163.3	190.4
AF.52	Mutual funds' shares										
AF.521	UK mutual funds' shares	NNVO	1.7	1.6	1.3	0.9	1.0	1.2	1.5	1.7	1.7
AF.5	Total shares and other equity	NNVA	70.9	113.2	117.0	101.3	144.2	205.9	261.1	340.7	341.4
AF.7	Other accounts receivable	NNVU	1.0	1.0	1.0	0.8	0.6	0.5	0.2	0.1	–
AF.A	**Total financial assets**	NNST	2 778.0	3 256.2	3 535.7	3 763.9	4 316.6	4 887.1	5 717.5	6 543.8	7 214.9

1 UK monetary financial institutions

4.2.9 Monetary financial institutions

ESA95 sectors S.121 Central bank & S.122 Other monetary financial institutions. Unconsolidated

£ billion

			1999	2000	2001	2002	2003	2004	2005	2006	2007
IV.3	**FINANCIAL BALANCE SHEET** continued at end of period										
AF.L	**Financial liabilities**										
AF.2	Currency and deposits										
AF.21	Currency	NNWC	35.1	35.6	36.3	37.9	40.8	46.3	47.2	49.0	50.0
AF.22	Transferable deposits										
AF.221	Deposits with UK MFIs[1]	NNWE	2 186.4	2 582.3	2 834.8	3 034.7	3 518.7	3 984.9	4 677.5	5 332.0	5 895.3
AF.2	Total currency and deposits	NNWB	2 221.6	2 617.9	2 871.2	3 072.5	3 559.6	4 031.2	4 724.7	5 381.0	5 945.4
AF.3	Securities other than shares										
AF.331	Short term: money market instruments										
AF.3315	Issued by UK MFIs[1]	NNWR	233.5	265.8	291.0	302.6	282.1	283.2	291.7	327.7	346.1
AF.332	Medium (1 to 5 year) and long term (over 5 year) bonds										
AF.3325	Medium term bonds issued by UK MFIs[1]	NNXD	67.7	74.6	77.6	81.0	107.0	134.7	175.4	205.8	285.3
AF.3326	Other medium & long term bonds issued by UK residents	NNXG	55.3	69.2	79.3	92.2	113.2	119.4	138.8	143.4	112.9
AF.34	Financial derivatives	NNXI	−0.4	−0.1	0.3	−	−	0.1	0.2	0.7	−0.5
AF.3	Total securities other than shares	NNWK	356.1	409.5	448.2	475.8	502.4	537.5	606.3	677.6	743.9
AF.4	Loans										
AF.41	Short term loans										
AF.411	Loans by UK MFIs[1], excluding loans secured on dwellings & financial leasing	NNXO	−	−	−	−	−	−	−	−	−
AF.42	Long term loans										
AF.421	Direct investment	NNXU	2.7	0.6	0.9	0.9	1.2	1.3	1.3	1.3	1.3
AF.423	Finance leasing	NNYB	1.1	1.1	1.2	1.5	1.7	1.8	1.9	2.0	2.1
AF.424	Other long-term loans by UK residents	NNYC	−	−	−	−	−	−	−	−	−
AF.4	Total loans	NNXM	3.9	1.7	2.2	2.4	2.9	3.1	3.2	3.3	3.3
AF.5	Shares and other equity										
AF.51	Shares and other equity, excluding mutual funds' shares										
AF.514	Quoted UK shares	NNYJ	63.4	39.1	28.3	19.4	20.8	14.0	11.3	13.5	5.0
AF.515	Unquoted UK shares	NNYK	58.4	94.2	104.5	109.1	108.0	119.8	124.5	126.8	133.3
AF.517	UK shares and bonds issued by other UK residents	NSQV	−	−	−	−	−	−	−	−	−
AF.5	Total shares and other equity	NNYE	121.8	133.4	132.7	128.5	128.8	133.8	135.7	140.2	138.3
AF.7	Other accounts payable	NNYY	3.9	4.8	4.4	3.9	4.0	4.9	5.8	6.3	7.6
AF.L	**Total financial liabilities**	NNVX	2 707.2	3 167.3	3 458.7	3 683.1	4 197.7	4 710.5	5 475.7	6 208.4	6 838.5
BF.90	**Net financial assets / liabilities**										
AF.A	Total financial assets	NNST	2 778.0	3 256.2	3 535.7	3 763.9	4 316.6	4 887.1	5 717.5	6 543.8	7 214.9
-AF.L	*less* Total financial liabilities	−NNVX	−2 707.2	−3 167.3	−3 458.7	−3 683.1	−4 197.7	−4 710.5	−5 475.7	−6 208.4	−6 838.5
BF.90	**Net financial assets (+) / liabilities (-)**	NYOL	70.8	88.9	77.0	80.8	118.9	176.6	241.9	335.4	376.4

1 UK monetary financial institutions

4.3.2 Other financial intermediaries and financial auxiliaries
ESA95 sectors S.123 Other financial intermediaries & S.124 Financial auxiliaries

£ million

			1999	2000	2001	2002	2003	2004	2005	2006
II	**DISTRIBUTION AND USE OF INCOME ACCOUNTS**									
II.1	**PRIMARY DISTRIBUTION OF INCOME ACCOUNT**									
II.1.1	**GENERATION OF INCOME ACCOUNT** before deduction of fixed capital consumption									
	Resources									
B.1g	**Total resources (Gross Value Added)**	**NHMH**	**10 106**	**7 413**	**8 556**	**12 784**	**12 975**	**13 429**	**15 286**	**16 352**
	Uses									
D.1	Compensation of employees									
D.11	Wages and salaries	**NHED**	7 797	8 432	8 965	9 373	9 181	10 732	11 975	14 884
D.12	Employers' social contributions	**NHEE**	1 221	1 390	1 439	1 520	1 880	2 546	3 062	3 095
D.1	Total	**NHLX**	9 018	9 822	10 404	10 893	11 061	13 278	15 037	17 979
D.2	Taxes on production and imports, paid									
D.29	Production taxes other than on products	**NHLY**	456	429	528	527	551	564	562	608
-D.3	*less* Subsidies, received									
-D.39	Production subsidies other than on products	**−NHLF**	–	–	–	–	–	–	–	–
B.2g	Operating surplus, gross	**NHBY**	632	−2 838	−2 376	1 364	1 363	−413	−313	−2 235
B.1g	**Total uses (Gross Value Added)**	**NHMH**	**10 106**	**7 413**	**8 556**	**12 784**	**12 975**	**13 429**	**15 286**	**16 352**

4.3.3 Other financial intermediaries and financial auxiliaries

ESA95 sectors S.123 Other financial intermediaries & S.124 Financial auxiliaries

£ million

			1999	2000	2001	2002	2003	2004	2005	2006	2007
II.1.2	**ALLOCATION OF PRIMARY INCOME ACCOUNT**										
	Resources										
B.2g	Operating surplus, gross	**NHBY**	632	−2 838	−2 376	1 364	1 363	−413	−313	−2 235	1 950
D.4	Property income, received										
D.41	Interest	**NHLQ**	17 686	22 243	23 421	18 172	18 159	24 669	34 719	46 212	61 159
D.42	Distributed income of corporations	**NHLR**	12 439	22 354	19 600	23 601	27 883	32 508	35 371	42 267	50 336
D.43	Reinvested earnings on direct foreign investment	**NHNS**	2 763	2 849	2 699	2 942	4 004	1 381	2 166	2 600	2 923
D.44	Property income attributed to insurance policy-holders	**NHMM**	11	8	9	8	9	9	15	13	10
D.45	Rent	**NHMN**	–	–	–	–	–	–	–	–	–
D.4	Total	**NHML**	32 899	47 454	45 729	44 723	50 055	58 567	72 271	91 092	114 428
Total	Total resources	**NRKX**	33 531	44 616	43 353	46 087	51 418	58 154	71 958	88 857	116 378
	Uses										
D.4	Property income										
D.41	Interest	**NHLS**	22 874	32 291	32 720	27 549	26 884	33 484	44 868	58 566	79 076
D.42	Distributed income of corporations	**NHLT**	13 028	15 528	25 626	21 007	21 609	24 323	26 360	31 494	36 607
D.43	Reinvested earnings on direct foreign investment	**NHNU**	767	1 485	−2 568	873	991	814	1 958	3 141	7 171
D.45	Rent	**NHMQ**	–	–	–	–	–	–	–	–	–
D.4	Total	**NHMO**	36 669	49 304	55 778	49 429	49 484	58 621	73 186	93 201	122 854
B.5g	**Balance of primary incomes, gross**	**NRKZ**	**−3 138**	**−4 688**	**−12 425**	**−3 342**	**1 934**	**−467**	**−1 228**	**−4 344**	**−6 476**
Total	Total uses	**NRKX**	33 531	44 616	43 353	46 087	51 418	58 154	71 958	88 857	116 378

4.3.4 Other financial intermediaries and financial auxiliaries
ESA95 sectors S.123 Other financial intermediaries & S.124 Financial auxiliaries

£ million

			1999	2000	2001	2002	2003	2004	2005	2006	2007
II.2	**SECONDARY DISTRIBUTION OF INCOME ACCOUNT**										
	Resources										
B.5g	**Balance of primary incomes, gross**	NRKZ	−3 138	−4 688	−12 425	−3 342	1 934	−467	−1 228	−4 344	−6 476
D.61	Social contributions										
D.612	Imputed social contributions	NHMX	143	153	154	172	158	168	173	179	182
D.7	Other current transfers										
D.72	Non-life insurance claims	NHMT	91	123	89	134	139	141	179	183	139
D.75	Miscellaneous current transfers	NRLD	–	–	–	–	–	–	–	–	–
D.7	Total	NRLE	91	123	89	134	139	141	179	183	139
Total	Total resources	NRLF	−2 904	−4 412	−12 182	−3 036	2 231	−158	−876	−3 982	−6 155
	Uses										
D.5	Current taxes on income, wealth etc.										
D.51	Taxes on income	NHMU	3 299	4 859	9 290	5 042	1 499	268	−359	6 472	5 302
D.62	Social benefits other than social transfers in kind	NHMW	143	153	154	172	158	168	173	179	182
D.7	Other current transfers										
D.71	Net non-life insurance premiums	NHNA	91	123	89	134	139	141	179	183	139
D.75	Miscellaneous current transfers	NHNQ	23	24	24	24	24	24	24	24	24
D.7	Total	NHMZ	114	147	113	158	163	165	203	207	163
B.6g	**Gross Disposable Income**	NRLG	−6 460	−9 571	−21 739	−8 408	411	−759	−893	−10 840	−11 802
Total	Total uses	NRLF	−2 904	−4 412	−12 182	−3 036	2 231	−158	−876	−3 982	−6 155

4.3.6 Other financial intermediaries and financial auxiliaries
ESA95 sectors S.123 Other financial intermediaries & S.124 Financial auxiliaries

£ million

			1999	2000	2001	2002	2003	2004	2005	2006	2007
II.4.1	**USE OF DISPOSABLE INCOME ACCOUNT**										
	Resources										
B.6g	**Total resources (Gross Disposable Income)**	NRLG	−6 460	−9 571	−21 739	−8 408	411	−759	−893	−10 840	−11 802
	Uses										
B.8g	**Total uses (Gross Saving)**	NRLJ	−6 460	−9 571	−21 739	−8 408	411	−759	−893	−10 840	−11 802

4.3.7 Other financial intermediaries and financial auxiliaries

ESA95 sectors S.123 Other financial intermediaries & S.124 Financial auxiliaries

£ million

			1999	2000	2001	2002	2003	2004	2005	2006	2007
III	**ACCUMULATION ACCOUNTS**										
III.1	**CAPITAL ACCOUNT**										
III.1.1	**CHANGE IN NET WORTH DUE TO SAVING & CAPITAL TRANSFERS ACCOUNT**										
	Changes in liabilities and net worth										
B.8g	**Gross Saving**	**NRLJ**	−6 460	−9 571	−21 739	−8 408	411	−759	−893	−10 840	−11 802
D.9	Capital transfers receivable										
D.92	Investment grants	**NHNG**	–	–	–	–	–	–	–	–	–
D.99	Other capital transfers	**NHNH**	–	–	–	–	–	–	–	–	–
D.9	Total	**NHNF**	–	–	–	–	–	–	–	–	–
-D.9	*less* Capital transfers payable										
-D.91	Capital taxes	**−NRXX**	–	–	–	–	–	–	–	–	–
-D.99	Other capital transfers	**−NHLH**	–	–	–	–	–	–	–	–	–
-D.9	Total	**−NHNI**	–	–	–	–	–	–	–	–	–
B.10.1g	Total change in liabilities and net worth	**NRMI**	−6 460	−9 571	−21 739	−8 408	411	−759	−893	−10 840	−11 802
	Changes in assets										
B.10.1g	Change in net worth due to saving and capital transfers before deduction of fixed capital consumption	**NRMI**	−6 460	−9 571	−21 739	−8 408	411	−759	−893	−10 840	−11 802
III.1.2	**ACQUISITION OF NON-FINANCIAL ASSETS ACCOUNT**										
B.10.1g	**Total changes in liabilities and net worth due to saving and capital transfers**	**NRMI**	−6 460	−9 571	−21 739	−8 408	411	−759	−893	−10 840	−11 802
	Changes in assets										
P.5	Gross capital formation										
P.51	Gross fixed capital formation	**NHLP**	2 298	2 310	1 546	1 379	1 162	725	1 108	1 366	1 518
P.52	Changes in inventories	**NHLO**	–	–	–	–	–	–	–	–	–
P.53	Acquisitions less disposals of valuables	**NHNN**	–	–	–	–	–	–	–	–	–
P.5	Total	**NHNM**	2 298	2 310	1 546	1 379	1 162	725	1 108	1 366	1 518
K.2	Acquisitions less disposals of non-produced non-financial assets	**NHNO**	–	–	–	6	11	18	20	20	20
B.9	**Net lending (+) / net borrowing (-)**	**NHLW**	−8 758	−11 881	−23 285	−9 793	−762	−1 502	−2 021	−12 226	−13 340
Total	Total change in assets	**NRMI**	−6 460	−9 571	−21 739	−8 408	411	−759	−893	−10 840	−11 802

4.3.8 Other financial intermediaries and financial auxiliaries
ESA95 sectors S.123 and S.124 Unconsolidated

£ million

		1999	2000	2001	2002	2003	2004	2005	2006	2007
III.2	**FINANCIAL ACCOUNT**									
F.A	**Net acquisition of financial assets**									
F.2	Currency and deposits									
F.21	Currency	NFJD	–	–	–	–	–	–	–	–	–
F.22	Transferable deposits									
F.2211	Sterling deposits with UK banks	NFJG	−12 555	20 176	8 653	6 101	2 788	26 511	70 628	70 119	56 110
F.2212	Foreign currency deposits with UK banks	NFJH	2 601	19 659	29 439	−970	26 864	15 439	30 777	38 938	48 879
F.2213	Sterling deposits with UK building societies	NFJI	454	141	326	102	1 298	177	255	153	2 893
F.229	Deposits with rest of the world monetary financial institutions	NFJJ	47 109	46 983	58 040	−12 963	52 104	37 303	167 116	50 338	36 409
F.29	Other deposits	NFJK	–	2 691	−1 567	1 265	−1 063	1 393	1 392	−2 083	2 259
F.2	Total currency and deposits	NFJC	37 609	89 650	94 891	−6 465	81 991	80 823	270 168	157 465	146 550
F.3	Securities other than shares									
F.331	Short term: money market instruments									
F.3311	Issued by UK central government	NFJN	−650	−59	1 071	−413	2 492	1 075	−2 053	1 041	1 258
F.3312	Issued by UK local government	NFJR	–	–	–	–	–	–	–	–	–
F.3315	Issued by UK monetary financial institutions	NFJS	6 431	2 651	−6 807	4 125	−1 155	−4 508	471	−3 377	6 913
F.3316	Issued by other UK residents	NFJX	191	486	−1 037	−429	118	341	−102	−228	183
F.3319	Issued by the rest of the world	NFJY	3 579	−4 144	2 093	−2 018	1 911	665	1 273	3 920	−3 618
F.332	Medium (1 to 5 year) and long term (over 5 year) bonds									
F.3321	Issued by UK central government	NFKA	9 712	12 347	−9 855	5 932	2 024	4 236	−6 011	15 758	24 174
F.3322	Issued by UK local government	NFKD	16	28	22	39	9	8	–	–	–
F.3325	Medium term bonds issued by UK MFIs[1]	NFKE	604	−422	576	839	2 191	2 189	3 312	3 565	4 802
F.3326	Other medium & long term bonds issued by UK residents	NFKH	12 475	15 573	11 126	4 064	15 705	8 649	9 623	−4 421	3 788
F.3329	Long term bonds issued by the rest of the world	NFKI	−27 709	−1 307	−18 168	−464	12 422	23 431	14 666	−18 987	−14 561
F.3	Total securities other than shares	NFJL	4 649	25 153	−20 979	11 675	35 717	36 086	21 179	−2 729	22 939
F.4	Loans									
F.42	Long term loans									
F.421	Direct investment	NFKV	493	253	1 142	3 705	−2 731	2 031	2 575	862	2 569
F.422	Loans secured on dwellings	NFKY	6 298	13 608	16 256	23 641	35 070	42 268	43 823	63 435	80 549
F.423	Finance leasing	NFLC	−303	−251	321	750	745	722	565	670	622
F.424	Other long-term loans by UK residents	NFLD	3 070	5	2 776	4 253	4 978	2 338	9 991	5 153	58 363
F.4	Total loans	NFKN	9 558	13 615	20 495	32 349	38 062	47 359	56 954	70 120	142 103
F.5	Shares and other equity									
F.51	Shares and other equity, excluding mutual funds' shares									
F.514	Quoted UK shares	NFLK	14 402	1 157	69 605	10 921	11 619	16 629	1 953	6 956	34 819
F.515	Unquoted UK shares	NFLL	−3 460	15 761	−1 181	−876	−585	−1 103	1 842	−635	−55
F.517	UK shares and bonds issued by other UK residents	NSPJ	–	–	–	–	–	–	–	–	–
F.519	Shares and other equity issued by the rest of the world	NFLP	20 549	32 127	30 906	−5 177	13 651	13 219	−9 410	−2 762	36 379
F.52	Mutual funds' shares									
F.521	UK mutual funds' shares	NFLT	29	118	−12	41	16	76	143	131	42
F.5	Total shares and other equity	NFLF	31 520	49 163	99 318	4 909	24 701	28 821	−5 472	3 690	71 185
F.6	Insurance technical reserves									
F.62	Prepayments of insurance premiums and reserves for outstanding claims	NFLY	−22	15	−20	20	10	48	52	66	−1
F.7	Other accounts receivable	NFLZ	706	657	393	618	605	644	643	645	645
F.A	**Total net acquisition of financial assets**	NFIY	84 020	178 253	194 098	43 106	181 086	193 781	343 524	229 257	383 421

1 UK monetary financial institutions

4.3.8 Other financial intermediaries and financial auxiliaries
ESA95 sectors S.123 and S.124 Unconsolidated

continued   £ million

		1999	2000	2001	2002	2003	2004	2005	2006	2007
III.2	**FINANCIAL ACCOUNT** continued									
F.L	**Net acquisition of financial liabilities**									
F.2	Currency and deposits	NFMG	–	2 919	–2 578	476	–536	18	550	–12	4 299
F.3	Securities other than shares										
F.331	Short term: money market instruments										
F.3316	Issued by UK residents other than monetary financial institutions and government	NFNB	31	–16	–	267	–567	122	237	1 422	–287
F.332	Medium (1 to 5 year) and long term (over 5 year) bonds										
F.3326	Other medium & long term bonds issued by UK residents institutions and government	NFNL	17 162	24 073	23 255	20 662	53 255	70 726	83 767	117 570	137 678
F.3	Total securities other than shares	NFMP	17 193	24 057	23 255	20 929	52 688	70 848	84 004	118 992	137 391
F.4	Loans										
F.41	Short term loans										
F.4111	Sterling loans by UK banks	NFNU	14 075	20 952	4 114	9 983	16 291	29 086	32 625	46 791	114 915
F.4112	Foreign currency loans by the UK banks	NFNV	–2 768	30 383	26 528	16 548	40 304	33 707	16 587	60 687	80 350
F.4113	Sterling loans by building societies	NFNW	1 958	2 215	1 606	1 892	4 937	3 832	6 683	8 466	6 746
F.419	Loans by rest of the world monetary financial institutions	NFNX	54 877	55 555	77 118	–34 727	31 085	71 096	209 344	–23 043	52 111
F.42	Long term loans										
F.421	Direct investment	NFNZ	1 283	601	11 060	6 554	2 200	1 872	–7 370	11	6 288
F.423	Finance leasing	NFOG	–155	–66	128	136	104	95	71	81	79
F.424	Other long-term loans by UK residents	NFOH	–954	13 400	6 224	708	–5 216	810	17 150	40 239	–6 053
F.429	Other long-term loans by the rest of the world	NFOI	46	–30	6	–21	–42	10	29	–	26
F.4	Total loans	NFNR	68 362	123 010	126 784	1 073	89 663	140 508	275 119	133 232	254 462
F.5	Shares and other equity										
F.51	Shares and other equity, excluding mutual funds' shares										
F.514	Quoted UK shares	NFOO	2 276	5 273	10 297	–809	10 711	7 490	6 799	14 905	2 058
F.515	Unquoted UK shares	NFOP	7 633	23 337	12 119	7 234	12 217	18 487	23 534	35 751	35 937
F.517	UK shares and bonds issued by other UK residents	NSPK	–	–	–	–	–	–	–	–	–
F.52	Mutual funds' shares										
F.521	UK mutual funds' shares	NFOX	14 719	14 102	9 338	6 259	8 212	3 489	8 300	14 445	–2 032
F.5	Total shares and other equity	NFOJ	24 628	42 712	31 754	12 684	31 140	29 466	38 633	65 101	35 963
F.7	Other accounts payable	NFPD	13	10	–2	500	–614	–179	141	110	–1 029
F.L	**Total net acquisition of financial liabilities**	NFMC	110 196	192 708	179 213	35 662	172 341	240 661	398 447	317 423	431 086
B.9	**Net lending / borrowing**										
F.A	Total net acquisition of financial assets	NFIY	84 020	178 253	194 098	43 106	181 086	193 781	343 524	229 257	383 421
-F.L	*less* Total net acquisition of financial liabilities	–NFMC	–110 196	–192 708	–179 213	–35 662	–172 341	–240 661	–398 447	–317 423	–431 086
B.9f	Net lending (+) / net borrowing (-), from financial account	NYNM	–26 176	–14 455	14 885	7 444	8 745	–46 880	–54 923	–88 166	–47 665
dB.9f	Statistical discrepancy	NYOY	17 418	2 574	–38 170	–17 237	–9 507	45 378	52 902	75 940	34 325
B.9	**Net lending (+) / net borrowing (-), from capital account**	NHLW	**–8 758**	**–11 881**	**–23 285**	**–9 793**	**–762**	**–1 502**	**–2 021**	**–12 226**	**–13 340**

4.3.9 Other financial intermediaries and financial auxiliaries
ESA95 sectors S.123 and S.124 Unconsolidated

£ billion

			1999	2000	2001	2002	2003	2004	2005	2006	2007
IV.3	**FINANCIAL BALANCE SHEET** at end of period										
AF.A	**Financial assets**										
AF.2	Currency and deposits										
AF.21	Currency	**NLPM**	0.1	0.1	0.1	0.1	0.1	0.1	0.1	0.1	0.1
AF.22	Transferable deposits										
AF.2211	Sterling deposits with UK banks	**NLPP**	81.2	103.7	112.6	117.2	117.1	140.7	209.8	279.9	335.1
AF.2212	Foreign currency deposits with UK banks	**NLPQ**	60.4	83.3	112.3	103.7	128.2	140.9	173.0	200.9	264.5
AF.2213	Sterling deposits with UK building societies	**NLPR**	1.4	0.8	1.1	1.2	2.5	2.7	2.9	3.1	6.0
AF.229	Deposits with rest of the world monetary financial institutions	**NLPS**	158.8	212.2	267.6	248.5	296.2	324.8	506.9	514.8	569.4
AF.29	Other deposits	**NLPT**	–	2.7	1.1	1.8	0.8	2.2	3.5	1.5	3.7
AF.2	Total currency and deposits	**NLPL**	301.9	402.7	494.8	472.5	545.0	611.3	896.3	1 000.2	1 178.8
AF.3	Securities other than shares										
AF.331	Short term: money market instruments										
AF.3311	Issued by UK central government	**NLPW**	–	–	1.7	0.9	3.1	4.0	1.9	2.9	4.1
AF.3312	Issued by UK local government	**NLQA**	–	–	–	–	–	–	–	–	–
AF.3315	Issued by UK monetary financial institutions	**NLQB**	26.6	29.2	22.8	27.1	25.6	22.3	23.1	22.1	26.4
AF.3316	Issued by other UK residents	**NLQG**	2.9	2.7	1.4	0.9	0.7	1.3	1.1	0.8	1.0
AF.3319	Issued by the rest of the world	**NLQH**	7.5	3.8	6.0	5.6	7.8	8.5	7.5	10.5	7.6
AF.332	Medium (1 to 5 year) and long term (over 5 year) bonds										
AF.3321	Issued by UK central government	**NLQJ**	21.6	33.1	22.7	27.3	31.3	31.1	44.9	63.4	92.5
AF.3322	Issued by UK local government	**NLQM**	–	–	–	–	–	–	–	–	–
AF.3325	Medium term bonds issued by UK MFIs[1]	**NLQN**	4.6	3.8	4.3	5.0	8.2	10.2	13.8	16.6	23.2
AF.3326	Other medium & long term bonds issued by UK residents	**NLQQ**	29.3	40.2	51.6	56.0	69.7	79.5	89.9	96.9	99.5
AF.3329	Long term bonds issued by the rest of the world	**NLQR**	51.7	52.1	43.3	38.8	50.3	71.8	95.4	71.5	53.0
AF.3	Total securities other than shares	**NLPU**	144.3	165.0	153.8	161.5	196.7	228.8	277.6	284.8	307.2
AF.4	Loans										
AF.42	Long term loans										
AF.421	Direct investment	**NLRE**	2.1	2.2	3.5	7.1	11.3	18.4	20.7	17.3	19.8
AF.422	Loans secured on dwellings	**NLRH**	32.6	39.8	56.1	76.1	117.1	170.1	214.1	279.3	348.8
AF.423	Finance leasing	**NLRL**	20.6	20.7	21.0	21.8	22.5	23.2	23.8	24.5	25.1
AF.424	Other long-term loans by UK residents	**NLRM**	6.4	7.6	4.9	4.8	6.3	3.0	1.3	5.0	14.6
AF.4	Total loans	**NLQW**	61.7	70.3	85.6	109.8	157.2	214.8	259.8	326.1	408.4
AF.5	Shares and other equity										
AF.51	Shares and other equity, excluding mutual funds' shares										
AF.514	Quoted UK shares	**NLRT**	106.5	98.3	153.7	131.9	173.0	201.6	250.0	289.6	316.9
AF.515	Unquoted UK shares	**NLRU**	59.4	98.0	121.3	131.1	135.6	150.6	161.5	176.2	186.4
AF.517	UK shares and bonds issued by other UK residents	**NSOH**	–	–	–	–	–	–	–	–	–
AF.519	Shares and other equity issued by the rest of the world	**NLRY**	159.6	184.4	173.1	142.7	169.9	183.6	202.7	223.4	279.1
AF.52	Mutual funds' shares										
AF.521	UK mutual funds' shares	**NLSC**	4.7	4.4	3.4	2.4	2.9	3.2	4.2	4.6	4.5
AF.5	Total shares and other equity	**NLRO**	330.2	385.1	451.6	408.1	481.4	539.0	618.4	693.8	786.9
AF.6	Insurance technical reserves										
AF.62	Prepayments of insurance premiums and reserves for outstanding claims	**NLSH**	0.8	0.7	0.6	0.7	0.8	0.9	0.9	0.8	0.9
AF.7	Other accounts receivable	**NLSI**	8.8	9.8	10.4	11.4	11.9	12.4	13.1	13.2	15.2
AF.A	**Total financial assets**	**NLPH**	847.7	1 033.6	1 196.8	1 163.9	1 393.0	1 607.2	2 066.1	2 318.9	2 697.4

1 UK monetary financial institutions

4.3.9 Other financial intermediaries and financial auxiliaries
ESA95 sectors S.123 and S.124 Unconsolidated

continued

£ billion

			1999	2000	2001	2002	2003	2004	2005	2006	2007
IV.3	**FINANCIAL BALANCE SHEET** continued at end of period											
AF.L	**Financial liabilities**											
AF.2	Currency and deposits	**NLSP**	–	2.9	0.3	0.8	0.3	0.3	1.8	1.6	5.9
AF.3 AF.331 AF.3316	Securities other than shares Short term: money market instruments Issued by UK residents other than monetary financial institutions and government	**NLTK**	15.6	21.4	23.3	21.1	19.4	20.2	26.2	42.8	46.8
AF.332 AF.3326	Medium (1 to 5 year) and long term (over 5 year) bonds Other medium & long term bonds issued by UK residents institutions and government	**NLTU**	115.6	138.2	165.2	189.4	243.6	333.3	430.7	513.3	639.2
AF.3	Total securities other than shares	**NLSY**	131.2	159.6	188.5	210.5	263.1	353.5	456.9	556.0	686.0
AF.4 AF.41 AF.4111 AF.4112 AF.4113 AF.419 AF.42 AF.421 AF.423 AF.424 AF.429	Loans Short term loans Sterling loans by UK banks Foreign currency loans by UK banks Sterling loans by UK building societies Loans by rest of the world monetary financial institutions Long term loans Direct investment Finance leasing Other long-term loans by UK residents Other long-term loans by the rest of the world	**NLUD** **NLUE** **NLUF** **NLUG** **NLUI** **NLUP** **NLUQ** **NLUR**	148.1 80.3 9.4 275.0 6.6 1.2 13.5 0.5	164.9 119.8 8.4 316.1 8.1 1.1 13.3 0.5	166.4 146.0 10.0 390.4 20.0 1.3 13.9 0.5	173.8 163.5 11.3 357.8 25.6 1.4 14.6 0.5	193.5 202.9 16.4 384.3 29.9 1.5 15.8 0.5	235.3 226.7 19.8 446.2 44.6 1.6 19.7 0.5	266.0 253.1 26.5 670.3 38.6 1.7 26.2 0.5	314.4 289.4 32.8 602.3 38.8 1.7 30.9 0.5	446.9 382.4 41.2 673.5 45.1 1.8 19.8 0.5
AF.4	Total loans	**NLUA**	534.5	632.1	748.4	748.6	844.8	994.3	1 282.8	1 310.9	1 611.3
AF.5 AF.51 AF.514 AF.515 AF.517 AF.52 AF.521	Shares and other equity Shares and other equity, excluding mutual funds' shares Quoted UK shares Unquoted UK shares UK shares and bonds issued by other UK residents Mutual funds' shares UK mutual funds' shares	**NLUX** **NLUY** **NSOI** **NLVG**	220.5 106.3 – 298.7	270.7 135.2 – 304.5	275.0 143.8 – 268.2	215.6 135.9 – 215.8	274.2 155.3 – 266.3	303.7 176.0 – 303.9	341.0 204.0 – 385.0	399.2 244.1 – 452.4	353.4 243.1 – 507.5
AF.5	Total shares and other equity	**NLUS**	625.4	710.4	687.0	567.3	695.8	783.6	930.0	1 095.8	1 103.9
AF.7	Other accounts payable	**NLVM**	0.8	0.8	0.8	1.8	2.3	2.2	2.1	2.5	2.5
AF.L	**Total financial liabilities**	**NLSL**	1 291.9	1 505.8	1 624.9	1 528.9	1 806.3	2 133.9	2 673.5	2 966.9	3 409.7
BF.90	**Net financial assets / liabilities**											
AF.A -AF.L	Total financial assets *less* Total financial liabilities	**NLPH** **−NLSL**	847.7 −1 291.9	1 033.6 −1 505.8	1 196.8 −1 624.9	1 163.9 −1 528.9	1 393.0 −1 806.3	1 607.2 −2 133.9	2 066.1 −2 673.5	2 318.9 −2 966.9	2 697.4 −3 409.7
BF.90	**Net financial assets (+) / liabilities (-)**	**NYOF**	−444.2	−472.1	−428.1	−365.0	−413.3	−526.7	−607.4	−648.0	−712.3

4.4.2 Insurance corporations and pension funds
ESA95 sector S.125

£ million

			1999	2000	2001	2002	2003	2004	2005	2006
II	**DISTRIBUTION AND USE OF INCOME ACCOUNTS**									
II.1	**PRIMARY DISTRIBUTION OF INCOME ACCOUNT**									
II.1.1	**GENERATION OF INCOME ACCOUNT**									
	Resources									
B.1g	**Total resources (Gross Value Added)**	NRHH	**12 530**	**9 872**	**9 884**	**17 534**	**20 377**	**18 364**	**17 443**	**18 174**
	Uses									
D.1	Compensation of employees									
D.11	Wages and salaries	NHEJ	5 990	6 691	6 907	6 937	7 176	6 130	6 159	6 245
D.12	Employers' social contributions	NHEL	792	899	930	971	1 164	1 451	1 585	1 300
D.1	Total	NSCV	6 782	7 590	7 837	7 908	8 340	7 581	7 744	7 545
D.2	Taxes on production and imports, paid									
D.29	Production taxes other than on products	NHOS	251	310	324	337	346	353	366	384
-D.3	*less* Subsidies, received									
-D.39	Production subsidies other than on products	−NHNZ	−	−	−	−	−	−	−	−
B.2g	Operating surplus, gross	NHBZ	5 497	1 972	1 723	9 289	11 691	10 430	9 333	10 245
B.1g	**Total uses (Gross Value Added)**	NRHH	**12 530**	**9 872**	**9 884**	**17 534**	**20 377**	**18 364**	**17 443**	**18 174**

4.4.3 Insurance corporations and pension funds
ESA95 sector S.125

£ million

			1999	2000	2001	2002	2003	2004	2005	2006	2007
II.1.2	**ALLOCATION OF PRIMARY INCOME ACCOUNT**										
	Resources										
B.2g	Operating surplus, gross	NHBZ	5 497	1 972	1 723	9 289	11 691	10 430	9 333	10 245	12 931
D.4	Property income, received										
D.41	Interest	NHOK	23 135	26 189	24 556	23 473	25 460	28 364	27 400	27 865	34 146
D.42	Distributed income of corporations	NHOL	24 440	19 258	22 944	21 729	20 513	21 940	24 304	27 110	27 538
D.43	Reinvested earnings on direct foreign investment	NHQM	976	542	−899	−75	1 572	2 697	3 108	2 615	2 897
D.44	Property income attributed to insurance policy-holders	NHPG	28	19	19	18	24	21	34	33	24
D.45	Rent	NHPH	29	29	29	30	30	31	31	31	32
D.4	Total	NHPF	48 608	46 037	46 649	45 175	47 599	53 053	54 877	57 654	64 637
Total	Total resources	NRMN	54 105	48 009	48 372	54 464	59 290	63 483	64 210	67 899	77 568
	Uses										
D.4	Property income										
D.41	Interest	NHOM	808	1 074	912	1 017	963	1 402	1 972	2 200	2 740
D.42	Distributed income of corporations	NHON	3 244	4 352	4 170	2 801	3 144	4 258	3 920	4 905	7 245
D.43	Reinvested earnings on direct foreign investment	NHQO	78	44	−1 120	−55	535	920	868	1 500	−161
D.44	Property income attributed to insurance policy-holders	NQCG	54 903	54 494	54 795	53 652	56 715	56 150	65 805	68 349	74 084
D.45	Rent	NHPK	−	−	−	−	−	−	−	−	−
D.4	Total	NHPT	59 033	59 964	58 757	57 415	61 357	62 730	72 565	76 954	83 908

4.4.4 Insurance corporations and pension funds
ESA95 sector S.125

£ million

			1999	2000	2001	2002	2003	2004	2005	2006	2007
II.2	**SECONDARY DISTRIBUTION OF INCOME ACCOUNT**										
	Resources										
B.5g	**Balance of primary incomes, gross**	NRMO	−4 928	−11 955	−10 385	−2 951	−2 067	753	−8 355	−9 055	−6 340
D.61	Social contributions										
D.611	Actual social contributions										
D.6111	Employers' actual contributions	NSAR	19 128	20 891	21 836	26 025	32 504	38 473	42 963	47 527	45 995
D.6112	Employees social contributions	NSAS	30 878	31 569	31 933	32 967	32 158	31 652	36 786	39 807	41 425
D.6113	Social contributions by the self-employed	NSAT	–	–	–	–	–	–	–	–	–
D.611	Total	NSCN	50 006	52 460	53 769	58 992	64 662	70 125	79 749	87 334	87 420
D.612	Imputed social contributions	NHPR	110	118	115	125	120	97	89	76	70
D.61	Total	NRMP	50 116	52 578	53 884	59 117	64 782	70 222	79 838	87 410	87 490
D.7	Other current transfers										
D.71	Net non-life insurance premiums	NSCT	22 894	24 550	19 553	26 620	23 000	28 148	31 711	36 531	27 745
D.72	Non-life insurance claims	NHPN	228	345	211	320	346	366	417	476	361
D.7	Total	NRMR	23 122	24 895	19 764	26 940	23 346	28 514	32 128	37 007	28 106
Total	Total resources	NRMS	68 310	65 518	63 263	83 106	86 061	99 489	103 611	115 362	109 256
	Uses										
D.5	Current taxes on income, wealth, etc.										
D.51	Taxes on income	NHPO	2 687	1 614	−1 567	−2 346	1 884	3 575	5 174	3 779	1 400
D.62	Social benefits other than social transfers in kind										
D.622	Private funded social benefits	SBDW	35 992	38 310	37 736	41 209	43 297	40 668	46 916	55 629	45 514
D.623	Unfunded employee social benefits	NHPR	110	118	115	125	120	97	89	76	70
D.62	Total	NHPQ	36 102	38 428	37 851	41 334	43 417	40 765	47 005	55 705	45 584
D.7	Other current transfers										
D.71	Net non-life insurance premiums	NHPU	228	345	211	320	346	366	417	476	361
D.72	Non-life insurance claims	NSCS	22 894	24 550	19 553	26 620	23 000	28 148	31 711	36 531	27 745
D.75	Miscellaneous current transfers	NHQK	–	–	–	–	–	–	–	–	–
D.7	Total	NHPT	23 122	24 895	19 764	26 940	23 346	28 514	32 128	37 007	28 106
B.6g	**Gross Disposable Income**	NRMT	**6 399**	**581**	**7 215**	**17 178**	**17 414**	**26 635**	**19 304**	**18 871**	**34 166**
Total	Total uses	NRMS	68 310	65 518	63 263	83 106	86 061	99 489	103 611	115 362	109 256

4.4.6 Insurance corporations and pension funds
ESA95 sector S.125

£ million

			1999	2000	2001	2002	2003	2004	2005	2006	2007
II.4.1	**USE OF DISPOSABLE INCOME ACCOUNT**										
	Resources										
B.6g	**Total resources (Gross Disposable Income)**	**NRMT**	6 399	581	7 215	17 178	17 414	26 635	19 304	18 871	34 166
	Uses										
D.8	Adjustment for the change in net equity of households in pension funds	**NRYH**	14 014	14 150	16 033	17 783	21 365	29 457	32 833	31 705	41 906
B.8g	**Gross Saving**	**NRMV**	−7 615	−13 569	−8 818	−605	−3 951	−2 822	−13 529	−12 834	−7 740
B.6g	**Total uses (Gross Disposable Income)**	**NRMT**	6 399	581	7 215	17 178	17 414	26 635	19 304	18 871	34 166

4.4.7 Insurance corporations and pension funds
ESA95 sector S.125

£ million

			1999	2000	2001	2002	2003	2004	2005	2006	2007
III	**ACCUMULATION ACCOUNTS**										
III.1	**CAPITAL ACCOUNT**										
III.1.1	**CHANGE IN NET WORTH DUE TO SAVING & CAPITAL TRANSFERS**										
	Changes in liabilities and net worth										
B.8g	**Gross Saving**	**NRMV**	−7 615	−13 569	−8 818	−605	−3 951	−2 822	−13 529	−12 834	−7 740
D.9	Capital transfers receivable										
D.92	Investment grants	**NHQA**	–	–	–	–	–	–	–	–	–
D.99	Other capital transfers	**NHQB**	–	–	412	412	391	328	321	446	388
D.9	Total	**NHPZ**	–	–	412	412	391	328	321	446	388
-D.9	*less* Capital transfers payable										
-D.91	Capital taxes	**−NHNW**	–	–	–	–	–	–	–	–	–
-D.99	Other capital transfers	**−NHOB**	–	–	−412	−412	−391	−328	−321	−446	−388
-D.9	Total	**−NHQD**	–	–	−412	−412	−391	−328	−321	−446	−388
B.10.1g	Total change in liabilities and net worth	**NRYI**	−7 615	−13 569	−8 818	−605	−3 951	−2 822	−13 529	−12 834	−7 740
	Changes in assets										
B.10.1g	Change in net worth due to saving and capital transfers before deduction of fixed capital consumption	**NRYI**	−7 615	−13 569	−8 818	−605	−3 951	−2 822	−13 529	−12 834	−7 740
III.1.2	**ACQUISITION OF NON-FINANCIAL ASSETS ACCOUNT**										
B.10.1g	**Total changes in liabilities and net worth due to saving and capital transfers**	**NRYI**	−7 615	−13 569	−8 818	−605	−3 951	−2 822	−13 529	−12 834	−7 740
	Changes in assets										
P.5	Gross capital formation										
P.51	Gross fixed capital formation	**NHOJ**	3 337	5 705	2 809	1 936	−464	360	378	2 412	778
P.52	Changes in inventories	**NHOI**	–	–	–	–	–	–	–	–	–
P.53	Acquisitions less disposals of valuables	**NHQH**	−28	−127	–	−74	−166	−173	−299	−74	−35
P.5	Total	**NHQG**	3 309	5 578	2 809	1 862	−630	187	79	2 338	743
K.2	Acquisitions less disposals of non-produced non-financial assets	**NHQI**	−37	−45	−43	−42	−14	−24	−21	−14	−16
B.9	**Net lending (+) / net borrowing (-)**	**NHOQ**	**−10 887**	**−19 102**	**−11 584**	**−2 425**	**−3 307**	**−2 985**	**−13 587**	**−15 158**	**−8 467**
Total	Total change in assets	**NRYI**	−7 615	−13 569	−8 818	−605	−3 951	−2 822	−13 529	−12 834	−7 740

4.4.8 Insurance corporations and pension funds
ESA95 sector S.125. Unconsolidated

£ million

			1999	2000	2001	2002	2003	2004	2005	2006	2007
III.2	**FINANCIAL ACCOUNT**										
F.A	**Net acquisition of financial assets**										
F.2	Currency and deposits										
F.22	Transferable deposits										
F.2211	Sterling deposits with UK banks	NBSK	−1 389	4 432	−458	−1 046	−1 185	5 081	−3 471	5 853	14 977
F.2212	Foreign Currency Deposits with UK Banks	IE2X	−624	1 319	−799	−2 241	1 509	842	−786	2 384	1 561
F.2213	Sterling deposits with UK building societies	NBSM	1 154	−76	384	357	−266	327	−53	453	869
F.229	Deposits with rest of the world monetary financial institutions	NBSN	723	1 769	2 456	1 497	7 626	8 201	5 093	7 278	11 741
F.29	Other deposits	NBSO	–	–	–	–	–	–	–	–	–
F.2	Total currency and deposits	NBSG	−136	7 444	1 583	−1 433	7 684	14 451	783	15 968	29 148
F.3	Securities other than shares										
F.331	Short term: money market instruments										
F.3311	Issued by UK central government	NBSR	−530	169	376	266	−359	376	−537	224	−15
F.3315	Issued by UK monetary financial institutions	NBSW	1 149	788	3 554	2 683	3 102	2 006	−1 703	4 208	3 963
F.3316	Issued by other UK residents	NBTB	901	75	461	51	129	−1 934	3 445	−2 032	513
F.3319	Issued by the rest of the world	NBTC	243	−106	−159	333	70	602	1 419	−556	857
F.332	Medium (1 to 5 year) and long term (over 5 year) bonds										
F.3321	Issued by UK central government	NBTE	3 059	−27 594	−3 322	3 237	19 771	20 084	27 148	20 519	−4 159
F.3322	Issued by UK local government	NBTH	−52	32	−69	20	5	−100	139	230	−29
F.33251	Medium term bonds issued by UK banks	NBTJ	1 443	−1 261	738	1 329	5 191	5 451	8 310	10 591	13 471
F.33252	Medium term bonds issued by UK building societies	NBTK	413	−11	−179	1 113	1 248	921	1 448	−65	742
F.3326	Other medium & long term bonds issued by UK residents	NBTL	18 760	32 137	25 747	21 745	14 128	11 837	842	4 592	1 210
F.3329	Long term bonds issued by the rest of the world	NBTM	9 986	10 608	9 196	4 829	996	4 056	6 241	22 244	36 894
F.3	Total securities other than shares	NBSP	35 372	14 837	36 343	35 606	44 281	43 299	46 752	59 955	53 447
F.4	Loans										
F.42	Long term loans										
F.421	Direct investment	NBTZ	−30	1 234	1 214	1 040	1 969	1 169	748	526	660
F.422	Loans secured on dwellings	NBUC	−646	168	43	−165	209	34	−428	−212	−15
F.424	Other long-term loans by UK residents	NBUH	16 280	9 158	−1 530	1 562	6 229	7 768	9 276	4 784	−4 059
F.4	Total loans	NBTR	15 604	10 560	−273	2 437	8 407	8 971	9 596	5 098	−3 414
F.5	Shares and other equity										
F.51	Shares and other equity, excluding mutual funds' shares										
F.514	Quoted UK shares	NBUO	−11 132	19 953	−42 601	−14 238	−19 588	−17 605	−52 397	−26 370	−28 188
F.515	Unquoted UK shares	NBUP	−389	−2 241	−301	321	−1 232	189	−887	−1 065	−337
F.517	UK shares and bonds issued by other UK residents	NSPC	–	–	–	–	–	–	–	–	–
F.519	Shares and other equity issued by the rest of the world	NBUT	2 497	−15 768	17 770	19 519	2 511	16 089	31 419	10 382	11 895
F.52	Mutual funds' shares										
F.521	UK mutual funds' shares	NBUX	5 597	7 100	1 921	3 321	881	287	11 652	9 590	−1 387
F.5	Total shares and other equity	NBUJ	−3 427	9 044	−23 211	8 923	−17 428	−1 040	−10 213	−7 463	−18 017
F.6	Insurance technical reserves										
F.62	Prepayments of insurance premiums and reserves for outstanding claims	NBVC	−24	21	−21	22	10	54	55	78	1
F.7	Other accounts receivable	NBVD	2 594	−3 151	8 686	15 259	7 977	3 770	2 766	40 315	12 898
F.A	**Total net acquisition of financial assets**	NBSC	49 983	38 755	23 107	60 814	50 931	69 505	49 739	113 951	74 063

4.4.8 Insurance corporations and pension funds

ESA95 sector S.125. Unconsolidated

continued   £ million

			1999	2000	2001	2002	2003	2004	2005	2006	2007
III.2	**FINANCIAL ACCOUNT** continued										
F.L	**Net acquisition of financial liabilities**										
F.3	Securities other than shares										
F.332	Medium (1 to 5 year) and long term (over 5 year) bonds										
F.3326	Other medium & long term bonds issued by UK residents institutions and government	**NBWP**	1 126	219	2 484	339	2 347	1 595	1 232	61	714
F.3	Total securities other than shares	**NBVT**	1 126	219	2 484	339	2 347	1 595	1 232	61	714
F.4	Loans										
F.41	Short term loans										
F.411	Loans by UK monetary financial institutions, excluding loans secured on dwellings & financial leasing	**NBWX**	2 536	1 301	−715	−1 457	650	5 096	−1 990	658	−4 223
F.419	Loans by rest of the world monetary financial institutions	**ZMFP**	452	−3 331	4 113	2 454	3 551	6 360	456	10 544	832
F.42	Long term loans										
F.421	Direct investment	**NBXD**	1 790	72	2 028	181	394	678	2 011	1 780	−1 120
F.424	Other long-term loans by UK residents	**NBXL**	9 772	4 919	2 973	2 766	10 774	4 917	7 693	1 815	−9 368
F.4	Total loans	**NBWV**	14 550	2 961	8 399	3 944	15 369	17 051	8 170	14 797	−13 879
F.5	Shares and other equity										
F.51	Shares and other equity, excluding mutual funds' shares										
F.514	Quoted UK shares	**NBXS**	393	8 586	49	1 141	1 233	1 934	866	10 289	933
F.515	Unquoted UK shares	**NBXT**	32	2 520	171	2 184	746	1 578	711	1 731	587
F.5	Total shares and other equity	**NBXN**	425	11 106	220	3 325	1 979	3 512	1 577	12 020	1 520
F.6	Insurance technical reserves										
F.61	Net equity of households in life assurance and pension funds' reserves	**NBYD**	34 689	29 712	35 846	46 180	34 437	44 942	53 672	55 989	72 701
F.62	Prepayments of insurance premiums and reserves for outstanding claims	**NBYG**	−1 601	1 466	−1 753	1 781	687	3 778	3 969	6 011	39
F.6	Total insurance technical reserves	**NPWC**	33 088	31 178	34 093	47 961	35 124	48 720	57 641	62 000	72 740
F.7	Other accounts payable	**NBYH**	4 928	6 164	3 627	7 269	660	8 026	1 981	34 414	10 370
F.L	**Total net acquisition of financial liabilities**	**NBVG**	54 117	51 628	48 823	62 838	55 479	78 904	70 601	123 292	71 465
B.9	**Net lending / borrowing**										
F.A	Total net acquisition of financial assets	**NBSC**	49 983	38 755	23 107	60 814	50 931	69 505	49 739	113 951	74 063
-F.L	*less* Total net acquisition of financial liabilities	**−NBVG**	−54 117	−51 628	−48 823	−62 838	−55 479	−78 904	−70 601	−123 292	−71 465
B.9f	Net lending (+) / net borrowing (-), from financial account	**NYNN**	−4 134	−12 873	−25 716	−2 024	−4 548	−9 399	−20 862	−9 341	2 598
dB.9f	Statistical discrepancy	**NYPB**	−6 753	−6 229	14 132	−401	1 241	6 414	7 275	−5 817	−11 065
B.9	**Net lending (+) / net borrowing (-), from capital account**	**NHOQ**	**−10 887**	**−19 102**	**−11 584**	**−2 425**	**−3 307**	**−2 985**	**−13 587**	**−15 158**	**−8 467**

4.4.9 Insurance corporations and pension funds

ESA95 sector S.125. Unconsolidated

£ billion

			1999	2000	2001	2002	2003	2004	2005	2006	2007
IV.3	**FINANCIAL BALANCE SHEET** at end of period										
AF.A	**Financial assets**										
AF.2	Currency and deposits										
AF.22	Transferable deposits										
AF.2211	Sterling deposits with UK banks	NIYH	49.4	54.1	53.8	53.1	49.5	55.3	51.5	56.5	71.4
AF.2212	Foreign currency deposits with UK Banks	IE2Y	5.0	6.3	5.5	3.3	4.8	5.6	4.8	7.2	8.8
AF.2213	Sterling deposits with UK building societies	NIYJ	4.3	2.7	3.0	3.4	3.1	3.5	3.4	3.9	4.7
AF.229	Deposits with rest of the world monetary financial institutions	NIYK	5.7	6.9	8.2	8.1	15.5	25.3	33.9	37.4	46.0
AF.29	Other deposits	NIYL	–	–	–	–	–	–	–	–	–
AF.2	Total currency and deposits	NIYD	64.3	69.9	70.6	67.9	72.9	89.7	93.7	104.9	130.9
AF.3	Securities other than shares										
AF.331	Short term: money market instruments										
AF.3311	Issued by UK central government	NIYO	0.6	0.6	0.6	0.8	0.5	1.0	0.4	0.7	0.6
AF.3315	Issued by UK monetary financial institutions	NIYT	14.5	15.3	18.8	21.5	24.6	26.6	24.9	29.1	33.1
AF.3316	Issued by other UK residents	NIYY	2.7	2.8	3.2	3.3	3.4	1.5	4.9	2.9	3.4
AF.3319	Issued by the rest of the world	NIYZ	1.4	1.3	1.1	1.4	1.5	2.1	3.5	3.0	3.8
AF.332	Medium (1 to 5 year) and long term (over 5 year) bonds										
AF.3321	Issued by UK central government	NIZB	192.1	189.8	171.3	184.3	202.4	224.6	231.0	241.1	242.4
AF.3322	Issued by UK local government	NIZE	0.6	0.5	0.5	0.5	0.4	0.3	0.4	0.5	0.5
AF.3325	Medium term bonds issued by UK MFIs[1]	NIZF	11.5	11.4	11.8	13.7	23.1	29.1	39.5	47.9	67.5
AF.3326	Other medium & long term bonds issued by UK residents	NIZI	88.2	120.3	137.6	171.1	174.2	175.4	186.4	178.2	182.4
AF.3329	Long term bonds issued by the rest of the world	NIZJ	75.8	85.3	106.2	109.3	118.6	142.3	168.3	212.2	259.5
AF.3	Total securities other than shares	NIYM	387.2	427.2	451.1	505.8	548.7	603.0	659.4	715.5	793.2
AF.4	Loans										
AF.42	Long term loans										
AF.421	Direct investment	NIZW	2.1	5.7	7.4	5.7	4.8	6.9	8.2	5.0	5.7
AF.422	Loans secured on dwellings	NIZZ	1.1	1.3	1.3	1.2	1.4	1.4	1.0	0.8	0.8
AF.424	Other long-term loans by UK residents	NJAE	43.0	41.7	48.6	51.4	65.1	84.7	86.3	107.3	98.6
AF.4	Total loans	NIZO	46.2	48.7	57.3	58.3	71.3	93.0	95.5	113.2	105.0
AF.5	Shares and other equity										
AF.51	Shares and other equity, excluding mutual funds' shares										
AF.514	Quoted UK shares	NJAL	724.1	683.5	538.6	397.7	443.3	467.8	486.0	493.6	459.0
AF.515	Unquoted UK shares	NJAM	5.6	6.7	7.2	7.7	6.7	4.5	5.2	2.9	3.3
AF.517	UK shares and bonds issued by other UK residents	NSOC	–	–	–	–	–	–	–	–	–
AF.519	Shares and other equity issued by the rest of the world	NJAQ	283.9	258.8	255.7	207.3	227.6	255.4	350.4	383.7	417.9
AF.52	Mutual funds' shares										
AF.521	UK mutual funds' shares	NJAU	139.2	144.5	125.8	103.1	142.0	159.8	237.6	279.7	282.4
AF.5	Total shares and other equity	NJAG	1 152.9	1 093.5	927.3	715.8	819.7	887.5	1 079.2	1 159.9	1 162.6
AF.6	Insurance technical reserves										
AF.62	Prepayments of insurance premiums and reserves for outstanding claims	NJAZ	0.9	0.9	0.7	0.8	0.9	0.9	1.0	1.0	1.0
AF.7	Other accounts receivable	NJBA	16.0	17.2	18.4	35.5	50.7	49.5	50.2	85.6	97.4
AF.A	**Total financial assets**	NIZN	1 667.5	1 657.3	1 525.5	1 384.0	1 564.2	1 723.7	1 979.0	2 180.1	2 290.2

1 UK monetary financial institutions

4.4.9 Insurance corporations and pension funds
ESA95 sector S.125. Unconsolidated

continued

£ billion

			1999	2000	2001	2002	2003	2004	2005	2006	2007
IV.3	**FINANCIAL BALANCE SHEET** continued at end of period											
AF.L	**Financial liabilities**											
AF.3 AF.332 AF.3326	Securities other than shares Medium (1 to 5 year) and long term (over 5 year) bonds Other medium & long term bonds issued by UK residents institutions and government	**NJCM**	0.1	0.7	0.5	0.1	0.3	0.6	0.3	0.5	1.5
AF.3	Total securities other than shares	**NJBQ**	0.1	0.7	0.5	0.1	0.3	0.6	0.3	0.5	1.5
AF.4 AF.41 AF.411	Loans Short term loans Loans by UK monetary financial institutions, excluding loans secured on dwellings & financial leasing	**NJCU**	9.4	10.7	10.0	8.5	9.1	14.2	12.3	12.9	8.7
AF.419 AF.42	Loans by Rest of World monetary financial institutions Long term loans	**C657**	8.9	5.5	8.5	10.9	15.3	21.6	23.3	35.2	36.4
AF.421	Direct investment	**NJDA**	6.8	6.9	9.6	7.6	7.9	8.6	10.4	11.0	9.9
AF.424	Other long-term loans by UK residents	**NJDI**	0.5	0.5	0.5	0.5	0.5	0.5	0.5	0.5	0.5
AF.4	Total loans	**NJCS**	25.6	23.6	28.5	27.5	32.8	44.9	46.4	59.6	55.5
AF.5 AF.51 AF.514	Shares and other equity Shares and other equity, excluding mutual funds' shares Quoted UK shares	**NJDP**	72.8	69.0	56.3	33.4	37.0	43.8	56.9	73.1	67.3
AF.515	Unquoted UK shares	**NJDQ**	9.6	9.8	10.0	11.7	13.6	9.8	9.9	18.0	19.2
AF.517	UK shares and bonds issued by other UK residents	**NSOD**	–	–	–	–	–	–	–	–	–
AF.5	Total shares and other equity	**NJDK**	82.5	78.8	66.4	45.1	50.6	53.6	66.9	91.1	86.5
AF.6 AF.61	Insurance technical reserves Net equity of households in life assurance and pension funds' reserves	**NJEA**	1 631.5	1 599.2	1 531.5	1 384.3	1 509.4	1 603.4	1 894.5	2 071.9	2 186.9
AF.62	Prepayments of insurance premiums and reserves for outstanding claims	**NJED**	58.9	62.8	59.0	62.8	63.5	67.2	71.2	77.2	77.3
AF.6	Total insurance technical reserves	**NPXS**	1 690.4	1 662.0	1 590.5	1 447.1	1 572.9	1 670.6	1 965.7	2 149.1	2 264.2
AF.7	Other accounts payable	**NJEE**	18.2	23.0	26.4	28.1	35.5	42.3	44.4	73.8	85.1
AF.L	**Total financial liabilities**	**NJCR**	1 816.8	1 788.1	1 712.4	1 547.9	1 692.1	1 812.0	2 123.7	2 374.1	2 492.7
BF.90	**Net financial assets / liabilities**											
AF.A	Total financial assets	**NIZN**	1 667.5	1 657.3	1 525.5	1 384.0	1 564.2	1 723.7	1 979.0	2 180.1	2 290.2
-AF.L	*less* Total financial liabilities	**-NJCR**	−1 816.8	−1 788.1	−1 712.4	−1 547.9	−1 692.1	−1 812.0	−2 123.7	−2 374.1	−2 492.7
BF.90	**Net financial assets (+) / liabilities (-)**	**NYOI**	−149.3	−130.8	−186.9	−163.9	−127.9	−88.3	−144.7	−194.0	−202.5

167

4.5 Financial derivatives:
Gross positions of UK banks, securities dealers and other institutions by counterparty

£ million

	MFIs[1]		Other Financial[2]		Other UK[3]		Rest of World		
	Sterling	Other currencies	Sterling	Other currencies	Sterling	Other currencies	Sterling	Other currencies	Total
2001									
FINANCIAL BALANCE SHEET									
Assets									
UK banks[4]	29 077	112 464	11 899	65 799	5 126	4 247	43 496	480 990	753 098
Securities dealers[5]	5 535	29 861	2 559	5 208	1 302	1 021	13 194	51 901	110 581
Total	34 612	142 325	14 458	71 007	6 428	5 268	56 690	532 891	863 679
Liabilities									
UK banks[4]	26 870	114 279	16 376	64 844	4 120	4 463	43 811	485 773	760 536
Securities dealers[5]	6 899	27 845	4 384	6 673	723	215	13 588	50 204	110 531
Total	33 769	142 124	20 760	71 517	4 843	4 678	57 399	535 977	871 067

	UK	Rest of World	Total
2001			
FINANCIAL BALANCE SHEET			
Assets			
Insurance[6]	6 809	994	7 803
Pension Funds[7]	3 050	753	3 803
Insurance and Pension Funds Total	9 859	1 747	11 606
Other Financial Intermediaries[8]	1 703	220	1 923
Total	11 562	1 967	13 529
Liabilities			
Insurance[6]	2 077	203	2 280
Pension Funds[7]	722	738	1 460
Insurance and Pension Funds Total	2 799	941	3 740
Other Financial Intermediaries[8]	1 822	8	1 830
Total	4 621	949	5 570

KEY:

Source: ONS, Bank of England and Financial Services Authority

These data are not included in the aggregates shown in the main tables.

1 MFIs = Monetary financial institutions covers banks and building societies.
2 Other Financial = Other financial institutions and insurance corporations and pension funds.
3 Other UK = Government, private and public non-financial corporations and households.
4 UK banks = Collected by the Bank of England.
5 Securities dealers = Collected by ONS.
6 Insurance = Includes both general and long-term insurance, and are collected by ONS.
7 Pension Funds = Relates to self administered pension funds only, and are collected by ONS.
8 Other Financial Intermediaries = This does not include securities dealers (see above), includes unit trusts, investment trusts, OEICS, finance leasing, credit grantors and factoring companies all collected by ONS. This also includes Building Societies data collected by the Financial Services Authority.

Further information about the data on financial derivatives collected by ONS, including transactions, can be obtained from an article in the May 2005 edition of Economic Trends.

4.5 Financial derivatives:
Gross positions of UK banks, securities dealers and other institutions by counterparty

continued   £ million

	MFIs[1]		Other Financial[2]		Other UK[3]		Rest of World		Total
	Sterling	Other currencies	Sterling	Other currencies	Sterling	Other currencies	Sterling	Other currencies	
2002									
FINANCIAL BALANCE SHEET									
Assets									
UK banks[4]	46 219	187 463	19 391	83 408	8 131	3 645	56 656	626 158	1 031 071
Securities dealers[5]	5 849	20 716	6 272	43 187	1 139	2 436	16 214	70 901	166 714
Total	52 068	208 179	25 663	126 595	9 270	6 081	72 870	697 059	1 197 785
Liabilities									
UK banks[4]	41 139	192 769	20 830	82 738	4 500	7 013	57 118	631 538	1 037 645
Securities dealers[5]	7 551	21 701	9 382	41 798	1 003	1 782	17 188	73 745	174 150
Total	48 690	214 470	30 212	124 536	5 503	8 795	74 306	705 283	1 211 795

	UK	Rest of World	Total
2002			
FINANCIAL BALANCE SHEET			
Assets			
Insurance[6]	5 491	791	6 282
Pension Funds[7]	1 775	696	2 471
Insurance and Pension Funds Total	7 266	1 487	8 753
Other Financial Intermediaries[8]	2 035	359	2 394
Total	9 301	1 846	11 147
Liabilities			
Insurance[6]	20	531	551
Pension Funds[7]	1 282	392	1 674
Insurance and Pension Funds Total	1 302	923	2 225
Other Financial Intermediaries[8]	1 296	69	1 365
Total	2 598	992	3 590

Source: ONS, Bank of England and Financial Services Authority

KEY:

These data are not included in the aggregates shown in the main tables.

1 MFIs = Monetary financial institutions covers banks and building societies.
2 Other Financial = Other financial institutions and insurance corporations and pension funds.
3 Other UK = Government, private and public non-financial corporations and households.
4 UK banks = Collected by the Bank of England.
5 Securities dealers = Collected by ONS.
6 Insurance = Includes both general and long-term insurance, and are collected by ONS.
7 Pension Funds = Relates to self administered pension funds only, and are collected by ONS.
8 Other Financial Intermediaries = This does not include securities dealers (see above), includes unit trusts, investment trusts, OEICS, finance leasing, credit grantors and factoring companies all collected by ONS. This also includes Building Societies data collected by the Financial Services Authority.

Further information about the data on financial derivatives collected by ONS, including transactions, can be obtained from an article in the May 2005 edition of Economic Trends.

4.5 Financial derivatives:
Gross positions of UK banks, securities dealers and other institutions by counterparty

continued

£ million

	MFIs[1]		Other Financial[2]		Other UK[3]		Rest of World		
	Sterling	Other currencies	Sterling	Other currencies	Sterling	Other currencies	Sterling	Other currencies	Total
2003									
FINANCIAL BALANCE SHEET									
Assets									
UK banks[4]	40 068	155 012	21 256	101 044	9 185	4 983	44 141	579 275	954 964
Securities dealers[5]	6 201	19 410	9 367	17 133	511	474	10 640	144 041	207 777
Total	46 269	174 422	30 623	118 177	9 696	5 457	54 781	723 316	1 162 741
Liabilities									
UK banks[4]	28 991	164 651	20 418	100 278	6 023	7 812	32 391	600 008	960 572
Securities dealers[5]	8 048	23 431	13 619	18 402	540	244	13 971	149 960	228 215
Total	37 039	188 082	34 037	118 680	6 563	8 056	46 362	749 968	1 188 787

	UK	Rest of World	Total
2003			
FINANCIAL BALANCE SHEET			
Assets			
Insurance[6]	4 445	204	4 649
Pension Funds[7]	3 089	561	3 650
Insurance and Pension Funds Total	7 534	765	8 299
Other Financial Intermediaries[8]	5 253	572	5 825
Total	12 787	1 337	14 124
Liabilities			
Insurance[6]	877	215	1 092
Pension Funds[7]	1 817	437	2 254
Insurance and Pension Funds Total	2 694	652	3 346
Other Financial Intermediaries[8]	2 838	700	3 538
Total	5 532	1 352	6 884

KEY:

Source: ONS, Bank of England and Financial Services Authority

These data are not included in the aggregates shown in the main tables.

1 MFIs = Monetary financial institutions covers banks and building societies.
2 Other Financial = Other financial institutions and insurance corporations and pension funds.
3 Other UK = Government, private and public non-financial corporations and households.
4 UK banks = Collected by the Bank of England.
5 Securities dealers = Collected by ONS.
6 Insurance = Includes both general and long-term insurance, and are collected by ONS.
7 Pension Funds = Relates to self administered pension funds only, and are collected by ONS.
8 Other Financial Intermediaries = This does not include securities dealers (see above), includes unit trusts, investment trusts, OEICS, finance leasing, credit grantors and factoring companies all collected by ONS. This also includes Building Societies data collected by the Financial Services Authority.

Further information about the data on financial derivatives collected by ONS, including transactions, can be obtained from an article in the May 2005 edition of Economic Trends.

4.5 Financial derivatives:
Gross positions of UK banks, securities dealers and other institutions by counterparty

continued

£ million

	MFIs[1]		Other Financial[2]		Other UK[3]		Rest of World		
	Sterling	Other currencies	Sterling	Other currencies	Sterling	Other currencies	Sterling	Other currencies	Total
2004									
FINANCIAL BALANCE SHEET									
Assets									
UK banks[4]	37 727	207 204	35 908	154 678	10 803	4 755	46 078	663 302	1 160 455
Securities dealers[5]	11 669	54 662	7 350	13 764	507	347	11 485	104 670	204 454
Total	49 396	261 866	43 258	168 442	11 310	5 102	57 563	767 972	1 364 909
Liabilities									
UK banks[4]	27 833	223 191	34 316	152 452	6 506	7 695	36 268	678 753	1 167 014
Securities dealers[5]	17 958	61 129	8 642	11 592	712	517	14 034	112 155	226 739
Total	45 791	284 320	42 958	164 044	7 218	8 212	50 302	790 908	1 393 753

	UK	Rest of World	Total
2004			
FINANCIAL BALANCE SHEET			
Assets			
Insurance[6]	3 862	3	3 865
Pension Funds[7]	10 235	2 962	13 197
Insurance and Pension Funds Total	14 097	2 965	17 062
Other Financial Intermediaries[8]	3 490	408	3 898
Total	17 587	3 373	20 960
Liabilities			
Insurance[6]	692	141	833
Pension Funds[7]	7 873	3 082	10 955
Insurance and Pension Funds Total	8 565	3 223	11 788
Other Financial Intermediaries[8]	2 641	137	2 778
Total	11 206	3 360	14 566

KEY:

Source: ONS, Bank of England and Financial Services Authority

These data are not included in the aggregates shown in the main tables.

1 MFIs = Monetary financial institutions covers banks and building societies.
2 Other Financial = Other financial institutions and insurance corporations and pension funds.
3 Other UK = Government, private and public non-financial corporations and households.
4 UK banks = Collected by the Bank of England.
5 Securities dealers = Collected by ONS.
6 Insurance = Includes both general and long-term insurance, and are collected by ONS.
7 Pension Funds = Relates to self administered pension funds only, and are collected by ONS.
8 Other Financial Intermediaries = This does not include securities dealers (see above), includes unit trusts, investment trusts, OEICS, finance leasing, credit grantors and factoring companies all collected by ONS. This also includes Building Societies data collected by the Financial Services Authority.

Further information about the data on financial derivatives collected by ONS, including transactions, can be obtained from an article in the May 2005 edition of Economic Trends.

4.5 Financial derivatives:
Gross positions of UK banks, securities dealers and other institutions by counterparty

continued

£ million

	MFIs[1]		Other Financial[2]		Other UK[3]		Rest of World		
	Sterling	Other currencies	Sterling	Other currencies	Sterling	Other currencies	Sterling	Other currencies	Total
2005									
FINANCIAL BALANCE SHEET									
Assets									
UK banks[4]	51 702	262 038	36 522	195 784	14 750	7 762	51 327	768 752	1 388 637
Securities dealers[5]	11 869	102 410	6 509	20 674	1 048	1 168	15 002	186 531	345 211
Total	63 571	364 448	43 031	216 458	15 798	8 930	66 329	955 283	1 733 848
Liabilities									
UK banks[4]	59 243	272 352	30 422	193 338	10 667	8 666	66 286	764 817	1 405 791
Securities dealers[5]	24 491	119 426	12 739	18 797	1 368	11 487	18 190	183 147	389 645
Total	83 734	391 778	43 161	212 135	12 035	20 153	84 476	947 964	1 795 436

	UK	Rest of World	Total
2005			
FINANCIAL BALANCE SHEET			
Assets			
Insurance[6]	5 830	–47	5 783
Pension Funds[7]	22 157	2 668	24 825
Insurance and Pension Funds Total	27 987	2 621	30 608
Other Financial Intermediaries[8]	6 141	538	6 679
Total	34 128	3 159	37 287
Liabilities			
Insurance[6]	773	12	785
Pension Funds[7]	16 818	2 785	19 603
Insurance and Pension Funds Total	17 591	2 797	20 388
Other Financial Intermediaries[8]	3 815	111	3 926
Total	21 406	2 908	24 314

KEY:

Source: ONS, Bank of England and Financial Services Authority

These data are not included in the aggregates shown in the main tables.

1 MFIs = Monetary financial institutions covers banks and building societies.
2 Other Financial = Other financial institutions and insurance corporations and pension funds.
3 Other UK = Government, private and public non-financial corporations and households.
4 UK banks = Collected by the Bank of England.
5 Securities dealers = Collected by ONS.
6 Insurance = Includes both general and long-term insurance, and are collected by ONS.
7 Pension Funds = Relates to self administered pension funds only, and are collected by ONS.
8 Other Financial Intermediaries = This does not include securities dealers (see above), includes unit trusts, investment trusts, OEICS, finance leasing, credit grantors and factoring companies all collected by ONS. This also includes Building Societies data collected by the Financial Services Authority.

Further information about the data on financial derivatives collected by ONS, including transactions, can be obtained from an article in the May 2005 edition of Economic Trends.

4.5 Financial derivatives:
Gross positions of UK banks, securities dealers and other institutions by counterparty

continued   £ million

	MFIs[1]		Other Financial[2]		Other UK[3]		Rest of World		
	Sterling	Other currencies	Sterling	Other currencies	Sterling	Other currencies	Sterling	Other currencies	Total
2006									
FINANCIAL BALANCE SHEET									
Assets									
UK banks[4]	65 931	281 076	44 398	197 161	18 263	5 570	62 865	790 853	1 466 117
Securities dealers[5]	16 415	45 918	19 134	33 419	2 630	2 111	28 596	234 529	382 752
Total	82 346	326 994	63 532	230 580	20 893	7 681	91 461	1 025 382	1 848 869
Liabilities									
UK banks[4]	61 786	299 782	30 659	194 813	11 620	8 840	62 364	828 112	1 497 976
Securities dealers[5]	23 552	85 572	13 407	28 463	1 676	2 884	23 625	234 353	413 532
Total	85 338	385 354	44 066	223 276	13 296	11 724	85 989	1 062 465	1 911 508

	UK	Rest of World	Total
2006			
FINANCIAL BALANCE SHEET			
Assets			
Insurance[6]	..	..	..
Pension Funds[7]	..	..	..
Insurance and Pension Funds Total	..	..	..
Other Financial Intermediaries[8]	..	..	..
Total	..	..	..
Liabilities			
Insurance[6]	..	..	..
Pension Funds[7]	..	..	..
Insurance and Pension Funds Total	..	..	..
Other Financial Intermediaries[8]	..	..	..
Total	..	..	..

Source: ONS, Bank of England and Financial Services Authority

KEY:

These data are not included in the aggregates shown in the main tables.

1 MFIs = Monetary financial institutions covers banks and building societies.
2 Other Financial = Other financial institutions and insurance corporations and pension funds.
3 Other UK = Government, private and public non-financial corporations and households.
4 UK banks = Collected by the Bank of England.
5 Securities dealers = Collected by ONS.
6 Insurance = Includes both general and long-term insurance, and are collected by ONS.
7 Pension Funds = Relates to self administered pension funds only, and are collected by ONS.
8 Other Financial Intermediaries = This does not include securities dealers (see above), includes unit trusts, investment trusts, OEICS, finance leasing, credit grantors and factoring companies all collected by ONS. This also includes Building Societies data collected by the Financial Services Authority.

Further information about the data on financial derivatives collected by ONS, including transactions, can be obtained from an article in the May 2005 edition of Economic Trends.

Gross Positions for Insurance, Pension Funds and Other Financial Intermediaries are collected annually, 2007 data currently not available.

Chapter 5
General government

5.1.1 General government
ESA95 sector S.13 Unconsolidated

£ million

			1999	2000	2001	2002	2003	2004	2005	2006
I	**PRODUCTION ACCOUNT**									
	Resources									
P.1	Output									
P.11	Market output	NMXJ	13 568	14 930	17 438	19 464	20 780	26 509	30 630	33 038
P.12	Output for own final use	NMXK	448	430	407	428	451	172	176	183
P.13	Other non-market output	NMYK	169 652	181 972	194 584	212 577	232 819	251 769	268 638	285 669
P.1	Total resources	NMXL	183 668	197 332	212 429	232 469	254 050	278 450	299 444	318 890
	Uses									
P.2	Intermediate consumption	NMXM	84 687	92 254	99 232	110 828	121 618	135 010	146 242	158 519
B.1g	**Gross Value Added**	NMXN	**98 981**	**105 078**	**113 197**	**121 641**	**132 432**	**143 440**	**153 202**	**160 371**
Total	Total uses	NMXL	183 668	197 332	212 429	232 469	254 050	278 450	299 444	318 890
B.1g	**Gross Value Added**	NMXN	**98 981**	**105 078**	**113 197**	**121 641**	**132 432**	**143 440**	**153 202**	**160 371**
K.1	*less* Consumption of fixed capital	−NMXO	−9 262	−9 542	−9 796	−10 289	−10 807	−11 429	−12 174	−12 931
B.1n	Value added, net of fixed capital consumption	NMXP	89 719	95 536	103 401	111 352	121 625	132 011	141 028	147 440

5.1.2 General government
ESA95 sector S.13 Unconsolidated

£ million

			1999	2000	2001	2002	2003	2004	2005	2006
II	**DISTRIBUTION AND USE OF INCOME ACCOUNTS**									
II.1	**PRIMARY DISTRIBUTION OF INCOME ACCOUNT**									
II.1.1	**GENERATION OF INCOME ACCOUNT**									
	Resources									
B.1g	**Total resources (Gross Value Added)**	NMXN	**98 981**	**105 078**	**113 197**	**121 641**	**132 432**	**143 440**	**153 202**	**160 371**
	Uses									
D.1	Compensation of employees									
D.11	Wages and salaries	NMXQ	73 190	77 871	85 183	91 355	100 475	111 311	116 624	122 159
D.12	Employers' social contributions	NMXR	16 529	17 665	18 218	19 997	21 150	20 700	24 404	25 281
D.1	Total	NMXS	89 719	95 536	103 401	111 352	121 625	132 011	141 028	147 440
D.2	Taxes on production and imports, paid									
D.29	Production taxes other than on products	NMXT	–	–	–	–	–	–	–	–
D.3	*less* Subsidies, received									
D.39	Production subsidies other than on products	−NMXU	–	–	–	–	–	–	–	–
B.2g	Operating surplus, gross	NMXV	9 262	9 542	9 796	10 289	10 807	11 429	12 174	12 931
B.1g	**Total uses (Gross Value Added)**	NMXN	**98 981**	**105 078**	**113 197**	**121 641**	**132 432**	**143 440**	**153 202**	**160 371**
K.1	After deduction of fixed capital consumption	−NMXO	−9 262	−9 542	−9 796	−10 289	−10 807	−11 429	−12 174	−12 931
B.2n	Operating surplus, net	NMXW	–	–	–	–	–	–	–	–

5.1.3 General government
ESA95 sector S.13 Unconsolidated

£ million

			1999	2000	2001	2002	2003	2004	2005	2006	2007
II.1.2	**ALLOCATION OF PRIMARY INCOME ACCOUNT**										
	Resources										
B.2g	Operating surplus, gross	NMXV	9 262	9 542	9 796	10 289	10 807	11 429	12 174	12 931	14 523
D.2	Taxes on production and imports, received										
D.21	Taxes on products										
D.211	Value added tax (VAT)	NZGF	57 701	59 985	63 522	68 251	74 595	79 761	81 416	85 586	89 681
D.212	Taxes and duties on imports excluding VAT										
D.2121	Import duties	NMXZ	–	–	–	–	–	–	–	–	–
D.2122	Taxes on imports excluding VAT and import duties	NMBT	–	–	–	–	–	–	–	–	–
D.214	Taxes on products excluding VAT and import duties	NMYB	48 442	51 956	50 745	52 001	52 858	56 137	56 906	60 540	64 292
D.21	Total taxes on products	NVCC	106 143	111 941	114 267	120 252	127 453	135 898	138 322	146 126	153 973
D.29	Other taxes on production	NMYD	16 503	17 083	17 565	18 113	18 517	18 853	19 706	20 831	21 558
D.2	Total taxes on production and imports, received	NMYE	122 646	129 024	131 832	138 365	145 970	154 751	158 028	166 957	175 531
-D.3	*less* Subsidies, paid										
-D.31	Subsidies on products	–NMYF	–3 625	–3 791	–3 953	–4 672	–5 311	–5 111	–5 198	–5 994	–5 383
-D.39	Other subsidies on production	–LIUF	–663	–574	–662	–954	–1 434	–1 562	–2 449	–3 093	–3 753
-D.3	Total	–NMRL	–4 288	–4 365	–4 615	–5 626	–6 745	–6 673	–7 647	–9 087	–9 136
D.4	Property income, received										
D.41	Total Interest	NMYL	7 388	7 403	7 359	6 683	7 131	6 804	6 458	7 109	8 107
D.42	Distributed income of corporations	NMYM	5 280	5 480	4 710	3 290	3 027	2 763	2 866	2 541	3 032
D.44	Property income attributed to insurance policy holders	NMYO	33	54	24	18	19	19	27	25	19
D.45	Rent from sectors other than general government	NMYR	529	1 289	1 919	1 901	1 565	1 182	1 229	1 226	1 242
D.4	Total	NMYU	13 230	14 226	14 012	11 892	11 742	10 768	10 580	10 901	12 400
Total	Total resources	NMYV	140 850	148 427	151 025	154 920	161 774	170 275	173 135	181 702	193 318
	Uses										
D.4	Property income, paid										
D.41	Total interest	NRKB	30 620	30 585	27 911	25 410	26 913	27 013	29 469	30 392	34 232
D.4	Total	NMYY	30 620	30 585	27 911	25 410	26 913	27 013	29 469	30 392	34 232
B.5g	**Balance of primary incomes, gross**	NMZH	**110 230**	**117 842**	**123 114**	**129 510**	**134 861**	**143 262**	**143 666**	**151 310**	**159 086**
Total	Total uses	NMYV	140 850	148 427	151 025	154 920	161 774	170 275	173 135	181 702	193 318
K.1	After deduction of fixed capital consumption	–NMXO	–9 262	–9 542	–9 796	–10 289	–10 807	–11 429	–12 174	–12 931	–13 816
B.5n	Balance of primary incomes, net	NMZI	100 968	108 300	113 318	119 221	124 054	131 833	131 492	138 379	145 270

5.1.4 General government
ESA95 sector S.13 Unconsolidated

£ million

			1999	2000	2001	2002	2003	2004	2005	2006	2007
II.2	**SECONDARY DISTRIBUTION OF INCOME ACCOUNT**										
	Resources										
B.5g	Balance of primary incomes, gross	NMZH	110 230	117 842	123 114	129 510	134 861	143 262	143 666	151 310	159 086
D.5	Current taxes on income, wealth, etc.										
D.51	Taxes on income	NMZJ	129 553	140 002	147 264	142 842	144 234	154 127	172 498	192 812	199 289
D.59	Other current taxes	NVCM	19 519	20 287	22 068	23 664	26 016	28 001	29 444	30 906	32 627
D.5	Total	NMZL	149 072	160 289	169 332	166 506	170 250	182 128	201 942	223 718	231 916
D.61	Social contributions										
D.611	Actual social contributions										
D.6111	Employers' actual social contributions	NMZM	33 401	36 397	38 460	38 780	45 067	49 202	52 769	56 024	59 303
D.6112	Employees' social contributions	NMZN	26 645	27 293	28 725	29 568	34 376	38 835	41 768	44 378	46 088
D.6113	Social contributions by self- and non-employed persons	NMZO	1 883	2 049	2 183	2 318	2 595	2 727	2 825	2 930	3 013
D.611	Total	NMZP	61 929	65 739	69 368	70 666	82 038	90 764	97 362	103 332	108 404
D.612	Imputed social contributions	NMZQ	6 927	7 395	7 577	8 348	6 456	6 219	7 383	7 289	7 788
D.61	Total	NMZR	68 856	73 134	76 945	79 014	88 494	96 983	104 745	110 621	116 192
D.7	Other current transfers										
D.72	Non-life insurance claims	NMZS	436	393	265	320	276	338	328	366	277
D.73	Current transfers within general government	NMZT	64 446	66 187	72 522	77 592	85 224	94 720	101 369	110 407	113 046
D.74	Current international cooperation	NMZU	3 176	2 084	4 568	3 112	3 570	3 673	3 726	3 674	3 573
D.75	Miscellaneous current transfers from sectors other than general government	NMZX	392	447	460	502	562	721	728	612	584
D.7	Other current transfers	NNAA	68 450	69 111	77 815	81 526	89 632	99 452	106 151	115 059	117 480
Total	Total resources	NNAB	396 608	420 376	447 206	456 556	483 237	521 825	556 504	600 708	624 674
	Uses										
D.59	Other current taxes	EBFQ	861	860	902	876	842	924	1 022	1 075	1 111
D.62	Social benefits other than social transfers in kind	NNAD	117 685	120 163	129 591	136 801	146 066	154 332	161 425	167 053	177 645
D.7	Other current transfers										
D.71	Net non-life insurance premiums	NNAE	436	393	265	320	276	338	328	366	277
D.73	Current transfers within general government	NNAF	64 446	66 187	72 522	77 592	85 224	94 720	101 369	110 407	113 046
D.74	Current international cooperation	NNAG	1 456	2 181	2 190	2 362	2 433	3 080	3 255	3 632	3 909
D.75	Miscellaneous current transfers to sectors other than general government	NNAI	18 466	20 913	22 131	27 351	30 275	31 178	34 355	34 695	36 173
	Of which: GNP based fourth own resource	NMFH	4 632	4 379	3 858	5 335	6 772	7 549	8 732	8 521	8 323
D.7	Other current transfers	NNAN	84 804	89 674	97 108	107 625	118 208	129 316	139 307	149 100	153 405
B.6g	**Gross Disposable Income**	NNAO	**193 258**	**209 679**	**219 605**	**211 254**	**218 121**	**237 253**	**254 750**	**283 480**	**292 513**
Total	Total uses	NNAB	396 608	420 376	447 206	456 556	483 237	521 825	556 504	600 708	624 674
K.1	After deduction of fixed capital consumption	−NMXO	−9 262	−9 542	−9 796	−10 289	−10 807	−11 429	−12 174	−12 931	−13 816
B.6n	Disposable income, net	NNAP	183 996	200 137	209 809	200 965	207 314	225 824	242 576	270 549	278 697

5.1.5 General government
ESA95 sector S.13 Unconsolidated

£ million

			1999	2000	2001	2002	2003	2004	2005	2006	2007
II.3	**REDISTRIBUTION OF INCOME IN KIND ACCOUNT**										
	Resources										
B.6g	**Total resources (Gross Disposable Income)**	**NNAO**	**193 258**	**209 679**	**219 605**	**211 254**	**218 121**	**237 253**	**254 750**	**283 480**	**292 513**
	Uses										
D.63	Social transfers in kind										
D.632	Transfers of individual non-market goods and services	**NSZE**	102 742	109 297	118 458	130 816	143 954	148 944	160 456	173 115	183 031
B.7g	Adjusted disposable income, gross	**NSZI**	90 516	100 382	101 147	80 438	74 167	88 309	94 294	110 365	109 482
B.6g	**Total uses (Gross Disposable Income)**	**NNAO**	**193 258**	**209 679**	**219 605**	**211 254**	**218 121**	**237 253**	**254 750**	**283 480**	**292 513**

5.1.6 General government
ESA95 sector S.13 Unconsolidated

£ million

		1999	2000	2001	2002	2003	2004	2005	2006	2007
II.4	**USE OF INCOME ACCOUNT**									
II.4.1	**USE OF DISPOSABLE INCOME ACCOUNT**									
	Resources									
B.6g	**Total resources (Gross Disposable Income)**	**NNAO**								
		193 258	209 679	219 605	211 254	218 121	237 253	254 750	283 480	292 513
	Uses									
P.3	Final consumption expenditure									
P.31	Individual consumption expenditure	**NNAQ**	102 742	109 297	118 458	130 816	143 954	148 944	160 456	173 115	183 031
P.32	Collective consumption expenditure	**NQEP**	66 910	72 675	76 126	81 761	88 865	102 825	108 182	112 554	113 869
P.3	Total	**NMRK**	169 652	181 972	194 584	212 577	232 819	251 769	268 638	285 669	296 900
B.8g	**Gross Saving**	**NNAU**	**23 606**	**27 707**	**25 021**	**−1 323**	**−14 698**	**−14 516**	**−13 888**	**−2 189**	**−4 387**
B.6g	**Total uses (Gross Disposable Income)**	**NNAO**	193 258	209 679	219 605	211 254	218 121	237 253	254 750	283 480	292 513
-K.1	After deduction of fixed capital consumption	**−NMXO**	−9 262	−9 542	−9 796	−10 289	−10 807	−11 429	−12 174	−12 931	−13 816
B.8n	Saving, net	**NNAV**	14 344	18 165	15 225	−11 612	−25 505	−25 945	−26 062	−15 120	−18 203
II.4.2	**USE OF ADJUSTED DISPOSABLE INCOME ACCOUNT**									
	Resources									
B.7g	Total resources, adjusted disposable income, gross	**NSZI**	90 516	100 382	101 147	80 438	74 167	88 309	94 294	110 365	109 482
	Uses									
P.4	Actual final consumption									
P.42	Actual collective consumption	**NRMZ**	66 910	72 675	76 126	81 761	88 865	102 825	108 182	112 554	113 869
B.8g	**Gross Saving**	**NNAU**	**23 606**	**27 707**	**25 021**	**−1 323**	**−14 698**	**−14 516**	**−13 888**	**−2 189**	**−4 387**
Total	Total uses	**NSZI**	90 516	100 382	101 147	80 438	74 167	88 309	94 294	110 365	109 482

5.1.7 General government

ESA95 sector S.13 Unconsolidated

£ million

			1999	2000	2001	2002	2003	2004	2005	2006	2007
III	ACCUMULATION ACCOUNTS										
III.1	CAPITAL ACCOUNT										
III.1.1	CHANGE IN NET WORTH DUE TO SAVING & CAPITAL TRANSFERS										
	Changes in liabilities and net worth										
B.8g	**Gross Saving**	NNAU	23 606	27 707	25 021	−1 323	−14 698	−14 516	−13 888	−2 189	−4 387
D.9	Capital transfers receivable										
D.91	Capital taxes										
	from sectors other than general government	NMGI	1 951	2 215	2 396	2 381	2 416	2 871	3 150	3 575	3 890
D.92	Investment grants	NSZF	3 298	4 105	4 652	6 328	7 360	6 804	7 582	8 515	9 878
D.99	Other capital transfers	NNAX	205	411	828	1 147	5 161	3 961	4 475	2 562	3 096
D.9	Total capital transfers receivable	NNAY	5 454	6 731	7 876	9 856	14 937	13 636	15 207	14 652	16 864
-D.9	*less* Capital transfers payable										
-D.92	Investment grants	−NNAW	−8 774	−8 821	−11 313	−13 646	−17 335	−16 176	−19 990	−21 163	−24 056
-D.99	Other capital transfers	−NNBB	−210	−340	−1 302	−683	−4 494	−3 896	−16 172	−3 526	−2 659
-D.9	Total capital transfers payable	−NNBC	−8 984	−9 161	−12 615	−14 329	−21 829	−20 072	−36 162	−24 689	−26 715
B.10.1g	Total change in liabilities and net worth	NMWG	20 076	25 277	20 282	−5 796	−21 590	−20 952	−34 843	−12 226	−14 238
	Changes in assets										
B.10.1g	Changes in net worth due to gross saving and capital transfers	NMWG	20 076	25 277	20 282	−5 796	−21 590	−20 952	−34 843	−12 226	−14 238
K.1	After deduction of fixed capital consumption	−NMXO	−9 262	−9 542	−9 796	−10 289	−10 807	−11 429	−12 174	−12 931	−13 816
B.10.1n	Changes in net worth due to net saving and capital transfers	NNBD	10 814	15 735	10 486	−16 085	−32 397	−32 381	−47 017	−25 157	−28 054
III.1.2	ACQUISITION OF NON-FINANCIAL ASSETS ACCOUNT										
	Changes in liabilities and net worth										
B.10.1n	Changes in net worth due to net saving and capital transfers	NNBD	10 814	15 735	10 486	−16 085	−32 397	−32 381	−47 017	−25 157	−28 054
K.1	Consumption of fixed capital	NMXO	9 262	9 542	9 796	10 289	10 807	11 429	12 174	12 931	13 816
B.10.1g	Total change in liabilities and net worth	NMWG	20 076	25 277	20 282	−5 796	−21 590	−20 952	−34 843	−12 226	−14 238
	Changes in assets										
P.5	Gross capital formation										
P.51	Gross fixed capital formation	NNBF	12 599	12 227	13 533	15 452	20 509	23 219	7 091	23 667	25 210
P.52	Changes in inventories	NNBG	−268	−140	−18	–	15	−46	−6	−4	−20
P.53	Acquisitions less disposals of valuables	NPOZ	10	12	22	22	16	20	16	14	18
P.5	Total	NNBI	12 341	12 099	13 537	15 474	20 540	23 193	7 101	23 677	25 208
K.2	Acquisitions less disposals of non-produced non-financial assets	NNBJ	−888	−776	−915	−1 087	−957	−1 084	−1 166	−1 037	−1 124
B.9g	**Net lending(+) / net borrowing(-)**	NNBK	8 623	13 954	7 660	−20 183	−41 173	−43 061	−40 778	−34 866	−38 322
Total	Total change in assets	NMWG	20 076	25 277	20 282	−5 796	−21 590	−20 952	−34 843	−12 226	−14 238

5.1.8 General government
ESA95 sector S.13 Unconsolidated

£ million

			1999	2000	2001	2002	2003	2004	2005	2006	2007
III.2	**FINANCIAL ACCOUNT**										
F.A	**Net acquisition of financial assets**										
F.1	Monetary gold and special drawing rights (SDRs)	**NFPH**	−374	−956	−808	−240	−2	−37	−8	47	−50
F.2	Currency and deposits										
F.22	Transferable deposits with monetary financial institutions										
F.221	UK institutions	**NFPN**	−144	15 799	−9 098	−3 479	2 476	1 397	334	7 631	6 363
F.229	Rest of the world institutions	**NFPR**	3 177	−840	−261	−299	−916	−1 407	−1 516	−671	−550
F.29	Other deposits	**NFPS**	−	3 009	−2 637	644	−546	−67	−75	−47	4 342
F.2	Total currency and deposits	**NFPK**	3 033	17 968	−11 996	−3 134	1 014	−77	−1 257	6 913	10 155
F.3	Securities other than shares										
F.331	Short term: money market instruments										
F.3311	Issued by UK central government	**NFPV**	204	−218	119	−141	−38	−59	14	−18	−51
F.3312	Issued by UK local government	**NFPZ**	−	−	−	−	−	−	−	−	−
F.3315	Issued by UK monetary financial institutions	**NFQA**	565	1 850	−1 305	−233	−75	519	54	801	−2 991
F.3316	Issued by other UK residents	**NFQF**	−34	59	366	741	−1 067	10	197	1 917	−472
F.3319	Issued by the rest of the world	**NFQG**	−337	244	273	−1 576	−987	106	1 465	1 363	2 125
F.332	Medium (1 to 5 year) and long term (over 5 year) bonds										
F.3321	Issued by UK central government	**NFQI**	−17	−195	191	−264	−101	−98	7	75	−126
F.3326	Other medium & long term bonds issued by UK residents	**NFQP**	−387	11	−49	−17	−	−	1 071	−620	−42
F.3329	Long term bonds issued by the rest of the world	**NFQQ**	−3 105	5 418	−1 838	2 280	−390	1 551	370	−854	2 127
F.34	Financial derivatives	**NFQR**	−	185	102	−238	−136	−173	137	−419	−343
F.3	Total securities other than shares	**NFPT**	−3 111	7 354	−2 141	552	−2 794	1 856	3 315	2 245	227
F.4	Loans										
F.42	Long term loans										
F.422	Loans secured on dwellings	**NFRG**	106	11	97	206	186	−26	252	340	423
F.424	Other long-term loans by UK residents	**NFRL**	2 803	3 736	3 771	−314	−994	2 530	4 923	4 154	4 061
F.429	Other long-term loans by the rest of the world	**NFRM**	−	−	−	−	−	−	−	−	−
F.4	Total loans	**NFQV**	2 909	3 747	3 868	−108	−808	2 504	5 175	4 494	4 484
F.5	Shares and other equity										
F.51	Shares and other equity, excluding mutual funds' shares										
F.514	Quoted UK shares	**NFRS**	−316	54	−54	−218	45	−117	138	192	−2 484
F.515	Unquoted UK shares	**NFRT**	−	−	−811	−	−29	−	−550	−	−2 188
F.516	Other UK equity (including direct investment in property)	**NFRU**	−2 072	−2 350	−2 508	−3 064	−5 504	−3 803	−3 850	−3 543	−2 171
F.517	UK shares and bonds issued by other UK residents	**NSPW**	−	−	−	−	−	−	−	−	−
F.519	Shares and other equity issued by the rest of the world	**NFRX**	302	290	256	409	234	283	656	810	725
F.5	Total shares and other equity	**NFRN**	−2 086	−2 006	−3 117	−2 873	−5 254	−3 637	−3 606	−2 541	−6 118
F.6	Insurance technical reserves										
F.62	Prepayments of insurance premiums and reserves for outstanding claims	**NFSG**	−30	24	−26	27	8	42	44	61	−
F.7	Other accounts receivable	**NFSH**	7 679	1 235	391	−1 819	3 058	2 276	5 517	2 897	−1 741
F.A	**Total net acquisition of financial assets**	**NFPG**	8 020	27 366	−13 829	−7 595	−4 778	2 927	9 180	14 116	6 957

5.1.8 General government
ESA95 sector S.13 Unconsolidated

continued

£ million

			1999	2000	2001	2002	2003	2004	2005	2006	2007
III.2	**FINANCIAL ACCOUNT** continued										
F.L	**Net acquisition of financial liabilities**										
F.2	Currency and deposits										
F.21	Currency	**NFSP**	191	226	228	180	216	171	180	154	123
F.29	Non-transferable deposits	**NFSW**	−907	2 578	−3 084	1 946	3 266	2 423	5 502	5 240	7 930
F.2	Total currency and deposits	**NFSO**	−716	2 804	−2 856	2 126	3 482	2 594	5 682	5 394	8 053
F.3	Securities other than shares										
F.331	Short term: money market instruments										
F.3311	Issued by UK central government	**NFSZ**	−404	−1 652	8 623	10 330	2 592	999	−3 902	−1 752	−1 367
F.3312	Issued by UK local government	**NFTD**	−	−	−	−	−	−	−	−	−
F.332	Medium (1 to 5 year) and long term (over 5 year) bonds										
F.3321	Issued by UK central government	**NFTM**	−4 560	−12 700	−17 219	1 555	31 474	34 219	39 917	41 013	38 951
F.3322	Issued by UK local government	**NFTP**	−2	−12	−	47	18	−226	213	360	−9
F.3	Total securities other than shares	**NFSX**	−4 966	−14 364	−8 596	11 932	34 084	34 992	36 228	39 621	37 575
F.4	Loans										
F.41	Short term loans										
F.411	Loans by UK monetary financial institutions, excluding loans secured on dwellings & financial leasing	**NFUB**	5 270	−337	−6 615	1 731	1 109	7 406	3 070	−1 825	386
F.419	Loans by rest of the world monetary financial institutions	**NFUF**	−45	−39	−36	−14	−7	−6	−3	−1	−
F.42	Long term loans										
F.423	Finance leasing	**NFUO**	563	432	229	277	512	474	507	304	442
F.424	Other long-term loans by UK residents	**NFUP**	1 870	1 419	−212	−1 727	−3 912	507	2 608	2 638	1 266
F.429	Other long-term loans by the rest of the world	**NFUQ**	−166	−263	11	−9	166	611	72	240	−32
F.4	Total loans	**NFTZ**	7 492	1 212	−6 623	258	−2 132	8 992	6 254	1 356	2 062
F.7	Other accounts payable	**NFVL**	−1 215	23 438	−2 627	−848	423	−1 181	2 777	1 953	−1 442
F.L	**Total net acquisition of financial liabilities**	**NFSK**	595	13 090	−20 702	13 468	35 857	45 397	50 941	48 324	46 248
B.9	**Net lending / borrowing**										
F.A	Total net acquisition of financial assets	**NFPG**	8 020	27 366	−13 829	−7 595	−4 778	2 927	9 180	14 116	6 957
-F.L	*less* Total net acquisition of financial liabilities	**−NFSK**	−595	−13 090	20 702	−13 468	−35 857	−45 397	−50 941	−48 324	−46 248
B.9f	Net lending (+) / net borrowing (-), from financial account	**NYNO**	7 425	14 276	6 873	−21 063	−40 635	−42 470	−41 761	−34 208	−39 291
dB.9f	Statistical discrepancy	**NYOZ**	1 198	−322	787	880	−538	−591	983	−658	969
B.9g	**Net lending (+) / net borrowing (-), from capital account**	**NNBK**	8 623	13 954	7 660	−20 183	−41 173	−43 061	−40 778	−34 866	−38 322

5.1.9 General government
ESA95 sector S.13 Unconsolidated

£ billion

			1999	2000	2001	2002	2003	2004	2005	2006	2007
IV.3	**FINANCIAL BALANCE SHEET** at end of period										
AN	**Non-financial assets**	CGIX	385.3	440.7	490.3	505.3	545.9	600.6	657.0	706.1	757.0
AF.A	**Financial assets**										
AF.1	Monetary gold and special drawing rights (SDRs)	NIFC	4.0	3.1	2.4	2.4	2.6	2.5	3.2	3.4	4.3
AF.2	Currency and deposits										
AF.22	Transferable deposits										
AF.221	Deposits with UK monetary financial institutions	NLVW	14.5	32.2	23.1	20.3	23.9	26.9	27.1	34.5	41.0
AF.229	Deposits with rest of the world monetary financial institutions	NLWA	8.7	6.6	6.3	5.9	4.9	3.3	2.0	1.2	1.0
AF.29	Other deposits	NLWB	–	3.0	0.3	1.0	0.4	0.4	0.4	0.2	4.6
AF.2	Total currency and deposits	NLUT	23.2	41.8	29.7	27.1	29.2	30.6	29.4	35.9	46.6
AF.3	Securities other than shares										
AF.331	Short term: money market instruments										
AF.3311	Issued by UK central government	NLWE	0.5	0.2	0.4	0.2	0.2	0.1	0.1	0.1	0.1
AF.3312	Issued by UK local government	NLWI	–	–	–	–	–	–	–	–	–
AF.3315	Issued by UK monetary financial institutions	NLWJ	3.0	5.4	4.0	3.9	3.9	4.4	4.5	5.2	2.3
AF.3316	Issued by other UK residents	NLWO	0.1	0.2	0.5	1.3	0.2	0.2	0.3	2.1	1.3
AF.3319	Issued by the rest of the world	NLWP	1.8	2.3	2.6	1.2	0.2	0.3	1.7	3.0	5.5
AF.332	Medium (1 to 5 year) and long term (over 5 year) bonds										
AF.3321	Issued by UK central government	NLWR	0.7	0.5	0.7	0.4	0.3	0.2	0.2	0.2	0.1
AF.3322	Issued by UK local government	NLWU	–	–	–	–	–	–	–	–	–
AF.3326	Other medium & long term bonds issued by UK residents	NLWY	0.2	0.1	0.1	0.1	0.1	0.1	1.1	0.5	0.5
AF.3329	Long term bonds issued by the rest of the world	NLWZ	7.6	16.7	14.4	16.8	16.2	17.1	17.5	15.3	18.2
AF.34	Financial derivatives	NLXA	–0.4	–	0.7	0.2	–	0.2	0.6	0.7	–0.4
AF.3	Total securities other than shares	NLWC	13.5	25.3	23.4	24.0	20.9	22.5	26.0	27.2	27.6
AF.4	Loans										
AF.42	Long term loans										
AF.422	Loans secured on dwellings	NLXP	0.6	0.6	0.7	0.9	1.1	1.1	1.3	1.7	2.1
AF.424	Other long-term loans by UK residents	NLXU	62.8	66.1	69.2	68.6	66.9	69.6	74.3	78.5	82.1
AF.4	Total loans	NLXE	63.4	66.8	69.9	69.6	68.0	70.7	75.7	80.2	84.2
AF.5	Shares and other equity										
AF.51	Shares and other equity, excluding mutual funds' shares										
AF.514	Quoted UK shares	NLYB	2.3	1.4	1.2	1.0	1.2	1.2	1.5	2.0	1.8
AF.515	Unquoted UK shares	NLYC	0.5	0.5	1.3	1.3	1.3	1.8	1.2	1.2	–0.9
AF.516	Other UK equity	H4O9	83.3	82.3	88.4	95.8	104.4	114.6	130.0	121.7	118.8
AF.517	UK shares and bonds issued by other UK residents	NSQP	–	–	–	–	–	–	–	–	–
AF.519	Shares and other equity issued by the rest of the world	NLYG	6.6	6.8	7.1	7.5	7.7	8.0	8.7	9.5	10.3
AF.5	Total shares and other equity	NLXW	92.8	91.1	97.9	105.6	114.7	125.6	141.4	134.3	130.0
AF.6	Insurance technical reserves										
AF.62	Prepayments of insurance premiums and reserves for outstanding claims	NLYP	1.1	1.0	0.9	0.9	0.8	0.7	0.8	0.8	0.8
AF.7	Other accounts receivable	NLYQ	41.0	42.0	42.8	41.5	45.4	47.8	53.1	55.9	54.4
AF.A	**Total financial assets**	NPUP	239.0	271.1	267.0	271.2	281.5	300.3	329.6	337.7	348.0

5.1.9 General government
ESA95 sector S.13 Unconsolidated

continued

£ billion

			1999	2000	2001	2002	2003	2004	2005	2006	2007
IV.3	**FINANCIAL BALANCE SHEET** continued at end of period											
AF.L	**Financial liabilities**											
AF.2	Currency and deposits											
AF.21	Currency	NLYY	2.8	3.0	3.2	3.3	3.4	3.5	3.7	3.8	3.9
AF.29	Non-transferable deposits	NLZF	72.3	75.1	72.5	74.5	76.7	79.1	84.7	89.9	97.8
AF.2	Total currency and deposits	NLYX	75.1	78.1	75.6	77.8	80.1	82.7	88.4	93.7	101.6
AF.3	Securities other than shares											
AF.331	Short term: money market instruments											
AF.3311	Issued by UK central government	NLZI	4.2	2.6	11.2	21.4	24.0	25.0	21.1	19.4	18.0
AF.3312	Issued by UK local government	NLZM	–	–	–	–	–	–	–	–	–
AF.332	Medium (1 to 5 year) and long term (over 5 year) bonds											
AF.3321	Issued by UK central government	NLZV	334.0	329.2	300.5	311.1	331.9	372.9	424.2	451.3	492.8
AF.3322	Issued by UK local government	NLZY	0.8	0.8	0.8	0.8	0.8	0.6	0.8	1.2	1.2
AF.3	Total securities other than shares	NLZG	339.0	332.6	312.5	333.4	356.8	398.5	446.1	471.8	512.0
AF.4	Loans											
AF.41	Short term loans											
AF.411	Loans by UK monetary financial institutions, excluding loans secured on dwellings & financial leasing	NNKY	22.0	26.0	20.2	22.8	25.0	32.6	35.7	34.1	34.7
AF.419	Loans by rest of the world monetary financial institutions	NNLC	0.2	0.1	–	–	–	–	–	–	–
AF.42	Long term loans											
AF.423	Finance leasing	NNLL	1.3	1.8	2.0	2.3	2.8	3.3	3.8	4.1	4.5
AF.424	Other long-term loans by UK residents	NNLM	49.1	50.1	50.1	48.3	44.5	45.6	48.0	50.6	51.1
AF.429	Other long-term loans by the rest of the world	NNLN	1.2	1.3	1.3	1.2	1.3	1.9	1.9	2.1	2.1
AF.4	Total loans	NNKW	73.9	79.2	73.6	74.7	73.7	83.3	89.4	90.8	92.4
AF.7	Other accounts payable	NNMI	19.3	42.2	41.8	39.3	42.6	44.7	46.1	48.7	47.8
AF.L	**Total financial liabilities**	NPVQ	507.3	532.0	503.5	525.2	553.1	609.2	670.0	705.0	753.8
AF.A	Total financial assets	NPUP	239.0	271.1	267.0	271.2	281.5	300.3	329.6	337.7	348.0
-AF.L	*less* Total financial liabilities	-NPVQ	-507.3	-532.0	-503.5	-525.2	-553.1	-609.2	-670.0	-705.0	-753.8
BF.90	**Net financial assets (+) / liabilities (-)**	NYOG	-268.3	-260.9	-236.4	-254.0	-271.6	-308.9	-340.4	-367.3	-405.9
	Net worth											
AN	Non-financial assets	CGIX	385.3	440.7	490.3	505.3	545.9	600.6	657.0	706.1	757.0
BF.90	Net financial assets (+) / liabilities (-)	NYOG	-268.3	-260.9	-236.4	-254.0	-271.6	-308.9	-340.4	-367.3	-405.9
BF.90	**Net worth**	CGRX	117.0	179.8	253.9	251.4	274.3	291.7	316.6	338.8	351.1

5.2.1 Central government
ESA95 sector S.1311

£ million

			1999	2000	2001	2002	2003	2004	2005	2006
I	**PRODUCTION ACCOUNT**									
	Resources									
P.1	Output									
P.11	Market output	NMIW	2 606	2 535	3 075	3 480	3 514	6 971	8 880	9 380
P.12	Output for own final use	QYJV	134	86	44	42	44	–	–	3
P.13	Other non-market output	NMBJ	103 594	110 829	118 778	130 348	142 658	152 563	161 800	173 905
P.1	Total resources	NMAE	106 334	113 450	121 897	133 870	146 216	159 534	170 680	183 288
	Uses									
P.2	Intermediate consumption	NMAF	53 864	58 077	61 659	68 890	74 383	81 694	88 570	97 096
B.1g	**Gross Value Added**	NMBR	**52 470**	**55 373**	**60 238**	**64 980**	**71 833**	**77 840**	**82 110**	**86 192**
Total	Total uses	NMAE	106 334	113 450	121 897	133 870	146 216	159 534	170 680	183 288
B.1g	**Gross Value Added**	NMBR	**52 470**	**55 373**	**60 238**	**64 980**	**71 833**	**77 840**	**82 110**	**86 192**
-K.1	*less* Consumption of fixed capital	−NSRN	−5 396	−5 495	−5 483	−5 636	−5 902	−6 115	−6 355	−6 566
B.1n	Value added, net of fixed capital consumption	NMAH	47 074	49 878	54 755	59 344	65 931	71 725	75 755	79 626

5.2.2 Central government
ESA95 sector S.1311

£ million

			1999	2000	2001	2002	2003	2004	2005	2006
II	**DISTRIBUTION AND USE OF INCOME ACCOUNTS**									
II.1	**PRIMARY DISTRIBUTION OF INCOME ACCOUNT**									
II.1.1	**GENERATION OF INCOME ACCOUNT**									
	Resources									
B.1g	**Total resources (Gross Value Added)**	NMBR	**52 470**	**55 373**	**60 238**	**64 980**	**71 833**	**77 840**	**82 110**	**86 192**
	Uses									
D.1	Compensation of employees									
D.11	Wages and salaries	NMAI	38 346	40 437	45 292	48 648	54 514	61 404	62 290	65 724
D.12	Employers' social contributions	NMAL	8 728	9 441	9 463	10 696	11 417	10 321	13 465	13 902
D.1	Total	NMBG	47 074	49 878	54 755	59 344	65 931	71 725	75 755	79 626
D.2	Taxes on production and imports, paid									
D.29	Production taxes other than on products	NMAN	–	–	–	–	–	–	–	–
-D.3	*less* Subsidies, received									
-D.39	Production subsidies other than on products	−NMAO	–	–	–	–	–	–	–	–
B.2g	Operating surplus, gross	NRLN	5 396	5 495	5 483	5 636	5 902	6 115	6 355	6 566
B.1g	**Total uses (Gross Value Added)**	NMBR	**52 470**	**55 373**	**60 238**	**64 980**	**71 833**	**77 840**	**82 110**	**86 192**
-K.1	After deduction of fixed capital consumption	−NSRN	−5 396	−5 495	−5 483	−5 636	−5 902	−6 115	−6 355	−6 566
B.2n	Operating surplus, net	NMAP	–	–	–	–	–	–	–	–

5.2.3 Central government
ESA95 sector S.1311

£ million

			1999	2000	2001	2002	2003	2004	2005	2006	2007
II.1.2	**ALLOCATION OF PRIMARY INCOME ACCOUNT**										
	Resources										
B.2g	Operating surplus, gross	**NRLN**	5 396	5 495	5 483	5 636	5 902	6 115	6 355	6 566	7 803
D.2	Taxes on production and imports, received										
D.21	Taxes on products										
D.211	Value added tax (VAT)	**NZGF**	57 701	59 985	63 522	68 251	74 595	79 761	81 416	85 586	89 681
D.212	Taxes and duties on imports excluding VAT										
D.2121	Import duties	**NMXZ**	–	–	–	–	–	–	–	–	–
D.2122	Taxes on imports excluding VAT and import duties	**NMBT**	–	–	–	–	–	–	–	–	–
D.214	Taxes on products excluding VAT and import duties	**NMYB**	48 442	51 956	50 745	52 001	52 858	56 137	56 906	60 540	64 292
D.21	Total taxes on products	**NMYC**	106 143	111 941	114 267	120 252	127 453	135 898	138 322	146 126	153 973
D.29	Other taxes on production	**NMBX**	16 361	16 934	17 408	17 940	18 329	18 690	19 524	20 629	21 333
D.2	Total taxes on production and imports, received	**NMBY**	122 504	128 875	131 675	138 192	145 782	154 588	157 846	166 755	175 306
-D.3	*less* Subsidies, paid										
-D.31	Subsidies on products	**–NMCB**	–2 976	–3 083	–3 096	–3 634	–4 030	–3 525	–3 507	–4 258	–3 615
-D.39	Other subsidies on production	**–NMCC**	–647	–553	–653	–937	–1 416	–1 323	–1 383	–1 432	–1 952
-D.3	Total	**–NMCD**	–3 623	–3 636	–3 749	–4 571	–5 446	–4 848	–4 890	–5 690	–5 567
D.4	Property income										
D.41	Total Interest	**NMCE**	6 495	6 365	6 482	5 865	6 331	5 705	5 351	5 864	6 467
D.42	Distributed income of corporations	**NMCH**	2 045	2 358	2 392	1 789	1 773	2 074	2 164	1 866	2 434
D.45	Rent from sectors other than general government	**NMCK**	529	1 289	1 919	1 901	1 565	1 182	1 229	1 226	1 242
D.4	Total	**NMCL**	9 069	10 012	10 793	9 555	9 669	8 961	8 744	8 956	10 143
Total	Total resources	**NMCM**	133 346	140 746	144 202	148 812	155 907	164 816	168 055	176 587	187 685
	Uses										
D.4	Property income										
D.41	Total Interest	**RVFK**	26 265	26 382	23 661	21 429	22 421	23 252	26 000	26 738	30 506
D.4	Total property income	**NUHA**	26 265	26 382	23 661	21 429	22 421	23 252	26 000	26 738	30 506
B.5g	**Balance of primary incomes, gross**	**NRLP**	**107 081**	**114 364**	**120 541**	**127 383**	**133 486**	**141 564**	**142 055**	**149 849**	**157 179**
Total	Total uses	**NMCM**	133 346	140 746	144 202	148 812	155 907	164 816	168 055	176 587	187 685
-K.1	After deduction of fixed capital consumption	**–NSRN**	–5 396	–5 495	–5 483	–5 636	–5 902	–6 115	–6 355	–6 566	–6 843
B.5n	Balance of primary incomes, net	**NMCT**	101 685	108 869	115 058	121 747	127 584	135 449	135 700	143 283	150 336

5.2.4 Central government
ESA95 sector S.1311

£ million

			1999	2000	2001	2002	2003	2004	2005	2006	2007
II.2	**SECONDARY DISTRIBUTION OF INCOME ACCOUNT**										
	Resources										
B.5g	**Balance of primary incomes, gross**	NRLP	**107 081**	**114 364**	**120 541**	**127 383**	**133 486**	**141 564**	**142 055**	**149 849**	**157 179**
D.5	Current taxes on income, wealth, etc.										
D.51	Taxes on income	NMCU	129 553	140 002	147 264	142 842	144 234	154 127	172 498	192 812	199 289
D.59	Other current taxes	NMCV	6 753	6 369	6 920	7 133	7 534	7 991	8 331	8 687	9 321
D.5	Total	NMCP	136 306	146 371	154 184	149 975	151 768	162 118	180 829	201 499	208 610
D.61	Social contributions										
D.611	Actual social contributions										
D.6111	Employers' actual social contributions	NMCY	33 401	36 397	38 460	38 780	45 067	49 202	52 769	56 024	59 303
D.6112	Employees' social contributions	NMDB	26 062	26 715	28 116	28 931	33 717	38 132	41 010	43 581	45 247
D.6113	Social contributions by self- and non-employed persons	NMDE	1 883	2 049	2 183	2 318	2 595	2 727	2 825	2 930	3 013
D.611	Total	NMCX	61 346	65 161	68 759	70 029	81 379	90 061	96 604	102 535	107 563
D.612	Imputed social contributions	QYJS	5 213	5 538	5 620	6 282	4 311	3 997	5 073	4 863	5 251
D.61	Total	NMCW	66 559	70 699	74 379	76 311	85 690	94 058	101 677	107 398	112 814
D.7	Other current transfers										
D.72	Non-life insurance claims	NMDJ	–	–	–	–	–	–	–	–	–
D.73	Current transfers within general government	NMDK	–	–	–	–	–	–	–	–	–
D.74	Current international cooperation	NMDL	3 176	2 084	4 568	3 112	3 570	3 604	3 668	3 594	3 527
D.75	Miscellaneous current transfers from sectors other than general government	NMEZ	392	447	460	502	562	721	728	612	584
D.7	Other current transfers	NMDI	3 568	2 531	5 028	3 614	4 132	4 325	4 396	4 206	4 111
Total	Total resources	NMDN	313 514	333 965	354 132	357 283	375 076	402 065	428 957	462 952	482 714
	Uses										
D.62	Social benefits other than social transfers in kind	NMDR	102 867	105 672	114 509	120 938	129 606	137 379	143 507	147 998	157 397
D.7	Other current transfers										
D.71	Net non-life insurance premiums	NMDX	–	–	–	–	–	–	–	–	–
D.73	Current transfers within general government	QYJR	64 446	66 187	72 522	77 592	85 224	94 720	101 369	110 407	113 046
D.74	Current international cooperation	NMDZ	1 456	2 181	2 190	2 362	2 433	3 080	3 255	3 632	3 909
D.75	Miscellaneous current transfers to sectors other than general government										
	GNP based fourth own resource	NMFH	4 632	4 379	3 858	5 335	6 772	7 549	8 732	8 521	8 323
	NHS trusts compensation payments	MJTI	274	582	648	572	606	758	863	850	733
	Misc grants to non profit institutions	DFT8	13 535	15 920	17 602	21 421	22 873	22 842	24 735	25 299	27 092
D.75	Total	NMFC	18 441	20 881	22 108	27 328	30 251	31 149	34 330	34 670	36 148
D.7	Other current transfers	NMDW	84 343	89 249	96 820	107 282	117 908	128 949	138 954	148 709	153 103
B.6g	**Gross Disposable Income**	NRLR	**126 304**	**139 044**	**142 803**	**129 063**	**127 562**	**135 737**	**146 496**	**166 245**	**172 214**
Total	Total uses	NMDN	313 514	333 965	354 132	357 283	375 076	402 065	428 957	462 952	482 714
-K.1	After deduction of fixed capital consumption	-NSRN	-5 396	-5 495	-5 483	-5 636	-5 902	-6 115	-6 355	-6 566	-6 843
B.6n	Disposable income, net	NMEB	120 908	133 549	137 320	123 427	121 660	129 622	140 141	159 679	165 371

5.2.4S Central government
Social contributions and benefits

ESA95 sector S.1311

£ million

Part			1999	2000	2001	2002	2003	2004	2005	2006	2007
	SECONDARY DISTRIBUTION OF INCOME (further detail of certain items)										
	Resources										
D.61	Social contributions										
	National Insurance Contributions (NICs)										
D.611	Actual social contributions										
D.61111	Employers' NICs	CEAN	31 286	34 028	35 706	35 735	39 890	43 586	46 741	49 552	52 300
D.61121	Employees' NICs	GCSE	23 573	24 175	25 236	25 357	29 055	32 396	34 742	37 039	38 474
D.61131	Self- and non-employed persons' NICs	NMDE	1 883	2 049	2 183	2 318	2 595	2 727	2 825	2 930	3 013
D.61	Total national insurance contributions	AIIH	56 742	60 252	63 125	63 410	71 540	78 709	84 308	89 521	93 787
	Pension schemes[1]										
D.611	Actual social contributions										
D.61112	Employers' contributions	GCMP	2 115	2 369	2 754	3 045	5 177	5 616	6 028	6 472	7 003
D.61122	Employees' contributions	CX3X	2 489	2 540	2 880	3 574	4 662	5 736	6 268	6 542	6 773
D.612	Imputed social contributions	QYJS	5 213	5 538	5 620	6 282	4 311	3 997	5 073	4 863	5 251
D.61	Total pension schemes	FAD5	9 817	10 447	11 254	12 901	14 150	15 349	17 369	17 877	19 027
D.61	Total social contributions	NMCW	66 559	70 699	74 379	76 311	85 690	94 058	101 677	107 398	112 814
	Uses										
D.62	Social benefits										
D.621	Social security benefits in cash										
	National insurance fund										
	Retirement pensions	CSDG	37 319	38 686	41 323	43 967	46 098	48 495	50 929	53 228	56 630
	Widows' and guardians' allowances	CSDH	970	984	1 080	1 096	1 027	939	882	807	755
	Unemployment benefit	CSDI	−1	−1	–	−2	–	−1	−4	–	–
	Jobseeker's allowance	CJTJ	473	436	454	512	519	454	486	474	428
	Sickness benefit	CSDJ	–	–	–	–	–	–	–	–	–
	Invalidity benefit	CSDK	–	–	–	–	–	–	–	–	–
	Incapacity benefit	CUNL	6 925	6 705	6 736	6 754	6 792	6 674	6 618	6 545	6 655
	Maternity benefit	CSDL	40	42	55	66	107	146	162	172	215
	Death grant	CSDM	–	–	–	–	–	–	–	–	–
	Statutory sick pay	CSDQ	29	28	25	19	58	75	78	83	98
	Statutory maternity pay	GTKZ	580	610	663	711	1 130	1 336	1 249	1 319	1 512
	Payment in lieu of benefits foregone	GTKV	–	–	–	–	–	–	–	–	–
	Total national insurance fund benefits	ACHH	46 335	47 490	50 336	53 123	55 731	58 118	60 400	62 628	66 293
	Redundancy fund benefit	GTKN	137	167	198	278	245	169	274	200	178
	Maternity fund benefit	GTKO	–	–	–	–	–	–	–	–	–
	Social fund benefit	GTLQ	1 087	1 753	1 885	1 910	2 135	2 240	2 232	2 253	2 348
	Benefits paid to overseas residents	FJVZ	1 123	1 161	1 239	1 338	1 404	1 539	1 596	1 648	1 774
D.621	Total social security benefits in cash	QYRJ	48 682	50 571	53 658	56 649	59 515	62 066	64 502	66 729	70 593
D.623	Total unfunded social benefits	QYJT	11 647	12 439	13 027	14 744	15 602	16 615	17 617	18 744	21 176
D.624	Social assistance benefits in cash										
	War pensions and allowances	CSDD	1 255	1 214	1 200	1 173	1 108	1 079	1 018	995	966
	Income support	CSDE	12 068	12 830	13 901	14 400	14 986	15 946	15 595	15 633	15 860
	Income tax credits and reliefs	RYCQ	1 863	4 532	5 586	6 344	8 805	11 329	12 418	14 006	15 253
	Child Benefit	EKY3	10 366	8 631	8 728	8 906	9 281	9 623	9 627	10 124	10 415
	Non-contributory job seekers' allowance	EKY4	2 900	2 529	2 175	2 112	2 098	1 931	1 848	2 067	2 306
	Care allowances	EKY5	2 790	2 911	4 579	5 174	5 379	5 839	6 123	6 427	6 809
	Disability benefits	EKY6	5 544	5 919	7 016	7 716	8 249	8 716	9 248	9 841	10 486
	Other benefits	EKY7	5 692	4 039	4 586	3 670	4 535	4 178	5 457	3 380	3 478
	Benefits paid to overseas residents	RNNF	60	57	53	50	48	57	54	52	55
D.624	Total social assistance benefits in cash	NZGO	42 538	42 662	47 824	49 545	54 489	58 698	61 388	62 525	65 628
D.62	Total social benefits	NMDR	102 867	105 672	114 509	120 938	129 606	137 379	143 507	147 998	157 397

1 Mainly civil service, armed forces', teachers' and NHS pension schemes

5.2.5 Central government
ESA95 sector S.1311

£ million

			1999	2000	2001	2002	2003	2004	2005	2006	2007
II.3	**REDISTRIBUTION OF INCOME IN KIND ACCOUNT**										
	Resources										
B.6g	Total resources (Gross Disposable Income)	**NRLR**	126 304	139 044	142 803	129 063	127 562	135 737	146 496	166 245	172 214
	Uses										
D.63	Social transfers in kind										
D.631	Social benefits in kind										
D.632	Transfers of individual non-market goods and services	**NMED**	59 909	63 042	68 211	75 408	83 215	83 577	89 807	98 532	104 834
B.7g	Adjusted disposable income, gross	**NSVS**	66 395	76 002	74 592	53 655	44 347	52 160	56 689	67 713	67 380
B.6g	**Total uses (Gross Disposable Income)**	**NRLR**	126 304	139 044	142 803	129 063	127 562	135 737	146 496	166 245	172 214

5.2.6 Central government
ESA95 sector S.1311

£ million

			1999	2000	2001	2002	2003	2004	2005	2006	2007
II.4	**USE OF INCOME ACCOUNT**										
II.4.1	**USE OF DISPOSABLE INCOME ACCOUNT**										
	Resources										
B.6g	Total resources (Gross Disposable Income)	**NRLR**	126 304	139 044	142 803	129 063	127 562	135 737	146 496	166 245	172 214
	Uses										
P.3	Final consumption expenditure										
P.31	Individual consumption expenditure	**NMED**	59 909	63 042	68 211	75 408	83 215	83 577	89 807	98 532	104 834
P.32	Collective consumption expenditure	**NMEE**	43 685	47 787	50 567	54 940	59 443	68 986	71 993	75 373	75 712
P.3	Total	**NMBJ**	103 594	110 829	118 778	130 348	142 658	152 563	161 800	173 905	180 546
B.8g	**Gross Saving**	**NRLS**	22 710	28 215	24 025	–1 285	–15 096	–16 826	–15 304	–7 660	–8 332
B.6g	**Total uses (Gross Disposable Income)**	**NRLR**	126 304	139 044	142 803	129 063	127 562	135 737	146 496	166 245	172 214
-K.1	After deduction of fixed capital consumption	**–NSRN**	–5 396	–5 495	–5 483	–5 636	–5 902	–6 115	–6 355	–6 566	–6 843
B.8n	Saving, net	**NMEG**	17 314	22 720	18 542	–6 921	–20 998	–22 941	–21 659	–14 226	–15 175
II.4.2	**USE OF ADJUSTED DISPOSABLE INCOME ACCOUNT**										
	Resources										
B.7g	Total resources, adjusted disposable income, gross	**NSVS**	66 395	76 002	74 592	53 655	44 347	52 160	56 689	67 713	67 380
	Uses										
P.4	Actual final consumption										
P.42	Actual collective consumption	**NMEE**	43 685	47 787	50 567	54 940	59 443	68 986	71 993	75 373	75 712
B.8g	**Gross Saving**	**NRLS**	22 710	28 215	24 025	–1 285	–15 096	–16 826	–15 304	–7 660	–8 332
Total	Total uses	**NSVS**	66 395	76 002	74 592	53 655	44 347	52 160	56 689	67 713	67 380

5.2.7 Central government
ESA95 sector S.1311

£ million

			1999	2000	2001	2002	2003	2004	2005	2006	2007
III	ACCUMULATION ACCOUNTS										
III.1	CAPITAL ACCOUNT										
III.1.1	CHANGE IN NET WORTH DUE TO SAVINGS AND CAPITAL TRANSFERS										
	Changes in liabilities and net worth										
B.8g	**Gross Saving**	**NRLS**	**22 710**	**28 215**	**24 025**	**−1 285**	**−15 096**	**−16 826**	**−15 304**	**−7 660**	**−8 332**
D.9	Capital transfers receivable										
D.91	Capital taxes										
	from sectors other than general government	**NMGI**	1 951	2 215	2 396	2 381	2 416	2 871	3 150	3 575	3 890
D.92	Investment grants	**GCMT**	–	–	–	–	–	–	–	–	–
D.99	Other capital transfers	**NMEK**	–	–	412	412	391	1 679	2 497	1 488	1 388
D.9	Total capital transfers receivable	**NMEH**	1 951	2 215	2 808	2 793	2 807	4 550	5 647	5 063	5 278
-D.9	*less* Capital transfers payable										
-D.92	Investment grants	**−NMEN**	−7 618	−7 821	−10 396	−12 807	−16 170	−15 049	−18 427	−19 528	−22 217
-D.99	Other capital transfers	**−NMEO**	−210	−340	−1 302	−678	−4 489	−2 649	−14 847	−2 641	−1 661
-D.9	Total capital transfers payable	**−NMEL**	−7 828	−8 161	−11 698	−13 485	−20 659	−17 698	−33 274	−22 169	−23 878
B.10.1g	Total change in liabilities and net worth	**NMEP**	16 833	22 269	15 135	−11 977	−32 948	−29 974	−42 931	−24 766	−26 932
	Changes in assets										
B.10.1g	Changes in net worth due to gross saving and capital transfers	**NMEP**	16 833	22 269	15 135	−11 977	−32 948	−29 974	−42 931	−24 766	−26 932
-K.1	After deduction of fixed capital consumption	**−NSRN**	−5 396	−5 495	−5 483	−5 636	−5 902	−6 115	−6 355	−6 566	−6 843
B.10.1n	Changes in net worth due to net saving and capital transfers	**NMEQ**	11 437	16 774	9 652	−17 613	−38 850	−36 089	−49 286	−31 332	−33 775
III.1.2	ACQUISITION OF NON-FINANCIAL ASSETS ACCOUNT										
	Changes in liabilities and net worth										
B.10.1n	Changes in net worth due to saving and capital transfers	**NMEQ**	11 437	16 774	9 652	−17 613	−38 850	−36 089	−49 286	−31 332	−33 775
K.1	Consumption of fixed capital	**NSRN**	5 396	5 495	5 483	5 636	5 902	6 115	6 355	6 566	6 843
B.10.1g	Total changes in liabilities and net worth	**NMEP**	16 833	22 269	15 135	−11 977	−32 948	−29 974	−42 931	−24 766	−26 932
	Changes in assets										
P.5	Gross capital formation										
P.51	Gross fixed capital formation	**NMES**	6 356	5 675	5 964	7 506	6 372	8 328	−6 425	9 860	10 828
P.52	Changes in inventories	**NMFE**	−268	−140	−18	–	15	−46	−6	−4	−20
P.53	Acquisitions less disposals of valuables	**NPPD**	10	12	22	22	16	20	16	14	18
P.5	Total	**NMER**	6 098	5 547	5 968	7 528	6 403	8 302	−6 415	9 870	10 826
K.2	Acquisitions less disposals of non-produced non-financial assets	**NMFG**	−173	−187	−196	−327	−157	−227	−264	−90	−196
B.9g	**Net lending(+) / net borrowing(-)**	**NMFJ**	**10 908**	**16 909**	**9 363**	**−19 178**	**−39 194**	**−38 049**	**−36 252**	**−34 546**	**−37 562**
Total	Total change in assets	**NMEP**	16 833	22 269	15 135	−11 977	−32 948	−29 974	−42 931	−24 766	−26 932

5.2.8 Central government
ESA95 sector S.1311 Unconsolidated

£ million

			1999	2000	2001	2002	2003	2004	2005	2006	2007
III.2	**FINANCIAL ACCOUNT**										
F.A	**Net acquisition of financial assets**										
F.1	Monetary gold and special drawing rights (SDRs)	NWXM	−374	−956	−808	−240	−2	−37	−8	47	−50
F.2	Currency and deposits										
F.22	Transferable deposits										
F.2211	Sterling deposits with UK banks	NAUB	−78	15 063	−8 521	−4 516	1 200	−1 506	538	1 656	1 721
F.2212	Foreign currency deposits with UK banks	NARV	12	120	−1 270	−356	−41	−947	−329	542	297
F.2213	Sterling deposits with UK building societies	NARW	−4	11	5	63	4	−35	47	48	6
F.229	Deposits with rest of the world monetary financial institutions	NARX	3 177	−840	−261	−299	−916	−1 407	−1 516	−671	−550
F.29	Other deposits national savings & tax	RYWO	−	2 919	−2 578	376	−681	−	−	161	3 761
F.2	Total currency and deposits	NARQ	3 107	17 273	−12 625	−4 732	−434	−3 895	−1 260	1 736	5 235
F.3	Securities other than shares										
F.331	Short term: money market instruments										
F.3315	Issued by UK MFI's	NSUN	−	1 435	−1 285	−720	−99	751	213	1 768	−2 038
F.3316	Issued by other UK residents	NSRI	−	−	325	730	−1 029	−	−	1 192	−1 142
F.3319	Issued by the rest of the world	NASM	−337	244	273	−1 576	−987	106	1 465	1 363	2 125
F.332	Medium (1 to 5 year) and long term (over 5 year) bonds										
F.3326	Other medium & long term bonds issued by UK residents	NASV	−387	11	−49	−17	−	−	856	−620	−42
F.3329	Long term bonds issued by the rest of the world	NASW	−3 105	5 418	−1 838	2 280	−390	1 551	370	−854	2 127
F.34	Financial derivatives	−CFZG	−	185	102	−238	−136	−173	137	−419	−343
F.3	Total securities other than shares	NARZ	−3 829	7 293	−2 472	459	−2 641	2 235	3 041	2 430	687
F.4	Loans										
F.42	Long term loans										
F.422	Loans secured on dwellings	NATM	−1	−1	−	−	−	−	−	−	−
F.424	Other long-term loans by UK residents	NATR	2 786	3 767	3 847	−231	−976	2 568	4 711	4 176	4 360
F.429	Other long-term loans by the rest of the world	NATS	−	−	−	−	−	−	−	−	−
F.4	Total loans	NATB	2 785	3 766	3 847	−231	−976	2 568	4 711	4 176	4 360
F.5	Shares and other equity										
F.51	Shares and other equity, excluding mutual funds' shares										
F.514	Quoted UK shares	NATY	−12	−103	−	−	−	−	295	32	−2 316
F.515	Unquoted UK shares	NATZ	−	−	−518	−	−29	−	−550	−	−2 060
F.516	Other UK equity (including direct investment in property)	NAUA	−49	−55	−103	−204	−25	−117	−1 249	−1 356	−76
F.517	UK shares and bonds issued by other UK residents	NSOX	−	−	−	−	−	−	−	−	−
F.519	Shares and other equity issued by the rest of the world	NAUD	302	290	256	409	234	283	656	810	725
F.5	Total shares and other equity	NATT	241	132	−365	205	180	166	−848	−514	−3 727
F.7	Other accounts receivable	NAUN	7 873	1 290	815	−696	2 777	2 310	5 339	2 898	−1 684
F.A	**Total net acquisition of financial assets**	NARM	9 803	28 798	−11 608	−5 235	−1 096	3 347	10 975	10 773	4 821

5.2.8 Central government
ESA95 sector S.1311 Unconsolidated

continued   £ million

			1999	2000	2001	2002	2003	2004	2005	2006	2007
III.2	**FINANCIAL ACCOUNT** continued										
F.L	**Net acquisition of financial liabilities**										
F.2	Currency and deposits										
F.21	Currency	**NAUV**	191	226	228	180	216	171	180	154	123
F.29	Non-transferable deposits	**NAVC**	−907	2 578	−3 084	1 946	3 266	2 423	5 502	5 240	7 930
F.2	Total currency and deposits	**NAUU**	−716	2 804	−2 856	2 126	3 482	2 594	5 682	5 394	8 053
F.3	Securities other than shares										
F.331	Short term: money market instruments										
F.3311	Issued by UK central government	**NAVF**	−404	−1 652	8 623	10 330	2 592	999	−3 902	−1 752	−1 367
F.332	Medium (1 to 5 year) and long term (over 5 year) bonds										
F.33211	British government securities	**NAVT**	−4 504	−12 684	−11 568	4 701	29 748	34 205	39 900	40 998	38 936
F.33212	Other central government bonds	**NAVU**	−56	−16	−5 651	−3 146	1 726	14	17	15	15
F.3	Total securities other than shares	**NAVD**	−4 964	−14 352	−8 596	11 885	34 066	35 218	36 015	39 261	37 584
F.4	Loans										
F.41	Short term loans										
F.411	Loans by UK monetary financial institutions, excluding loans secured on dwellings & financial leasing	**NAWH**	6 087	−55	−6 615	915	−53	5 878	2 336	−2 996	−1 068
F.419	Loans by rest of the world monetary financial institutions	**NAWL**	−1	–	−2	−1	–	–	–	–	–
F.42	Long term loans										
F.423	Finance leasing	**NAWV**	563	432	229	259	497	450	502	301	442
F.424	Other long-term loans by UK residents	**NAWV**	−38	−25	−23	−18	−19	−14	−12	−7	−6
F.429	Other long-term loans by the rest of the world	**NAWW**	−105	−114	−45	−48	−45	−46	−65	7	−3
F.4	Total loans	**NAWF**	6 506	238	−6 456	1 107	380	6 268	2 761	−2 695	−635
F.7	Other accounts payable	**NAXR**	−1 405	23 709	−2 987	−356	281	−2 319	3 139	2 680	−1 658
F.L	**Total net acquisition of financial liabilities**	**NAUQ**	−579	12 399	−20 895	14 762	38 209	41 761	47 597	44 640	43 344
B.9	**Net lending / borrowing**										
F.A	Total net acquisition of financial assets	**NARM**	9 803	28 798	−11 608	−5 235	−1 096	3 347	10 975	10 773	4 821
-F.L	*less* Total net acquisition of financial liabilities	**−NAUQ**	579	−12 399	20 895	−14 762	−38 209	−41 761	−47 597	−44 640	−43 344
B.9f	Net lending (+) / net borrowing (-), from financial account	**NZDX**	10 382	16 399	9 287	−19 997	−39 305	−38 414	−36 622	−33 867	−38 523
dB.9f	Statistical discrepancy	**NZDW**	526	510	76	819	111	365	370	−679	961
B.9g	**Net lending (+) / net borrowing (-), from capital account**	**NMFJ**	**10 908**	**16 909**	**9 363**	**−19 178**	**−39 194**	**−38 049**	**−36 252**	**−34 546**	**−37 562**

5.2.9 Central government
ESA95 sector S.1311 Unconsolidated

£ billion

			1999	2000	2001	2002	2003	2004	2005	2006	2007
IV.3	**FINANCIAL BALANCE SHEET** at end of period										
AN	**Non-financial assets**	CGIY	157.4	182.6	189.0	197.8	211.8	221.1	250.6	269.1	281.4
AF.A	**Financial assets**										
AF.1	Monetary gold and special drawing rights (SDRs)	NIFC	4.0	3.1	2.4	2.4	2.6	2.5	3.2	3.4	4.3
AF.2 AF.22 AF.221	Currency and deposits Transferable deposits Deposits with UK monetary financial institutions	NIFI	1.8	18.9	9.1	4.6	6.8	5.5	5.6	7.7	9.8
AF.229	Deposits with rest of the world monetary financial institutions	NIFM	8.7	6.6	6.3	5.9	4.9	3.3	2.0	1.2	1.0
AF.29	Other deposits	NIFN	–	2.9	0.3	0.7	–	–	–	–	3.8
AF.2	Total currency and deposits	NIFF	10.6	28.5	15.8	11.2	11.7	8.8	7.6	8.9	14.6
AF.3 AF.331 AF.3315	Securities other than shares Short term: money market instruments Issued by UK MFI's	NSUO	–	2.0	0.8	0.1	–	0.8	1.0	2.7	0.8
AF.3316	Issued by other UK residents	NSRH	–	–	0.3	1.1	–	–	–	1.2	0.1
AF.3319	Issued by the rest of the world	NIGB	1.8	2.3	2.6	1.2	0.2	0.3	1.7	3.0	5.5
AF.332 AF.3322	Medium (1 to 5 year) and long term (over 5 year) bonds Issued by UK local government	NIGG	–	–	–	–	–	–	–	–	–
AF.3326	Other medium & long term bonds issued by UK residents	NIGK	0.2	0.1	0.1	0.1	0.1	0.1	0.9	0.3	0.3
AF.3329	Long term bonds issued by the rest of the world	NIGL	7.6	16.7	14.4	16.8	16.2	17.1	17.5	15.3	18.2
AF.34	Financial derivatives	ZYBQ	–0.4	–	0.7	0.2	–	0.2	0.6	0.7	–0.4
AF.3	Total securities other than shares	NIFO	9.3	21.1	18.9	19.4	16.4	18.4	21.8	23.3	24.4
AF.4 AF.42 AF.422	Loans Long term loans Loans secured on dwellings	NIHB	0.1	0.1	0.1	0.1	0.1	0.1	0.1	0.1	0.1
AF.424	Other long-term loans by UK residents	NIHG	62.5	65.8	68.9	68.4	66.6	69.4	74.1	78.3	81.9
AF.4	Total loans	NIGQ	62.6	65.9	69.0	68.4	66.7	69.5	74.2	78.4	82.0
AF.5 AF.51 AF.514	Shares and other equity Shares and other equity, excluding mutual funds' shares Quoted UK shares	NIHN	0.2	0.1	–	–	–	–	0.3	0.6	0.6
AF.515	Unquoted UK shares	NIHO	0.1	0.1	0.9	0.9	0.9	1.4	0.8	0.8	–1.3
AF.516	Other UK equity	H4O7	11.0	10.6	10.0	9.8	9.3	8.4	13.3	10.8	7.4
AF.517	UK shares and bonds issued by other UK residents	NSNX	–	–	–	–	–	–	–	–	–
AF.519	Shares and other equity issued by the rest of the world	NIHS	6.6	6.8	7.1	7.5	7.7	8.0	8.7	9.5	10.3
AF.5	Total shares and other equity	NIHI	17.9	17.6	18.0	18.2	18.0	17.8	23.1	21.6	17.0
AF.7	Other accounts receivable	NIIC	39.2	40.4	41.5	41.2	44.5	46.7	51.8	54.6	53.1
AF.A	**Total financial assets**	NIGP	143.4	176.6	165.6	160.8	159.9	163.6	181.6	190.2	195.4

5.2.9 Central government
ESA95 sector S.1311 Unconsolidated

continued

£ billion

			1999	2000	2001	2002	2003	2004	2005	2006	2007
IV.3	**FINANCIAL BALANCE SHEET** continued										
	at end of period										
AF.L	**Financial liabilities**										
AF.2	Currency and deposits										
AF.21	Currency	**NIIK**	2.8	3.0	3.2	3.3	3.4	3.5	3.7	3.8	3.9
AF.29	Non-transferable deposits	**NIIR**	72.3	75.1	72.5	74.5	76.7	79.1	84.7	89.9	97.8
AF.2	Total currency and deposits	**NIIJ**	75.1	78.1	75.6	77.8	80.1	82.7	88.4	93.7	101.6
AF.3	Securities other than shares										
AF.331	Short term: money market instruments										
AF.33111	Sterling Treasury bills	**NIIV**	4.2	2.6	11.2	21.4	24.0	25.0	21.1	19.4	18.0
AF.33112	ECU Treasury bills	**NIIW**	–	–	–	–	–	–	–	–	–
AF.332	Medium (1 to 5 year) and long term (over 5 year) bonds										
AF.33211	British government securities	**NIJI**	324.3	318.9	296.0	309.3	330.3	370.1	421.3	448.4	490.0
AF.33212	Other central government bonds	**NIJJ**	9.7	10.3	4.5	1.8	1.6	2.8	3.0	2.9	2.8
AF.3	Total securities other than shares	**NIIS**	338.2	331.8	311.7	332.5	355.9	397.9	445.3	470.6	510.8
AF.4	Loans										
AF.41	Short term loans										
AF.411	Loans by UK monetary financial institutions, excluding loans secured on dwellings & financial leasing	**NIJW**	19.6	24.3	18.2	20.0	20.8	26.3	28.1	25.0	24.4
AF.419	Loans by rest of the world monetary financial institutions	**ZMFG**	–	–	–	–	–	–	–	–	–
AF.42	Long term loans										
AF.423	Finance leasing	**NIKJ**	1.3	1.8	2.0	2.3	2.8	3.2	3.7	4.0	4.5
AF.424	Other long-term loans by UK residents	**NIKK**	0.2	–	–	–	0.1	0.1	0.1	0.1	–
AF.429	Other long-term loans by the rest of the world	**NIKL**	0.4	0.5	0.5	0.4	0.2	0.1	0.1	–	–
AF.4	Total loans	**NIJU**	21.5	26.6	20.7	22.6	23.8	29.8	31.9	29.1	28.9
AF.7	Other accounts payable	**NILG**	9.6	32.9	31.8	30.0	32.8	33.9	35.2	37.4	37.0
AF.L	**Total financial liabilities**	**NIJT**	444.4	469.4	439.9	462.9	492.7	544.3	600.8	630.8	678.3
BF.90	**Net financial assets / liabilities**										
AF.A	Total financial assets	**NIGP**	143.4	176.6	165.6	160.8	159.9	163.6	181.6	190.2	195.4
-AF.L	*less* Total financial liabilities	**-NIJT**	–444.4	–469.4	–439.9	–462.9	–492.7	–544.3	–600.8	–630.8	–678.3
BF.90	**Net financial assets (+) / liabilities (-)**	**NZDZ**	–301.0	–292.8	–274.3	–302.1	–332.8	–380.7	–419.2	–440.6	–482.9
	Net worth										
AN	Non-financial assets	**CGIY**	157.4	182.6	189.0	197.8	211.8	221.1	250.6	269.1	281.4
BF.90	Net financial assets (+) / liabilities (-)	**NZDZ**	–301.0	–292.8	–274.3	–302.1	–332.8	–380.7	–419.2	–440.6	–482.9
BF.90	**Net worth**	**CGRY**	–143.6	–110.2	–85.3	–104.3	–121.0	–159.7	–168.6	–171.5	–201.5

5.3.1 Local government
ESA95 sector S.1313

£ million

			1999	2000	2001	2002	2003	2004	2005	2006
I	**PRODUCTION ACCOUNT**									
	Resources									
P.1	Output									
P.11	Market output	**NMIX**	10 962	12 395	14 363	15 984	17 266	19 538	21 750	23 658
P.12	Output for own final use	**QYJW**	314	344	363	386	407	172	176	180
P.13	Other non-market output	**NMMT**	66 058	71 143	75 806	82 229	90 161	99 206	106 838	111 764
P.1	Total resources	**NMIZ**	77 334	83 882	90 532	98 599	107 834	118 916	128 764	135 602
	Uses									
P.2	Intermediate consumption	**NMJA**	30 823	34 177	37 573	41 938	47 235	53 316	57 672	61 423
B.1g	**Gross Value Added**	**NMJB**	**46 511**	**49 705**	**52 959**	**56 661**	**60 599**	**65 600**	**71 092**	**74 179**
Total	Total uses	**NMIZ**	77 334	83 882	90 532	98 599	107 834	118 916	128 764	135 602
B.1g	**Gross Value Added**	**NMJB**	**46 511**	**49 705**	**52 959**	**56 661**	**60 599**	**65 600**	**71 092**	**74 179**
-K.1	*less* Consumption of fixed capital	**-NSRO**	−3 866	−4 047	−4 313	−4 653	−4 905	−5 314	−5 819	−6 365
B.1n	Value added, net of fixed capital consumption	**NMJD**	42 645	45 658	48 646	52 008	55 694	60 286	65 273	67 814

5.3.2 Local government
ESA95 sector S.1313

£ million

			1999	2000	2001	2002	2003	2004	2005	2006
II	**DISTRIBUTION AND USE OF INCOME ACCOUNTS**									
II.1	**PRIMARY DISTRIBUTION OF INCOME ACCOUNT**									
II.1.1	**GENERATION OF INCOME ACCOUNT**									
	Resources									
B.1g	**Total resources (Gross Value Added)**	**NMJB**	**46 511**	**49 705**	**52 959**	**56 661**	**60 599**	**65 600**	**71 092**	**74 179**
	Uses									
D.1	Compensation of employees									
D.11	Wages and salaries	**NMJF**	34 844	37 434	39 891	42 707	45 961	49 907	54 334	56 435
D.12	Employers' social contributions	**NMJG**	7 801	8 224	8 755	9 301	9 733	10 379	10 939	11 379
D.1	Total	**NMJE**	42 645	45 658	48 646	52 008	55 694	60 286	65 273	67 814
D.2	Taxes on production and imports, paid									
D.29	Production taxes other than on products	**NMHY**	–	–	–	–	–	–	–	–
-D.3	*less* Subsidies, received									
-D.39	Production subsidies other than on products	**-NMJL**	–	–	–	–	–	–	–	–
B.2g	Operating surplus, gross	**NRLT**	3 866	4 047	4 313	4 653	4 905	5 314	5 819	6 365
B.1g	**Total uses (Gross Valued Added)**	**NMJB**	**46 511**	**49 705**	**52 959**	**56 661**	**60 599**	**65 600**	**71 092**	**74 179**
-K.1	After deduction of fixed capital consumption	**-NSRO**	−3 866	−4 047	−4 313	−4 653	−4 905	−5 314	−5 819	−6 365
B.2n	Operating surplus, net	**NMJM**	–	–	–	–	–	–	–	–

5.3.3 Local government
ESA95 sector S.1313

£ million

			1999	2000	2001	2002	2003	2004	2005	2006	2007
II.1.2	**ALLOCATION OF PRIMARY INCOME ACCOUNT**										
	Resources										
B.2g	Operating surplus, gross	**NRLT**	3 866	4 047	4 313	4 653	4 905	5 314	5 819	6 365	6 720
D.2	Taxes on production and imports, received										
D.29	Taxes on production other than on products	**NMYH**	142	149	157	173	188	163	182	202	225
-D.3	*less* Subsidies, paid										
-D.31	Subsidies on products	**−LIUA**	−649	−708	−857	−1 038	−1 281	−1 586	−1 691	−1 736	−1 768
-D.39	Other subsidies on production	**−LIUC**	−16	−21	−9	−17	−18	−239	−1 066	−1 661	−1 801
D.4	Property income										
D.41	Total interest	**NMKB**	893	1 038	877	818	800	1 099	1 107	1 245	1 640
D.42	Distributed income of corporations	**FDDA**	3 235	3 122	2 318	1 501	1 254	689	702	675	598
D.44	Property income attributed to insurance policy holders	**NMKK**	33	54	24	18	19	19	27	25	19
D.45	Rent										
	from sectors other than general government	**NMKM**	–	–	–	–	–	–	–	–	–
D.4	Total property income	**NMJZ**	4 161	4 214	3 219	2 337	2 073	1 807	1 836	1 945	2 257
Total	Total resources	**NMKN**	7 504	7 681	6 823	6 108	5 867	5 459	5 080	5 115	5 633
	Uses										
D.4	Property income										
D.41	Total interest	**NCBW**	4 355	4 203	4 250	3 981	4 492	3 761	3 469	3 654	3 726
D.4	Total property income	**NUHI**	4 355	4 203	4 250	3 981	4 492	3 761	3 469	3 654	3 726
B.5g	**Balance of primary incomes, gross**	**NRLU**	**3 149**	**3 478**	**2 573**	**2 127**	**1 375**	**1 698**	**1 611**	**1 461**	**1 907**
Total	Total uses	**NMKN**	7 504	7 681	6 823	6 108	5 867	5 459	5 080	5 115	5 633
-K.1	After deduction of fixed capital consumption	**−NSRO**	−3 866	−4 047	−4 313	−4 653	−4 905	−5 314	−5 819	−6 365	−6 973
B.5n	Balance of primary incomes, net	**NMKZ**	−717	−569	−1 740	−2 526	−3 530	−3 616	−4 208	−4 904	−5 066

5.3.4 Local government
ESA95 sector S.1313

£ million

			1999	2000	2001	2002	2003	2004	2005	2006	2007
II.2	**SECONDARY DISTRIBUTION OF INCOME ACCOUNT**										
	Resources										
B.5g	**Balance of primary incomes, gross**	NRLU	**3 149**	**3 478**	**2 573**	**2 127**	**1 375**	**1 698**	**1 611**	**1 461**	**1 907**
D.5	Current taxes on income, wealth etc.										
D.59	Current taxes other than on income	NMIS	12 766	13 918	15 148	16 531	18 482	20 010	21 113	22 219	23 306
D.61	Social contributions										
D.611	Actual social contributions										
D.6112	Employees' social contributions	NMWM	583	578	609	637	659	703	758	797	841
D.612	Imputed social contributions	GCMN	1 714	1 857	1 957	2 066	2 145	2 222	2 310	2 426	2 537
D.61	Total	NSMM	2 297	2 435	2 566	2 703	2 804	2 925	3 068	3 223	3 378
D.7	Other current transfers										
D.72	Non-life insurance claims	NMLR	436	393	265	320	276	338	328	366	277
D.73	Current transfers within general government	QYJR	64 446	66 187	72 522	77 592	85 224	94 720	101 369	110 407	113 046
D.74	Current Grants from Rest of the World	GNK8	–	–	–	–	–	69	58	80	46
D.7	Other current transfers	NMLO	64 882	66 580	72 787	77 912	85 500	95 127	101 755	110 853	113 369
Total	Total resources	NMLX	83 094	86 411	93 074	99 273	108 161	119 760	127 547	137 756	141 960
	Uses										
D.59	Other current taxes	EBFS	861	860	902	876	842	924	1 022	1 075	1 111
D.62	Social benefits other than social transfers in kind	NSMN	14 818	14 491	15 082	15 863	16 460	16 953	17 918	19 055	20 248
D.7	Other current transfers										
D.71	Net non-life insurance premiums	NMMI	436	393	265	320	276	338	328	366	277
D.73	Current transfers within general government	NMDK	–	–	–	–	–	–	–	–	–
D.75	Miscellaneous current transfers	EBFE	25	32	23	23	24	29	25	25	25
D.7	Other current transfers	NMMF	461	425	288	343	300	367	353	391	302
B.6g	**Gross Disposable Income**	NRLW	**66 954**	**70 635**	**76 802**	**82 191**	**90 559**	**101 516**	**108 254**	**117 235**	**120 299**
Total	Total uses	NMLX	83 094	86 411	93 074	99 273	108 161	119 760	127 547	137 756	141 960
-K.1	After deduction of fixed capital consumption	–NSRO	–3 866	–4 047	–4 313	–4 653	–4 905	–5 314	–5 819	–6 365	–6 973
B.6n	Disposable income, net	NMMQ	63 088	66 588	72 489	77 538	85 654	96 202	102 435	110 870	113 326

5.3.4S Local government
Social contributions and benefits

ESA95 sector S.1313

£ million

			1999	2000	2001	2002	2003	2004	2005	2006	2007
Part	**SECONDARY DISTRIBUTION OF INCOME** (further detail of certain items)										
	Resources										
D.61	Social contributions										
	Unfunded pension schemes[1]										
D.611	Actual social contributions										
D.61122	Employees' voluntary contributions	NMWM	583	578	609	637	659	703	758	797	841
D.612	Imputed social contributions										
D.612	Employers' contributions	GCMN	1 714	1 857	1 957	2 066	2 145	2 222	2 310	2 426	2 537
D.61	Total social contributions	NSMM	2 297	2 435	2 566	2 703	2 804	2 925	3 068	3 223	3 378
	Uses										
D.62	Social benefits										
D.623	Unfunded employee social benefits										
	Unfunded pensions paid[1]	NMWK	1 863	1 975	2 083	2 192	2 317	2 446	2 585	2 736	2 887
	Other unfunded employee benefits	EWRN	434	460	483	511	487	479	483	487	491
D.623	Total unfunded social benefits	GCMO	2 297	2 435	2 566	2 703	2 804	2 925	3 068	3 223	3 378
D.624	Social assistance benefits in cash										
	Student grants	GCSI	1 407	848	996	1 082	1 208	1 037	1 094	1 207	1 334
	Rent rebates	CTML	5 350	5 284	5 277	5 232	5 120	5 167	5 246	5 339	5 412
	Rent allowances	GCSR	5 752	5 921	6 241	6 846	7 328	7 824	8 510	9 286	10 124
	Total other transfers	ZXHZ	12	3	2	–	–	–	–	–	–
D.624	Total social assistance benefits in cash	ADAL	12 521	12 056	12 516	13 160	13 656	14 028	14 850	15 832	16 870
D.62	Total social benefits	NSMN	14 818	14 491	15 082	15 863	16 460	16 953	17 918	19 055	20 248

1 Mainly police and firefighters' schemes

5.3.5 Local government
ESA95 sector S.1313

£ million

			1999	2000	2001	2002	2003	2004	2005	2006	2007
II.3	**REDISTRIBUTION OF INCOME IN KIND ACCOUNT**										
	Resources										
B.6g	**Total resources (Gross Disposable Income)**	**NRLW**	66 954	70 635	76 802	82 191	90 559	101 516	108 254	117 235	120 299
	Uses										
D.63	Social transfers in kind										
D.631	Social benefits in kind										
D.632	Transfers of individual non-market goods and services	**NMMU**	42 833	46 255	50 247	55 408	60 739	65 367	70 649	74 583	78 197
B.7g	Adjusted disposable income, gross	**NSXL**	24 121	24 380	26 555	26 783	29 820	36 149	37 605	42 652	42 102
B.6g	**Total uses (Gross Disposable Income)**	**NRLW**	66 954	70 635	76 802	82 191	90 559	101 516	108 254	117 235	120 299

5.3.6 Local government
ESA95 sector S.1313

£ million

			1999	2000	2001	2002	2003	2004	2005	2006	2007
II.4	**USE OF INCOME ACCOUNT**										
II.4.1	**USE OF DISPOSABLE INCOME ACCOUNT**										
	Resources										
B.6g	**Total resources (Gross Disposable Income)**	**NRLW**	66 954	70 635	76 802	82 191	90 559	101 516	108 254	117 235	120 299
	Uses										
P.3	Final consumption expenditure										
P.31	Individual consumption expenditure	**NMMU**	42 833	46 255	50 247	55 408	60 739	65 367	70 649	74 583	78 197
P.32	Collective consumption expenditure	**NMMV**	23 225	24 888	25 559	26 821	29 422	33 839	36 189	37 181	38 157
P.3	Total	**NMMT**	66 058	71 143	75 806	82 229	90 161	99 206	106 838	111 764	116 354
B.8g	**Gross Saving**	**NRLX**	**896**	**−508**	**996**	**−38**	**398**	**2 310**	**1 416**	**5 471**	**3 945**
B.6g	**Total uses (Gross Disposable Income)**	**NRLW**	66 954	70 635	76 802	82 191	90 559	101 516	108 254	117 235	120 299
-K.1	After deduction of fixed capital consumption	**−NSRO**	−3 866	−4 047	−4 313	−4 653	−4 905	−5 314	−5 819	−6 365	−6 973
B.8n	Saving, net	**NMMX**	−2 970	−4 555	−3 317	−4 691	−4 507	−3 004	−4 403	−894	−3 028
II.4.2	**USE OF ADJUSTED DISPOSABLE INCOME ACCOUNT**										
	Resources										
B.7g	Total resources, adjusted disposable income, gross	**NSXL**	24 121	24 380	26 555	26 783	29 820	36 149	37 605	42 652	42 102
	Uses										
P.4	Actual final consumption										
P.42	Actual collective consumption	**NMMV**	23 225	24 888	25 559	26 821	29 422	33 839	36 189	37 181	38 157
B.8g	**Gross Saving**	**NRLX**	**896**	**−508**	**996**	**−38**	**398**	**2 310**	**1 416**	**5 471**	**3 945**
Total	Total uses	**NSXL**	24 121	24 380	26 555	26 783	29 820	36 149	37 605	42 652	42 102

5.3.7 Local government
ESA95 sector S.1313

£ million

			1999	2000	2001	2002	2003	2004	2005	2006	2007
III	**ACCUMULATION ACCOUNTS**										
III.1	**CAPITAL ACCOUNT**										
III.1.1	**CHANGE IN NET WORTH DUE TO SAVINGS AND CAPITAL TRANSFERS**										
	Changes in liabilities and net worth										
B.8g	**Gross Saving**	NRLX	**896**	**−508**	**996**	**−38**	**398**	**2 310**	**1 416**	**5 471**	**3 945**
D.9	Capital transfers receivable										
D.92	Investment grants	NMNE	3 298	4 105	4 652	6 328	7 360	6 804	7 582	8 515	9 878
D.99	Other capital transfers	NMNH	205	411	416	735	4 770	2 282	1 978	1 074	1 708
D.9	Total capital transfers receivable	NMMY	3 503	4 516	5 068	7 063	12 130	9 086	9 560	9 589	11 586
-D.9	*less* Capital transfers payable										
-D.92	Investment grants	−NMNR	−1 156	−1 000	−917	−839	−1 165	−1 127	−1 563	−1 635	−1 839
-D.99	Other capital transfers	−NMNU	–	–	–	−5	−5	−1 247	−1 325	−885	−998
-D.9	Total capital transfers payable	−NMNL	−1 156	−1 000	−917	−844	−1 170	−2 374	−2 888	−2 520	−2 837
B.10.1g	Total change in liabilities and net worth	NRMJ	3 243	3 008	5 147	6 181	11 358	9 022	8 088	12 540	12 694
	Changes in assets										
B.10.1g	Changes in net worth due to gross saving and capital transfers	NRMJ	3 243	3 008	5 147	6 181	11 358	9 022	8 088	12 540	12 694
-K.1	After deduction of fixed capital consumption	−NSRO	−3 866	−4 047	−4 313	−4 653	−4 905	−5 314	−5 819	−6 365	−6 973
B.10.1n	Changes in net worth due to net saving and capital transfers	NMNX	−623	−1 039	834	1 528	6 453	3 708	2 269	6 175	5 721
III.1.2	**ACQUISITION OF NON-FINANCIAL ASSETS ACCOUNT**										
	Changes in liabilities and net worth										
B.10.1n	Changes in net worth due to saving and capital transfers	NMNX	−623	−1 039	834	1 528	6 453	3 708	2 269	6 175	5 721
K.1	Consumption of fixed capital	NSRO	3 866	4 047	4 313	4 653	4 905	5 314	5 819	6 365	6 973
B.10.1g	Total changes in liabilities and net worth	NRMJ	3 243	3 008	5 147	6 181	11 358	9 022	8 088	12 540	12 694
	Changes in assets										
P.5	Gross capital formation										
P.51	Gross fixed capital formation	NMOA	6 243	6 552	7 569	7 946	14 137	14 891	13 516	13 807	14 382
P.52	Changes in inventories	NMOB	–	–	–	–	–	–	–	–	–
P.5	Total	NMNZ	6 243	6 552	7 569	7 946	14 137	14 891	13 516	13 807	14 382
K.2	Acquisitions less disposals of non-produced non-financial assets	NMOD	−715	−589	−719	−760	−800	−857	−902	−947	−928
B.9g	**Net lending(+) / net borrowing(-)**	NMOE	**−2 285**	**−2 955**	**−1 703**	**−1 005**	**−1 979**	**−5 012**	**−4 526**	**−320**	**−760**
Total	Total change in assets	NRMJ	3 243	3 008	5 147	6 181	11 358	9 022	8 088	12 540	12 694

5.3.8 Local government
ESA95 sector S.1313 Unconsolidated

£ million

			1999	2000	2001	2002	2003	2004	2005	2006	2007
III.2	**FINANCIAL ACCOUNT**										
F.A	Net acquisition of financial assets										
F.2	Currency and deposits										
F.22	Transferable deposits										
F.2211	Sterling deposits with UK banks	NBYS	−728	207	256	894	234	2 770	275	3 774	1 693
F.2212	Foreign currency deposits with UK banks	NBYT	−25	14	−7	−1	−9	1	28	−20	2
F.2213	Sterling deposits with building societies	NBYU	679	384	439	437	1 088	1 114	−225	1 631	2 644
F.29	Other deposits	NBYW	–	90	−59	268	135	−67	−75	−208	581
F.2	Total currency and deposits	NBYO	−74	695	629	1 598	1 448	3 818	3	5 177	4 920
F.3	Securities other than shares										
F.331	Short term: money market instruments										
F.3311	Issued by UK central government	NBYZ	204	−218	119	−141	−38	−59	14	−18	−51
F.3315	Issued by UK monetary financial institutions	NBZE	565	415	−20	487	24	−232	−159	−967	−953
F.3316	Issued by other UK residents	NBZJ	−34	59	41	11	−38	10	197	725	670
F.332	Medium (1 to 5 year) and long term (over 5 year) bonds										
F.3321	Issued by UK central government	NBZM	−17	−195	191	−264	−101	−98	7	75	−126
F.3326	Issued by other UK residents	E55E	–	–	–	–	–	–	215	–	–
F.3	Total securities other than shares	NBYX	718	61	331	93	−153	−379	274	−185	−460
F.4	Loans										
F.42	Long term loans										
F.422	Loans secured on dwellings	NCAK	107	12	97	206	186	−26	252	340	423
F.424	Other long-term loans by UK residents	NCAP	17	−31	−76	−83	−18	−38	212	−22	−299
F.4	Total loans	NBZZ	124	−19	21	123	168	−64	464	318	124
F.5	Shares and other equity										
F.51	Shares and other equity, excluding mutual funds' shares										
F.514	Quoted UK shares	NCAW	−304	157	−54	−218	45	−117	−157	160	−168
F.515	Unquoted UK shares	NCAX	–	–	−293	–	–	–	–	–	−128
F.516	Other UK equity	HN68	−2 023	−2 295	−2 405	−2 860	−5 479	−3 686	−2 601	−2 187	−2 095
F.517	UK shares and bonds issued by other UK residents	NSPE	–	–	–	–	–	–	–	–	–
F.5	Total shares and other equity	NCAR	−2 327	−2 138	−2 752	−3 078	−5 434	−3 803	−2 758	−2 027	−2 391
F.6	Insurance technical reserves										
F.62	Prepayments of insurance premiums and reserves for outstanding claims	NCBK	−30	24	−26	27	8	42	44	61	–
F.7	Other accounts receivable	NCBL	−194	−55	−424	−1 123	281	−34	178	−1	−57
F.A	**Total net acquisition of financial assets**	NBYK	−1 783	−1 432	−2 221	−2 360	−3 682	−420	−1 795	3 343	2 136

5.3.8 Local government
ESA95 sector S.1313 Unconsolidated

			1999	2000	2001	2002	2003	2004	2005	2006	2007
III.2	**FINANCIAL ACCOUNT** continued										
F.L	**Net acquisition of financial liabilities**										
F.3	Securities other than shares										
F.331	Short term: money market instruments										
F.3312	Issued by UK local government	**NCCH**	–	–	–	–	–	–	–	–	–
F.332	Medium (1 to 5 year) and long term (over 5 year) bonds										
F.3322	Issued by UK local authorities	**NCCT**	−2	−12	–	47	18	−226	213	360	−9
F.3	Total securities other than shares	**NCCB**	−2	−12	–	47	18	−226	213	360	−9
F.4	Loans										
F.41	Short term loans										
F.411	Loans by UK monetary financial institutions, excluding loans secured on dwellings & financial leasing	**NCDF**	−817	−282	–	816	1 162	1 528	734	1 171	1 454
F.419	Loans by rest of the world monetary financial institutions	**NCDJ**	−44	−39	−34	−13	−7	−6	−3	−1	–
F.42	Long term loans										
F.423	Finance leasing	**NCDS**	–	–	–	18	15	24	5	3	–
F.424	Other long-term loans by UK residents	**NCDT**	1 908	1 444	−189	−1 709	−3 893	521	2 620	2 645	1 272
F.429	Other long-term loans by the rest of the world	**NCDU**	−61	−149	56	39	211	657	137	233	−29
F.4	Total loans	**NCDD**	986	974	−167	−849	−2 512	2 724	3 493	4 051	2 697
F.7	Other accounts payable	**NCEP**	190	−271	360	−492	142	1 138	−362	−727	216
F.L	**Total net acquisition of financial liabilities**	**NCBO**	1 174	691	193	−1 294	−2 352	3 636	3 344	3 684	2 904
B.9	**Net lending / borrowing**										
F.A	Total net acquisition of financial assets	**NBYK**	−1 783	−1 432	−2 221	−2 360	−3 682	−420	−1 795	3 343	2 136
-F.L	*less* Total net acquisition of financial liabilities	**−NCBO**	−1 174	−691	−193	1 294	2 352	−3 636	−3 344	−3 684	−2 904
B.9f	Net lending (+) / net borrowing (-), from financial account	**NYNQ**	−2 957	−2 123	−2 414	−1 066	−1 330	−4 056	−5 139	−341	−768
dB.9f	Statistical discrepancy	**NYPC**	672	−832	711	61	−649	−956	613	21	8
B.9g	**Net lending (+) / net borrowing (-), from capital account**	**NMOE**	**−2 285**	**−2 955**	**−1 703**	**−1 005**	**−1 979**	**−5 012**	**−4 526**	**−320**	**−760**

5.3.9 Local government
ESA95 sector S.1313 Unconsolidated

£ billion

			1999	2000	2001	2002	2003	2004	2005	2006	2007
IV.3	**FINANCIAL BALANCE SHEET** at end of period										
AN	**Non-financial assets**	CGIZ	228.0	258.1	301.3	307.5	334.1	379.6	406.4	437.0	475.6
AF.A	**Financial assets**										
AF.2	Currency and deposits										
AF.22	Transferable deposits										
AF.2211	Sterling deposits with UK banks	NJEP	8.3	8.7	8.9	10.2	10.6	13.6	13.9	17.6	19.2
AF.2212	Foreign currency deposits with UK banks	NJEQ	–	–	–	–	–	–	–	–	–
AF.2213	Sterling deposits with UK building societies	NJER	4.4	4.6	5.0	5.4	6.5	7.8	7.6	9.2	11.9
AF.29	Other deposits	NJET	–	0.1	–	0.3	0.4	0.4	0.4	0.2	0.8
AF.2	Total currency and deposits	NJEL	12.7	13.4	14.0	15.9	17.6	21.8	21.9	27.0	32.0
AF.3	Securities other than shares										
AF.331	Short term: money market instruments										
AF.3311	Issued by UK central government	NJEW	0.5	0.2	0.4	0.2	0.2	0.1	0.1	0.1	0.1
AF.3315	Issued by UK monetary financial institutions	NJFB	3.0	3.4	3.3	3.8	3.9	3.6	3.5	2.5	1.6
AF.3316	Issued by other UK residents	NJFG	0.1	0.2	0.2	0.2	0.2	0.1	0.3	0.8	1.3
AF.332	Medium (1 to 5 year) and long term (over 5 year) bonds										
AF.3321	Issued by UK central government	NJFJ	0.7	0.5	0.7	0.4	0.3	0.2	0.2	0.2	0.1
AF.3326	Issued by other UK residents	E55D	–	–	–	–	–	–	0.2	0.2	0.2
AF.3	Total securities other than shares	NJEU	4.2	4.3	4.5	4.7	4.5	4.1	4.3	3.9	3.2
AF.4	Loans										
AF.42	Long term loans										
AF.422	Loans secured on dwellings	NJGH	0.5	0.5	0.6	0.8	1.0	1.0	1.3	1.6	2.0
AF.424	Other long-term loans by UK residents	NJGM	0.3	0.3	0.3	0.3	0.3	0.3	0.3	0.2	0.3
AF.4	Total loans	NJFW	0.8	0.8	0.9	1.1	1.3	1.3	1.5	1.8	2.3
AF.5	Shares and other equity										
AF.51	Shares and other equity, excluding mutual funds' shares										
AF.514	Quoted UK shares	NJGT	2.1	1.4	1.2	1.0	1.2	1.2	1.2	1.4	1.2
AF.515	Unquoted UK shares	NJGU	0.4	0.4	0.4	0.4	0.4	0.4	0.4	0.4	0.4
AF.516	Other UK equity	HN69	72.4	71.7	78.4	86.0	95.1	106.2	116.7	110.9	111.4
AF.517	UK shares and bonds issued by other UK residents	NSOE	–	–	–	–	–	–	–	–	–
AF.5	Total shares and other equity	NJGO	74.9	73.5	79.9	87.4	96.7	107.7	118.3	112.7	113.0
AF.6	Insurance technical reserves										
AF.62	Prepayments of insurance premiums and reserves for outstanding claims	NJHH	1.1	1.0	0.9	0.9	0.8	0.7	0.8	0.8	0.8
AF.7	Other accounts receivable	NJHI	1.8	1.6	1.3	0.3	0.8	1.1	1.3	1.3	1.3
AF.A	**Total financial assets**	NJFV	95.5	94.5	101.5	110.4	121.7	136.8	148.1	147.5	152.5

5.3.9 Local government
ESA95 sector S.1313 Unconsolidated

continued

£ billion

			1999	2000	2001	2002	2003	2004	2005	2006	2007
IV.3	**FINANCIAL BALANCE SHEET** continued										
	at end of period										
AF.L	**Financial liabilities**										
AF.3	Securities other than shares										
AF.331	Short term: money market instruments										
AF.3312	Issued by UK local government	NJIE	–	–	–	–	–	–	–	–	–
AF.332	Medium (1 to 5 year) and long term (over 5 year) bonds										
AF.3322	Issued by UK local government	NJIQ	0.8	0.8	0.8	0.8	0.8	0.6	0.8	1.2	1.2
AF.3326	Issued by UK residents	IH3I	–	–	–	–	–	–	–	–	–
AF.3	Total securities other than shares	NJHY	0.8	0.8	0.8	0.8	0.8	0.6	0.8	1.2	1.2
AF.4	Loans										
AF.41	Short term loans										
AF.411	Loans by UK monetary financial institutions, excluding										
	loans secured on dwellings & financial leasing	NJJC	2.4	1.7	1.9	2.9	4.3	6.3	7.6	9.1	10.3
AF.419	Loans by rest of the world monetary financial institutions	ZMFC	0.2	0.1	–	–	–	–	–	–	–
AF.42	Long term loans										
AF.423	Finance leasing	NJJP	–	–	–	–	–	0.1	0.1	0.1	0.1
AF.424	Other long-term loans by UK residents	NJJQ	48.9	50.1	50.1	48.4	44.5	45.5	48.0	50.5	51.1
AF.429	Other long-term loans by the rest of the world	NJJR	0.9	0.7	0.8	0.8	1.1	1.7	1.9	2.1	2.1
AF.4	Total loans	NJJA	52.4	52.6	52.9	52.1	49.9	53.6	57.5	61.8	63.5
AF.7	Other accounts payable	NJKM	9.7	9.2	9.9	9.3	9.7	10.8	10.9	11.3	10.8
AF.L	**Total financial liabilities**	NJIZ	62.9	62.6	63.6	62.2	60.4	64.9	69.2	74.2	75.5
BF.90	**Net financial assets / liabilities**										
AF.A	Total financial assets	NJFV	95.5	94.5	101.5	110.4	121.7	136.8	148.1	147.5	152.5
-AF.L	*less* Total financial liabilities	-NJIZ	−62.9	−62.6	−63.6	−62.2	−60.4	−64.9	−69.2	−74.2	−75.5
BF.90	**Net financial assets (+) / liabilities (-)**	NYOJ	32.7	31.9	37.9	48.2	61.3	71.8	78.8	73.3	77.0
	Net worth										
AN	Non-financial assets	CGIZ	228.0	258.1	301.3	307.5	334.1	379.6	406.4	437.0	475.6
BF.90	Net financial assets (+) / liabilities (-)	NYOJ	32.7	31.9	37.9	48.2	61.3	71.8	78.8	73.3	77.0
BF.90	**Net worth**	CGRZ	260.6	290.0	339.3	355.7	395.3	451.4	485.2	510.3	552.6

Chapter 6

Households and non-profit institutions serving households (NPISH)

6.1.1 Households and non-profit institutions serving households
ESA95 sectors S.14 and S.15

£ million

			1999	2000	2001	2002	2003	2004	2005	2006
I	**PRODUCTION ACCOUNT**									
	Resources									
P.1	Output									
P.11	Market output	QWLF	185 862	195 741	209 723	220 913	232 646	234 957	247 520	261 088
P.12	Output for own final use	QWLG	54 649	57 758	63 215	66 856	72 869	75 068	80 208	85 571
P.13	Other non-market output	QWLH	22 185	23 531	25 111	26 422	27 668	28 748	30 402	32 209
P.1	Total resources	QWLI	262 696	277 030	298 049	314 191	333 183	338 773	358 130	378 868
	Uses									
P.2	Intermediate consumption	QWLJ	117 521	122 385	132 144	139 280	146 526	141 708	155 235	166 044
B.1g	**Gross Value Added**	QWLK	**145 175**	**154 645**	**165 905**	**174 911**	**186 657**	**197 065**	**202 895**	**212 824**
Total	Total uses	QWLI	262 696	277 030	298 049	314 191	333 183	338 773	358 130	378 868
B.1g	**Gross Value Added**	QWLK	**145 175**	**154 645**	**165 905**	**174 911**	**186 657**	**197 065**	**202 895**	**212 824**
-K.1	*less* Consumption of fixed capital	-QWLL	-27 976	-30 518	-32 908	-36 043	-36 903	-42 509	-43 257	-48 623
B.1n	Value added, net	QWLM	117 199	124 127	132 997	138 868	149 754	154 556	159 638	164 201

6.1.2 Households and non-profit institutions serving households
ESA95 sectors S.14 and S.15

£ million

			1999	2000	2001	2002	2003	2004	2005	2006
II	**DISTRIBUTION AND USE OF INCOME ACCOUNTS**									
II.1	**PRIMARY DISTRIBUTION OF INCOME ACCOUNT**									
II.1.1	**GENERATION OF INCOME ACCOUNT**									
	before deduction of fixed capital consumption									
	Resources									
B.1g	**Total resources (Gross Value Added)**	QWLK	145 175	154 645	165 905	174 911	186 657	197 065	202 895	212 824
	Uses									
D.1	Compensation of employees									
D.11	Wages and salaries	QWLN	40 080	43 029	45 975	48 035	49 939	48 998	51 110	52 335
D.12	Employers' social contributions	QWLO	5 285	5 792	6 183	6 723	7 941	10 597	11 635	12 787
D.1	Total	QWLP	45 365	48 821	52 158	54 758	57 880	59 595	62 745	65 122
D.2	Taxes on production and imports, paid									
D.29	Production taxes other than on products	QWLQ	72	56	47	58	61	64	68	51
-D.3	*less* Subsidies received									
-D.39	Production subsidies other than on products	-QWLR	-338	-335	-582	-519	-592	-592	-3 408	-3 220
B.2g	Operating surplus, gross	QWLS	45 134	49 172	53 000	55 647	60 984	65 182	68 632	71 963
B.3g	Mixed income, gross	QWLT	54 942	56 931	61 282	64 967	68 324	72 816	74 858	78 908
B.1g	**Total uses (Gross Value Added)**	QWLK	**145 175**	**154 645**	**165 905**	**174 911**	**186 657**	**197 065**	**202 895**	**212 824**
-K.1	After deduction of fixed capital consumption	-QWLL	-27 976	-30 518	-32 908	-36 043	-36 903	-42 509	-43 257	-48 623
B.2n	Operating surplus, net	QWLU	28 390	30 890	33 438	34 994	39 443	42 589	44 881	46 959
B.3n	Mixed income, net	QWLV	43 710	44 695	47 936	49 577	52 962	52 900	55 352	55 289

6.1.3 Households and non-profit institutions serving households
ESA95 sectors S.14 and S.15

£ million

			1999	2000	2001	2002	2003	2004	2005	2006	2007
II.1.2	**ALLOCATION OF PRIMARY INCOME ACCOUNT** before deduction of fixed capital consumption										
	Resources										
B.2g	Operating surplus, gross	QWLS	45 134	49 172	53 000	55 647	60 984	65 182	68 632	71 963	79 858
B.3g	Mixed income, gross	QWLT	54 942	56 931	61 282	64 967	68 324	72 816	74 858	78 908	83 628
D.1	Compensation of employees										
D.11	Wages and salaries	QWLW	431 795	462 505	491 044	508 681	527 689	548 899	573 932	599 461	626 566
D.12	Employers' social contributions	QWLX	64 199	69 824	73 216	78 782	89 263	98 706	107 663	115 290	117 626
D.1	Total	QWLY	495 994	532 329	564 260	587 463	616 952	647 605	681 595	714 751	744 192
D.4	Property income, received										
D.41	Interest	QWLZ	30 188	35 488	31 957	26 658	27 251	34 550	40 007	42 706	53 507
D.42	Distributed income of corporations	QWMA	41 035	43 755	49 894	43 787	45 248	45 862	50 704	47 957	44 864
D.44	Attributed property income of insurance policy holders	QWMC	53 346	53 081	53 277	52 104	55 008	54 623	64 028	66 640	72 750
D.45	Rent	QWMD	105	105	105	106	108	110	110	112	112
D.4	Total	QWME	124 674	132 429	135 233	122 655	127 615	135 145	154 849	157 415	171 233
Total	Total resources	QWMF	720 744	770 861	813 775	830 732	873 875	920 748	979 934	1 023 037	1 078 911
	Uses										
D.4	Property income, paid										
D.41	Interest	QWMG	29 540	36 968	33 752	30 512	32 001	43 207	46 739	49 046	66 225
D.45	Rent	QWMH	215	215	215	216	220	224	224	228	228
D.4	Total	QWMI	29 755	37 183	33 967	30 728	32 221	43 431	46 963	49 274	66 453
B.5g	**Balance of primary incomes, gross**	QWMJ	**690 989**	**733 678**	**779 808**	**800 004**	**841 654**	**877 317**	**932 971**	**973 763**	**1 012 458**
Total	Total uses	QWMF	720 744	770 861	813 775	830 732	873 875	920 748	979 934	1 023 037	1 078 911
-K.1	After deduction of fixed capital consumption	-QWLL	−27 976	−30 518	−32 908	−36 043	−36 903	−42 509	−43 257	−48 623	−54 663
B.5n	Balance of primary incomes, net	QWMK	663 013	703 160	746 900	763 961	804 751	834 808	889 714	925 140	957 795

6.1.4 Households and non-profit institutions serving households
ESA95 sectors S.14 and S.15

£ million

			1999	2000	2001	2002	2003	2004	2005	2006	2007
II.2	**SECONDARY DISTRIBUTION OF INCOME ACCOUNT**										
	Resources										
B.5g	**Balance of primary incomes, gross**	QWMJ	**690 989**	**733 678**	**779 808**	**800 004**	**841 654**	**877 317**	**932 971**	**973 763**	**1 012 458**
D.612	Imputed social contributions	RVFH	450	476	502	530	505	499	506	514	518
D.62	Social benefits other than social transfers in kind	QWML	157 647	162 833	171 814	182 673	193 596	198 680	211 686	225 891	226 334
D.7	Other current transfers										
D.72	Non-life insurance claims	QWMM	15 775	15 713	11 723	17 327	13 890	17 479	17 199	20 346	15 455
D.75	Miscellaneous current transfers	QWMN	24 392	27 520	29 080	33 041	34 687	34 845	37 840	38 708	39 850
D.7	Total	QWMO	40 167	43 233	40 803	50 368	48 577	52 324	55 039	59 054	55 305
	Total resources	QWMP	889 253	940 220	992 927	1 033 575	1 084 332	1 128 820	1 200 202	1 259 222	1 294 615
	Uses										
D.5	Current taxes on income, wealth, etc										
D.51	Taxes on income	QWMQ	96 528	105 299	111 888	112 171	113 087	119 591	130 200	139 969	150 989
D.59	Other current taxes	NVCO	18 658	19 427	21 166	22 788	25 174	27 077	28 422	29 831	31 516
D.5	Total	QWMS	115 186	124 726	133 054	134 959	138 261	146 668	158 622	169 800	182 505
D.61	Social contributions										
D.611	Actual social contributions										
D.6111	Employers' actual social contributions	QWMT	52 529	57 288	60 296	64 805	77 571	87 675	95 732	103 551	105 298
D.6112	Employees' social contributions	QWMU	57 434	58 807	60 599	62 458	66 490	70 451	78 540	84 129	87 487
D.6113	Social contributions by self- and non-employed	QWMV	1 883	2 049	2 183	2 318	2 595	2 727	2 825	2 930	3 013
D.611	Total	QWMW	111 846	118 144	123 078	129 581	146 656	160 853	177 097	190 610	195 798
D.612	Imputed social contributions	QWMX	11 670	12 536	12 920	13 977	11 692	11 031	11 931	11 739	12 328
D.61	Total	QWMY	123 516	130 680	135 998	143 558	158 348	171 884	189 028	202 349	208 126
D.62	Social benefits other than social transfers in kind	QWMZ	922	948	977	1 006	987	988	1 000	1 010	1 014
D.7	Other current transfers										
D.71	Net non-life insurance premiums	QWNA	15 775	15 713	11 723	17 327	13 890	17 479	17 199	20 346	15 455
D.75	Miscellaneous current transfers	QWNB	10 117	10 865	11 081	11 458	11 930	12 462	13 442	13 274	13 484
D.7	Total	QWNC	25 892	26 578	22 804	28 785	25 820	29 941	30 641	33 620	28 939
B.6g	**Gross Disposable Income**[1]	QWND	**623 737**	**657 288**	**700 094**	**725 267**	**760 916**	**779 339**	**820 911**	**852 443**	**874 031**
	Total uses	QWMP	889 253	940 220	992 927	1 033 575	1 084 332	1 128 820	1 200 202	1 259 222	1 294 615
-K.1	After deduction of fixed capital consumption	-QWLL	-27 976	-30 518	-32 908	-36 043	-36 903	-42 509	-43 257	-48 623	-54 663
B.6n	Disposable income, net	QWNE	595 761	626 770	667 186	689 224	724 013	736 830	777 654	803 820	819 368

1 Gross household disposable income revalued by the implied households and NPISH's final consumption expenditure deflator is as follows:

		1999	2000	2001	2002	2003	2004	2005	2006	2007
Real household disposable income: (Chained volume measures)										
£ million (Reference year 2003)	RVGK	665 374	693 322	724 114	738 900	760 916	767 096	788 338	799 898	800 676
Index (2003 = 100)	OSXR	87.4	91.1	95.2	97.1	100.0	100.8	103.6	105.1	105.2

6.1.4S   Households and non-profit institutions serving households
Social benefits and contributions

ESA95 sectors S.14 and S.15   £ million

Part			1999	2000	2001	2002	2003	2004	2005	2006	2007
	SECONDARY DISTRIBUTION OF INCOME (further detail of certain items)										
	Benefits										
	Resources										
D.62	Social benefits										
D.621	Social security benefits in cash										
	National insurance fund benefits[1]	ACHH	46 335	47 490	50 336	53 123	55 731	58 118	60 400	62 628	66 293
	Redundancy fund benefit	GTKN	137	167	198	278	245	169	274	200	178
	Social fund benefit	GTLQ	1 087	1 753	1 885	1 910	2 135	2 240	2 232	2 253	2 348
	Maternity fund benefits	GTKO	–	–	–	–	–	–	–	–	–
D.621	Total social security benefits in cash	HAYQ	47 559	49 410	52 419	55 311	58 111	60 527	62 906	65 081	68 819
D.622	Private funded social benefits										
	Funded social benefits	D3N3	35 428	37 817	37 107	40 224	42 120	39 374	45 469	54 134	43 980
	Employee benefits from employers' liability insurance	NRXD	502	458	591	930	1 143	1 269	1 400	1 458	1 502
D.622	Total private funded social benefits	HAYR	35 930	38 275	37 697	41 155	43 264	40 643	46 869	55 592	45 482
D.623	Unfunded employee social benefits										
	Unfunded central government pensions paid[2]	E8AF	11 295	12 076	12 645	14 345	15 221	16 240	17 238	18 361	20 791
	Unfunded local government pensions paid[3]	NMWK	1 863	1 975	2 083	2 192	2 317	2 446	2 585	2 736	2 887
	Other unfunded employee benefits[4]	EWRM	5 529	5 964	6 208	6 539	6 104	5 666	5 410	5 320	5 416
D.623	Total unfunded social benefits	RVFF	18 687	20 015	20 936	23 076	23 642	24 352	25 233	26 417	29 094
D.624	Social assistance benefits in cash										
	Received from central government	LNJT	42 478	42 605	47 771	49 495	54 441	58 641	61 334	62 473	65 573
	Received from local government	ADAL	12 521	12 056	12 516	13 160	13 656	14 028	14 850	15 832	16 870
	Received from NPISHs	HABJ	472	472	475	476	482	489	494	496	496
D.624	Total social assistance benefits in cash	HAYU	55 471	55 133	60 762	63 131	68 579	73 158	76 678	78 801	82 939
D.62	Total social benefits	QWML	157 647	162 833	171 814	182 673	193 596	198 680	211 686	225 891	226 334
	Uses										
D.62	Social benefits	QWMZ	922	948	977	1 006	987	988	1 000	1 010	1 014
	Contributions										
	Resources										
D.612	Imputed social contributions	RVFH	450	476	502	530	505	499	506	514	518
	Uses										
D.61	Social Contributions										
D.611	Actual social contributions										
D.6111	Employers' actual social contributions										
	National Insurance contributions	CEAN	31 286	34 028	35 706	35 735	39 890	43 586	46 741	49 552	52 300
	Notionally funded pension schemes	GCMP	2 115	2 369	2 754	3 045	5 177	5 616	6 028	6 472	7 003
	Funded pension schemes	RIUO	19 128	20 891	21 836	26 025	32 504	38 473	42 963	47 527	45 995
D.6111	Total employers' actual social contributions	QWMT	52 529	57 288	60 296	64 805	77 571	87 675	95 732	103 551	105 298
D.6112	Employees' actual social contributions										
	National Insurance contributions	GCSE	23 573	24 175	25 236	25 357	29 055	32 396	34 742	37 039	38 474
	Unfunded central government pension schemes	E8AA	2 460	2 516	2 855	3 550	4 639	5 714	6 246	6 514	6 742
	Unfunded local government pension schemes	NMWM	583	578	609	637	659	703	758	797	841
	Funded pension schemes	GCRR	30 818	31 538	31 899	32 914	32 137	31 638	36 794	39 779	41 430
D.6112	Total employees' actual social contributions	QWMU	57 434	58 807	60 599	62 458	66 490	70 451	78 540	84 129	87 487
D.6113	Social contributions by self and non-employed	QWMV	1 883	2 049	2 183	2 318	2 595	2 727	2 825	2 930	3 013
D.611	Total actual social contributions	QWMW	111 846	118 144	123 078	129 581	146 656	160 853	177 097	190 610	195 798
D.612	Imputed social contributions										
	Employers imputed contributions to unfunded central government pension schemes	E8AC	4 861	5 175	5 238	5 883	3 930	3 622	4 694	4 480	4 866
	Employers imputed contributions to unfunded local government pension schemes	NMWL	1 280	1 397	1 474	1 555	1 658	1 743	1 827	1 939	2 046
	Other imputed unfunded employers' contributions	EWRM	5 529	5 964	6 208	6 539	6 104	5 666	5 410	5 320	5 416
D.612	Total imputed social contributions	QWMX	11 670	12 536	12 920	13 977	11 692	11 031	11 931	11 739	12 328
D.61	Total social contributions	QWMY	123 516	130 680	135 998	143 558	158 348	171 884	189 028	202 349	208 126

1 For a more detailed analysis see table 5.2.4S
2 Mainly civil service, armed forces', teachers' and NHS staff
3 Mainly police and fire fighters
4 Such as payments whilst absent from work due to illness

6.1.5 Households and non-profit institutions serving households
ESA95 sectors S.14 and S.15

£ million

			1999	2000	2001	2002	2003	2004	2005	2006	2007
II.3	**REDISTRIBUTION OF INCOME IN KIND ACCOUNT**										
	Resources										
B.6g	**Gross Disposable Income**	QWND	623 737	657 288	700 094	725 267	760 916	779 339	820 911	852 443	874 031
D.63	Social transfers in kind										
D.631	Social benefits in kind										
D.6313	Social assistance benefits in kind	QWNH	–	–	–	–	–	–	–	–	–
D.632	Transfers of individual non-market goods and services	NSSA	124 927	132 828	143 569	157 238	171 622	177 692	190 858	205 324	217 618
D.63	Total social transfers in kind	NSSB	124 927	132 828	143 569	157 238	171 622	177 692	190 858	205 324	217 618
Total	Total resources	NSSC	748 664	790 116	843 663	882 505	932 538	957 031	1 011 769	1 057 767	1 091 649
	Uses										
D.63	Social transfers in kind										
D.631	Social benefits in kind										
D.6313	Social assistance benefits in kind	HAEJ	–	–	–	–	–	–	–	–	–
D.632	Transfers of individual non-market goods and services	HABK	22 185	23 531	25 111	26 422	27 668	28 748	30 402	32 209	34 587
D.63	Total social transfers in kind	HAEK	22 185	23 531	25 111	26 422	27 668	28 748	30 402	32 209	34 587
B.7g	Adjusted disposable income, gross	NSSD	726 479	766 585	818 552	856 083	904 870	928 283	981 367	1 025 558	1 057 062
Total	Total uses	NSSC	748 664	790 116	843 663	882 505	932 538	957 031	1 011 769	1 057 767	1 091 649

6.1.6 Households and non-profit institutions serving households
ESA95 sectors S.14 and S.15

£ million

			1999	2000	2001	2002	2003	2004	2005	2006	2007
II.4	**USE OF INCOME ACCOUNT**										
II.4.1	**USE OF DISPOSABLE INCOME ACCOUNT**										
	Resources										
B.6g	**Gross Disposable Income**	QWND	623 737	657 288	700 094	725 267	760 916	779 339	820 911	852 443	874 031
D.8	Adjustment for the change in net equity of households in pension funds	NSSE	14 016	14 154	16 038	17 784	21 377	29 468	32 888	31 714	41 943
Total	Total resources	NSSF	637 753	671 442	716 132	743 051	782 293	808 807	853 799	884 157	915 974
	Uses										
P.3	Final consumption expenditure										
P.31	Individual consumption expenditure	NSSG	604 556	640 089	672 889	707 386	742 276	776 250	810 667	846 868	893 414
B.8g	**Gross Saving**	NSSH	**33 197**	**31 353**	**43 243**	**35 665**	**40 017**	**32 557**	**43 132**	**37 289**	**22 560**
Total	Total uses	NSSF	637 753	671 442	716 132	743 051	782 293	808 807	853 799	884 157	915 974
-K.1	After deduction of fixed capital consumption	-QWLL	-27 976	-30 518	-32 908	-36 043	-36 903	-42 509	-43 257	-48 623	-54 663
B.8n	Saving, net	NSSI	5 221	836	10 334	-378	3 114	-9 952	-125	-11 334	-32 103
II.4.2	**USE OF ADJUSTED DISPOSABLE INCOME ACCOUNT**										
	Resources										
B.7g	Adjusted disposable income, gross	NSSD	726 479	766 585	818 552	856 083	904 870	928 283	981 367	1 025 558	1 057 062
D.8	Adjustment for the change in net equity of households in pension funds	NSSE	14 016	14 154	16 038	17 784	21 377	29 468	32 888	31 714	41 943
Total	Total resources	NSSJ	740 495	780 739	834 590	873 867	926 247	957 751	1 014 255	1 057 272	1 099 005
	Uses										
P.4	Actual final consumption										
P.41	Actual individual consumption	NQEO	707 298	749 386	791 347	838 202	886 230	925 194	971 123	1 019 983	1 076 445
B.8g	**Gross Saving**[1]	NSSH	**33 197**	**31 353**	**43 243**	**35 665**	**40 017**	**32 557**	**43 132**	**37 289**	**22 560**
Total	Total uses	NSSJ	740 495	780 739	834 590	873 867	926 247	957 751	1 014 255	1 057 272	1 099 005

1 Households' saving as a percentage of total available households' resources is as follows:

		1999	2000	2001	2002	2003	2004	2005	2006	2007
Households' saving ratio (per cent)	RVGL	5.2	4.7	6.0	4.8	5.1	4.0	5.1	4.2	2.5

6.1.7 Households and non-profit institutions serving households
ESA95 sectors S.14 and S.15

£ million

			1999	2000	2001	2002	2003	2004	2005	2006	2007
III	**ACCUMULATION ACCOUNTS**										
III.1	**CAPITAL ACCOUNT**										
III.1.1	**CHANGE IN NET WORTH DUE TO SAVING & CAPITAL TRANSFERS ACCOUNT**										
	Changes in liabilities and net worth										
B.8g	**Gross Saving**	**NSSH**	**33 197**	**31 353**	**43 243**	**35 665**	**40 017**	**32 557**	**43 132**	**37 289**	**22 560**
D.9	Capital transfers receivable										
D.92	Investment grants	**NSSL**	2 645	2 727	3 148	3 456	4 691	4 371	6 695	5 255	6 339
D.99	Other capital transfers	**NSSM**	1 144	1 371	2 639	1 869	1 956	2 831	2 755	2 989	3 440
D.9	Total	**NSSN**	3 789	4 098	5 787	5 325	6 647	7 202	9 450	8 244	9 779
-D.9	*less* Capital transfers payable										
-D.91	Capital taxes	**−NSSO**	−1 951	−2 215	−2 396	−2 381	−2 416	−2 871	−3 150	−3 575	−3 890
-D.99	Other capital transfers	**−NSSQ**	−499	−461	−1 712	−994	−938	−952	−927	−1 157	−1 127
-D.9	Total	**−NSSR**	−2 450	−2 676	−4 108	−3 375	−3 354	−3 823	−4 077	−4 732	−5 017
B.10.1g	Total change in liabilities and net worth	**NSSS**	34 536	32 775	44 922	37 615	43 310	35 936	48 505	40 801	27 322
	Changes in assets										
B.10.1g	Changes in net worth due to gross saving and capital transfers	**NSSS**	34 536	32 775	44 922	37 615	43 310	35 936	48 505	40 801	27 322
-K.1	After deduction of fixed capital consumption	**−QWLL**	−27 976	−30 518	−32 908	−36 043	−36 903	−42 509	−43 257	−48 623	−54 663
B.10.1n	Changes in net worth due to saving and capital transfers	**NSST**	6 560	2 257	12 014	1 572	6 407	−6 573	5 248	−7 822	−27 341
III.1.2	**ACQUISITION OF NON-FINANCIAL ASSETS ACCOUNT**										
	Changes in liabilities and net worth										
B.10.1n	Changes in net worth due to saving and capital transfers	**NSST**	6 560	2 257	12 014	1 572	6 407	−6 573	5 248	−7 822	−27 341
K.1	Consumption of fixed capital	**QWLL**	27 976	30 518	32 908	36 043	36 903	42 509	43 257	48 623	54 663
B.10.1g	Total change in liabilities and net worth	**NSSS**	34 536	32 775	44 922	37 615	43 310	35 936	48 505	40 801	27 322
	Changes in assets										
P.5	Gross capital formation										
P.51	Gross fixed capital formation	**NSSU**	38 234	39 018	43 457	49 764	55 226	65 404	66 739	74 430	82 049
P.52	Changes in inventories	**NSSV**	227	67	199	195	175	126	−260	−15	294
P.53	Acquisitions less disposals of valuables	**NSSW**	264	193	374	309	210	215	77	387	413
P.5	Total gross capital formation	**NSSX**	38 725	39 278	44 030	50 268	55 611	65 745	66 556	74 802	82 756
K.2	Acquisitions less disposals of non-produced non-financial assets	**NSSY**	−138	−67	−152	−176	−210	−276	−320	−358	−340
B.9	**Net lending (+) / net borrowing (-)**	**NSSZ**	**−4 051**	**−6 436**	**1 044**	**−12 477**	**−12 091**	**−29 533**	**−17 731**	**−33 643**	**−55 094**
Total	Total change in assets	**NSSS**	34 536	32 775	44 922	37 615	43 310	35 936	48 505	40 801	27 322

6.1.8 Households and non-profit institutions serving households
ESA95 sectors S.14 and S.15 Unconsolidated

£ million

			1999	2000	2001	2002	2003	2004	2005	2006	2007
III.2	**FINANCIAL ACCOUNT**										
F.A	**Net acquisition of financial assets**										
F.2	Currency and deposits										
F.21	Currency	NFVT	2 219	1 694	2 022	1 505	1 882	2 520	1 997	1 845	2 249
F.22	Transferable deposits										
F.2211	Sterling deposits with UK banks	NFVW	16 485	18 841	27 589	33 677	42 099	43 431	43 490	50 651	22 865
F.2212	Foreign currency deposits with UK banks	NFVX	8	165	119	62	489	602	101	811	1 052
F.2213	Sterling deposits with UK building societies	NFVY	11 206	11 517	13 796	12 330	8 443	12 856	14 109	14 228	22 917
F.229	Deposits with rest of the world monetary financial institutions	NFVZ	1 643	1 745	4 845	2 375	5 365	7 975	3 693	6 563	12 493
F.29	Other deposits	NFWA	−867	−445	−681	−552	4 506	1 544	4 129	6 166	5 824
F.2	Total currency and deposits	NFVS	30 694	33 517	47 690	49 397	62 784	68 928	67 519	80 264	67 400
F.3	Securities other than shares										
F.331	Short term: money market instruments										
F.3311	Issued by UK central government	NFWD	−17	7	−6	−	−	−	−	−	−
F.3312	Issued by UK local authorities	NFWH	−	−	−	−	−	−	−	−	−
F.3315	Issued by UK monetary financial institutions	NFWI	710	−418	1 956	−496	−152	144	−730	1 588	689
F.3316	Issued by other UK residents	NFWN	−	−	1	1	2	−	1	−	2
F.332	Medium (1 to 5 year) and long term (over 5 year) bonds										
F.3321	Issued by UK central government	NFWQ	−5 109	9 764	1 817	942	3 948	−7 774	−9 705	−13 651	−9 054
F.3322	Issued by UK local authorities	NFWT	34	−72	47	−12	4	−134	74	130	20
F.3326	Other medium & long term bonds issued by UK residents	NFWX	36	168	676	213	39	183	218	224	−242
F.3329	Long term bonds issued by the rest of the world	NFWY	−380	256	88	88	88	88	88	88	88
F.34	Financial derivatives	NFWZ	−	−	−	−	−	−	−	−	−
F.3	Total securities other than shares	NFWB	−4 726	9 705	4 579	736	3 929	−7 493	−10 054	−11 621	−8 497
F.4	Loans										
F.42	Long term loans										
F.424	Other long-term loans by UK residents	NFXT	3 805	186	3 489	1 932	5 538	−1 604	2 391	−2 662	−7 558
F.4	Total loans	NFXD	3 805	186	3 489	1 932	5 538	−1 604	2 391	−2 662	−7 558
F.5	Shares and other equity										
F.51	Shares and other equity, excluding mutual funds' shares										
F.514	Quoted UK shares	NFYA	−25 823	−13 533	−20 348	16 109	−1 979	2 491	−24 019	−12 783	−35 868
F.515	Unquoted UK shares	NFYB	−31	−8 989	−5 665	−5 190	−1 768	−4 912	−11 648	−10 255	−14 052
F.516	Other UK equity (including direct investment in property)	NFYC	20	−24	−12	−	−	−	−	−	−
F.517	UK shares and bonds issued by other UK residents	NSPY	−	−	−	−	−	−	−	−	−
F.519	Shares and other equity issued by the rest of the world	NFYF	1 122	−224	1 626	640	3 638	4 333	9 089	1 793	3 380
F.52	Mutual funds' shares										
F.521	UK mutual funds' shares	NFYJ	9 086	6 784	7 417	2 878	7 306	3 061	−3 610	4 607	−738
F.529	Rest of the world mutual funds' shares	NFYK	70	63	33	−8	41	536	1 810	783	−110
F.5	Total shares and other equity	NFXV	−15 556	−15 923	−16 949	14 429	7 238	5 509	−28 378	−15 855	−47 388
F.6	Insurance technical reserves										
F.61	Net equity of households in life assurance and pension funds' reserves	NFYL	34 691	29 716	35 851	46 181	34 449	44 953	53 727	55 998	72 738
F.62	Prepayments of insurance premiums and reserves for outstanding claims	NFYO	−632	120	−1 159	1 014	1 860	2 446	2 128	3 252	49
F.6	Total insurance technical reserves	NPWX	34 059	29 836	34 692	47 195	36 309	47 399	55 855	59 250	72 787
F.7	Other accounts receivable	NFYP	4 754	6 701	1 716	3 185	−1 351	9 224	3 269	30 875	10 007
F.A	**Total net acquisition of financial assets**	NFVO	53 030	64 022	75 217	116 874	114 447	121 963	90 602	140 251	86 751

6.1.8 Households and non-profit institutions serving households
ESA95 sectors S.14 and S.15 Unconsolidated

continued   £ million

			1999	2000	2001	2002	2003	2004	2005	2006	2007
III.2	**FINANCIAL ACCOUNT** continued										
F.L	**Net acquisition of financial liabilities**										
F.3	Securities other than shares										
F.331	Short term: money market instruments										
F.3316	Issued by UK residents other than monetary financial institutions and general government	**NFZR**	−18	55	54	40	−73	−4	157	707	631
F.332	Medium (1 to 5 year) and long term (over 5 year) bonds										
F.3326	Other medium & long term bonds issued by UK residents institutions and general government	**NGAB**	–	–	48	–	200	67	31	400	–
F.34	Financial derivatives	**NGAD**	–	–	–	–	–	–	–	–	–
F.3	Total securities other than shares	**NFZF**	−18	55	102	40	127	63	188	1 107	631
F.4	Loans										
F.41	Short term loans										
F.4111	Sterling loans by UK banks	**NGAK**	12 536	15 887	17 338	20 049	17 642	22 991	16 904	15 556	10 498
F.4112	Foreign currency loans by UK banks	**NGAL**	37	158	13	141	82	178	103	336	241
F.4113	Sterling loans by UK building societies	**NGAM**	−54	100	72	279	348	445	470	−14	42
F.419	Loans by rest of the world monetary financial institutions	**NGAN**	−849	−1 715	3 802	1 310	3 839	6 767	88	7 102	210
F.42	Long term loans										
F.4221	Loans secured on dwellings by banks	**NGAT**	21 492	19 482	31 094	48 928	47 579	42 844	30 990	28 056	10 669
F.4222	Loans secured on dwellings by building societies	**NGAU**	10 651	8 938	6 833	11 034	18 950	17 160	12 662	15 255	11 820
F.4229	Loans secured on dwellings by others	**NGAV**	5 757	13 786	16 396	23 682	35 465	42 276	43 705	62 870	81 356
F.424	Other long-term loans by UK residents	**NGAX**	13 104	8 292	76	5 610	5 036	5 117	8 212	3 406	5 756
F.4	Total loans	**NGAH**	62 674	64 928	75 624	111 033	128 941	137 778	113 134	132 567	120 592
F.7	Other accounts payable	**NGBT**	1 284	−1 400	7 795	10 302	7 027	4 924	3 621	36 180	10 892
F.L	**Total net acquisition of financial liabilities**	**NFYS**	63 940	63 583	83 521	121 375	136 095	142 765	116 943	169 854	132 115
B.9	**Net lending / borrowing**										
F.A	Total net acquisition of financial assets	**NFVO**	53 030	64 022	75 217	116 874	114 447	121 963	90 602	140 251	86 751
-F.L	*less* Total net acquisition of financial liabilities	**−NFYS**	−63 940	−63 583	−83 521	−121 375	−136 095	−142 765	−116 943	−169 854	−132 115
B.9f	Net lending (+) / net borrowing (-), from financial account	**NZDY**	−10 910	439	−8 304	−4 501	−21 648	−20 802	−26 341	−29 603	−45 364
dB.9f	Statistical discrepancy	**NZDV**	6 859	−6 875	9 348	−7 976	9 557	−8 731	8 610	−4 040	−9 730
B.9	**Net lending (+) / net borrowing (-), from capital account**	**NSSZ**	−4 051	−6 436	1 044	−12 477	−12 091	−29 533	−17 731	−33 643	−55 094

6.1.9 Households and non-profit institutions serving households
ESA95 sectors S.14 and S.15 Unconsolidated

£ billion

			1999	2000	2001	2002	2003	2004	2005	2006	2007
IV.3	**FINANCIAL BALANCE SHEET** at end of period										
AN.2	**Non-financial assets**	CGCZ	2 137.3	2 430.7	2 607.3	3 135.0	3 491.6	3 902.0	4 045.5	4 470.3	4 916.4
AF.A	**Financial assets**										
AF.2	Currency and deposits										
AF.21	Currency	NNMQ	24.1	25.8	27.9	29.3	31.2	33.6	35.6	37.4	39.6
AF.22	Transferable deposits										
AF.2211	Sterling deposits with UK banks	NNMT	373.7	408.5	436.2	468.9	510.3	553.5	592.1	643.0	686.6
AF.2212	Foreign currency deposits with UK banks	NNMU	1.9	2.1	2.2	2.2	2.6	3.1	3.4	3.9	4.9
AF.2213	Sterling deposits with UK building societies	NNMV	111.2	109.2	123.0	135.0	143.5	156.3	174.8	189.1	212.0
AF.229	Deposits with rest of the world monetary financial institutions	NNMW	26.4	28.4	31.8	32.7	40.7	50.8	57.7	63.3	74.9
AF.29	Other deposits	NNMX	63.1	62.7	62.4	62.7	67.2	68.7	72.8	78.9	84.8
AF.2	Total currency and deposits	NNMP	600.3	636.7	683.6	731.0	795.5	866.1	936.4	1 015.7	1 102.7
AF.3	Securities other than shares										
AF.331	Short term: money market instruments										
AF.3311	Issued by UK central government	NNNA	–	–	–	–	–	–	–	–	–
AF.3312	Issued by UK local authorities	NNNE	–	–	–	–	–	–	–	–	–
AF.3315	Issued by UK monetary financial institutions	NNNF	2.5	2.2	2.6	2.3	2.3	2.5	1.9	3.2	4.2
AF.3316	Issued by other UK residents	NNNK	0.2	0.5	0.4	0.5	0.5	0.5	0.4	0.5	0.4
AF.332	Medium (1 to 5 year) and long term (over 5 year) bonds										
AF.3321	Issued by UK central government	NNNN	39.0	30.8	38.8	40.3	35.0	31.0	37.5	18.0	3.9
AF.3322	Issued by UK local authorities	NNNQ	0.2	0.2	0.2	0.3	0.4	0.3	0.4	0.7	0.7
AF.3326	Other medium & long term bonds issued by UK residents	NNNV	3.9	4.1	4.3	4.5	4.7	4.9	5.1	5.3	5.5
AF.3329	Long term bonds issued by the rest of the world	NNNV	6.9	7.5	7.6	7.8	7.7	7.7	7.7	7.5	7.6
AF.34	Financial derivatives	NNNW									
AF.3	Total securities other than shares	NNMY	52.8	45.3	54.1	55.7	50.6	47.0	53.0	35.3	22.3
AF.4	Loans										
AF.42	Long term loans										
AF.424	Other long-term loans by UK residents	NNOQ	6.6	6.7	6.8	6.7	6.8	7.0	7.0	7.3	3.4
AF.4	Total loans	NNOA	6.6	6.7	6.8	6.7	6.8	7.0	7.0	7.3	3.4
AF.5	Shares and other equity										
AF.51	Shares and other equity, excluding mutual funds' shares										
AF.514	Quoted UK shares	NNOX	280.5	289.5	229.1	164.7	196.9	203.6	216.5	224.8	186.2
AF.515	Unquoted UK shares	NNOY	263.6	242.5	179.9	122.5	135.1	139.8	164.7	151.4	162.0
AF.516	Other UK equity (including direct investment in property)	NNOZ	1.4	1.4	1.4	1.4	1.4	1.4	1.4	1.4	1.4
AF.517	UK shares and bonds issued by other UK residents	NSQR	–	–	–	–	–	–	–	–	–
AF.519	Shares and other equity issued by the rest of the world	NNPC	24.8	25.2	25.2	25.1	33.8	43.6	64.2	73.2	82.0
AF.52	Mutual funds' shares										
AF.521	UK mutual funds' shares	NNPG	150.8	151.8	136.1	108.3	118.9	138.2	139.7	164.1	216.6
AF.529	Rest of the world mutual funds' shares	NNPH	2.1	1.7	1.7	1.4	1.4	1.7	4.1	6.0	3.5
AF.5	Total shares and other equity	NNOS	723.3	712.1	573.3	423.4	487.5	528.3	590.5	620.8	651.6
AF.6	Insurance technical reserves										
AF.61	Net equity of households in life assurance and pension funds' reserves	NNPI	1 631.3	1 599.0	1 531.3	1 384.1	1 509.2	1 603.2	1 894.3	2 071.7	2 186.7
AF.62	Prepayments of insurance premiums and reserves for outstanding claims	NNPL	31.4	34.8	33.7	34.9	35.1	36.3	37.0	38.8	38.9
AF.6	Total insurance technical reserves	NPYL	1 662.7	1 633.7	1 564.9	1 419.0	1 544.3	1 639.5	1 931.3	2 110.5	2 225.6
AF.7	Other accounts receivable	NNPM	76.1	82.8	86.3	84.7	90.0	98.7	101.4	128.9	140.2
AF.A	**Total financial assets**	NNML	3 121.8	3 117.4	2 968.9	2 720.5	2 974.7	3 186.5	3 619.7	3 918.4	4 145.8

6.1.9 Households and non-profit institutions serving households

ESA95 sectors S.14 and S.15 Unconsolidated

continued

£ billion

			1999	2000	2001	2002	2003	2004	2005	2006	2007
IV.3		**FINANCIAL BALANCE SHEET** continued at end of period									
AF.L		**Financial liabilities**									
AF.3		Securities other than shares									
AF.331		Short term: money market instruments									
AF.3316		Issued by other UK residents	NNQO	–	0.1	0.1	0.2	0.1	0.1	0.1	0.8	1.2
AF.332		Medium (1 to 5 year) and long term (over 5 year) bonds									
AF.3326		Other medium & long term bonds issued by UK residents	NNQY	2.7	2.8	2.8	2.8	3.0	3.1	3.1	3.2	3.2
AF.34		Financial derivatives	NNRA	–	–	–	–	–	–	–	–	–
AF.3		Total securities other than shares	NNQC	2.8	2.9	3.0	3.0	3.1	3.2	3.3	3.9	4.4
AF.4		Loans									
AF.41		Short term loans									
AF.411		Loans by UK monetary financial institutions, excluding loans secured on dwellings & financial leasing	NNRG	103.3	117.7	132.4	148.5	152.4	169.7	179.3	185.6	191.5
AF.419		Loans by rest of the world monetary financial institutions	NNRK	6.9	5.2	7.8	9.1	13.8	20.4	21.8	30.2	30.8
AF.42		Long term loans									
AF.4221		Loans secured on dwellings by banks	NNRQ	345.0	386.3	418.6	467.6	511.0	543.1	558.6	586.6	604.7
AF.4222		Loans secured on dwellings by building societies	NNRR	113.5	107.0	113.4	123.6	142.3	165.4	167.0	182.4	194.3
AF.4229		Loans secured on dwellings by others	NNRS	34.3	41.7	58.2	78.2	119.6	172.6	212.6	277.3	347.6
AF.424		Other long-term loans by UK residents	NNRU	15.6	16.0	18.1	20.9	21.8	24.0	25.8	28.7	32.3
AF.4		Total loans	NNRE	618.7	674.0	748.6	847.9	960.9	1 095.2	1 165.2	1 290.8	1 401.2
AF.7		Other accounts payable	NNSQ	55.7	57.1	58.7	72.4	85.8	86.1	88.2	121.4	133.2
AF.L		**Total financial liabilities**	NNPP	677.2	734.0	810.3	923.3	1 049.9	1 184.5	1 256.7	1 416.1	1 538.8
BF.90		**Net financial assets / liabilities**									
AF.A		Total financial assets	NNML	3 121.8	3 117.4	2 968.9	2 720.5	2 974.7	3 186.5	3 619.7	3 918.4	4 145.8
-AF.L		*less* Total financial liabilities	–NNPP	–677.2	–734.0	–810.3	–923.3	–1 049.9	–1 184.5	–1 256.7	–1 416.1	–1 538.8
BF.90		**Net financial assets (+) / liabilities (-)**	NZEA	2 444.6	2 383.4	2 158.6	1 797.3	1 924.9	2 001.9	2 363.0	2 502.3	2 607.0
		Total net worth									
AN		Non-financial assets	CGCZ	2 137.3	2 430.7	2 607.3	3 135.0	3 491.6	3 902.0	4 045.5	4 470.3	4 916.4
BF.90		Net financial assets (+) / liabilities (-)	NZEA	2 444.6	2 383.4	2 158.6	1 797.3	1 924.9	2 001.9	2 363.0	2 502.3	2 607.0
BF.90		**Net worth**	CGRC	4 582.0	4 814.1	4 765.9	4 932.3	5 416.5	5 903.9	6 408.5	6 972.6	7 523.4

6.2 Households final consumption expenditure: classified by purpose
At current market prices

£ million

			1999	2000	2001	2002	2003	2004	2005	2006	2007
P.31	**FINAL CONSUMPTION EXPENDITURE OF HOUSEHOLDS**										
	Durable goods										
	Furnishings, household equipment and										
05.	routine maintenance of the house	LLIJ	16 566	18 006	19 275	20 470	21 595	22 316	22 976	23 622	24 960
06.	Health	LLIK	1 881	1 997	2 109	2 411	2 604	2 467	2 368	2 650	2 714
07.	Transport	LLIL	31 888	33 291	35 864	36 574	38 016	38 643	38 361	39 047	40 893
08.	Communication	LLIM	512	601	636	644	810	850	900	900	926
09.	Recreation and culture	LLIN	14 262	14 878	15 970	16 471	17 752	19 058	20 180	21 012	21 439
12.	Miscellaneous goods and services	LLIO	3 398	3 403	3 750	4 204	4 284	4 739	4 636	5 283	5 507
D	Total durable goods	UTIA	68 507	72 176	77 604	80 774	85 061	88 073	89 421	92 514	96 439
	Semi-durable goods										
03.	Clothing and footwear	LLJL	32 661	34 759	36 092	38 351	40 389	42 114	42 999	44 178	45 801
	Furnishings, household equipment and										
05.	routine maintenance of the house	LLJM	10 577	11 677	12 400	13 361	13 932	13 502	13 396	13 987	13 795
07.	Transport	LLJN	3 018	2 772	2 783	3 112	3 423	3 048	3 444	3 438	3 567
09.	Recreation and culture	LLJO	19 049	20 405	21 606	23 910	26 009	26 544	26 659	26 671	26 983
12.	Miscellaneous goods and services	LLJP	1 926	2 018	2 427	2 886	3 356	3 477	3 278	3 448	3 659
SD	Total semi-durable goods	UTIQ	67 231	71 631	75 308	81 620	87 109	88 685	89 776	91 722	93 805
	Non-durable goods										
01.	Food & drink	ABZV	57 040	58 628	59 804	61 310	63 174	64 830	67 187	69 410	77 094
02.	Alcohol & tobacco	ADFL	24 458	24 617	25 158	25 966	27 297	28 101	28 437	30 061	31 073
	Housing, water, electricity, gas and										
04.	other fuels	LLIX	21 800	22 265	23 076	23 444	24 241	27 439	29 375	33 936	35 793
	Furnishings, household equipment and										
05.	routine maintenance of the house	LLIY	2 657	2 786	2 972	3 169	3 338	3 879	3 873	4 091	4 097
06.	Health	LLIZ	3 111	3 268	3 613	3 855	3 938	4 457	4 525	4 491	4 601
07.	Transport	LLJA	18 210	19 987	19 391	19 129	20 072	21 161	24 183	25 089	26 356
09.	Recreation and culture	LLJB	12 665	12 959	13 107	13 392	13 507	13 976	14 359	14 879	15 308
12.	Miscellaneous goods and services	LLJC	9 121	9 463	9 884	11 272	12 602	13 187	13 276	14 208	15 552
ND	Total non-durable goods	UTII	149 062	153 973	157 005	161 537	168 169	177 030	185 215	196 165	209 874
	Total goods	UTIE	284 800	297 780	309 917	323 931	340 339	353 788	364 412	380 401	400 118
	Services										
03.	Clothing and footwear	LLJD	714	720	730	741	766	682	760	824	847
	Housing, water, electricity, gas and										
04.	other fuels	LLJE	81 393	85 785	92 829	97 794	104 810	110 605	117 947	125 760	133 779
	Furnishings, household equipment and										
05.	routine maintenance of the house	LLJF	3 046	3 206	3 327	3 448	3 601	3 772	4 084	3 791	3 682
06.	Health	LLJG	3 783	3 943	4 254	4 512	4 793	5 105	5 413	5 603	6 183
07.	Transport	LLJH	34 121	37 002	38 397	41 332	43 058	45 604	48 180	50 923	53 295
08.	Communication	LLJI	11 493	12 755	13 521	14 031	14 844	15 944	16 308	16 532	17 114
09.	Recreation and culture	LLJJ	21 505	21 912	22 769	25 349	27 118	29 263	31 218	32 528	34 739
10.	Education	ADIE	8 943	9 534	9 409	9 381	9 610	11 094	11 762	12 432	13 255
11.	Restaurants and hotels	ADIF	64 387	68 557	71 620	76 426	78 902	82 476	84 808	86 729	90 699
12.	Miscellaneous goods and services	LLJK	62 808	68 423	71 481	73 456	74 609	77 229	83 414	87 259	92 059
S	Total services	UTIM	292 193	311 837	328 337	346 470	362 111	381 774	403 894	422 381	445 652
	Final consumption expenditure in the UK										
	by resident and non-resident households										
0.	**(domestic concept)**	ABQI	576 993	609 617	638 254	670 401	702 450	735 562	768 306	802 782	845 770
P.33	Final consumption expenditure outside the UK by UK resident households	ABTA	19 690	21 654	22 907	24 435	26 314	27 550	29 028	30 389	32 098
-P.34	*Less* Final consumption expenditure in the UK by households resident in the rest of the world	CDFD	−14 312	−14 713	−13 383	−13 872	−14 156	−15 610	−17 069	−18 512	−19 041
	Final consumption expenditure by UK resident										
	households in the UK and abroad										
P.31	**(national concept)**	ABPB	582 371	616 558	647 778	680 964	714 608	747 502	780 265	814 659	858 827

Additional detail is published in *Consumer Trends* and table A7 of *UK Economic Accounts*, available from the ONS website (www.statistics.gov.uk/consumertrends).

6.3 Households final consumption expenditure: classified by purpose
Chained volume measures (reference year 2003)

£ million

			1999	2000	2001	2002	2003	2004	2005	2006	2007
P.31	**FINAL CONSUMPTION EXPENDITURE OF HOUSEHOLDS**										
	Durable goods										
05.	Furnishings, household equipment and routine maintenance of the house	LLME	16 764	18 442	19 542	20 603	21 595	21 974	22 325	22 753	23 227
06.	Health	LLMF	2 585	2 455	2 337	2 421	2 604	2 361	2 239	2 519	2 536
07.	Transport	LLMG	29 455	31 680	35 100	36 057	38 016	38 962	39 617	40 792	42 629
08.	Communication	LLMH	428	536	582	640	810	824	957	1 030	1 296
09.	Recreation and culture	LLMI	9 657	11 243	13 344	14 911	17 752	21 053	25 553	30 063	36 478
12.	Miscellaneous goods and services	LLMJ	3 656	3 618	3 932	4 360	4 284	4 636	4 493	4 821	4 791
D	Total durable goods	UTIC	61 603	67 366	74 551	78 825	85 061	89 810	95 184	101 978	110 957
	Semi-durable goods										
03.	Clothing and footwear	LLNG	27 921	30 969	33 712	37 727	40 389	43 400	45 405	47 006	49 230
05.	Furnishings, household equipment and routine maintenance of the house	LLNH	10 177	11 473	12 221	13 215	13 932	13 507	13 679	14 364	14 087
07.	Transport	LLNI	3 136	2 856	2 880	3 172	3 423	2 989	3 279	3 167	3 239
09.	Recreation and culture	LLNJ	17 229	19 175	20 339	23 040	26 009	27 340	27 997	28 461	28 683
12.	Miscellaneous goods and services	LLNK	1 932	2 053	2 438	2 920	3 356	3 489	3 196	3 315	3 410
SD	Total semi-durable goods	UTIS	60 277	66 478	71 563	80 058	87 109	90 725	93 556	96 313	98 649
	Non-durable goods										
01.	Food & drink	ADIP	59 904	61 944	61 048	62 143	63 174	64 473	65 855	66 499	70 579
02.	Alcohol & tobacco	ADIS	27 623	26 704	26 497	26 884	27 297	27 861	27 735	28 463	28 807
04.	Housing, water, electricity, gas and other fuels	LLMS	22 594	23 189	23 958	23 881	24 241	26 157	25 521	24 932	24 436
05.	Furnishings, household equipment and routine maintenance of the house	LLMT	2 492	2 666	2 878	3 101	3 338	4 033	4 025	4 108	4 029
06.	Health	LLMU	3 314	3 397	3 686	3 895	3 938	4 473	4 583	4 577	4 617
07.	Transport	LLMV	19 691	19 114	19 550	19 825	20 072	20 058	21 132	20 826	21 260
09.	Recreation and culture	LLMW	13 713	13 657	13 537	13 681	13 507	13 794	14 102	14 282	14 497
12.	Miscellaneous goods and services	LLMX	8 669	9 248	9 586	11 124	12 602	13 335	13 550	14 997	15 962
ND	Total non-durable goods	UTIK	157 573	159 677	160 597	164 482	168 169	174 184	176 503	178 684	184 187
	Total goods	UTIG	277 468	292 390	306 198	323 179	340 339	354 719	365 243	376 975	393 793
	Services										
03.	Clothing and footwear	LLMY	819	805	790	775	766	658	696	721	707
04.	Housing, water, electricity, gas and other fuels	LLMZ	101 184	102 168	102 778	104 106	104 810	106 095	106 834	109 156	109 433
05.	Furnishings, household equipment and routine maintenance of the house	LLNA	3 874	3 821	3 718	3 646	3 601	3 562	3 661	3 251	3 009
06.	Health	LLNB	4 531	4 612	4 683	4 665	4 793	5 005	5 195	5 187	5 559
07.	Transport	LLNC	41 413	43 153	40 971	42 611	43 058	43 872	44 357	45 288	45 828
08.	Communication	LLND	10 527	12 167	13 877	14 158	14 844	15 837	16 547	16 787	17 925
09.	Recreation and culture	LLNE	24 795	25 101	25 960	26 216	27 118	28 381	29 166	28 948	29 718
10.	Education	ADMJ	11 394	11 489	10 692	10 091	9 610	10 591	10 717	10 832	11 052
11.	Restaurants and hotels	ADMK	74 191	76 252	76 434	78 303	78 902	80 651	80 051	78 868	79 647
12.	Miscellaneous goods and services	LLNF	66 738	69 846	72 526	73 631	74 609	74 702	77 207	78 887	79 364
S	Total services	UTIO	338 130	348 641	352 299	358 149	362 111	369 354	374 431	377 925	382 242
0.	Final consumption expenditure in the UK by resident and non-resident households (domestic concept)	ABQJ	613 617	639 565	657 752	681 082	702 450	724 073	739 674	754 900	776 035
P.33	Final consumption expenditure outside the UK by UK resident households	ABTC	21 899	24 189	24 897	26 376	26 314	27 994	27 675	28 339	29 909
-P.34	Less Final consumption expenditure in the UK by households resident in the rest of the world	CCHX	−16 031	−16 038	−14 164	−14 292	−14 156	−15 210	−16 061	−16 861	−16 781
P.3	Final consumption expenditure by UK resident households in the UK and abroad (national concept)	ABPF	619 651	647 796	668 482	693 124	714 608	736 857	751 288	766 378	789 163

Additional detail is published in *Consumer Trends* and table A7 of *UK Economic Accounts*, available from the ONS website (www.statistics.gov.uk/consumertrends).

6.4 Individual consumption expenditure at current market prices by households, non-profit institutions serving households and general government

Classified by function (COICOP/COPNI/COFOG)[1]

£ million

		1999	2000	2001	2002	2003	2004	2005	2006	2007
P.31	**FINAL CONSUMPTION EXPENDITURE OF HOUSEHOLDS**									
01.	**Food and non-alcoholic beverages** ABZV	57 040	58 628	59 804	61 310	63 174	64 830	67 187	69 410	77 094
01.1	Food ABZW	50 685	51 905	52 742	53 984	55 507	56 667	58 690	60 627	67 084
01.2	Non-alcoholic beverages ADFK	6 355	6 723	7 062	7 326	7 667	8 163	8 497	8 783	10 010
02.	**Alcoholic beverages and tobacco** ADFL	24 458	24 617	25 158	25 966	27 297	28 101	28 437	30 061	31 073
02.1	Alcoholic beverages ADFM	10 166	10 395	10 700	11 344	12 027	13 035	13 065	13 924	15 053
02.2	Tobacco ADFN	14 292	14 222	14 458	14 622	15 270	15 066	15 372	16 137	16 020
03.	**Clothing and footwear** ADFP	33 375	35 479	36 822	39 092	41 155	42 796	43 759	45 002	46 648
03.1	Clothing ADFQ	28 932	31 048	32 103	33 927	35 689	36 770	37 609	38 419	39 723
03.2	Footwear ADFR	4 443	4 431	4 719	5 165	5 466	6 026	6 150	6 583	6 925
04.	**Housing, water, electricity, gas and other fuels** ADFS	103 193	108 050	115 905	121 238	129 051	138 044	147 322	159 696	169 572
04.1	Actual rentals for housing ADFT	22 584	23 595	25 302	25 828	27 610	29 205	30 142	32 716	34 629
04.2	Imputed rentals for housing ADFU	51 401	54 378	59 581	63 279	68 458	72 179	78 179	82 388	87 769
04.3	Maintenance and repair of the dwelling ADFV	10 234	10 512	11 340	12 306	12 615	13 956	13 538	13 287	14 233
04.4	Water supply and miscellaneous dwelling services ADFW	5 201	5 033	5 059	5 222	5 438	5 831	6 279	6 820	7 228
04.5	Electricity, gas and other fuels ADFX	13 773	14 532	14 623	14 603	14 930	16 873	19 184	24 485	25 713
05.	**Furnishings, household equipment and routine maintenance of the house** ADFY	32 846	35 675	37 974	40 448	42 466	43 469	44 329	45 491	46 534
05.1	Furniture, furnishings, carpets and other floor coverings ADFZ	12 437	13 758	14 362	15 591	16 789	17 168	17 309	17 702	18 815
05.2	Household textiles ADGG	3 972	4 465	4 636	5 086	5 452	5 299	4 916	5 146	5 431
05.3	Household appliances ADGL	5 038	5 156	5 758	5 715	5 578	6 028	6 391	6 704	6 727
05.4	Glassware, tableware and household utensils ADGM	3 722	4 231	4 609	4 710	4 701	3 870	4 210	4 122	3 493
05.5	Tools and equipment for house and garden ADGN	2 586	2 722	2 977	3 355	3 589	4 006	4 090	4 445	4 739
05.6	Goods and services for routine household maintenance ADGO	5 091	5 343	5 632	5 991	6 357	7 098	7 413	7 372	7 329
06.	**Health** ADGP	8 775	9 208	9 976	10 778	11 335	12 029	12 306	12 744	13 498
06.1	Medical products, appliances and equipment ADGQ	4 992	5 265	5 722	6 266	6 542	6 924	6 893	7 141	7 315
06.2	Out-patient services ADGR	2 107	2 178	2 344	2 422	2 553	2 747	2 909	2 983	3 459
06.3	Hospital services ADGS	1 676	1 765	1 910	2 090	2 240	2 358	2 504	2 620	2 724
07.	**Transport** ADGT	87 237	93 052	96 435	100 147	104 569	108 456	114 168	118 497	124 111
07.1	Purchase of vehicles ADGU	31 888	33 291	35 864	36 574	38 016	38 643	38 361	39 047	40 893
07.2	Operation of personal transport equipment ADGV	34 450	37 059	37 028	38 816	40 507	42 848	47 205	49 059	51 224
07.3	Transport services ADGW	20 899	22 702	23 543	24 757	26 046	26 965	28 602	30 391	31 994
08.	**Communication** ADGX	12 005	13 356	14 157	14 675	15 654	16 794	17 208	17 432	18 040
08.1	Postal services CDEF	899	873	870	878	890	961	1 017	1 005	1 043
08.2	Telephone & telefax equipment ADWO	512	601	636	644	810	850	900	900	926
08.3	Telephone & telefax services ADWP	10 594	11 882	12 651	13 153	13 954	14 983	15 291	15 527	16 071
09.	**Recreation and culture** ADGY	67 481	70 154	73 452	79 122	84 386	88 841	92 416	95 090	98 469
09.1	Audio-visual, photographic and information processing equipment ADGZ	16 312	17 034	17 580	18 051	19 408	20 603	21 234	20 927	20 608
09.2	Other major durables for recreation and culture ADHL	3 582	3 944	4 325	4 672	5 126	5 271	5 711	6 019	6 149
09.3	Other recreational items and equipment; flowers, garden and pets ADHZ	17 655	18 636	20 216	22 475	23 894	24 349	24 769	25 723	27 364
09.4	Recreational and cultural services ADIA	19 876	20 272	21 034	23 555	25 278	27 313	28 830	30 272	32 142
09.5	Newspapers, books and stationery ADIC	10 056	10 268	10 297	10 369	10 680	11 305	11 872	12 149	12 206
09.6	Package holidays[2] ADID	–	–	–	–	–	–	–	–	–
10.	**Education**									
10.	Education services ADIE	8 943	9 534	9 409	9 381	9 610	11 094	11 762	12 432	13 255
11.	**Restaurants and hotels** ADIF	64 387	68 557	71 620	76 426	78 902	82 476	84 808	86 729	90 699
11.1	Catering services ADIG	55 164	59 019	62 449	66 701	68 839	72 399	74 294	75 501	78 382
11.2	Accommodation services ADIH	9 223	9 538	9 171	9 725	10 063	10 077	10 514	11 228	12 317
12.	**Miscellaneous goods and services** ADII	77 253	83 307	87 542	91 818	94 851	98 632	104 604	110 198	116 777
12.1	Personal care ADIJ	13 229	13 883	14 626	16 444	18 181	19 538	20 022	21 020	22 595
12.3	Personal effects n.e.c. ADIK	4 673	4 748	5 455	6 140	6 462	6 819	6 647	7 652	7 987
12.4	Social protection ADIL	8 446	8 643	8 963	9 219	9 501	8 745	8 918	9 452	10 140
12.5	Insurance ADIM	20 257	22 238	25 423	25 456	24 373	23 345	25 407	25 100	26 744
12.6	Financial services n.e.c. ADIN	24 386	27 706	26 990	28 384	29 977	33 173	35 758	39 289	41 663
12.7	Other services n.e.c. ADIO	6 262	6 089	6 085	6 175	6 357	7 012	7 852	7 685	7 648
0.	**Final consumption expenditure in the UK by resident and non-resident households (domestic concept)** ABQI	576 993	609 617	638 254	670 401	702 450	735 562	768 306	802 782	845 770
P.33	Final consumption expenditure outside the UK by UK resident households ABTA	19 690	21 654	22 907	24 435	26 314	27 550	29 028	30 389	32 098
-P.34	*less* Final consumption expenditure in the UK by households resident in the rest of the world CDFD	−14 312	−14 713	−13 383	−13 872	−14 156	−15 610	−17 069	−18 512	−19 041
P.31	**Final consumption expenditure by UK resident households in the UK and abroad (national concept)** ABPB	582 371	616 558	647 778	680 964	714 608	747 502	780 265	814 659	858 827

6.4 Individual consumption expenditure at current market prices by households, non-profit institutions serving households and general government

continued   **Classified by function (COICOP/COPNI/COFOG)[1]**   £ million

		1999	2000	2001	2002	2003	2004	2005	2006	2007
P.31 CONSUMPTION EXPENDITURE OF UK RESIDENT HOUSEHOLDS										
P.31 Final consumption expenditure of UK resident households in the UK and abroad	**ABPB**	582 371	616 558	647 778	680 964	714 608	747 502	780 265	814 659	858 827
13. FINAL INDIVIDUAL CONSUMPTION EXPENDITURE OF NPISH										
P.31 Final individual consumption expenditure of NPISH	**ABNV**	22 185	23 531	25 111	26 422	27 668	28 748	30 402	32 209	34 587
14. FINAL INDIVIDUAL CONSUMPTION EXPENDITURE OF OF GENERAL GOVERNMENT										
14.1 Health	**IWX5**	50 254	53 236	58 032	63 388	69 888	76 307	82 068	89 744	95 209
14.2 Recreation and culture	**IWX6**	6 104	6 240	6 665	7 404	7 800	5 150	5 518	5 777	5 997
14.3 Education	**IWX7**	29 570	31 682	34 174	37 533	40 423	42 487	46 045	48 958	51 990
14.4 Social protection	**IWX8**	16 814	18 139	19 587	22 491	25 843	25 000	26 825	28 636	29 835
14.5 Housing	**QYXO**	–	–	–	–	–	–	–	–	–
P.31 Final individual consumption expenditure of general government	**NNAQ**	102 742	109 297	118 458	130 816	143 954	148 944	160 456	173 115	183 031
P.31 Total, individual consumption expenditure/ P.41 actual individual consumption	**NQEO**	707 298	749 386	791 347	838 202	886 230	925 194	971 123	1 019 983	1 076 445

1 "Purpose" or "function" classifications are designed to indicate the "socio-economic objectives" that institutional units aim to achieve through various kinds of outlays. COICOP is the Classification of Individual Consumption by Purpose and applies to households. COPNI is the Classification of the Purposes of Non-profit Institutions Serving Households and COFOG the Classification of the Functions of Government. The introduction of ESA95 coincides with the redefinition of these classifications and data will be available on a consistent basis for all European Union member states.

2 Package holidays data are dispersed between components (transport etc)

6.5 Individual consumption expenditure by households, NPISH and general government Chained volume measures (reference year 2003)

Classified by function (COICOP/COPNI/COFOG)[1]

£ million

			1999	2000	2001	2002	2003	2004	2005	2006	2007
P.31	**FINAL CONSUMPTION EXPENDITURE OF HOUSEHOLDS**										
01.	**Food and non-alcoholic beverages**	ADIP	59 904	61 944	61 048	62 143	63 174	64 473	65 855	66 499	70 579
01.1	Food	ADIQ	53 697	55 255	53 992	54 835	55 507	56 240	57 305	57 969	61 239
01.2	Non-alcoholic beverages	ADIR	6 260	6 725	7 063	7 312	7 667	8 233	8 550	8 530	9 340
02.	**Alcoholic beverages and tobacco**	ADIS	27 623	26 704	26 497	26 884	27 297	27 861	27 735	28 463	28 807
02.1	Alcoholic beverages	ADIT	10 309	10 476	10 831	11 516	12 027	13 204	13 331	14 005	15 047
02.2	Tobacco	ADIU	17 541	16 341	15 716	15 380	15 270	14 657	14 404	14 458	13 760
03.	**Clothing and footwear**	ADIW	28 689	31 744	34 485	38 499	41 155	44 058	46 101	47 727	49 937
03.1	Clothing	ADIX	24 424	27 394	29 827	33 315	35 689	37 924	39 688	40 823	42 770
03.2	Footwear	ADIY	4 324	4 360	4 660	5 185	5 466	6 134	6 413	6 904	7 167
04.	**Housing, water, electricity, gas and other fuels**	ADIZ	123 662	125 299	126 749	127 979	129 051	132 252	132 355	134 088	133 869
04.1	Actual rentals for housing	ADJA	27 366	27 345	27 418	27 084	27 610	27 933	27 644	29 071	28 929
04.2	Imputed rentals for housing	ADJB	64 980	65 704	66 495	67 872	68 458	69 438	70 672	71 154	71 456
04.3	Maintenance and repair of the dwelling	ADJC	11 791	11 675	12 139	12 702	12 615	13 581	12 793	12 115	12 399
04.4	Water supply and miscellaneous dwelling services	ADJD	5 228	5 386	5 379	5 424	5 438	5 537	5 429	5 521	5 505
04.5	Electricity, gas and other fuels	ADJE	14 363	15 149	15 277	14 891	14 930	15 763	15 817	16 227	15 580
05.	**Furnishings, household equipment and routine maintenance of the house**	ADJF	33 130	36 305	38 310	40 552	42 466	43 076	43 690	44 476	44 352
05.1	Furniture, furnishings, carpets and other floor coverings	ADJG	13 120	14 514	14 860	15 896	16 789	16 751	16 425	16 419	16 797
05.2	Household textiles	ADJH	3 743	4 361	4 534	5 043	5 452	5 202	4 944	5 283	5 627
05.3	Household appliances	ADJI	4 648	4 922	5 549	5 566	5 578	6 059	6 527	7 033	6 894
05.4	Glassware, tableware and household utensils	ADJJ	3 699	4 266	4 655	4 717	4 701	3 866	4 317	4 231	3 554
05.5	Tools and equipment for house and garden	ADJK	2 435	2 590	2 856	3 238	3 589	4 136	4 293	4 611	4 841
05.6	Goods and services for routine household maintenance	ADJL	5 556	5 708	5 859	6 092	6 357	7 062	7 184	6 899	6 639
06.	**Health**	ADJM	10 362	10 421	10 697	10 980	11 335	11 839	12 017	12 283	12 712
06.1	Medical products, appliances and equipment	ADJN	5 839	5 819	6 020	6 315	6 542	6 834	6 822	7 096	7 153
06.2	Out-patient services	ADJO	2 556	2 528	2 560	2 492	2 553	2 712	2 829	2 780	3 128
06.3	Hospital services	ADJP	1 976	2 082	2 122	2 173	2 240	2 293	2 366	2 407	2 431
07.	**Transport**	ADJQ	92 969	96 209	98 485	101 621	104 569	105 881	108 385	110 073	112 956
07.1	Purchase of vehicles	ADJR	29 455	31 680	35 100	36 057	38 016	38 962	39 617	40 792	42 629
07.2	Operation of personal transport equipment	ADJS	39 617	39 124	39 225	40 668	40 507	40 508	41 553	40 907	41 074
07.3	Transport services	ADJT	24 661	25 913	24 214	24 965	26 046	26 411	27 215	28 374	29 253
08.	**Communication**	ADJU	10 948	12 698	14 452	14 796	15 654	16 661	17 504	17 817	19 221
08.1	Postal services	CCGZ	960	916	901	906	890	932	1 034	1 120	1 289
08.2	Telephone & telefax equipment	ADQF	428	536	582	640	810	824	957	1 030	1 296
08.3	Telephone & telefax services	ADQG	9 604	11 264	12 978	13 254	13 954	14 905	15 513	15 667	16 636
09.	**Recreation and culture**	ADJV	63 601	68 038	72 552	77 597	84 386	90 568	96 818	101 754	109 376
09.1	Audio-visual, photographic and information processing equipment	ADJW	11 178	13 022	14 690	16 301	19 408	23 041	27 358	30 782	36 314
09.2	Other major durables for recreation and culture	ADJX	3 798	4 182	4 560	4 817	5 126	5 117	5 419	5 678	5 837
09.3	Other recreational items and equipment; flowers, gardens and pets	ADJY	16 190	17 455	18 980	21 642	23 894	24 842	25 541	26 943	28 518
09.4	Recreational and cultural services	ADJZ	22 827	23 206	24 049	24 333	25 278	26 522	26 995	26 977	27 547
09.5	Newspapers, books and stationery	ADKM	11 242	11 181	10 910	10 756	10 680	11 046	11 505	11 374	11 160
09.6	Package holidays[2]	ADMI	–	–	–	–	–	–	–	–	–
10.	**Education**										
10.	Education services	ADMJ	11 394	11 489	10 692	10 091	9 610	10 591	10 717	10 832	11 052
11.	**Restaurants and Hotels**	ADMK	74 191	76 252	76 434	78 303	78 902	80 651	80 051	78 868	79 647
11.1	Catering services	ADML	63 354	65 644	66 815	68 462	68 839	70 766	70 248	68 896	69 088
11.2	Accommodation services	ADMM	10 851	10 610	9 620	9 843	10 063	9 885	9 803	9 972	10 559
12.	**Miscellaneous goods and services**	ADMN	80 917	84 709	88 415	92 015	94 851	96 162	98 446	102 020	103 527
12.1	Personal care	ADMO	13 497	14 251	14 719	16 526	18 181	19 451	19 747	21 035	21 989
12.3	Personal effects n.e.c.	ADMP	4 871	4 922	5 607	6 289	6 462	6 730	6 481	7 134	7 134
12.4	Social protection	ADMQ	10 778	10 357	10 058	9 760	9 501	8 416	8 062	8 013	8 263
12.5	Insurance	ADMR	22 511	23 526	25 453	24 880	24 373	22 633	23 523	24 125	23 752
12.6	Financial services n.e.c.	ADMS	22 140	24 666	25 875	28 040	29 977	32 391	33 760	35 338	36 260
12.7	Other services n.e.c.	ADMT	7 937	7 336	6 827	6 536	6 357	6 545	6 870	6 377	6 129
0.	**Final consumption expenditure in the UK by resident and non-resident households (domestic concept)**	ABQJ	613 617	639 565	657 752	681 082	702 450	724 073	739 674	754 900	776 035
P.33	Final consumption expenditure outside the UK by UK resident households	ABTC	21 899	24 189	24 897	26 376	26 314	27 994	27 675	28 339	29 909
-P.34	*less* Final consumption expenditure in the UK by households resident in the rest of the world	CCHX	−16 031	−16 038	−14 164	−14 292	−14 156	−15 210	−16 061	−16 861	−16 781
P.31	**Final consumption expenditure by UK resident households in the UK and abroad (national concept)**	ABPF	619 651	647 796	668 482	693 124	714 608	736 857	751 288	766 378	789 163

6.5 Individual consumption expenditure by households, NPISH and general government Chained volume measures (reference year 2003)

continued   **Classified by function (COICOP/COPNI/COFOG)[1]**   £ million

		1999	2000	2001	2002	2003	2004	2005	2006	2007
P.31 CONSUMPTION EXPENDITURE OF UK RESIDENT HOUSEHOLDS										
P.31 Final consumption expenditure of UK resident households in the UK and abroad	ABPF	619 651	647 796	668 482	693 124	714 608	736 857	751 288	766 378	789 163
13. FINAL INDIVIDUAL CONSUMPTION EXPENDITURE OF NPISH										
P.31 Final individual consumption expenditure of NPISH	ABNU	25 341	27 536	27 567	27 576	27 668	27 198	27 212	28 289	29 269
14. FINAL INDIVIDUAL CONSUMPTION EXPENDITURE OF GENERAL GOVERNMENT										
14.1 Health	EMOA	60 466	62 289	64 952	67 350	69 888	72 862	75 013	77 175	80 211
14.2 Recreation and culture	QYXK	6 340	6 361	6 611	7 162	7 800	8 132	8 570	8 598	8 888
14.3 Education	EMOB	39 122	39 504	39 743	40 210	40 423	40 453	40 263	40 107	40 049
14.4 Social protection	QYXM	23 359	23 454	23 645	24 864	25 843	27 213	27 203	27 347	27 602
14.5 Housing	QYXN	–	–	–	–	–	–	–	–	–
P.31 Final individual consumption expenditure of general government	NSZK	129 050	131 426	134 867	139 546	143 954	148 660	151 049	153 227	156 750
P.31 Total, individual consumption expenditure/ **P.41 actual individual consumption**	YBIO	773 446	806 541	830 840	860 237	886 230	912 715	929 549	947 894	975 182

1 "Purpose" or "function" classifications are designed to indicate the "socio-economic objectives" that institutional units aim to achieve through various kinds of outlays. COICOP is the Classification of Individual Consumption by Purpose and applies to households. COPNI is the Classification of the Purposes of Non-profit Institutions Serving Households and COFOG the Classification of the Functions of Government. The introduction of ESA95 coincides with the redefinition of these classifications and data will be available on a consistent basis for all European Union member states.

2 Package holidays data are dispersed between components (transport etc)

Chapter 7

Rest of the world

7.1.0 Rest of the world
ESA95 sector S.2

£ million

			1999	2000	2001	2002	2003	2004	2005	2006	2007
V.I	**EXTERNAL ACCOUNT OF GOODS AND SERVICES**										
	Resources										
P.7	Imports of goods and services										
P.71	Imports of goods	**LQBL**	195 217	220 912	230 305	234 229	236 927	251 774	280 197	319 947	309 955
P.72	Imports of services	**KTMR**	60 963	66 881	70 573	74 380	79 745	84 372	93 545	99 641	105 862
P.7	Total resources, total imports	**KTMX**	256 180	287 793	300 878	308 609	316 672	336 146	373 742	419 588	415 817
	Uses										
P.6	Exports of goods and services										
P.61	Exports of goods	**LQAD**	166 166	187 936	189 093	186 524	188 320	190 874	211 608	243 635	220 703
P.62	Exports of services	**KTMQ**	76 525	81 883	87 773	94 012	102 357	112 518	119 420	132 749	147 634
P.6	Total exports	**KTMW**	242 691	269 819	276 866	280 536	290 677	303 392	331 028	376 384	368 337
B.11	**External balance of goods and services**	**–KTMY**	**13 489**	**17 974**	**24 012**	**28 073**	**25 995**	**32 754**	**42 714**	**43 204**	**47 480**
P.7	Total uses	**KTMX**	256 180	287 793	300 878	308 609	316 672	336 146	373 742	419 588	415 817

7.1.2 Rest of the world
ESA95 sector S.2

£ million

£ million

			1999	2000	2001	2002	2003	2004	2005	2006	2007
V.II	**EXTERNAL ACCOUNT OF PRIMARY INCOMES AND CURRENT TRANSFERS**										
	Resources										
B.11	**External balance of goods and services**	**–KTMY**	**13 489**	**17 974**	**24 012**	**28 073**	**25 995**	**32 754**	**42 714**	**43 204**	**47 480**
D.1	Compensation of employees										
D.11	Wages and salaries	**KTMO**	759	882	1 021	1 054	1 057	1 425	1 584	1 803	1 824
D.2	Taxes on production and imports, received										
D.21	Taxes on products										
D.211	Value added type taxes (VAT)	**FJKM**	3 811	4 204	3 575	2 808	2 740	1 789	1 999	2 167	2 319
D.212	Taxes and duties on imports excluding VAT										
D.2121	Import duties	**FJWE**	2 024	2 086	2 069	1 919	1 937	2 145	2 237	2 329	2 412
D.2122	Taxes on imports excluding VAT and duties	**FJWF**	–	–	–	–	–	–	–	–	–
D.214	Taxes on products excluding VAT and import duties	**FJWG**	46	44	31	25	18	25	24	–	–
D.2	Total taxes on production and imports, received	**FJWB**	5 881	6 334	5 675	4 752	4 695	3 959	4 260	4 496	4 731
-D.3	*less* Subsidies, paid										
-D.31	Subsidies on products	**–FJWJ**	–2 443	–2 236	–1 755	–1 862	–2 099	–2 725	–	–	–
-D.39	Other subsidies on production	**–NHQR**	–338	–335	–582	–519	–592	–592	–3 408	–3 220	–2 943
-D.3	Total	**–FJWI**	–2 781	–2 571	–2 337	–2 381	–2 691	–3 317	–3 408	–3 220	–2 943
D.4	Property income, received										
D.41	Interest	**QYNG**	71 862	93 471	95 024	74 064	71 082	78 889	113 945	157 867	206 377
D.42	Distributed income of corporations	**QYNH**	24 375	24 797	32 932	23 417	24 851	30 510	37 735	44 776	34 979
D.43	Reinvested earnings on direct foreign investment	**QYNI**	4 607	10 788	–992	3 647	7 429	8 558	10 501	22 930	33 118
D.44	Property income attributed to insurance policy-holders	**NHRM**	1 133	1 034	1 124	1 196	1 243	1 101	1 102	1 033	841
D.4	Total	**HMBO**	101 977	130 090	128 088	102 324	104 605	119 058	163 283	226 606	275 315
D.5	Current taxes on income, wealth etc										
D.51	Taxes on income	**FJWM**	682	775	523	644	444	535	589	464	633
D.61	Social contributions										
D.611	Actual social contributions										
D.6112	Employees' social contributions	**FJWQ**	–	–	–	–	–	–	–	–	–
D.62	Social benefits other than social transfers in kind										
D.621	Social security benefits in cash	**FJVZ**	1 123	1 161	1 239	1 338	1 404	1 539	1 596	1 648	1 774
D.622	Private funded social benefits	**QZEM**	62	35	39	54	33	25	47	37	32
D.624	Social assistance benefits in cash	**RNNF**	60	57	53	50	48	57	54	52	55
D.62	Total	**FJKO**	1 245	1 253	1 331	1 442	1 485	1 621	1 697	1 737	1 861
D.7	Other current transfers										
D.71	Net non-life insurance premiums	**FJKS**	10	18	25	19	19	47	16	39	50
D.72	Non-life insurance claims	**NHRR**	2 495	2 086	3 471	3 008	2 208	3 181	6 133	6 612	5 021
D.74	Current international cooperation	**FJWT**	1 456	2 181	2 190	2 362	2 433	3 080	3 255	3 632	3 909
D.75	Miscellaneous current transfers	**FJWU**	7 607	7 615	7 222	8 878	10 610	11 631	13 354	13 176	13 191
	of which GNP based fourth own resource	**NMFH**	4 632	4 379	3 858	5 335	6 772	7 549	8 732	8 521	8 323
D.7	Total	**FJWR**	11 568	11 900	12 908	14 267	15 270	17 939	22 758	23 459	22 171
D.8	Adjustment for the change in net equity of households in pension funds	**QZEP**	–2	–4	–5	–1	–12	–11	–55	–9	–37
Total	Total resources	**NSUK**	132 818	166 633	171 216	150 174	150 848	173 963	233 422	298 540	351 035

7.1.2

Rest of the world

ESA95 sector S.2

£ million

			1999	2000	2001	2002	2003	2004	2005	2006	2007
V.II	**EXTERNAL ACCOUNT OF PRIMARY INCOMES AND CURRENT TRANSFERS** continued										
	Uses										
D.1	Compensation of employees										
D.11	Wages and salaries	KTMN	960	1 032	1 087	1 121	1 116	931	974	1 058	1 159
D.2	Taxes on production and imports, paid										
D.21	Taxes on products										
D.212	Taxes and duties on imports excluding VAT										
D.2121	Import duties	FJVQ	–	–	–	–	–	–	–	–	–
D.2122	Taxes on imports excluding VAT and duties	FJVR	–	–	–	–	–	–	–	–	–
D.214	Taxes on products excluding VAT and import duties	FJVS	–	–	–	–	–	–	–	–	–
D.21	Total taxes on products	FJVN	–	–	–	–	–	–	–	–	–
D.2	Total taxes on production and imports, paid	FJVM	–	–	–	–	–	–	–	–	–
D.4	Property income, paid										
D.41	Interest	QYNJ	61 231	79 584	82 969	59 788	57 624	64 454	92 618	135 421	177 647
D.42	Distributed income of corporations	QYNK	18 110	27 140	27 258	28 546	42 989	41 852	49 592	54 232	52 643
D.43	Reinvested earnings on direct foreign investment	QYNL	21 392	25 178	27 220	32 209	21 456	31 076	43 555	47 795	54 296
D.44	Property income attributed to insurance policy-holders										
D.4	Total	HMBN	100 733	131 902	137 447	120 543	122 069	137 382	185 765	237 448	284 586
D.5	Current taxes on income, wealth etc										
D.51	Taxes on income	NHRS	337	357	398	527	375	482	546	649	640
D.61	Social contributions										
D.6112	Employee's social contributions	FKAA	89	55	59	77	44	36	14	56	26
D.7	Other current transfers										
D.71	Net non-life insurance premiums	NHRX	2 495	2 086	3 471	3 008	2 208	3 181	6 133	6 612	5 021
D.72	Non-life insurance claims	FJTT	10	18	25	19	19	47	16	39	50
D.74	Current international cooperation	FJWA	3 176	2 084	4 568	3 112	3 570	3 673	3 726	3 674	3 573
D.75	Miscellaneous current transfers	NHSI	3 164	3 312	3 059	3 110	3 140	3 031	3 557	3 973	3 412
D.7	Total	NHRW	8 845	7 500	11 123	9 249	8 937	9 932	13 432	14 298	12 056
B.12	**Current external balance**	–HBOG	**21 854**	**25 787**	**21 102**	**18 657**	**18 307**	**25 200**	**32 691**	**45 031**	**52 568**
Total	Total uses	NSUK	132 818	166 633	171 216	150 174	150 848	173 963	233 422	298 540	351 035

7.1.7 Rest of the world

ESA95 sector S.2

£ million

			1999	2000	2001	2002	2003	2004	2005	2006	2007
V.III	**ACCUMULATION ACCOUNTS**										
V.III.1	**CAPITAL ACCOUNT**										
	Changes in liabilities and net worth										
B.12	**Current external balance**	–HBOG	**21 854**	**25 787**	**21 102**	**18 657**	**18 307**	**25 200**	**32 691**	**45 031**	**52 568**
D.9	Capital transfers receivable										
D.92	Investment grants	NHSA	171	225	237	263	345	389	396	388	405
D.99	Other capital transfers	NHSB	570	538	1 506	833	693	637	1 816	2 038	784
D.9	Total	NHRZ	741	763	1 743	1 096	1 038	1 026	2 212	2 426	1 189
-D.9	*less* Capital transfers payable										
-D.92	Investment grants	–NHQQ	–332	–1 071	–569	–296	–624	–1 111	–1 482	–668	–857
-D.99	Other capital transfers	–NHQS	–1 144	–1 371	–2 589	–1 864	–1 951	–2 298	–2 491	–2 725	–2 953
-D.9	Total	–NHSC	–1 476	–2 442	–3 158	–2 160	–2 575	–3 409	–3 973	–3 393	–3 810
B.10.1	Total, change in net worth due to saving (current external balance)and capital transfers	NHSD	21 119	24 108	19 687	17 593	16 770	22 817	30 930	44 064	49 947
	Changes in assets										
K.2	Acquisitions less disposals of non-produced non-financial assets	NHSG	12	24	–97	–132	–71	–319	–258	8	20
B.9	**Net lending(+)/net borrowing(-)**	NHRB	**21 107**	**24 084**	**19 784**	**17 725**	**16 841**	**23 136**	**31 188**	**44 056**	**49 927**
Total	Total change in assets	NHSD	21 119	24 108	19 687	17 593	16 770	22 817	30 930	44 064	49 947

7.1.8 Rest of the world
ESA95 sector S.2 Unconsolidated

£ million

			1999	2000	2001	2002	2003	2004	2005	2006	2007
III.2	**FINANCIAL ACCOUNT**										
F.A	**Net acquisition of financial assets**										
F.1	Monetary gold and special drawing rights	NEWJ	374	956	808	240	2	37	8	−47	50
F.2	Currency and deposits										
F.21	Currency	NEWN	85	75	−57	86	81	133	64	87	47
F.22	Transferable deposits										
F.2211	Sterling deposits with UK banks	NWXP	19 212	32 466	16 297	10 992	22 840	26 775	45 858	56 878	216 324
F.2212	Foreign currency deposits with UK banks	NFAS	−13 158	166 168	104 862	77 472	148 376	261 474	232 394	276 418	471 475
F.2213	Sterling deposits with UK building societies	NEWS	542	567	523	308	487	305	1 296	621	261
F.29	Other deposits	NEWU	693	528	−178	−24	232	−877	−57	474	−299
F.2	Total currency and deposits	NEWM	7 374	199 804	121 447	88 834	172 016	287 810	279 555	334 478	687 808
F.3	Securities other than shares										
F.331	Short term: money market instruments										
F.3311	Issued by UK central government	NEWX	410	−251	304	−180	2 150	1 973	−1 023	747	3 546
F.3315	Issued by UK monetary financial institutions	NEXC	13 540	38 265	19 079	18 960	335	7 976	−4 521	45 243	14 942
F.3316	Issued by other UK residents	NEXH	1 783	2 700	237	10 819	−4 323	183	−2 624	−3 471	2 904
F.332	Medium (1 to 5 year) and long term (over 5 year) bonds										
F.3321	Issued by UK central government	NEXK	−5 281	−300	−674	−3 636	11 197	12 617	30 689	24 895	25 322
F.3322	Issued by UK local authorities	NEXN	–	–	–	–	–	–	–	–	–
F.33251	Medium term bonds issued by UK banks	NEXP	4 244	891	3 425	1 706	12 117	16 525	19 240	26 148	34 587
F.33252	Medium term bonds issued by building societies	NEXQ	252	1 814	630	69	1 754	2 222	3 498	−113	1 910
F.3326	Other medium & long term bonds issued by UK residents	NEXR	27 080	8 284	2 845	20 316	63 687	56 301	80 002	75 328	113 279
F.3	Total securities other than shares	NEWV	42 028	51 403	25 846	48 054	86 917	97 797	125 261	168 777	196 490
F.4	Loans										
F.41	Short term loans										
F.4191	Loans by rest of the world monetary financial institutions	NEYD	−671	−3 707	43 961	12 924	39 859	94 693	23 259	84 268	−860
F.4192	Other Short-term loans by Rest of the World	ZMDZ	47 453	38 924	71 767	−38 798	30 857	42 108	183 664	−37 885	46 908
F.42	Long term loans										
F.4211	Outward direct investment	NEYG	13 068	29 481	13 467	39 286	12 453	18 815	30 025	26 801	23 906
F.4212	Inward direct investment	NEYH	17 043	12 207	17 705	11 159	474	−461	14 383	9 709	2 369
F.429	Other long-term loans by the rest of the world	QYLT	−120	−293	17	−30	124	904	94	228	−12
F.4	Total loans	NEXX	76 773	76 612	146 917	24 541	83 767	156 059	251 425	83 121	72 311
F.5	Shares and other equity										
F.51	Shares and other equity, excluding mutual funds' shares										
F.514	Quoted UK shares	NEYU	88 999	129 926	8 507	2 754	12 891	4 370	60 809	32 480	30 938
F.515	Unquoted UK shares	NEYV	25 810	60 303	26 389	13 849	18 691	20 315	41 477	34 469	61 600
F.516	Other UK equity (including direct investment in property)	NEYW	813	1 629	791	748	395	623	597	467	2 358
F.517	UK shares and bonds issued by other UK residents	NSPR	–	–	–	–	–	–	–	–	–
F.52	Mutual funds' shares										
F.521	UK mutual funds' shares	NEZD	3	43	5	8	4	28	49	50	22
F.5	Total shares and other equity	NEYP	115 625	191 901	35 692	17 359	31 981	25 336	102 932	67 466	94 918
F.6	Insurance technical reserves										
F.61	Net equity of households in life assurance and pension funds' reserves	NEZF	−2	−4	−5	−1	−12	−11	−55	−9	−37
F.62	Prepayments of insurance premiums and reserves for outstanding claims	NEZI	−602	942	−157	335	−1 371	232	725	1 183	−20
F.6	Total insurance technical reserves	NPWP	−604	938	−162	334	−1 383	221	670	1 174	−57
F.7	Other accounts receivable	NEZJ	−135	−90	526	−613	58	−158	158	57	245
F.A	**Total net acquisition of financial assets**	NEWI	241 435	521 524	331 074	178 749	373 358	567 102	760 009	655 026	1 051 765

7.1.8 Rest of the world
ESA95 sector S.2 Unconsolidated

continued

£ million

		1999	2000	2001	2002	2003	2004	2005	2006	2007
III.2	**FINANCIAL ACCOUNT** continued									
F.L	**Net acquisition of financial liabilities**									
F.2	Currency and deposits									
F.21	Currency	NEZR	−23	−16	−3	54	30	46	14	137	10
F.22	Transferable deposits										
F.229	Deposits with rest of the world monetary financial institutions[1]	NEZX	27 280	187 527	122 793	53 299	190 273	212 831	367 335	278 279	508 210
F.2	Total currency and deposits	NEZQ	27 257	187 511	122 790	53 353	190 303	212 877	367 349	278 416	508 220
F.3	Securities other than shares										
F.331	Short term: money market instruments										
F.3319	Issued by the rest of the world[1]	NFAM	13 930	−2 551	11 493	−6 133	12 224	−2 634	7 377	14 543	−1 922
F.332	Medium (1 to 5 year) and long term (over 5 year) bonds										
F.3329	Long term bonds issued by the rest of the world	NFAW	−10 300	53 299	30 261	9 900	818	88 342	84 672	101 268	68 455
F.34	Financial derivatives	NSUL	−2 685	−1 503	−8 412	−1 159	5 211	7 857	−9 211	−7 759	18 980
F.3	Total securities other than shares	NEZZ	945	49 245	33 342	2 608	18 253	93 565	82 838	108 052	85 513
F.4	Loans										
F.41	Short term loans										
F.4111	Sterling loans by UK banks	NFBE	2 590	1 896	4 796	4 736	460	6 889	20 214	22 120	26 218
F.4112	Foreign currency loans by UK banks	NFBF	14 632	53 028	43 294	12 778	70 529	105 146	115 010	97 294	200 311
F.4113	Sterling loans by UK building societies	NFBG	–	–	1	3	2	3	2	−1	−1
F.42	Long term loans										
F.4211	Outward direct investment	NFBK	15 323	11 750	10 225	16 530	11 961	18 059	13 657	2 344	43 066
F.4212	Inward direct investment	NFBL	13 284	2 767	1 066	10 054	−3 049	2 916	12 013	12 806	7 261
F.423	Finance leasing	NFBQ	–	–	–	–	–	–	–	–	–
F.424	Other long-term loans by UK residents	NSRT	−347	−1 495	28	−1 458	−292	−122	−1 657	−3 356	−701
F.4	Total loans	NFBB	45 482	67 946	59 410	42 643	79 611	132 891	159 239	131 207	276 154
F.5	Shares and other equity										
F.51	Shares and other equity, excluding mutual funds' shares										
F.519	Shares and other equity issued by the rest of the world	NFCD	137 968	193 618	88 797	55 592	61 972	107 366	119 152	93 054	142 395
F.52	Mutual funds' shares										
F.529	Rest of the world mutual funds' shares	NFCI	70	63	33	−8	41	536	1 810	783	−110
F.5	Total shares and other equity	NFBT	138 038	193 681	88 830	55 584	62 013	107 902	120 962	93 837	142 285
F.7	Other accounts payable	NFCN	208	8	−492	357	625	303	−960	1 639	−237
F.L	**Total net acquisition of financial liabilities**	NEZM	211 930	498 391	303 880	154 545	350 805	547 538	729 428	613 151	1 011 935
B.9	**Net lending / borrowing**										
F.A	Total net acquisition of financial assets	NEWI	241 435	521 524	331 074	178 749	373 358	567 102	760 009	655 026	1 051 765
-F.L	*less* Total net acquisition of financial liabilities	−NEZM	−211 930	−498 391	−303 880	−154 545	−350 805	−547 538	−729 428	−613 151	−1 011 935
B.9f	Net lending (+) / net borrowing (-), from financial account	NYOD	29 505	23 133	27 194	24 204	22 553	19 564	30 581	41 875	39 830
dB.9f	Statistical discrepancy	NYPO	−8 398	951	−7 410	−6 479	−5 712	3 572	607	2 181	10 097
B.9	**Net lending (+) / net borrowing (-), from capital account**	NHRB	**21 107**	**24 084**	**19 784**	**17 725**	**16 841**	**23 136**	**31 188**	**44 056**	**49 927**

1 There is a discontinuity in this series between 1995 and 1996 because an instrument breakdown of offical reserves is not available prior to 1996

7.1.9 Rest of the world
ESA95 sector S.2 Unconsolidated

£ billion

			1999	2000	2001	2002	2003	2004	2005	2006	2007
IV.3	**FINANCIAL BALANCE SHEET** at end of period										
AF.A	**Financial assets**										
AF.2	Currency and deposits										
AF.21	Currency	NLCW	1.1	1.1	1.1	1.2	1.3	1.4	1.5	1.5	1.6
AF.22	Transferable deposits										
AF.2211	Sterling deposits with UK banks	NLCZ	167.5	200.5	215.9	228.0	251.7	279.6	331.3	389.0	604.6
AF.2212	Foreign curency deposits with UK banks	NLDA	859.4	1 060.0	1 152.4	1 206.5	1 348.1	1 570.0	1 861.5	1 974.2	2 531.0
AF.2213	Sterling deposits with UK building societies	NLDB	5.2	4.1	4.6	4.9	5.4	5.7	6.9	7.6	7.8
AF.29	Other deposits	NLDD	1.3	1.8	1.7	1.6	1.9	1.0	0.9	1.4	1.1
AF.2	Total currency and deposits	NLCV	1 034.5	1 267.5	1 375.6	1 442.2	1 608.4	1 857.7	2 202.1	2 373.7	3 146.1
AF.3	Securities other than shares										
AF.331	Short term: money market instruments										
AF.3311	Issued by UK central government	NLDG	0.1	–	0.1	0.2	1.9	3.8	2.8	3.5	7.2
AF.3315	Issued by UK monetary financial institutions	NLDL	67.2	111.0	133.1	140.3	130.6	130.7	136.1	162.5	182.0
AF.3316	Issued by other UK residents	NLDQ	17.8	21.7	22.5	30.6	23.7	22.5	22.2	16.3	19.1
AF.332	Medium (1 to 5 year) and long term (over 5 year) bonds										
AF.3321	Issued by UK central government	NLDT	60.9	62.4	59.9	56.4	66.1	83.8	110.7	135.5	158.2
AF.3322	Issued by UK local authorities	NLDW	–	–	–	–	–	–	–	–	–
AF.33251	Medium term bonds issued by UK banks	NLDY	33.5	35.8	39.2	40.4	49.5	64.5	85.6	105.0	155.2
AF.33252	Medium term bonds issued by UK building societies	NLDZ	1.2	2.6	3.3	3.2	4.2	6.4	9.9	9.9	11.7
AF.3326	Other medium & long term bonds issued by UK residents	NLEA	145.2	171.3	188.6	228.9	295.7	361.8	464.0	531.2	605.9
AF.3	Total securities other than shares	NLDE	326.0	404.8	446.6	499.9	571.8	673.6	831.2	963.8	1 139.4
AF.4	Loans										
AF.41	Short term loans										
AF.4191	Loans by rest of the world monetary financial institutions	NLEM	122.2	120.6	152.6	166.1	212.0	302.8	343.0	430.1	436.8
AF.4192	Other short-term loans by rest of the World	ZMEA	225.8	248.3	318.0	280.9	308.3	343.8	538.3	466.4	528.4
AF.42	Long term loans										
AF.4211	Outward direct investment	NLEP	64.4	84.3	97.4	128.4	127.7	149.0	184.5	189.8	213.7
AF.4212	Inward direct investment	NLEQ	102.8	112.2	142.5	155.6	152.9	156.1	174.2	186.6	188.9
AF.429	Other long-term loans by the rest of the world	NLEX	2.0	2.1	2.1	2.0	2.2	3.2	3.2	3.4	3.3
AF.4	Total loans	NLEG	517.1	567.5	712.5	733.0	803.0	954.9	1 243.2	1 276.2	1 371.2
AF.5	Shares and other equity										
AF.51	Shares and other equity, excluding mutual funds' shares										
AF.514	Quoted UK shares	NLFD	588.6	641.8	543.1	418.7	500.4	549.9	654.7	738.9	775.7
AF.515	Unquoted UK shares	NLFE	204.6	257.4	285.3	236.5	255.4	273.4	348.7	451.9	551.6
AF.516	Other UK equity (including direct investment in property)	NLFF	11.7	13.5	14.1	15.9	15.9	17.8	18.4	20.2	24.8
AF.517	UK shares and bonds issued by other UK residents	NSOP	–	–	–	–	–	–	–	–	–
AF.52	Mutual funds' shares										
AF.521	UK mutual funds' shares	NLFM	1.7	1.6	1.3	0.9	1.0	1.2	1.5	1.7	1.7
AF.5	Total shares and other equity	NLEY	806.5	914.3	843.8	671.9	772.8	842.3	1 023.2	1 212.7	1 353.7
AF.6	Insurance technical reserves										
AF.61	Net equity of households in life assurance and pension funds' reserves	NLFO	0.2	0.2	0.2	0.2	0.2	0.2	0.2	0.2	0.2
AF.62	Prepayments of insurance premiums and reserves for outstanding claims	NLFR	14.1	10.8	10.7	12.6	10.2	11.3	14.2	18.2	18.2
AF.6	Total insurance technical reserves	NPYF	14.3	11.0	10.9	12.9	10.4	11.5	14.4	18.4	18.4
AF.7	Other accounts receivable	NLFS	2.2	2.1	2.7	2.0	1.9	1.7	2.0	1.9	2.2
AF.A	**Total financial assets**	NLEF	2 700.6	3 167.3	3 392.2	3 361.9	3 768.3	4 341.8	5 316.2	5 846.7	7 031.0

7.1.9 Rest of the world
ESA95 sector S.2 Unconsolidated

continued

£ billion

			1999	2000	2001	2002	2003	2004	2005	2006	2007
IV.3	**FINANCIAL BALANCE SHEET** continued at end of period										
AF.L	**Financial liabilities**										
AF.2	Currency and deposits										
AF.21	Currency	**NLGA**	0.5	0.5	0.5	0.5	0.6	0.6	0.6	0.7	0.8
AF.22	Transferable deposits										
AF.229	Deposits with rest of the world monetary financial institutions[1]	**NLGG**	870.9	1 087.2	1 185.8	1 203.3	1 399.9	1 605.5	2 055.1	2 189.5	2 760.6
AF.2	Total currency and deposits	**NLFZ**	871.3	1 087.7	1 186.3	1 203.9	1 400.5	1 606.1	2 055.7	2 190.2	2 761.4
AF.3	Securities other than shares										
AF.331	Short term: money market instruments										
AF.3319	Issued by the rest of the world[1]	**NLGV**	44.3	45.3	56.7	48.7	62.0	58.5	64.1	75.6	77.1
AF.332	Medium (1 to 5 year) and long term (over 5 year) bonds										
AF.3329	Long term bonds issued by the rest of the world	**NLHF**	392.4	478.6	523.7	538.2	550.1	611.3	717.2	796.0	905.1
AF.34	Financial Derivatives	**NLEC**	–	0.1	0.4	0.2	–	0.1	0.4	–	0.1
AF.3	Total securities other than shares	**NLGI**	436.6	524.0	580.7	587.1	612.1	669.9	781.6	871.5	982.2
AF.4	Loans										
AF.41	Short term loans										
AF.4111	Sterling loans by UK banks	**NLHN**	26.1	27.5	32.2	37.4	40.2	47.4	66.9	87.7	113.1
AF.4112	Foreign currency loans by UK banks	**NLHO**	189.1	252.4	290.9	290.9	358.3	448.9	575.6	621.3	842.8
AF.4113	Sterling loans by UK building societies	**NLHP**	–	–	–	–	–	–	–	–	–
AF.42	Long term loans										
AF.4211	Outward direct investment	**NLHT**	81.6	88.6	101.2	114.5	116.3	144.5	145.6	148.2	191.3
AF.4212	Inward direct investment	**NLHU**	51.9	53.4	56.3	61.6	59.0	61.0	77.0	81.3	88.6
AF.423	Finance leasing	**NLHZ**	–	–	–	–	–	–	–	–	–
AF.424	Other long-term loans by UK residents	**NROS**	10.2	8.6	8.8	7.3	7.2	7.3	7.3	6.1	6.3
AF.4	Total loans	**NLHK**	359.0	430.6	489.4	511.8	580.9	709.2	872.3	944.6	1 242.1
AF.5	Shares and other equity										
AF.51	Shares and other equity, excluding mutual funds' shares										
AF.519	Shares and other equity issued by the rest of the world	**NLIM**	836.6	1 020.8	992.2	931.3	1 049.0	1 128.8	1 348.3	1 456.3	1 651.0
AF.52	Mutual funds' shares										
AF.529	Rest of the world mutual funds' shares	**NLIR**	2.1	1.7	1.7	1.4	1.4	1.7	4.1	6.0	3.5
AF.5	Total shares and other equity	**NLIC**	838.7	1 022.5	993.9	932.7	1 050.4	1 130.5	1 352.4	1 462.3	1 654.5
AF.7	Other accounts payable	**NLIW**	2.7	3.3	3.0	4.1	4.8	3.6	2.7	3.8	4.9
AF.L	**Total financial liabilities**	**NLHJ**	2 508.4	3 068.1	3 253.2	3 239.6	3 648.6	4 119.3	5 064.9	5 472.6	6 645.1
BF.90	**Net financial assets / liabilities**										
AF.A	Total financial assets	**NLEF**	2 700.6	3 167.3	3 392.2	3 361.9	3 768.3	4 341.8	5 316.2	5 846.7	7 031.0
-AF.L	less Total financial liabilities	**–NLHJ**	–2 508.4	–3 068.1	–3 253.2	–3 239.6	–3 648.6	–4 119.3	–5 064.9	–5 472.6	–6 645.1
BF.90	**Net financial assets (+) / liabilities (-)**	**NLFK**	192.2	99.2	138.9	122.4	119.7	222.4	251.3	374.1	385.9

1 There is a discontinuity in this series between 1995 and 1996 because an instrument breakdown of official reserves is not available prior to 1996

Other analyses and derived statistics

Part 4

Chapter 8

Percentage distributions and growth rates

8.1 Composition of UK gross domestic product at market prices
By category of expenditure[1]

Current prices

		1999	2000	2001	2002	2003	2004	2005	2006	2007
	Gross domestic product: expenditure approach									
P.3	Final consumption expenditure									
P.41	Actual individual consumption									
P.3	Household final consumption expenditure	62.7	63.1	63.4	63.3	62.7	62.3	62.3	61.6	61.3
P.3	Final consumption expenditure of NPISH	2.4	2.4	2.5	2.5	2.4	2.4	2.4	2.4	2.5
P.31	Individual government final consumption expenditure	11.1	11.2	11.6	12.2	12.6	12.4	12.8	13.1	13.1
P.41	Total actual individual consumption	76.2	76.7	77.4	77.9	77.8	77.1	77.5	77.2	76.8
P.32	Collective government final consumption expenditure	7.2	7.4	7.4	7.6	7.8	8.6	8.6	8.5	8.1
P.3	Total final consumption expenditure	83.4	84.2	84.9	85.5	85.6	85.6	86.2	85.7	85.0
P.3	Households and NPISH	65.1	65.5	65.9	65.8	65.1	64.7	64.7	64.1	63.8
P.3	Central government	11.2	11.3	11.6	12.1	12.5	12.7	12.9	13.2	12.9
P.3	Local government	7.1	7.3	7.4	7.6	7.9	8.3	8.5	8.5	8.3
P.5	Gross capital formation									
P.51	Gross fixed capital formation	17.4	17.1	16.8	16.8	16.4	16.7	16.9	17.2	17.8
P.52	Changes in inventories	0.7	0.5	0.6	0.3	0.3	0.4	0.4	0.3	0.6
P.53	Acquisitions less disposals of valuables	–	–	–	–	–	–	–	–	–
P.5	Total gross capital formation	18.1	17.7	17.5	17.1	16.7	17.1	17.2	17.6	18.4
P.6	Exports of goods and services	26.1	27.6	27.1	26.1	25.5	25.3	26.4	28.5	26.3
-P.7	*less* imports of goods and services	−27.6	−29.5	−29.4	−28.7	−27.8	−28.0	−29.8	−31.7	−29.7
B.11	External balance of goods and services	−1.5	−1.8	−2.3	−2.6	−2.3	−2.7	−3.4	−3.3	−3.4
de	Statistical discrepancy between expenditure components and GDP	–	–	–	–	–	–	–	–	–
B.1*g	Gross domestic product at market prices	100.0	100.0	100.0	100.0	100.0	100.0	100.0	100.0	100.0

1 Based on table 1.2

8.2 Composition of UK gross domestic product at market prices
By category of income[1,2]

		1999	2000	2001	2002	2003	2004	2005	2006	2007
B.2g	Total gross operating surplus									
	Public non-financial corporations	0.8	0.7	0.7	0.6	0.6	0.6	0.7	0.7	0.7
	Private non-financial corporations	19.0	18.6	17.9	17.5	17.6	17.9	17.7	17.9	18.1
	Financial corporations	1.9	1.1	1.3	2.5	2.9	2.7	2.6	2.8	3.3
	Central government	0.6	0.6	0.5	0.5	0.5	0.5	0.5	0.5	0.6
	Local government	0.4	0.4	0.4	0.4	0.4	0.4	0.5	0.5	0.5
	Households and NPISH	4.9	5.0	5.2	5.2	5.4	5.4	5.5	5.4	5.7
B.2g	Total gross operating surplus	27.6	26.5	26.0	26.8	27.5	27.6	27.5	27.9	28.8
B.3	Mixed income	5.9	5.8	6.0	6.0	6.0	6.1	6.0	6.0	6.0
D.1	Compensation of employees	53.4	54.5	55.2	54.6	54.1	54.0	54.5	54.1	53.2
D.2	Taxes on production and imports[2]	13.8	13.9	13.5	13.3	13.2	13.2	13.0	13.0	12.9
-D.3	Subsidies on products	−0.8	−0.7	−0.7	−0.7	−0.8	−0.8	−0.9	−0.9	−0.9
di	Statistical discrepancy between income components and GDP	–	–	–	–	–	–	–	–	0.1
B.1*g	Gross domestic product	100.0	100.0	100.0	100.0	100.0	100.0	100.0	100.0	100.0

1 Based on table 1.2
2 Includes taxes on products

8.3 Gross value added at current basic prices analysed by industry[1,2,3]

Percentage

	1999	2000	2001	2002	2003	2004	2005	2006
Agriculture, hunting, forestry and fishing	1.1	1.0	0.9	0.9	1.0	1.0	0.7	0.7
Mining and quarrying	2.1	2.8	2.5	2.3	2.1	2.1	2.5	2.7
Manufacturing	18.4	17.4	16.4	15.3	14.3	13.8	13.3	13.0
Electricity, gas and water supply	1.9	1.8	1.7	1.7	1.6	1.6	1.5	1.6
Construction	5.1	5.3	5.6	5.7	5.9	6.0	6.1	6.3
Wholesale and retail trade; repairs; hotels and restaurants	15.0	14.9	15.1	14.9	14.8	14.9	14.6	14.4
Transport, storage and communication	7.9	8.0	7.8	7.6	7.5	7.5	7.2	6.9
Financial intermediation, real estate, renting and business activities	27.0	27.0	27.8	29.1	29.9	30.1	30.4	31.0
Public administration, national defence and compulsory social security	5.0	4.9	5.0	5.0	5.1	5.2	5.4	5.4
Education, health and social work	11.7	12.0	12.3	12.5	12.7	12.7	13.0	12.8
Other services[4]	4.8	4.9	4.9	5.0	5.1	5.2	5.4	5.2
Gross value added at basic prices	100.0	100.0	100.0	100.0	100.0	100.0	100.0	100.0

1 Based on Table 2.2.
2 Before providing for consumption of fixed capital.
3 See footnote 2 to Table 2.3.
4 Comprising sections O,P, Q of the SIC(92).

8.4 Annual increases in categories of expenditure (chained volume measures)

Percentage increase over previous year

		1999	2000	2001	2002	2003	2004	2005	2006	2007
P.3	Household final consumption expenditure	5.4	4.5	3.2	3.7	3.1	3.1	2.0	2.0	3.0
P.3	NPISH final consumption expenditure	−0.2	8.7	0.1	–	0.3	−1.7	0.1	4.0	3.5
P.3	General government final consumption	3.6	3.1	2.4	3.4	3.5	3.4	1.7	1.6	1.8
P.5	Gross fixed capital formation:									
	Private sector	4.0	4.2	1.6	4.0	1.9	7.2	4.2	8.3	9.6
	Public non-financial corporations	−17.8	−13.2	35.2	20.3	−51.5	−32.1	1 533.0	−73.6	13.8
	General government	5.8	−3.0	10.7	14.2	32.7	13.2	−69.5	233.8	6.5
	Total	3.0	2.7	2.6	3.6	1.1	4.9	2.2	6.0	7.1
P.6	Exports of goods and services	3.7	9.1	3.0	1.0	1.8	4.8	8.1	11.0	−4.5
P.7	Imports of goods and services	7.9	8.9	4.8	4.9	2.2	6.8	7.0	9.6	−1.9
B.1*g	Gross domestic product at market prices	3.5	3.9	2.5	2.1	2.8	2.8	2.1	2.8	3.0

8.5 Aggregates related to gross national income[1]

Percentage of gross national income

		1999	2000	2001	2002	2003	2004	2005	2006	2007
D.2	Taxes on production and imports[2]	13.9	13.9	13.4	13.1	13.0	13.0	12.7	12.9	12.8
D.5	Current taxes on income wealth etc	16.1	16.4	16.5	15.3	14.7	15.0	15.9	16.8	16.5
D.61	Compulsory social contributions[3]	6.1	6.2	6.1	5.8	6.2	6.5	6.6	6.7	6.7
D.91	Capital taxes	0.2	0.2	0.2	0.2	0.2	0.2	0.2	0.3	0.3
	Paid to central government	34.3	34.6	34.2	32.4	32.2	32.7	33.5	34.7	34.2
	Paid to local government	1.4	1.4	1.5	1.5	1.6	1.7	1.7	1.7	1.7
	Paid to institutions of the European Union	0.6	0.6	0.6	0.4	0.4	0.3	0.3	0.3	0.3
	Total taxes	36.4	36.7	36.2	34.4	34.2	34.7	35.5	36.7	36.2
D.3	Subsidies	0.8	0.7	0.7	0.7	0.8	0.8	0.9	0.9	0.9

1 Based on tables 1.2, 11.1 and 7.1.8.
2 Including National Insurance surcharge.
3 Including employers', employees', self employed and non-employed persons contributions

8.6 Rates of change of gross domestic product at current market prices ('money GDP')

Percentage change, at annual rate

Terminal year

Initial year	1966	1967	1968	1969	1970	1971	1972	1973	1974	1975	1976	1977	1978	1979	1980	1981	1982	1983	1984	1985	1986
1965	6.4	5.9	6.7	7.0	7.6	8.2	8.8	9.6	10.0	11.5	12.1	12.5	12.7	13.0	13.3	13.1	12.9	12.7	12.4	12.2	12.0
1966		5.5	6.9	7.2	7.9	8.6	9.2	10.0	10.4	12.1	12.7	13.0	13.2	13.5	13.8	13.5	13.3	13.0	12.7	12.6	12.3
1967			8.4	8.0	8.7	9.4	9.9	10.8	11.2	13.0	13.5	13.8	13.9	14.2	14.5	14.1	13.8	13.5	13.2	13.0	12.7
1968				7.7	8.8	9.7	10.3	11.3	11.6	13.6	14.2	14.4	14.5	14.8	15.0	14.6	14.2	13.9	13.5	13.2	12.9
1969					9.9	10.7	11.2	12.2	12.4	14.6	15.2	15.3	15.3	15.5	15.7	15.2	14.7	14.3	13.9	13.6	13.2
1970						11.6	11.8	13.0	13.1	15.6	16.0	16.1	16.0	16.2	16.3	15.7	15.2	14.7	14.2	13.8	13.4
1971							12.1	13.7	13.6	16.6	17.0	16.9	16.6	16.8	16.8	16.1	15.5	15.0	14.4	14.0	13.6
1972								15.4	14.4	18.2	18.2	17.9	17.4	17.4	17.4	16.5	15.8	15.2	14.6	14.2	13.7
1973									13.4	19.6	19.2	18.5	17.8	17.8	17.7	16.7	15.9	15.2	14.6	14.1	13.6
1974										26.3	22.2	20.3	19.0	18.7	18.4	17.2	16.2	15.4	14.6	14.1	13.6
1975											18.3	17.4	16.6	16.9	16.9	15.7	14.8	14.1	13.4	13.0	12.5
1976												16.4	15.8	16.4	16.6	15.2	14.3	13.5	12.8	12.4	11.9
1977													15.2	16.4	16.6	14.9	13.8	13.1	12.2	11.9	11.4
1978														17.6	17.3	14.8	13.5	12.7	11.8	11.5	11.0
1979															17.0	13.4	12.2	11.4	10.6	10.5	10.0
1980																9.9	9.8	9.6	9.1	9.2	8.9
1981																	9.7	9.5	8.8	9.0	8.7
1982																		9.3	8.3	8.8	8.5
1983																			7.4	8.5	8.2
1984																				9.7	8.6
1985																					7.6

Terminal year

Initial year	1987	1988	1989	1990	1991	1992	1993	1994	1995	1996	1997	1998	1999	2000	2001	2002	2003	2004	2005	2006	2007
1965	11.9	11.9	11.8	11.7	11.4	11.1	10.9	10.7	10.6	10.4	10.3	10.2	10.0	9.9	9.7	9.6	9.5	9.4	9.3	9.2	9.1
1966	12.2	12.2	12.1	11.9	11.6	11.3	11.1	10.9	10.7	10.6	10.4	10.3	10.2	10.0	9.8	9.7	9.6	9.5	9.4	9.3	9.2
1967	12.6	12.5	12.4	12.2	11.9	11.6	11.3	11.1	10.9	10.8	10.6	10.5	10.3	10.1	10.0	9.8	9.7	9.6	9.5	9.4	9.3
1968	12.8	12.7	12.6	12.4	12.1	11.7	11.4	11.2	11.0	10.9	10.7	10.5	10.4	10.2	10.0	9.9	9.8	9.6	9.5	9.4	9.3
1969	13.1	13.0	12.8	12.6	12.3	11.9	11.6	11.4	11.1	11.0	10.8	10.6	10.5	10.3	10.1	9.9	9.8	9.7	9.5	9.4	9.3
1970	13.3	13.2	13.0	12.8	12.4	12.0	11.7	11.4	11.2	11.0	10.8	10.6	10.5	10.3	10.1	9.9	9.8	9.7	9.5	9.4	9.3
1971	13.4	13.3	13.1	12.8	12.4	12.0	11.7	11.4	11.0	11.0	10.8	10.6	10.4	10.2	10.1	9.9	9.8	9.6	9.5	9.4	9.3
1972	13.4	13.3	13.1	12.9	12.4	12.0	11.7	11.4	11.1	10.9	10.8	10.6	10.4	10.0	10.0	9.8	9.7	9.6	9.4	9.3	9.2
1973	13.3	13.2	13.0	12.7	12.3	11.8	11.5	11.2	11.0	10.8	10.6	10.4	10.2	10.0	9.8	9.6	9.5	9.4	9.2	9.1	9.0
1974	13.3	13.2	13.0	12.7	12.2	11.7	11.4	11.1	10.8	10.6	10.4	10.3	10.1	9.9	9.7	9.5	9.4	9.2	9.1	9.0	8.9
1975	12.3	12.2	12.1	11.8	11.4	10.9	10.6	10.3	10.1	9.9	9.8	9.6	9.4	9.3	9.1	8.9	8.8	8.7	8.6	8.5	8.4
1976	11.8	11.7	11.6	11.4	10.9	10.5	10.2	9.9	9.7	9.5	9.4	9.2	9.1	8.9	8.7	8.6	8.5	8.4	8.2	8.1	8.1
1977	11.3	11.3	11.2	11.0	10.6	10.1	9.8	9.6	9.3	9.2	9.0	8.9	8.7	8.6	8.4	8.3	8.2	8.1	8.0	7.9	7.8
1978	10.9	10.9	10.8	10.6	10.2	9.7	9.4	9.2	9.0	8.9	8.7	8.6	8.4	8.3	8.1	8.0	7.9	7.8	7.7	7.6	7.6
1979	10.1	10.2	10.2	10.0	9.6	9.2	8.9	8.7	8.5	8.4	8.3	8.1	8.0	7.9	7.7	7.6	7.5	7.4	7.3	7.3	7.2
1980	9.1	9.4	9.4	9.4	8.9	8.5	8.3	8.1	7.9	7.9	7.8	7.7	7.5	7.4	7.3	7.2	7.1	7.1	7.0	6.9	6.9
1981	9.0	9.3	9.4	9.3	8.9	8.4	8.1	8.0	7.8	7.7	7.6	7.5	7.4	7.3	7.2	7.1	7.0	6.9	6.8	6.8	6.8
1982	8.8	9.3	9.3	9.2	8.8	8.3	8.0	7.8	7.7	7.6	7.5	7.4	7.3	7.2	7.0	6.9	6.9	6.8	6.7	6.7	6.6
1983	8.7	9.3	9.4	9.2	8.7	8.2	7.9	7.7	7.5	7.4	7.4	7.3	7.2	7.0	6.9	6.8	6.8	6.7	6.6	6.6	6.5
1984	9.1	9.7	9.7	9.6	8.9	8.3	7.9	7.7	7.5	7.5	7.4	7.3	7.1	7.0	6.9	6.8	6.7	6.7	6.6	6.5	6.5
1985	8.9	9.8	9.8	9.5	8.8	8.1	7.7	7.5	7.3	7.3	7.2	7.1	7.0	6.8	6.7	6.6	6.6	6.5	6.4	6.4	6.3
1986	10.2	10.9	10.5	10.0	9.0	8.1	7.7	7.5	7.3	7.2	7.1	7.0	6.9	6.8	6.6	6.6	6.5	6.5	6.3	6.3	6.3
1987		11.6	10.7	10.0	8.7	7.7	7.3	7.1	6.9	6.9	6.8	6.7	6.7	6.5	6.4	6.3	6.3	6.2	6.1	6.1	6.1
1988			9.8	9.2	7.8	6.8	6.5	6.4	6.3	6.3	6.3	6.3	6.2	6.1	6.0	6.0	6.0	5.9	5.8	5.8	5.8
1989				8.6	6.8	5.8	5.6	5.7	5.8	5.9	5.9	5.9	5.9	5.8	5.7	5.7	5.7	5.7	5.6	5.6	5.6
1990					5.0	4.4	4.7	5.0	5.2	5.4	5.5	5.6	5.6	5.5	5.4	5.4	5.5	5.5	5.4	5.4	5.4
1991						3.9	4.5	5.0	5.2	5.5	5.6	5.6	5.6	5.6	5.5	5.5	5.5	5.5	5.4	5.4	5.5
1992							5.2	5.5	5.6	5.9	5.9	5.9	5.9	5.8	5.7	5.6	5.7	5.6	5.5	5.5	5.6
1993								5.9	6.1	6.1	6.1	6.0	5.9	5.7	5.7	5.7	5.7	5.6	5.6	5.6	5.6
1994									5.8	6.2	6.2	6.1	6.0	5.9	5.7	5.6	5.7	5.6	5.5	5.5	5.6
1995										6.6	6.4	6.2	6.1	5.9	5.7	5.6	5.7	5.6	5.5	5.5	5.5
1996											6.2	6.0	5.9	5.7	5.5	5.5	5.5	5.5	5.4	5.4	5.4
1997												5.9	5.8	5.6	5.3	5.3	5.4	5.4	5.3	5.3	5.4
1998													5.6	5.4	5.1	5.2	5.3	5.3	5.2	5.2	5.3
1999														5.1	4.9	5.0	5.3	5.3	5.1	5.2	5.3
2000															4.6	4.9	5.3	5.5	5.2	5.3	5.3
2001																5.3	5.6	5.5	5.2	5.3	5.4
2002																	6.0	5.7	5.2	5.3	5.4
2003																		5.3	4.8	5.1	5.3
2004																			4.3	4.9	5.3
2005																				5.5	5.8
2006																					6.0

8.7 Rates of change of gross domestic product (Chained volume measures)

Percentage change, at annual rate

Terminal year

Initial year	1966	1967	1968	1969	1970	1971	1972	1973	1974	1975	1976	1977	1978	1979	1980	1981	1982	1983	1984	1985	1986
1965	1.9	2.2	2.9	2.7	2.6	2.5	2.7	3.2	2.7	2.4	2.4	2.4	2.5	2.5	2.2	1.9	1.9	2.0	2.1	2.1	2.2
1966		2.5	3.3	2.9	2.7	2.6	2.8	3.4	2.8	2.4	2.4	2.4	2.5	2.5	2.2	1.9	1.9	2.0	2.1	2.2	2.3
1967			4.2	3.1	2.8	2.6	2.8	3.6	2.9	2.4	2.4	2.4	2.5	2.5	2.2	1.9	1.9	2.0	2.1	2.1	2.2
1968				2.1	2.2	2.1	2.5	3.4	2.6	2.2	2.2	2.2	2.3	2.4	2.0	1.7	1.8	1.9	1.9	2.0	2.1
1969					2.2	2.2	2.7	3.8	2.7	2.2	2.2	2.3	2.4	2.4	2.0	1.7	1.7	1.9	1.9	2.0	2.1
1970						2.1	2.9	4.3	2.9	2.2	2.2	2.3	2.4	2.4	2.0	1.6	1.7	1.8	1.9	2.0	2.1
1971							3.7	5.4	3.1	2.2	2.3	2.3	2.4	2.5	1.9	1.6	1.6	1.8	1.9	2.0	2.1
1972								7.2	2.9	1.7	1.9	2.0	2.2	2.3	1.7	1.4	1.5	1.6	1.7	1.9	2.0
1973									-1.3	-1.0	0.2	0.8	1.2	1.5	1.0	0.7	0.8	1.1	1.2	1.4	1.6
1974										-0.6	1.0	1.5	1.9	2.1	1.3	1.0	1.1	1.4	1.5	1.7	1.9
1975											2.6	2.5	2.7	2.7	1.7	1.2	1.4	1.6	1.7	1.9	2.1
1976												2.4	2.8	2.8	1.5	1.0	1.1	1.5	1.6	1.9	2.1
1977													3.2	3.0	1.2	0.6	0.9	1.3	1.5	1.8	2.0
1978														2.7	0.3	-0.3	0.3	1.0	1.3	1.6	1.9
1979															-2.1	-1.7	-0.5	0.6	1.0	1.4	1.8
1980																-1.3	0.4	1.4	1.7	2.1	2.4
1981																	2.1	2.9	2.8	3.0	3.2
1982																		3.6	3.1	3.3	3.5
1983																			2.7	3.1	3.4
1984																				3.6	3.8
1985																					4.0

Terminal year

Initial year	1987	1988	1989	1990	1991	1992	1993	1994	1995	1996	1997	1998	1999	2000	2001	2002	2003	2004	2005	2006	2007
1965	2.3	2.5	2.4	2.4	2.2	2.2	2.2	2.2	2.3	2.3	2.3	2.3	2.4	2.4	2.4	2.4	2.4	2.4	2.4	2.4	2.5
1966	2.4	2.5	2.5	2.4	2.2	2.2	2.2	2.2	2.3	2.3	2.3	2.4	2.4	2.4	2.4	2.4	2.4	2.5	2.4	2.5	2.5
1967	2.4	2.5	2.5	2.4	2.2	2.2	2.2	2.2	2.3	2.3	2.3	2.4	2.4	2.4	2.4	2.4	2.4	2.4	2.4	2.4	2.5
1968	2.3	2.4	2.4	2.3	2.2	2.1	2.1	2.2	2.2	2.2	2.3	2.3	2.3	2.4	2.4	2.4	2.4	2.4	2.4	2.4	2.4
1969	2.3	2.4	2.4	2.3	2.2	2.1	2.1	2.2	2.2	2.2	2.3	2.3	2.3	2.4	2.4	2.4	2.4	2.4	2.4	2.4	2.4
1970	2.3	2.4	2.4	2.3	2.2	2.1	2.1	2.2	2.2	2.2	2.3	2.3	2.3	2.4	2.4	2.4	2.4	2.4	2.4	2.4	2.4
1971	2.3	2.4	2.4	2.3	2.2	2.1	2.1	2.2	2.2	2.2	2.3	2.3	2.4	2.4	2.4	2.4	2.4	2.4	2.4	2.4	2.4
1972	2.2	2.4	2.4	2.3	2.1	2.0	2.0	2.1	2.1	2.2	2.2	2.3	2.3	2.4	2.4	2.4	2.4	2.4	2.4	2.4	2.4
1973	1.8	2.1	2.1	2.0	1.8	1.7	1.7	1.9	1.9	2.0	2.0	2.1	2.1	2.2	2.2	2.2	2.2	2.2	2.2	2.2	2.3
1974	2.1	2.3	2.3	2.2	2.0	1.9	1.9	2.0	2.1	2.1	2.2	2.2	2.3	2.3	2.3	2.3	2.3	2.4	2.3	2.4	2.4
1975	2.3	2.5	2.5	2.4	2.2	2.0	2.0	2.2	2.2	2.2	2.3	2.3	2.4	2.4	2.4	2.4	2.5	2.5	2.4	2.5	2.5
1976	2.3	2.5	2.5	2.4	2.1	2.0	2.0	2.1	2.2	2.2	2.3	2.3	2.4	2.4	2.4	2.4	2.4	2.5	2.4	2.5	2.5
1977	2.3	2.5	2.5	2.4	2.1	2.0	2.0	2.1	2.2	2.2	2.3	2.3	2.4	2.4	2.4	2.4	2.4	2.5	2.4	2.5	2.5
1978	2.2	2.5	2.4	2.3	2.0	1.9	1.9	2.1	2.1	2.2	2.2	2.3	2.3	2.4	2.4	2.4	2.4	2.4	2.4	2.4	2.4
1979	2.1	2.4	2.4	2.3	2.0	1.8	1.8	2.0	2.1	2.1	2.2	2.3	2.3	2.4	2.4	2.4	2.4	2.4	2.4	2.4	2.4
1980	2.7	3.0	2.9	2.7	2.3	2.2	2.2	2.3	2.4	2.4	2.4	2.5	2.6	2.6	2.6	2.6	2.6	2.6	2.6	2.6	2.6
1981	3.4	3.7	3.5	3.2	2.7	2.5	2.5	2.6	2.6	2.6	2.7	2.7	2.8	2.8	2.8	2.8	2.8	2.8	2.8	2.8	2.8
1982	3.7	3.9	3.7	3.3	2.8	2.5	2.5	2.6	2.7	2.7	2.7	2.8	2.8	2.9	2.9	2.8	2.8	2.8	2.8	2.8	2.8
1983	3.7	4.0	3.7	3.3	2.7	2.4	2.4	2.5	2.6	2.6	2.7	2.7	2.8	2.8	2.8	2.8	2.8	2.8	2.7	2.7	2.8
1984	4.1	4.3	3.9	3.4	2.7	2.4	2.3	2.5	2.6	2.6	2.7	2.7	2.8	2.8	2.8	2.8	2.8	2.8	2.7	2.8	2.8
1985	4.3	4.5	4.0	3.3	2.5	2.2	2.2	2.4	2.5	2.5	2.6	2.7	2.7	2.8	2.8	2.7	2.7	2.7	2.7	2.7	2.7
1986	4.6	4.8	4.0	3.1	2.2	1.9	1.9	2.2	2.3	2.4	2.5	2.6	2.7	2.7	2.7	2.7	2.7	2.7	2.6	2.6	2.7
1987		5.0	3.6	2.7	1.6	1.3	1.5	1.9	2.0	2.1	2.2	2.4	2.5	2.6	2.6	2.5	2.5	2.6	2.5	2.5	2.6
1988			2.3	1.5	0.5	0.4	0.8	1.4	1.6	1.8	1.9	2.1	2.2	2.4	2.4	2.4	2.4	2.4	2.4	2.4	2.4
1989				0.8	-0.3	-0.2	0.4	1.2	1.5	1.7	1.9	2.1	2.2	2.4	2.4	2.4	2.4	2.4	2.4	2.4	2.5
1990					-1.4	-0.6	0.3	1.3	1.6	1.8	2.1	2.2	2.4	2.5	2.5	2.5	2.5	2.5	2.5	2.5	2.6
1991						0.1	1.2	2.2	2.4	2.5	2.6	2.8	2.9	3.0	2.9	2.9	2.8	2.8	2.8	2.8	2.8
1992							2.2	3.2	3.2	3.1	3.1	3.2	3.3	3.3	3.2	3.1	3.1	3.1	3.0	3.0	3.0
1993								4.3	3.7	3.4	3.4	3.4	3.4	3.5	3.4	3.2	3.2	3.1	3.1	3.0	3.0
1994									3.0	3.1	3.1	3.2	3.3	3.4	3.2	3.1	3.1	3.0	2.9	2.9	2.9
1995										2.9	3.1	3.3	3.3	3.4	3.3	3.1	3.1	3.0	2.9	2.9	2.9
1996											3.3	3.5	3.5	3.6	3.4	3.1	3.1	3.1	2.9	2.9	2.9
1997												3.6	3.5	3.7	3.4	3.1	3.1	3.0	2.9	2.9	2.9
1998													3.5	3.7	3.3	3.0	3.0	2.9	2.8	2.8	2.8
1999														3.9	3.2	2.8	2.8	2.8	2.7	2.7	2.7
2000															2.5	2.3	2.5	2.5	2.4	2.5	2.6
2001																2.1	2.5	2.6	2.4	2.5	2.6
2002																	2.8	2.8	2.5	2.6	2.7
2003																		2.8	2.4	2.6	2.7
2004																			2.1	2.4	2.6
2005																				2.8	2.9
2006																					3.0

8.8 Rates of change of GDP at market prices (current prices) Per capita

Percentage change, at annual rate

Initial year	Terminal year																				
	1987	1988	1989	1990	1991	1992	1993	1994	1995	1996	1997	1998	1999	2000	2001	2002	2003	2004	2005	2006	2007
1986	9.9	10.7	10.3	9.8	8.7	7.9	7.4	7.2	7.0	6.9	6.9	6.7	6.6	6.5	6.3	6.3	6.2	6.1	6.0	6.0	5.9
1987		11.4	10.4	9.7	8.4	7.4	7.0	6.8	6.7	6.6	6.6	6.5	6.4	6.2	6.1	6.0	6.0	5.9	5.8	5.7	5.7
1988			9.5	8.9	7.4	6.5	6.2	6.1	6.0	6.0	6.0	6.0	5.9	5.8	5.7	5.6	5.6	5.6	5.5	5.4	5.4
1989				8.2	6.4	5.5	5.3	5.4	5.4	5.6	5.6	5.6	5.6	5.5	5.4	5.4	5.4	5.3	5.2	5.2	5.2
1990					4.6	4.1	4.4	4.7	4.9	5.1	5.2	5.3	5.3	5.2	5.1	5.1	5.2	5.1	5.0	5.0	5.0
1991						3.7	4.3	4.7	4.9	5.2	5.3	5.4	5.4	5.3	5.2	5.2	5.2	5.2	5.1	5.0	5.1
1992							4.9	5.3	5.4	5.6	5.7	5.7	5.6	5.5	5.4	5.3	5.3	5.3	5.2	5.1	5.2
1993								5.7	5.6	5.8	5.9	5.8	5.7	5.6	5.4	5.4	5.4	5.3	5.2	5.2	5.2
1994									5.5	5.9	5.9	5.8	5.7	5.6	5.4	5.3	5.3	5.3	5.1	5.1	5.1
1995										6.4	6.1	6.0	5.8	5.6	5.4	5.3	5.3	5.3	5.1	5.1	5.1
1996											5.9	5.8	5.6	5.4	5.2	5.1	5.2	5.1	5.0	5.0	5.0
1997												5.6	5.4	5.2	5.0	5.0	5.1	5.0	4.9	4.9	4.9
1998													5.3	5.0	4.8	4.8	4.9	4.9	4.7	4.8	4.8
1999														4.8	4.5	4.6	4.9	4.9	4.7	4.7	4.8
2000															4.2	4.6	4.9	4.9	4.6	4.7	4.8
2001																4.9	5.2	5.1	4.7	4.8	4.9
2002																	5.6	5.2	4.7	4.7	4.9
2003																		4.8	4.2	4.5	4.7
2004																			3.6	4.3	4.6
2005																				4.9	5.1
2006																					5.3

8.9 Rates of change of GDP at market prices (Chained volume measures) Per capita

Percentage change, at annual rate

Initial year	Terminal year																				
	1987	1988	1989	1990	1991	1992	1993	1994	1995	1996	1997	1998	1999	2000	2001	2002	2003	2004	2005	2006	2007
1986	4.3	4.6	3.7	2.9	2.0	1.6	1.7	2.0	2.0	2.1	2.2	2.3	2.3	2.4	2.4	2.4	2.4	2.4	2.3	2.3	2.3
1987		4.8	3.4	2.4	1.4	1.1	1.2	1.6	1.8	1.9	2.0	2.1	2.2	2.3	2.3	2.2	2.2	2.2	2.2	2.2	2.2
1988			2.0	1.2	0.2	0.2	0.5	1.1	1.3	1.5	1.7	1.8	1.9	2.1	2.1	2.1	2.1	2.1	2.0	2.1	2.1
1989				0.5	-0.6	-0.5	0.2	0.9	1.2	1.4	1.6	1.8	1.9	2.1	2.1	2.1	2.1	2.1	2.0	2.1	2.1
1990					-1.7	-0.9	0.0	1.0	1.4	1.6	1.8	2.0	2.1	2.2	2.2	2.2	2.2	2.2	2.2	2.2	2.2
1991						-0.1	0.9	2.0	2.2	2.2	2.4	2.5	2.6	2.7	2.6	2.6	2.5	2.5	2.4	2.4	2.4
1992							2.0	3.0	2.9	2.8	2.9	3.0	3.0	3.1	2.9	2.8	2.8	2.7	2.6	2.6	2.6
1993								4.0	3.4	3.1	3.1	3.1	3.1	3.2	3.1	2.9	2.9	2.8	2.7	2.7	2.6
1994									2.8	2.7	2.8	2.9	3.0	3.1	2.9	2.8	2.7	2.7	2.6	2.5	2.5
1995										2.6	2.8	3.0	3.0	3.1	3.0	2.8	2.7	2.7	2.6	2.5	2.5
1996											3.0	3.2	3.3	3.3	3.0	2.8	2.7	2.7	2.5	2.5	2.5
1997												3.3	3.2	3.3	3.0	2.8	2.7	2.6	2.5	2.5	2.4
1998													3.1	3.3	2.9	2.6	2.6	2.5	2.4	2.3	2.3
1999														3.6	2.8	2.5	2.4	2.4	2.2	2.2	2.3
2000															2.1	1.9	2.1	2.1	2.0	2.0	2.1
2001																1.7	2.1	2.1	1.9	2.0	2.1
2002																	2.4	2.3	2.0	2.1	2.1
2003																		2.3	1.8	2.0	2.1
2004																			1.4	1.8	2.0
2005																				2.2	2.3
2006																					2.4

8.10 Rates of change of household disposable income (Chained volume measures)
Total

Percentage change, at annual rate

Initial year \ Terminal year	1966	1967	1968	1969	1970	1971	1972	1973	1974	1975	1976	1977	1978	1979	1980	1981	1982	1983	1984	1985	1986
1965	2.3	1.9	1.9	1.7	2.1	1.9	2.8	3.2	2.8	2.6	2.3	1.9	2.3	2.5	2.5	2.3	2.2	2.2	2.2	2.3	2.4
1966		1.5	1.7	1.4	2.0	1.8	2.9	3.4	2.8	2.6	2.3	1.8	2.3	2.6	2.5	2.3	2.1	2.1	2.2	2.3	2.4
1967			1.9	1.4	2.2	1.9	3.2	3.7	3.0	2.7	2.4	1.9	2.4	2.6	2.6	2.4	2.2	2.2	2.3	2.3	2.4
1968				0.9	2.3	1.9	3.5	4.0	3.2	2.9	2.4	1.9	2.4	2.7	2.6	2.4	2.2	2.2	2.3	2.4	2.5
1969					3.7	2.4	4.3	4.8	3.7	3.2	2.6	2.0	2.6	2.9	2.8	2.5	2.3	2.3	2.4	2.5	2.6
1970						1.1	4.7	5.2	3.6	3.1	2.4	1.8	2.4	2.8	2.7	2.4	2.2	2.2	2.3	2.4	2.5
1971							8.3	7.3	4.5	3.5	2.7	1.9	2.6	3.0	2.9	2.5	2.3	2.3	2.4	2.5	2.6
1972								6.3	2.6	2.0	1.4	0.6	1.7	2.3	2.2	1.9	1.7	1.7	1.9	2.0	2.2
1973									-0.9	-0.2	-0.1	-0.8	0.8	1.6	1.6	1.4	1.2	1.3	1.5	1.7	1.9
1974										0.8	0.1	-0.7	1.2	2.1	2.0	1.7	1.5	1.5	1.8	1.9	2.1
1975											-0.6	-1.5	1.4	2.5	2.3	1.9	1.6	1.6	1.9	2.0	2.2
1976												-2.3	2.4	3.5	3.0	2.4	1.9	2.0	2.2	2.3	2.5
1977													7.3	6.5	4.9	3.6	2.8	2.7	2.9	2.9	3.1
1978														5.8	3.7	2.3	1.7	1.8	2.1	2.3	2.6
1979															1.7	0.6	0.4	0.8	1.4	1.8	2.1
1980																-0.4	-0.2	0.5	1.4	1.8	2.2
1981																	-0.1	1.0	1.9	2.3	2.7
1982																		2.1	3.0	3.1	3.4
1983																			3.8	3.7	3.8
1984																				3.5	3.9
1985																					4.2

Initial year \ Terminal year	1987	1988	1989	1990	1991	1992	1993	1994	1995	1996	1997	1998	1999	2000	2001	2002	2003	2004	2005	2006	2007
1965	2.4	2.5	2.6	2.7	2.6	2.6	2.7	2.6	2.6	2.6	2.7	2.7	2.7	2.7	2.8	2.7	2.7	2.7	2.7	2.7	2.6
1966	2.4	2.5	2.6	2.7	2.7	2.7	2.7	2.6	2.6	2.6	2.7	2.7	2.7	2.7	2.8	2.8	2.8	2.7	2.7	2.7	2.6
1967	2.4	2.6	2.7	2.7	2.7	2.7	2.7	2.7	2.7	2.7	2.7	2.7	2.7	2.8	2.8	2.8	2.8	2.7	2.7	2.7	2.6
1968	2.4	2.6	2.7	2.8	2.7	2.7	2.8	2.7	2.7	2.7	2.8	2.7	2.7	2.8	2.8	2.8	2.8	2.8	2.8	2.7	2.7
1969	2.5	2.7	2.8	2.9	2.8	2.8	2.8	2.8	2.8	2.8	2.8	2.8	2.8	2.8	2.9	2.9	2.9	2.8	2.8	2.8	2.7
1970	2.4	2.6	2.7	2.8	2.8	2.8	2.8	2.7	2.7	2.7	2.8	2.8	2.8	2.8	2.9	2.9	2.8	2.8	2.8	2.8	2.7
1971	2.7	2.7	2.8	2.9	2.9	2.9	2.9	2.8	2.8	2.8	2.9	2.8	2.8	2.9	2.9	2.9	2.9	2.8	2.8	2.8	2.7
1972	2.2	2.4	2.5	2.6	2.6	2.6	2.6	2.6	2.6	2.6	2.6	2.6	2.6	2.7	2.7	2.7	2.7	2.7	2.7	2.6	2.6
1973	1.9	2.1	2.3	2.4	2.4	2.4	2.4	2.4	2.4	2.4	2.5	2.5	2.5	2.6	2.6	2.6	2.6	2.6	2.6	2.5	2.5
1974	2.1	2.3	2.5	2.6	2.6	2.6	2.6	2.6	2.6	2.6	2.6	2.6	2.6	2.7	2.8	2.7	2.7	2.7	2.7	2.6	2.6
1975	2.2	2.5	2.6	2.7	2.7	2.7	2.7	2.6	2.6	2.6	2.7	2.7	2.7	2.7	2.8	2.8	2.8	2.8	2.7	2.7	2.6
1976	2.5	2.7	2.9	3.0	2.9	2.9	2.9	2.8	2.8	2.8	2.9	2.9	2.9	2.9	3.0	2.9	2.9	2.9	2.9	2.8	2.7
1977	2.9	3.2	3.3	3.4	3.3	3.3	3.2	3.1	3.1	3.1	3.2	3.1	3.1	3.1	3.2	3.2	3.1	3.1	3.0	3.0	2.9
1978	2.5	2.8	3.0	3.1	3.0	3.0	3.0	2.9	2.9	2.9	2.9	2.9	2.9	3.0	3.0	3.0	3.0	2.9	2.9	2.8	2.7
1979	2.1	2.4	2.7	2.8	2.8	2.8	2.8	2.7	2.7	2.7	2.8	2.8	2.8	2.8	2.9	2.9	2.9	2.8	2.8	2.7	2.6
1980	2.1	2.5	2.8	3.0	2.9	2.9	2.9	2.8	2.8	2.8	2.9	2.8	2.8	2.9	3.0	2.9	2.9	2.8	2.8	2.8	2.7
1981	2.5	3.0	3.2	3.3	3.2	3.2	3.1	3.0	3.0	3.0	3.1	3.0	3.0	3.1	3.1	3.1	3.1	3.0	3.0	3.0	2.8
1982	3.1	3.5	3.7	3.8	3.6	3.5	3.4	3.3	3.2	3.2	3.3	3.2	3.2	3.2	3.3	3.2	3.2	3.1	3.1	3.0	2.9
1983	3.3	3.8	3.9	4.0	3.8	3.6	3.6	3.4	3.3	3.3	3.4	3.3	3.3	3.3	3.4	3.3	3.3	3.2	3.1	3.1	2.9
1984	3.1	3.8	4.0	4.1	3.8	3.6	3.6	3.3	3.3	3.3	3.3	3.2	3.2	3.3	3.3	3.3	3.3	3.1	3.1	3.0	2.9
1985	3.0	3.8	4.1	4.2	3.8	3.6	3.6	3.3	3.2	3.2	3.3	3.2	3.2	3.3	3.3	3.3	3.2	3.1	3.1	3.0	2.9
1986	1.7	3.6	4.0	4.2	3.7	3.5	3.5	3.2	3.1	3.1	3.2	3.1	3.1	3.2	3.3	3.2	3.2	3.1	3.0	3.0	2.8
1987		5.6	5.2	5.0	4.2	3.9	3.8	3.4	3.3	3.3	3.4	3.3	3.2	3.3	3.4	3.3	3.3	3.1	3.1	3.0	2.9
1988			4.8	4.7	3.8	3.5	3.4	3.1	3.0	3.0	3.1	3.0	3.0	3.1	3.2	3.1	3.1	3.0	3.0	2.9	2.7
1989				4.6	3.2	3.1	3.1	2.7	2.7	2.8	2.9	2.8	2.8	3.0	3.1	3.0	3.0	2.9	2.9	2.8	2.7
1990					1.9	2.3	2.6	2.3	2.3	2.5	2.7	2.6	2.7	2.8	3.0	2.9	2.9	2.7	2.7	2.7	2.5
1991						2.7	2.9	2.4	2.4	2.6	2.8	2.7	2.7	2.9	3.1	3.0	3.0	2.8	2.8	2.7	2.5
1992							3.0	2.2	2.3	2.5	2.9	2.7	2.7	2.9	3.1	3.0	3.0	2.8	2.8	2.7	2.5
1993								1.4	2.0	2.3	2.8	2.7	2.7	2.9	3.1	3.0	3.0	2.8	2.8	2.7	2.5
1994									2.6	2.8	3.3	3.0	3.0	3.2	3.3	3.2	3.2	2.9	2.9	2.8	2.6
1995										3.1	3.6	3.1	3.1	3.3	3.5	3.3	3.2	3.0	2.9	2.8	2.6
1996											4.2	3.1	3.1	3.3	3.6	3.3	3.3	2.9	2.9	2.8	2.5
1997												2.1	2.5	3.0	3.4	3.1	3.1	2.8	2.8	2.6	2.4
1998													2.9	3.5	3.8	3.4	3.3	2.9	2.9	2.7	2.4
1999														4.2	4.3	3.6	3.4	2.9	2.9	2.7	2.3
2000															4.4	3.2	3.1	2.6	2.6	2.4	2.1
2001																2.0	2.5	1.9	2.1	2.0	1.7
2002																	3.0	1.9	2.2	2.0	1.6
2003																		0.8	1.8	1.7	1.3
2004																			2.8	2.1	1.4
2005																				1.5	0.8
2006																					0.1

8.11 Rates of change of household disposable income (Chained volume measures) Per capita

Percentage change, at annual rate

Terminal year

Initial year	1967	1968	1969	1970	1971	1972	1973	1974	1975	1976	1977	1978	1979	1980	1981	1982	1983	1984	1985	1986	1987
1966	0.9	1.2	0.9	1.6	1.4	2.4	2.9	2.4	2.3	2.0	1.6	2.0	2.3	2.3	2.1	2.0	2.0	2.1	2.1	2.2	2.2
1967		1.4	1.0	1.8	1.5	2.7	3.3	2.7	2.4	2.1	1.7	2.2	2.4	2.4	2.2	2.0	2.0	2.1	2.2	2.3	2.2
1968			0.5	1.9	1.5	3.1	3.7	2.9	2.6	2.2	1.7	2.2	2.5	2.4	2.2	2.1	2.1	2.2	2.2	2.3	2.3
1969				3.4	2.0	4.0	4.5	3.4	2.9	2.4	1.8	2.4	2.7	2.6	2.4	2.2	2.2	2.3	2.3	2.4	2.4
1970					0.6	4.2	4.8	3.3	2.8	2.3	1.6	2.3	2.7	2.6	2.3	2.1	2.1	2.2	2.3	2.4	2.3
1971						8.0	7.0	4.3	3.4	2.6	1.8	2.5	2.9	2.8	2.4	2.2	2.2	2.3	2.4	2.5	2.4
1972							6.0	2.5	1.9	1.3	0.6	1.7	2.2	2.1	1.9	1.7	1.7	1.9	2.0	2.1	2.1
1973								-1.0	-0.1	-0.2	-0.7	0.8	1.6	1.6	1.3	1.2	1.3	1.5	1.6	1.8	1.8
1974									0.8	0.1	-0.7	1.3	2.1	2.0	1.7	1.5	1.5	1.7	1.9	2.1	2.0
1975										-0.5	-1.4	1.4	2.5	2.3	1.8	1.6	1.6	1.9	2.0	2.2	2.1
1976											-2.2	2.4	3.5	3.0	2.3	1.9	2.0	2.2	2.3	2.5	2.4
1977												7.3	6.5	4.8	3.5	2.8	2.7	2.8	2.9	3.0	2.8
1978													5.7	3.6	2.2	1.7	1.8	2.1	2.2	2.5	2.4
1979														1.5	0.6	0.4	0.8	1.4	1.7	2.0	1.9
1980															-0.4	-0.2	0.6	1.3	1.7	2.1	2.0
1981																0.0	1.1	1.9	2.2	2.6	2.4
1982																	2.1	2.9	3.0	3.2	2.9
1983																		3.6	3.4	3.6	3.1
1984																			3.3	3.6	2.9
1985																				4.0	2.7
1986																					1.5

Terminal year

Initial year	1988	1989	1990	1991	1992	1993	1994	1995	1996	1997	1998	1999	2000	2001	2002	2003	2004	2005	2006	2007
1966	2.3	2.4	2.5	2.5	2.5	2.5	2.4	2.4	2.4	2.5	2.5	2.5	2.5	2.5	2.5	2.5	2.5	2.5	2.4	2.3
1967	2.4	2.5	2.6	2.5	2.5	2.5	2.5	2.5	2.5	2.5	2.5	2.5	2.5	2.6	2.6	2.6	2.5	2.5	2.5	2.4
1968	2.4	2.5	2.6	2.6	2.6	2.6	2.5	2.5	2.5	2.6	2.5	2.5	2.6	2.6	2.6	2.6	2.5	2.5	2.5	2.4
1969	2.5	2.6	2.7	2.7	2.7	2.7	2.6	2.6	2.6	2.6	2.6	2.6	2.7	2.7	2.7	2.7	2.6	2.6	2.5	2.5
1970	2.5	2.6	2.7	2.6	2.6	2.6	2.6	2.6	2.6	2.6	2.6	2.6	2.6	2.7	2.6	2.6	2.6	2.6	2.5	2.4
1971	2.6	2.7	2.8	2.7	2.7	2.7	2.7	2.6	2.6	2.7	2.7	2.7	2.7	2.7	2.7	2.7	2.6	2.6	2.6	2.5
1972	2.3	2.4	2.5	2.5	2.5	2.5	2.4	2.4	2.4	2.5	2.5	2.5	2.5	2.6	2.5	2.5	2.5	2.5	2.4	2.3
1973	2.0	2.2	2.3	2.3	2.3	2.3	2.2	2.3	2.3	2.3	2.3	2.3	2.4	2.4	2.4	2.4	2.4	2.3	2.3	2.2
1974	2.3	2.4	2.5	2.5	2.5	2.5	2.4	2.4	2.4	2.5	2.5	2.5	2.5	2.6	2.5	2.5	2.5	2.5	2.4	2.3
1975	2.4	2.5	2.6	2.6	2.6	2.6	2.5	2.5	2.5	2.6	2.5	2.5	2.6	2.6	2.6	2.6	2.5	2.5	2.5	2.4
1976	2.6	2.8	2.9	2.8	2.8	2.8	2.7	2.7	2.7	2.7	2.7	2.7	2.7	2.8	2.7	2.7	2.6	2.6	2.6	2.5
1977	3.1	3.2	3.3	3.1	3.1	3.1	3.0	2.9	2.9	3.0	2.9	2.9	2.9	3.0	2.9	2.9	2.8	2.8	2.7	2.6
1978	2.7	2.8	2.9	2.8	2.8	2.8	2.7	2.7	2.7	2.8	2.7	2.7	2.7	2.8	2.8	2.7	2.7	2.6	2.6	2.5
1979	2.3	2.5	2.7	2.6	2.6	2.6	2.5	2.5	2.5	2.6	2.6	2.5	2.6	2.7	2.6	2.6	2.5	2.5	2.5	2.3
1980	2.4	2.7	2.8	2.7	2.7	2.7	2.6	2.6	2.6	2.7	2.6	2.6	2.7	2.7	2.7	2.7	2.6	2.6	2.5	2.4
1981	2.8	3.0	3.2	3.0	3.0	2.9	2.8	2.8	2.8	2.8	2.8	2.8	2.8	2.9	2.8	2.8	2.7	2.7	2.6	2.5
1982	3.3	3.5	3.6	3.4	3.3	3.2	3.0	3.0	3.0	3.0	3.0	2.9	3.0	3.0	3.0	3.0	2.8	2.8	2.7	2.6
1983	3.5	3.7	3.8	3.5	3.4	3.3	3.1	3.1	3.0	3.1	3.0	3.0	3.0	3.1	3.0	3.0	2.9	2.8	2.7	2.6
1984	3.5	3.7	3.8	3.5	3.4	3.3	3.1	3.0	3.0	3.1	3.0	2.9	3.0	3.1	3.0	3.0	2.8	2.8	2.7	2.6
1985	3.6	3.8	3.9	3.5	3.4	3.3	3.1	3.0	3.0	3.1	3.0	2.9	3.0	3.0	3.0	2.9	2.8	2.8	2.7	2.5
1986	3.4	3.8	3.9	3.4	3.3	3.2	2.9	2.9	2.9	3.0	2.9	2.8	2.9	3.0	2.9	2.9	2.7	2.7	2.6	2.5
1987	5.4	5.0	4.7	3.9	3.6	3.5	3.2	3.0	3.0	3.1	3.0	3.0	3.0	3.1	3.0	3.0	2.8	2.8	2.7	2.5
1988		4.5	4.4	3.4	3.2	3.1	2.8	2.7	2.7	2.9	2.8	2.7	2.8	2.9	2.8	2.8	2.7	2.6	2.5	2.4
1989			4.3	2.9	2.8	2.8	2.4	2.4	2.5	2.7	2.6	2.6	2.7	2.8	2.7	2.7	2.5	2.5	2.4	2.2
1990				1.6	2.0	2.3	2.0	2.1	2.2	2.4	2.4	2.4	2.5	2.7	2.6	2.6	2.4	2.4	2.3	2.1
1991					2.5	2.6	2.1	2.2	2.3	2.6	2.5	2.5	2.6	2.8	2.7	2.7	2.5	2.4	2.3	2.2
1992						2.8	2.0	2.1	2.3	2.6	2.5	2.5	2.6	2.8	2.7	2.7	2.5	2.4	2.3	2.1
1993							1.1	1.7	2.1	2.5	2.4	2.4	2.6	2.8	2.7	2.7	2.4	2.4	2.3	2.1
1994								2.3	2.6	3.0	2.7	2.7	2.9	3.0	2.9	2.8	2.6	2.5	2.4	2.2
1995									2.8	3.4	2.8	2.8	3.0	3.2	2.9	2.9	2.6	2.6	2.4	2.2
1996										4.0	2.9	2.7	3.0	3.2	3.0	2.9	2.6	2.5	2.4	2.1
1997											1.8	2.1	2.7	3.0	2.8	2.7	2.4	2.4	2.2	1.9
1998												2.5	3.2	3.5	3.0	2.9	2.5	2.4	2.2	1.9
1999													3.8	3.9	3.2	3.0	2.5	2.4	2.2	1.9
2000														4.0	2.9	2.8	2.2	2.1	1.9	1.6
2001															1.7	2.1	1.5	1.7	1.5	1.2
2002																2.6	1.5	1.7	1.5	1.1
2003																	0.3	1.2	1.1	0.7
2004																		2.1	1.5	0.8
2005																			0.9	0.2
2006																				-0.5

Chapter 9

Fixed capital formation supplementary tables

9.1 Gross fixed capital formation at current purchasers' prices
Analysis by type of asset and sector

£ million

		1999	2000	2001	2002	2003	2004	2005	2006	2007
Dwellings, excluding land										
Public non-financial corporations	DEER	1 529	1 421	2 387	2 837	3 509	3 235	3 574	4 049	4 175
Private non-financial corporations	DLWG	279	303	324	374	414	502	543	623	1 124
Financial corporations	DFIX	–	–	–	–	–	–	–	–	–
Central government	DFIZ	250	369	334	207	149	137	71	9	31
Local government	DKQC	–	–	–	–	–	–	–	–	–
Households and NPISH	DLWK	23 642	25 301	26 761	31 081	34 390	40 425	43 302	48 650	51 468
Total	DFDK	25 700	27 394	29 806	34 499	38 462	44 299	47 490	53 331	56 798
Other buildings and structures										
Public non-financial corporations	DEES	1 692	1 775	1 854	2 304	2 236	1 493	2 111	1 830	1 587
Private non-financial corporations	DLWN	26 594	27 124	27 936	29 123	30 643	27 984	30 495	31 967	37 300
Financial corporations	GGBT	2 509	2 176	2 017	2 007	2 089	1 602	2 479	2 411	2 433
Central government	DLWP	3 990	3 390	3 610	4 717	5 663	6 072	7 712	8 770	10 116
Local government	DJYS	5 424	6 044	6 738	6 961	9 030	9 794	11 172	12 160	12 392
Households and NPISH	DLWR	2 725	2 666	2 777	2 450	2 634	3 641	3 398	3 669	4 268
Total	DLWS	42 934	43 175	44 932	47 562	52 295	50 586	57 367	60 807	68 096
Transport equipment										
Public non-financial corporations	DEEP	155	178	171	110	126	193	334	181	175
Private non-financial corporations	DLWU	12 348	11 701	12 721	14 376	13 575	11 964	12 548	13 011	13 420
Financial corporations	GGBR	591	334	159	178	109	106	63	–5	106
Central government	DLWW	384	353	355	372	505	638	221	88	67
Local government	DKPN	225	187	233	195	253	373	389	412	432
Households and NPISH	DLWY	980	824	1 017	1 083	1 024	1 065	1 207	1 193	1 188
Total	DLWZ	14 683	13 577	14 656	16 314	15 592	14 339	14 762	14 880	15 388
Other machinery and equipment and cultivated assets										
Public non-financial corporations	DEEQ	617	600	628	787	1 037	1 042	16 478	986	1 629
Private non-financial corporations	DLXD	50 297	52 829	50 058	45 145	42 881	47 240	48 053	49 476	54 990
Financial corporations	DLXE	3 275	3 723	3 550	3 846	2 945	2 561	3 159	3 436	3 689
Central government	DLXF	1 702	1 346	1 566	2 040	2 058	2 213	–13 828	1 113	1 174
Local government	DLXG	394	353	673	827	1 118	1 439	1 390	1 367	1 310
Households and NPISH	DLXH	4 385	4 684	4 454	4 507	4 402	5 337	5 135	5 427	6 056
Total	DLXI	60 670	63 535	60 929	57 152	54 441	59 832	60 387	61 805	68 848
Intangible fixed assets										
Public non-financial corporations	DLXJ	625	551	397	556	623	737	754	769	802
Private non-financial corporations	DLXK	6 965	7 429	8 151	8 939	9 886	10 142	10 401	11 293	11 549
Financial corporations	DLXL	1 814	2 064	2 165	2 455	2 630	2 534	2 552	2 650	2 936
Central government	DLXM	173	108	55	52	56	49	37	45	67
Local government	DLXN	223	259	279	306	328	351	267	373	272
Households and NPISH	DLXO	223	259	279	306	327	351	376	401	429
Total	DLXP	10 023	10 670	11 326	12 614	13 850	14 164	14 387	15 531	16 055
Costs associated with the transfer of ownership of non-produced assets										
Public non-financial corporations	DLXQ	–1 906	–2 171	–2 254	–2 764	–5 674	–5 440	–2 675	–2 375	–2 177
Private non-financial corporations	DLXR	2 506	2 211	3 937	5 225	6 456	7 703	8 419	9 363	9 574
Financial corporations	DLXS	999	3 679	591	–163	–2 520	–1 549	–1 800	158	–1 333
Central government	DLXT	–143	109	44	118	–2 059	–781	–638	–165	–627
Local government	DLXU	–23	–291	–354	–343	3 408	2 934	298	–505	–24
Households and NPISH	DLXV	6 279	5 284	8 169	10 337	12 449	14 585	13 321	15 090	18 640
Total	DFBH	7 712	8 821	10 133	12 410	12 060	17 452	16 925	21 566	24 053
P.51 Gross fixed capital formation										
S.11001 Public non-financial corporations	FCCJ	2 712	2 354	3 183	3 830	1 857	1 260	20 576	5 440	6 191
S.11002 Private non-financial corporations	FDBM	98 989	101 597	103 127	103 182	103 855	105 535	110 459	115 733	127 957
S.12 Financial corporations	NHCJ	9 188	11 976	8 482	8 323	5 253	5 254	6 453	8 650	7 831
S.1311 Central government	NMES	6 356	5 675	5 964	7 506	6 372	8 328	–6 425	9 860	10 828
S.1313 Local government	NMOA	6 243	6 552	7 569	7 946	14 137	14 891	13 516	13 807	14 382
S.14+S.15 Households and NPISH	NSSU	38 234	39 018	43 457	49 764	55 226	65 404	66 739	74 430	82 049
S.1, P.51 Total gross fixed capital formation	NPQX	161 722	167 172	171 782	180 551	186 700	200 672	211 318	227 920	249 239

1 Components may not sum to totals due to rounding.

9.2 Gross fixed capital formation at current purchasers' prices
Analysis by broad sector and type of asset

Total economy

£ million

			1999	2000	2001	2002	2003	2004	2005	2006	2007
	Private sector										
	New dwellings, excluding land	DFDF	23 921	25 604	27 085	31 455	34 804	40 927	43 845	49 273	52 592
	Other buildings and structures	EQBU	31 828	31 966	32 730	33 580	35 366	33 227	36 372	38 047	44 001
	Transport equipment	EQBV	13 919	12 859	13 897	15 637	14 708	13 135	13 818	14 199	14 714
	Other machinery and equipment and cultivated assets	EQBW	57 957	61 236	58 062	53 498	50 228	55 138	56 347	58 339	64 735
	Intangible fixed assets	EQBX	9 002	9 752	10 595	11 700	12 843	13 027	13 329	14 344	14 914
	Costs associated with the transfer of ownership of non-produced assets	EQBY	9 784	11 174	12 697	15 399	16 385	20 739	19 940	24 611	26 881
P.51	Total	EQBZ	146 411	152 591	155 066	161 269	164 334	176 193	183 651	198 813	217 837
S.11001	**Public non-financial corporations**										
	New dwellings, excluding land	DEER	1 529	1 421	2 387	2 837	3 509	3 235	3 574	4 049	4 175
	Other buildings and structures	DEES	1 692	1 775	1 854	2 304	2 236	1 493	2 111	1 830	1 587
	Transport equipment	DEEP	155	178	171	110	126	193	334	181	175
	Other machinery and equipment and cultivated assets	DEEQ	617	600	628	787	1 037	1 042	16 478	986	1 629
	Intangible fixed assets	DLXJ	625	551	397	556	623	737	754	769	802
	Costs associated with the transfer of ownership of non-produced assets	DLXQ	−1 906	−2 171	−2 254	−2 764	−5 674	−5 440	−2 675	−2 375	−2 177
P.51	Total	FCCJ	2 712	2 354	3 183	3 830	1 857	1 260	20 576	5 440	6 191
S.13	**General government**										
	New dwellings, excluding land	DFHW	250	369	334	207	149	137	71	9	31
	Other buildings and structures	EQCH	9 414	9 434	10 348	11 678	14 693	15 866	18 884	20 930	22 508
	Transport equipment	EQCI	609	540	588	567	758	1 011	610	500	499
	Other machinery and equipment and cultivated assets	EQCJ	2 096	1 699	2 239	2 867	3 176	3 652	−12 438	2 480	2 484
	Intangible fixed assets	EQCK	396	367	334	358	384	400	304	418	339
	Costs associated with the transfer of ownership of non-produced assets	EQCL	−166	−182	−310	−225	1 349	2 153	−340	−670	−651
P.51	Total	NNBF	12 599	12 227	13 533	15 452	20 509	23 219	7 091	23 667	25 210
P.51	Total gross fixed capital formation	NPQX	161 722	167 172	171 782	180 551	186 700	200 672	211 318	227 920	249 238

1 Components may not sum to totals due to rounding.

9.3 Gross fixed capital formation at current purchasers' prices
Analysis by type of asset

Total economy

£ million

		1999	2000	2001	2002	2003	2004	2005	2006	2007
Tangible fixed assets										
New dwellings, excluding land	DFDK	25 700	27 394	29 806	34 499	38 462	44 299	47 490	53 331	56 798
Other buildings and structures	DLWS	42 934	43 175	44 932	47 562	52 295	50 586	57 367	60 807	68 096
Transport equipment	DLWZ	14 683	13 577	14 656	16 314	15 592	14 339	14 762	14 880	15 388
Other machinery and equipment and cultivated assets	DLXI	60 670	63 535	60 929	57 152	54 441	59 832	60 387	61 805	68 848
Total	EQCQ	143 987	147 681	150 323	155 527	160 790	169 056	180 006	190 823	209 130
Intangible fixed assets	DLXP	10 023	10 670	11 326	12 614	13 850	14 164	14 387	15 531	16 055
Costs associated with the transfer of ownership of non-produced assets	DFBH	7 712	8 821	10 133	12 410	12 060	17 452	16 925	21 566	24 053
P.51 Total gross fixed capital formation	NPQX	161 722	167 172	171 782	180 551	186 700	200 672	211 318	227 920	249 238

1 Components may not sum to totals due to rounding.

9.4 Gross fixed capital formation[1]
Chained volume measures (reference year 2003)

Total economy: Analysis by broad sector and type of asset

£ million

			1999	2000	2001	2002	2003	2004	2005	2006	2007
	Private sector										
	New dwellings, excluding land	DFDP	30 928	31 041	31 318	33 748	34 804	38 302	38 380	41 650	43 767
	Other buildings and structures	EQCU	33 931	33 206	33 251	33 406	35 366	32 131	35 033	36 567	42 194
	Transport equipment	EQCV	13 778	12 713	13 863	15 708	14 708	13 090	13 598	13 807	14 223
	Other machinery and equipment and cultivated assets	EQCW	49 522	53 869	54 140	52 405	50 228	56 659	57 925	61 053	67 107
	Intangible fixed assets	EQCX	10 185	10 702	11 228	11 680	12 843	13 023	13 072	13 881	14 091
	Costs associated with the transfer of ownership of non-produced assets	EQCY	16 821	16 293	16 173	17 369	16 385	19 603	16 809	18 437	18 311
P.51	Total	EQCZ	154 580	158 347	160 569	164 304	164 334	172 808	174 817	185 395	199 693
S.11001	**Public non-financial corporations**										
	New dwellings, excluding land	DEEW	1 747	1 552	2 521	2 898	3 509	3 161	3 423	3 807	3 749
	Other buildings and structures	DEEX	1 890	1 939	1 961	2 342	2 236	1 426	1 928	1 575	1 303
	Transport equipment	DEEU	164	186	180	114	126	193	326	179	174
	Other machinery and equipment and cultivated assets	DEEV	504	516	588	765	1 037	1 063	16 172	1 018	1 638
	Intangible fixed assets	EQDE	684	586	415	572	623	714	711	703	701
	Costs associated with the transfer of ownership of non-produced assets	EQDF	–3 141	–3 093	–2 825	–3 092	–5 674	–5 561	–2 812	–1 869	–1 793
P.51	Total	EQDG	1 796	1 695	2 424	3 019	1 857	996	19 748	5 413	5 772
S.13	**General government**										
	New dwellings, excluding land	DFID	286	404	354	213	149	135	69	9	27
	Other buildings and structures	EQDI	10 792	10 513	11 107	12 115	14 693	14 877	16 506	17 397	17 597
	Transport equipment	EQDJ	676	606	672	586	758	809	751	813	826
	Other machinery and equipment and cultivated assets	EQDK	1 632	1 424	2 063	2 801	3 176	3 757	–11 905	3 045	3 158
	Intangible fixed assets	EQDL	241	219	196	211	384	397	294	394	313
	Costs associated with the transfer of ownership of non-produced assets	EQDM	–1 728	–542	–548	–261	1 349	2 004	–93	–321	–199
P.51	Total	EQDN	13 328	12 894	14 214	15 991	20 509	21 978	5 621	21 338	21 723
P.51	Total gross fixed capital formation	NPQR	169 117	173 710	178 203	184 701	186 700	195 782	200 187	212 146	227 188

1 For the years before 2003, totals differ from the sum of their components.
2 Components may not sum to totals due to rounding.

9.5 Gross fixed capital formation[1]
Chained volume measures (reference year 2003)

Total economy: Analysis by type of asset

£ million

		1999	2000	2001	2002	2003	2004	2005	2006	2007
Tangible fixed assets										
New dwellings, excluding land	DFDV	32 863	32 888	34 172	36 839	38 462	41 598	41 872	45 466	47 543
Other buildings and structures	EQDP	46 738	45 780	46 413	47 913	52 295	48 434	53 467	55 539	61 094
Transport equipment	DLWJ	14 602	13 489	14 698	16 414	15 592	14 092	14 675	14 799	15 223
Other machinery and equipment and cultivated assets	DLWM	51 667	55 774	56 780	55 971	54 441	61 479	62 192	65 116	71 903
Total	EQDS	145 621	148 509	152 571	157 257	160 790	165 602	172 205	180 921	195 763
Intangible fixed assets	EQDT	11 079	11 445	11 742	12 371	13 850	14 134	14 077	14 978	15 105
Costs associated with the transfer of ownership of non-produced assets	DFDW	13 088	12 810	12 960	14 097	12 060	16 046	13 904	16 247	16 319
P.51 Total gross fixed capital formation	NPQR	169 117	173 710	178 203	184 701	186 700	195 782	200 187	212 146	227 188

1 For the years before 2003, totals differ from the sum of their components.
2 Components may not sum to totals due to rounding.

Chapter 10
Non-financial balance sheets

The non-financial balance sheets show the market value of non-financial assets in the UK and as such are a measure of the wealth of the UK.

When financial assets are added to the value of the non-financial assets, the result, the net worth of the UK, is estimated at £6,998 billion in 2007 – an increase of £506 billion on the previous year. The non-financial balance sheets figures also show that the most valuable asset continues to be housing with a total value of £4,314 billion in 2007 – up 10 per cent on the previous year and equivalent to 62 per cent of the nation's total wealth. The housing stock belonging to the household and non-profit organisations sector was worth £4,077 billion, up 10 per cent on the previous year.

Non-financial assets include both tangible and intangible assets. Tangible assets consist of property, plant & machinery, agricultural assets, vehicles and also include certain types of farming stocks (mainly dairy cattle and orchards) and military equipment whose use is not solely destructive. Intangible assets consist of the value of computer software, patents, mineral exploration and artistic originals.

Data sources include:

- Other government departments and agencies
- Annual reports of public corporations and major businesses
- Industry publications
- Chartered Institute of Public Finance and Accountancy report on Local Authority Assets

Where non-financial asset market valuations are not readily available, the UK net capital stocks data modelled in the PIM within ONS is used as a proxy.

For Central Government data are taken from returns made by government departments to HM Treasury. Central Government assets also include the value of the electro-magnetic spectrum. The spectrum is treated as a tangible non-produced asset and the payments made by mobile phone companies as rent.

Local authority housing is shown in the public corporations sector. This is because government-owned market activities are always treated as being carried out by public corporations, either in their own right or via quasi-corporations.

This publication contains upward revisions in non-financial corporations and households and non-profit institutions serving households reflecting improved methodology for the measurement of civil engineering works, vehicles and commercial, industrial and other buildings in the transport sector. Other revisions in the data are due to ongoing improvements in the Non-Financial Balance Sheets system, started in 2005, which were continued during the year; the most prominent of these relates to the values for commercial, industrial and other buildings. Revisions to the financial accounts and balance sheets for this *Blue Book* have also been incorporated into the overall values for net worth.

10.1 National balance sheet
Sector totals: summary of net worth

£ billion at end year

			1999	2000	2001	2002	2003	2004	2005	2006	2007
	Non-financial corporations[2]										
S.11001	Public[4]	CGRW	49.5	50.0	55.7	60.5	60.1	58.9	50.6	58.9	63.0
S.11002	Private[2]	TMPN	−650.4	−499.0	−310.7	38.8	−52.2	−104.0	−372.4	−517.1	−546.4
S.11	Total	CGRV	−600.9	−449.0	−255.0	99.4	7.9	−45.1	−321.9	−458.2	−483.4
S.12	Financial corporations	CGRU	−408.7	−396.0	−416.6	−326.2	−293.7	−301.5	−368.4	−360.8	−392.6
	General government[4]										
S.1311	Central government	CGRY	−143.6	−110.2	−85.3	−104.3	−121.0	−159.7	−168.6	−171.5	−201.5
S.1313	Local government	CGRZ	260.6	290.0	339.3	355.7	395.3	451.4	485.2	510.3	552.6
S.13	Total	CGRX	117.0	179.8	253.9	251.4	274.3	291.7	316.6	338.8	351.1
S.14+S.15	Households and NPISH[3]	CGRC	4 582.0	4 814.1	4 765.9	4 932.3	5 416.5	5 903.9	6 408.5	6 972.6	7 523.4
S.1	Total net worth	CGDA	3 689.3	4 148.9	4 348.2	4 956.8	5 405.0	5 849.0	6 034.9	6 492.4	6 998.4

1 See footnotes in tables 10.2-10.11 for changes to allocations of assets
  between sectors.
2 Including quasi-corporations.
3 Non-profit institutions serving households
4 Public sector (General government plus public non-financial corporations)
  is as follows:-

		1999	2000	2001	2002	2003	2004	2005	2006	2007
Public sector	CGTY	166.5	229.8	309.6	311.9	334.4	350.7	367.2	397.7	414.1

10.2 National balance sheet
Asset totals

£ billion at end year

		1999	2000	2001	2002	2003	2004	2005	2006	2007
Non-financial assets										
Tangible assets:										
Residential buildings	CGLK	1 848.9	2 106.5	2 267.8	2 737.1	3 054.9	3 427.0	3 555.0	3 915.3	4 313.6
Agricultural assets	CGMP	53.3	54.0	53.2	53.8	54.7	54.8	54.6	54.2	53.9
Commercial, industrial and other buildings	CGMU	575.4	574.2	562.9	589.8	608.4	661.4	663.4	752.2	699.0
Civil engineering works	CGQZ	498.2	522.9	575.6	586.3	622.7	665.4	706.5	745.9	799.4
Plant and machinery	CGRA	352.0	363.0	368.3	366.9	371.8	376.5	385.3	400.6	413.7
Vehicles, including ships, aircraft, etc	CGRB	110.2	114.3	122.0	134.7	146.6	153.6	155.0	163.2	185.7
Stocks and work in progress	CGRD	167.2	174.9	174.7	180.4	184.8	197.3	207.8	215.8	229.8
Spectrum[2]	ZLDX	–	21.9	21.9	21.9	21.9	21.9	21.9	21.9	21.9
Total tangible assets	CGRE	3 605.2	3 931.7	4 146.3	4 671.0	5 065.8	5 558.0	5 749.5	6 269.1	6 717.1
Intangible assets:										
Non-marketable tenancy rights	CGRF	237.4	276.7	300.1	365.3	413.5	466.1	486.9	545.1	611.5
Other intangible assets	CGRG	34.9	36.7	38.4	40.5	42.9	44.9	46.6	48.9	51.4
Total intangible assets	CGRH	272.3	313.4	338.5	405.9	456.4	511.0	533.5	594.0	663.0
Total non-financial assets	CGJB	3 877.5	4 245.1	4 484.8	5 076.8	5 522.2	6 069.0	6 283.0	6 863.1	7 380.0
Total net financial assets/liabilities	NQFT	−188.2	−96.2	−136.5	−120.0	−117.2	−220.0	−248.2	−370.7	−381.6
Total net worth[1]	CGDA	3 689.3	4 148.9	4 348.2	4 956.8	5 405.0	5 849.0	6 034.9	6 492.4	6 998.4

1 Net worth was previously defined as *net wealth*.
2 Following the grant of licences to mobile phone companies, the electro-
  magnetic spectrum is included as an asset for the first time in 2000.

10.3 Non-financial corporations

£ billion at end year

Non-financial assets		1999	2000	2001	2002	2003	2004	2005	2006	2007
Tangible assets:										
Residential buildings[2]	CGUT	125.8	134.6	147.5	164.8	182.0	200.9	214.2	212.8	228.4
of which Local Authority housing	CGWM	69.7	71.0	79.6	86.5	96.3	107.9	118.1	107.2	111.8
Agricultural assets	CGUU	4.0	4.0	3.9	4.1	4.2	4.2	4.2	4.1	4.0
Commercial, industrial and other buildings	CGUV	309.0	297.8	276.4	292.0	290.7	319.2	285.1	354.4	293.6
Civil engineering works	CGUW	262.8	257.5	267.8	271.9	283.0	287.0	298.6	306.5	321.4
Plant and machinery	CGUX	310.8	319.9	325.0	323.4	324.2	329.6	337.2	346.9	360.3
Vehicles, including ships, aircraft, etc	CGUY	47.6	52.1	54.4	60.8	68.7	71.4	69.7	76.9	97.6
Stocks and work in progress	CGUZ	151.3	159.0	158.8	164.0	168.0	180.3	191.3	199.2	213.0
Total tangible assets	CGVA	1 211.3	1 224.9	1 233.9	1 281.0	1 320.9	1 392.7	1 400.3	1 500.8	1 518.2
Intangible non-financial assets										
Non-marketable tenancy rights	CGVB	–	–	–	–	–	–	–	–	–
Other intangible assets	CGVC	29.5	30.7	31.9	33.5	35.3	36.8	38.3	40.2	42.7
Total intangible assets	CGVE	29.5	30.7	31.9	33.5	35.3	36.8	38.3	40.2	42.7
Total non-financial assets	CGES	1 240.8	1 255.6	1 265.7	1 314.5	1 356.2	1 429.5	1 438.6	1 541.0	1 560.9
Total net financial assets/liabilities	NYOM	−1 841.7	−1 704.6	−1 520.8	−1 215.1	−1 348.2	−1 474.6	−1 760.4	−1 999.2	−2 044.3
Total net worth[1]	CGRV	−600.9	−449.0	−255.0	99.4	7.9	−45.1	−321.9	−458.2	−483.4

1 Net worth was previously defined as *net wealth*.
2 Residential buildings in this table now include both council housing and housing association properties. The latter were formally included in table 10.10 (Non-profit institutions serving households).

10.4 Public non-financial corporations

£ billion at end year

Non-financial assets		1999	2000	2001	2002	2003	2004	2005	2006	2007
Tangible assets:										
Residential buildings[2]	CGVF	73.6	74.9	83.9	91.0	101.1	111.9	122.3	111.8	116.7
of which Local authority housing	CGWM	69.7	71.0	79.6	86.5	96.3	107.9	118.1	107.2	111.8
Agricultural assets	CGVG	1.0	0.9	0.9	0.9	0.9	0.9	0.9	0.9	0.9
Commercial, industrial and other buildings	CGVH	25.7	22.0	20.5	25.7	23.8	25.4	26.4	26.9	24.9
Civil engineering works	CGVI	10.7	12.6	16.6	22.4	15.9	15.5	15.7	17.2	18.9
Plant and machinery	CGVJ	5.1	4.9	4.8	7.4	7.7	8.3	8.3	8.3	8.8
Vehicles, including ships, aircraft, etc	CGVK	1.7	1.6	1.7	1.6	1.4	1.7	2.1	2.3	2.3
Stocks and work in progress	CGVL	5.3	5.2	5.2	5.1	5.1	5.2	5.2	5.3	5.3
Total tangible assets	CGVM	123.2	122.1	133.4	154.1	156.1	168.9	180.9	172.6	177.7
Intangible non-financial assets										
Non-marketable tenancy rights	CGVN	–	–	–	–	–	–	–	–	–
Other intangible assets	CGVO	3.4	3.7	3.8	4.0	4.2	4.5	4.8	5.0	5.2
Total intangible assets	CGVP	3.4	3.7	3.8	4.0	4.2	4.5	4.8	5.0	5.2
Total non-financial assets	CGGN	126.6	125.8	137.2	158.1	160.3	173.4	185.6	177.6	183.0
Total net financial assets/liabilities	NYOP	−77.1	−75.8	−81.5	−97.6	−100.2	−114.4	−135.1	−118.7	−120.0
Total net worth[1]	CGRW	49.5	50.0	55.7	60.5	60.1	58.9	50.6	58.9	63.0

1 Net worth was previously defined as *net wealth*.
2 Residential buildings in this table now include council housing.

10.5 Private non-financial corporations

£ billion at end year

		1999	2000	2001	2002	2003	2004	2005	2006	2007
Non-financial assets										
Tangible assets:										
Residential buildings[2]	TMPB	52.2	59.6	63.6	73.8	80.8	89.0	92.0	101.0	111.7
Agricultural assets	TMPC	3.0	3.1	3.1	3.1	3.3	3.3	3.3	3.2	3.1
Commercial, industrial and other buildings	TMPD	283.3	275.8	255.9	266.3	266.9	293.8	258.7	327.5	268.7
Civil engineering works	TMPE	252.1	245.0	251.3	249.5	267.1	271.5	282.9	289.4	302.5
Plant and machinery	TMPF	305.7	315.0	320.2	316.1	316.5	321.4	328.9	338.5	351.5
Vehicles, including ships, aircraft, etc	TMPO	45.9	50.5	52.8	59.2	67.3	69.6	67.6	74.6	95.3
Stocks and work in progress	TMPG	146.0	153.9	153.6	158.9	162.9	175.1	186.1	193.9	207.7
Total tangible assets	TMPH	1 088.1	1 102.8	1 100.5	1 126.9	1 164.8	1 223.8	1 219.4	1 328.2	1 340.4
Intangible non-financial assets										
Non-marketable tenancy rights	TMPI	–	–	–	–	–	–	–	–	–
Other intangible assets	TMPJ	26.1	27.0	28.1	29.5	31.1	32.3	33.5	35.2	37.5
Total intangible assets	TMPK	26.1	27.0	28.1	29.5	31.1	32.3	33.5	35.2	37.5
Total non-financial assets	TMPL	1 114.2	1 129.8	1 128.6	1 156.4	1 195.9	1 256.2	1 253.0	1 363.3	1 377.9
Total net financial assets/liabilities	NYOT	−1 764.7	−1 628.8	−1 439.3	−1 117.6	−1 248.1	−1 360.2	−1 625.4	−1 880.4	−1 924.3
Total net worth[1]	TMPN	−650.4	−499.0	−310.7	38.8	−52.2	−104.0	−372.4	−517.1	−546.4

1 Net worth was previously defined as *net wealth*.
2 Residential buildings now include Housing Association properties. These were formally included in table 10.10 (Non profit institutions serving households).

10.6 Financial corporations

£ billion at end year

		1999	2000	2001	2002	2003	2004	2005	2006	2007
Non-financial assets										
Tangible assets:										
Residential buildings	CGUD	1.0	0.8	0.6	0.7	0.5	0.4	0.9	1.4	2.7
Agricultural assets	CGUE	0.9	0.9	0.9	0.9	0.9	0.9	0.9	0.9	0.9
Commercial, industrial and other buildings	CGUF	95.9	98.7	102.9	103.0	109.2	117.4	121.9	125.0	123.1
Civil engineering works	CGUG	–	–	–	–	–	–	–	–	–
Plant and machinery	CGUH	10.9	11.7	11.1	11.3	11.5	11.3	11.3	11.6	12.0
Vehicles, including ships, aircraft, etc	CGUI	1.3	1.4	0.9	0.7	0.5	0.6	0.5	0.2	0.3
Stocks and work in progress	CGUO	–	–	–	–	–	–	–	–	–
Total tangible assets	CGUP	110.0	113.5	116.4	116.5	122.6	130.6	135.4	139.1	138.9
Intangible non-financial assets										
Non-marketable tenancy rights	CGUQ	–	–	–	–	–	–	–	–	–
Other intangible assets	CGUR	4.0	4.5	5.0	5.4	5.9	6.2	6.5	6.7	6.8
Total intangible assets	CGUS	4.0	4.5	5.0	5.4	5.9	6.2	6.5	6.7	6.8
Total non-financial assets	CGDB	114.0	118.0	121.4	122.0	128.5	136.9	141.9	145.8	145.8
Total net financial assets/liabilities	NYOE	−522.7	−514.0	−538.0	−448.2	−422.2	−438.4	−510.3	−506.5	−538.4
Total net worth[1]	CGRU	−408.7	−396.0	−416.6	−326.2	−293.7	−301.5	−368.4	−360.8	−392.6

1 Net worth was previously defined as *net wealth*.

10.7 General government

£ billion at end year

		1999	2000	2001	2002	2003	2004	2005	2006	2007
Non-financial assets										
Tangible assets:										
Residential buildings[2]	CGVQ	3.2	3.2	3.2	3.5	3.3	4.3	3.8	4.8	5.3
Agricultural assets	CGVR	2.0	2.1	2.1	2.1	2.2	2.2	2.1	2.1	2.1
Commercial, industrial and other buildings	CGVS	126.2	131.0	137.2	146.0	157.9	174.2	200.5	212.8	226.6
Civil engineering works	CGVT	233.9	263.2	305.6	312.2	337.5	376.3	406.0	437.4	476.0
Plant and machinery	CGVU	15.2	14.9	15.0	14.2	17.6	16.0	16.1	19.9	17.4
Vehicles, including ships, aircraft, etc	CGVV	3.6	3.3	4.3	4.4	4.3	4.5	5.6	5.8	6.5
Stocks and work in progress	CGVW	0.3	0.2	0.1	0.1	0.2	0.2	0.2	0.2	0.1
Spectrum[3]	ZLDB	–	21.9	21.9	21.9	21.9	21.9	21.9	21.9	21.9
Total tangible assets	CGVX	384.4	439.8	489.4	504.4	544.9	599.7	656.1	705.0	756.0
Intangible non-financial assets										
Non-marketable tenancy rights	CGVY	–	–	–	–	–	–	–	–	–
Other intangible assets	CGVZ	0.9	0.9	0.9	0.9	0.9	1.0	1.0	1.0	1.0
Total intangible assets	CGWA	0.9	0.9	0.9	0.9	0.9	1.0	1.0	1.0	1.0
Total non-financial assets	CGIX	385.3	440.7	490.3	505.3	545.9	600.6	657.0	706.1	757.0
Total net financial assets/liabilities	NYOG	−268.3	−260.9	−236.4	−254.0	−271.6	−308.9	−340.4	−367.3	−405.9
Total net worth[1]	CGRX	117.0	179.8	253.9	251.4	274.3	291.7	316.6	338.8	351.1

1 Net worth was previously defined as *net wealth*.
2 Council housing has now been transferred from General Government to the Public non-financial corporations sector.
3 Following the grant of licences to mobile phone companies, the electro-magnetic spectrum is included as an asset for the first time in 2000.

10.8 Central government[1]

£ billion at end year

		1999	2000	2001	2002	2003	2004	2005	2006	2007
Non-financial assets										
Tangible assets:										
Residential buildings	CGWB	3.2	3.2	3.2	3.5	3.3	4.3	3.8	4.8	5.3
Agricultural assets	CGWC	0.1	0.1	0.1	0.1	0.1	0.1	0.1	0.1	0.1
Commercial, industrial and other buildings	CGWD	48.8	49.5	52.1	56.7	63.0	69.1	87.9	92.9	97.6
Civil engineering works	CGWE	89.6	92.8	95.9	100.1	105.2	109.9	121.1	130.2	139.9
Plant and machinery	CGWF	11.8	11.7	11.6	11.4	14.3	11.8	11.2	14.4	11.5
Vehicles, including ships, aircraft, etc	CGWG	3.1	2.8	3.7	3.6	3.6	3.6	4.3	4.4	4.8
Stocks and work in progress	CGWH	0.3	0.2	0.1	0.1	0.2	0.2	0.2	0.2	0.1
Spectrum[3]	ZLDA	–	21.9	21.9	21.9	21.9	21.9	21.9	21.9	21.9
Total tangible assets	CGWI	156.9	182.2	188.7	197.6	211.6	220.9	250.5	269.0	281.3
Intangible non-financial assets										
Non-marketable tenancy rights	CGWJ	–	–	–	–	–	–	–	–	–
Other intangible assets	CGWK	0.4	0.4	0.3	0.2	0.2	0.2	0.1	0.1	0.1
Total intangible assets	CGWL	0.4	0.4	0.3	0.2	0.2	0.2	0.1	0.1	0.1
Total non-financial assets	CGIY	157.4	182.6	189.0	197.8	211.8	221.1	250.6	269.1	281.4
Total net financial assets/liabilities	NZDZ	−301.0	−292.8	−274.3	−302.1	−332.8	−380.7	−419.2	−440.6	−482.9
Total net worth[2]	CGRY	−143.6	−110.2	−85.3	−104.3	−121.0	−159.7	−168.6	−171.5	−201.5

1 UK national accounts classification excludes fighting equipment from tangible assets.
2 Net worth was previously defined as *net wealth*.
3 Following the grant of licences to mobile phone companies, the electro-magnetic spectrum is included as an asset for the first time in 2000.

10.9 Local government

£ billion at end year

		1999	2000	2001	2002	2003	2004	2005	2006	2007
Non-financial assets										
Tangible assets:										
Local Authority housing[2]	ZLCS	–	–	–	–	2.1	2.1	–	–	–
Agricultural assets	CGWN	1.9	2.0	2.0	2.0	2.1	2.1	2.0	2.0	2.0
Commercial, industrial and other buildings	CGWO	77.4	81.5	85.1	89.3	94.9	105.1	112.5	119.9	129.0
Civil engineering works	CGWP	144.3	170.4	209.7	212.0	232.3	266.5	284.9	307.2	336.1
Plant and machinery	CGWQ	3.4	3.2	3.4	2.8	3.4	4.2	4.9	5.5	5.9
Vehicles, including ships, aircraft, etc	CGWR	0.5	0.5	0.6	0.7	0.7	0.9	1.2	1.5	1.7
Stocks and work in progress	CGWS	–	–	–	–	–	–	–	–	–
Total tangible assets	CGWT	227.5	257.6	300.7	306.8	333.3	378.8	405.5	436.1	474.7
Intangible non-financial assets										
Non-marketable tenancy rights	CGWU	–	–	–	–	–	–	–	–	–
Other intangible assets	CGWV	0.5	0.5	0.6	0.7	0.8	0.8	0.9	0.9	0.9
Total intangible assets	CGWW	0.5	0.5	0.6	0.7	0.8	0.8	0.9	0.9	0.9
Total non-financial assets	CGIZ	228.0	258.1	301.3	307.5	334.1	379.6	406.4	437.0	475.6
Total net financial assets/liabilities	NYOJ	32.7	31.9	37.9	48.2	61.3	71.8	78.8	73.3	77.0
Total net worth[1]	CGRZ	260.6	290.0	339.3	355.7	395.3	451.4	485.2	510.3	552.6

1 Net worth was previously defined as *net wealth*.
2 The value of council housing is now shown in table 10.4 (Public non-financial corporations).

10.10 Households & non-profit institutions serving households (NPISH)

£ billion at end year

		1999	2000	2001	2002	2003	2004	2005	2006	2007
Non-financial assets										
Tangible assets:										
Residential buildings[2]	CGRI	1 718.9	1 967.9	2 116.5	2 568.1	2 869.0	3 221.3	3 336.2	3 696.3	4 077.3
Agricultural assets	CGRJ	46.4	47.0	46.3	46.8	47.4	47.5	47.3	47.1	46.9
Commercial, industrial and other buildings	CGRK	44.3	46.7	46.4	48.9	50.6	50.6	55.9	60.0	55.7
Civil engineering works	CGRL	1.6	2.2	2.2	2.2	2.1	2.0	2.0	2.0	2.0
Plant and machinery	CGRM	15.1	16.4	17.1	18.0	18.5	19.6	20.7	22.2	23.9
Vehicles, including ships, aircraft, etc	CGRN	57.6	57.5	62.4	68.8	73.1	77.1	79.3	80.2	81.4
Stocks and work in progress	CGRO	15.6	15.8	15.8	16.2	16.7	16.8	16.3	16.4	16.7
Total tangible assets	CGRP	1 899.5	2 153.5	2 306.6	2 769.0	3 077.4	3 435.0	3 557.7	3 924.2	4 304.0
Intangible non-financial assets										
Non-marketable tenancy rights	CGRQ	237.4	276.7	300.1	365.3	413.5	466.1	486.9	545.1	611.5
Other intangible assets	CGRS	0.5	0.6	0.6	0.7	0.8	0.8	0.9	0.9	0.9
Total intangible assets	CGRT	237.8	277.2	300.7	366.0	414.2	466.9	487.8	546.1	612.4
Total non-financial assets	CGCZ	2 137.3	2 430.7	2 607.3	3 135.0	3 491.6	3 902.0	4 045.5	4 470.3	4 916.4
Total net financial assets/liabilities	NZEA	2 444.6	2 383.4	2 158.6	1 797.3	1 924.9	2 001.9	2 363.0	2 502.3	2 607.0
Total net worth[1]	CGRC	4 582.0	4 814.1	4 765.9	4 932.3	5 416.5	5 903.9	6 408.5	6 972.6	7 523.4

1 Net worth was previously defined as *net wealth*.
2 Figures for Housing association properties are now included in table 10.5 (Private non-financial corporations).

10.11 Public sector

£ billion at end year

		1999	2000	2001	2002	2003	2004	2005	2006	2007
Non-financial assets										
Tangible assets:										
Residential buildings	**CGWX**	76.8	78.1	87.1	94.5	104.4	116.3	126.0	116.6	122.0
Agricultural assets	**CGWY**	3.1	3.0	2.9	3.0	3.1	3.1	3.1	3.0	3.0
Commercial, industrial and other buildings	**CGWZ**	152.0	153.0	157.7	171.6	181.7	199.6	226.9	239.7	251.5
Civil engineering works	**CGXA**	244.6	275.8	322.1	334.6	353.5	391.9	421.7	454.6	494.9
Plant and machinery	**CGXB**	20.3	19.9	19.8	21.6	25.4	24.3	24.4	28.2	26.2
Vehicles, including ships, aircraft, etc	**CGXC**	5.3	4.9	5.9	6.0	5.7	6.2	7.6	8.1	8.8
Stocks and work in progress	**CGXD**	5.6	5.3	5.3	5.3	5.2	5.4	5.4	5.5	5.4
Spectrum[2]	**ZLDC**	–	21.9	21.9	21.9	21.9	21.9	21.9	21.9	21.9
Total tangible assets	**CGXE**	507.6	561.9	622.8	658.6	701.0	768.6	836.9	877.7	933.7
Intangible non-financial assets										
Non-marketable tenancy rights	**CGXF**	–	–	–	–	–	–	–	–	–
Other intangible assets	**CGXG**	4.3	4.6	4.7	4.9	5.1	5.4	5.8	6.0	6.2
Total intangible assets	**CGXH**	4.3	4.6	4.7	4.9	5.1	5.4	5.8	6.0	6.2
Total non-financial assets	**CGJA**	511.9	566.5	627.5	663.4	706.1	774.0	842.7	883.7	939.9
Total net financial assets/liabilities	**CGSA**	–345.4	–336.7	–317.9	–351.5	–371.8	–423.3	–475.5	–486.0	–525.9
Total net worth[1]	**CGTY**	166.5	229.8	309.6	311.9	334.4	350.7	367.2	397.7	414.1

1 Net worth was previously defined as *net wealth*.
2 Following the grant of licences to mobile phone companies, the electro-magnetic spectrum is included as an asset for the first time in 2000.

Chapter 11

Public sector supplementary tables

Introduction

The National Accounts are traditionally updated with long-period revisions once a year, and then published in the *Blue Book*. The 2008 edition has been restricted in the revisions taken on as a result of an ONS decision to divert resources elsewhere. The process of revision can be complex, particularly if the time series being revised forms part of GDP.

The Government's fiscal policy rules rely on statistical measures based on the National Accounts framework. The speed with which revisions could be taken on in the National Accounts is not adequate for the purposes of fiscal policy, which is based on an economic cycle and requires up to date information over the entire cycle. This has led to a separate revisions policy for the *Public Sector Finances*, where revisions are immediately implemented, with the National Accounts catching up as soon as possible. In normal circumstances this would be in the next *Blue Book*.

As a consequence of these different revisions policies, the version of Chapter 11 published here is consistent with the National Accounts, but not with the *Public Sector Finances*.

Table 11.3 (key fiscal aggregates) has been withdrawn from this *Blue Book* as it would be confusing to publish an alternative incorrect version of the key fiscal aggregates. The main part of this table is already published once a quarter and the other series will be updated once a year in the *Public Sector Finances*.

Table 11.2 (functional breakdown of General Government) has also been withdrawn from this year's *Blue Book*. We plan to publish these data in the December 2008 *Public Sector Finances*.

Tables 11.4, 11.5, and 11.6 (reconciliation of financial balance sheets and transactions for the General Government sector and the Central and Local Government sub-sectors) have been withdrawn from this year's *Blue Book*. We plan to publish these data in the November 2008 *Public Sector Finances*.

Table 11.7 (housing operating account) has also been withdrawn from this year's *Blue Book*. We plan to publish these data in the December 2008 *Public Sector Finances*.

Taxes payable by UK residents (Table 11.1)

This table is consistent with the National Accounts. A more up to date version consistent with the latest Public Sector Finance data, incorporating revisions, will be made available alongside Public Sector Finances release.

This table shows the taxes and national insurance contributions payable to central government, local government, and to the institutions of the European Union.

Taxes on production are included in GDP at market prices. Taxes on products are taxes levied on the sale of goods and services. Other taxes on production include taxes levied on inputs to production (for example non-domestic rates by businesses) and some compulsory unrequited levies that producers have to pay.

Taxes on income and wealth include income tax and corporation tax. Also included are some charges payable by households (for example local government taxes and motor vehicle duty), which are classified as taxes on production when payable by businesses. The totals are measured gross of any tax credits and reliefs recorded as expenditure in the National Accounts, such as working families and child tax credit.

ESA95 has a category called compulsory social contributions. In the UK accounts this category includes all national insurance contributions. Details of total social contributions and benefits are shown in Tables 5.2.4S and 5.3.4S of Chapter 5.

Some UK taxes are recorded as the resources of the European Union. These include taxes on imports and an amount calculated as the hypothetical yield from VAT at a standard rate on a harmonised base across the EU.

11.1 Taxes paid by UK residents to general government and the European Union
Total economy sector S.1

£ million

			1999	2000	2001	2002	2003	2004	2005	2006	2007
Part	**GENERATION OF INCOME**										
	Uses										
D.2	Taxes on production and imports										
D.21	Taxes on products and imports										
D.211	Value added tax (VAT)										
	Paid to central government	NZGF	57 701	59 985	63 522	68 251	74 595	79 761	81 416	85 586	89 681
	Paid to the European Union	FJKM	3 811	4 204	3 575	2 808	2 740	1 789	1 999	2 167	2 319
D.211	Total	QYRC	61 512	64 189	67 097	71 059	77 335	81 550	83 415	87 753	92 000
D.212	Taxes and duties on imports excluding VAT										
D.2121	Paid to CG: import duties[1]	NMXZ	–	–	–	–	–	–	–	–	–
D.2121	Paid to EU: import duties	FJWE	2 024	2 086	2 069	1 919	1 937	2 145	2 237	2 329	2 412
D.212	Total	QYRB	2 024	2 086	2 069	1 919	1 937	2 145	2 237	2 329	2 412
D.214	Taxes on products excluding VAT and import duties										
	Paid to central government										
	Customs & excise revenue										
	Beer	GTAM	2 792	2 813	2 888	2 934	3 035	3 111	3 072	3 065	3 042
	Wines, cider, perry & spirits	GTAN	3 595	3 751	4 025	4 333	4 491	4 761	4 802	4 779	5 008
	Tobacco	GTAO	7 693	7 666	7 638	7 947	8 079	8 097	8 021	8 089	8 051
	Hydrocarbon oils	GTAP	22 391	23 041	22 046	22 070	22 476	23 412	23 346	23 448	24 512
	Car tax	GTAT	–	–	–	–	–	–	–	–	–
	Betting, gaming & lottery	CJQY	1 521	1 522	1 406	997	933	872	864	958	959
	Air passenger duty	CWAA	884	940	824	814	781	856	896	961	1 883
	Insurance premium tax	CWAD	1 423	1 707	1 861	2 138	2 294	2 359	2 343	2 314	2 310
	Landfill tax	BKOF	430	461	502	541	607	672	733	804	877
	Other	ACDN	–	–	–	–	–	–	–	–	–
	Fossil fuel levy	CIQY	104	56	86	32	–	–	–	–	–
	Gas levy	GTAZ	–	–	–	–	–	–	–	–	–
	Stamp duties	GTBC	6 000	8 367	7 344	7 431	7 256	8 884	9 910	13 074	14 634
	Levies on exports (Third country trade)	CUDF									
	Camelot payments to National Lottery										
	Distribution Fund	LIYH	1 574	1 590	1 480	1 452	1 293	1 342	1 349	1 440	1 310
	Purchase Tax	EBDB	–	–	–	–	–	–	–	–	–
	Hydro-benefit	LITN	35	42	46	44	44	40	10	–	–
	Aggregates levy	MDUQ	–	–	–	213	340	328	327	321	339
	Milk super levy	DFT3	–	–	14	35	56	69	19	1	–
	Climate change levy	LSNT	–	–	585	825	828	756	747	711	690
	Channel 4 funding formula	EG9G	–	–	–	–	–	–	–	–	–
	Renewable energy obligations	EP89	–	–	–	195	345	373	369	450	462
	Rail franchise premia	LITT	–	–	–	–	–	205	98	125	215
	Other taxes and levies	GCSP	–	–	–	–	–	–	–	–	–
	Total paid to central government	NMYB	48 442	51 956	50 745	52 001	52 858	56 137	56 906	60 540	64 292
	Paid to the European Union										
	Sugar levy	GTBA	46	44	31	25	18	25	24	–	–
	European Coal & Steel Community levy	GTBB	–	–	–	–	–	–	–	–	–
	Total paid to the European Union	FJWG	46	44	31	25	18	25	24	–	–
D.214	Total taxes on products excluding VAT & import duties	QYRA	48 488	52 000	50 776	52 026	52 876	56 162	56 930	60 540	64 292
D.21	Total taxes on products and imports	NZGW	112 024	118 275	119 942	125 004	132 148	139 857	142 582	150 622	158 704
D.29	Production taxes other than on products										
	Paid to central government										
	Consumer Credit Act fees	CUDB	157	119	205	190	208	220	197	223	281
	National non-domestic rates	CUKY	14 208	14 954	15 979	16 604	16 891	17 099	17 919	18 919	19 478
	Northern Ireland non-domestic rates	NSEZ	126	128	133	134	139	263	286	318	359
	Levies paid to CG levy-funded bodies	LITK	226	217	215	195	193	214	235	232	261
	Selective employment tax	CSAH	–	–	–	–	–	–	–	–	–
	National insurance surcharge	GTAY	–	–	–	–	–	–	–	–	–
	London regional transport levy	GTBE	–	–	–	–	–	–	–	–	–
	IBA levy	GTAL	–	–	–	–	–	–	–	–	–
	Motor vehicle duties paid by businesses	EKED	1 565	1 415	778	724	797	808	809	865	878
	Regulator fees	GCSQ	79	101	98	93	101	86	78	72	76
	Tithe Act payments[2]	EBDD	–	–	–	–	–	–	–	–	–
	Total	NMBX	16 361	16 934	17 408	17 940	18 329	18 690	19 524	20 629	21 333
	Paid to local government										
	Non-domestic rates[3]	NMYH	142	149	157	173	188	163	182	202	225
D.29	Total production taxes other than on products	NMYD	16 503	17 083	17 565	18 113	18 517	18 853	19 706	20 831	21 558
D.2	Total taxes on production and imports, paid										
	Paid to central government	NMBY	122 504	128 875	131 675	138 192	145 782	154 588	157 846	166 755	175 306
	Paid to local government	NMYH	142	149	157	173	188	163	182	202	225
	Paid to the European Union	FJWB	5 881	6 334	5 675	4 752	4 695	3 959	4 260	4 496	4 731
D.2	Total	NZGX	128 527	135 358	137 507	143 117	150 665	158 710	162 288	171 453	180 262

1 These taxes existed before the UK's entry into the EEC in 1973
2 These taxes existed before 1969
3 From 190/1991 onwards thse series only contain rates paid in Northern Ireland

11.1 Taxes paid by UK residents to general government and the European Union
Total economy sector S.1

continued

£ million

			1999	2000	2001	2002	2003	2004	2005	2006	2007
Part	**SECONDARY DISTRIBUTION OF INCOME**										
	Uses										
D.5	Current taxes on income, wealth etc										
D.51	Taxes on income										
	Paid to central government										
	Household income taxes	DRWH	94 713	103 129	108 506	109 358	111 559	117 481	128 098	137 368	147 389
	Corporation Tax	ACCD	32 924	33 003	33 520	28 866	28 489	31 160	37 820	47 108	43 912
	Petroleum revenue tax	DBHA	472	1 540	1 526	946	1 146	1 166	1 799	2 546	1 387
	Windfall tax	EYNK	–	–	–	–	–	–	–	–	–
	Other taxes on income	BMNX	1 444	2 330	3 712	3 672	3 040	4 320	4 781	5 790	6 601
D.51	Total	NMCU	129 553	140 002	147 264	142 842	144 234	154 127	172 498	192 812	199 289
D.59	Other current taxes										
	Paid to central government										
	Motor vehicle duty paid by households	CDDZ	3 308	3 191	3 324	3 570	3 923	3 955	3 953	4 145	4 506
	Northern Ireland domestic rates	NSFA	115	112	107	106	101	225	233	244	250
	Boat licences	NSNP	8	4	–	–	–	–	–	–	–
	Fishing licences	NRQB	–	–	–	–	–	19	20	20	20
	National non-domestic rates paid by non-market sectors[1]	BMNY	994	1 000	1 047	1 029	996	1 082	1 191	1 260	1 306
	Passport fees	E8A6	77	107	140	148	185	220	279	322	377
	Television licence fee	DH7A	2 251	1 955	2 302	2 280	2 329	2 490	2 655	2 696	2 862
	Total	NMCV	6 753	6 369	6 920	7 133	7 534	7 991	8 331	8 687	9 321
	Paid to local government										
	Domestic rates[2]	NMHK	67	73	80	83	91	139	147	155	169
	Community charge	NMHL	–	–	–	–	–	–	–	–	–
	Council tax	NMHM	12 699	13 845	15 068	16 448	18 391	19 871	20 966	22 064	23 137
	Total	NMIS	12 766	13 918	15 148	16 531	18 482	20 010	21 113	22 219	23 306
D.59	Total	NVCM	19 519	20 287	22 068	23 664	26 016	28 001	29 444	30 906	32 627
D.5	Total current taxes on income, wealth etc										
	Paid to central government	NMCP	136 306	146 371	154 184	149 975	151 768	162 118	180 829	201 499	208 610
	Paid to local government	NMIS	12 766	13 918	15 148	16 531	18 482	20 010	21 113	22 219	23 306
D.5	Total	NMZL	149 072	160 289	169 332	166 506	170 250	182 128	201 942	223 718	231 916
D.61	Social contributions										
D.611	Actual social contributions										
	Paid to central government (National Insurance Contributions)										
D.61111	Employers' compulsory contributions	CEAN	31 286	34 028	35 706	35 735	39 890	43 586	46 741	49 552	52 300
D.61121	Employees' compulsory contributions	GCSE	23 573	24 175	25 236	25 357	29 055	32 396	34 742	37 039	38 474
D.61131	Self- and non-employed persons' compulsory contributions	NMDE	1 883	2 049	2 183	2 318	2 595	2 727	2 825	2 930	3 013
D.611	Total	AIIH	56 742	60 252	63 125	63 410	71 540	78 709	84 308	89 521	93 787
Part	**CAPITAL ACCOUNT**										
	Changes in liabilities and net worth										
D.91	Other capital taxes										
	Paid to central government										
	Inheritance tax	GILF	1 920	2 156	2 366	2 327	2 386	2 821	3 100	3 471	3 787
	Tax on other capital transfers	GILG	31	59	30	54	30	50	50	50	50
	Development land tax and other	GCSV	–	–	–	–	–	–	–	–	–
	Tax paid on LG equal pay settlements	C625	–	–	–	–	–	–	–	54	53
D.91	Total	NMGI	1 951	2 215	2 396	2 381	2 416	2 871	3 150	3 575	3 890
	TOTAL TAXES AND COMPULSORY SOCIAL CONTRIBUTIONS										
	Paid to central government	GCSS	317 503	337 713	351 380	353 958	371 506	398 286	426 133	461 350	481 593
	Paid to local government	GCST	12 908	14 067	15 305	16 704	18 670	20 173	21 295	22 421	23 531
	Paid to the European Union	FJWB	5 881	6 334	5 675	4 752	4 695	3 959	4 260	4 496	4 731
	Total	GCSU	336 292	358 114	372 360	375 414	394 871	422 418	451 688	488 267	509 855

1 Up until 1995/96 these payments are included in national non-domestic rates under production taxes other than on products
2 From 1990/1991 onwards these series only contain rates paid in Northern Ireland

Chapter 12

Statistics for European Union purposes

The European Union uses National Accounts data for a number of administrative and economic purposes. Gross National Product (GNP), calculated in accordance with the European System of Accounts 1979 (ESA79), has been used in setting a ceiling on the EU budget and calculating part of Member States' contributions to the budget.

However, from 2002, the calculation reflects the move to the new European System of Accounts 1995 (ESA95) and the progression to Gross National Income (GNI) from GNP.[1] ESA95 is the basis on which most UK statistical information is now supplied to the EU.

ESA95 differs from the ESA79 in a number of ways, for example, the recording of interest payments, and the treatment of software in gross fixed capital formation and roads and bridges in the consumption of fixed capital formation.[2]

Data supplied for EU budgetary purposes

The GNP/GNI measure[3] is one component in the calculation of Member States' contributions to the EU Budget.

GNP data up to and including 2001 have been frozen, or 'closed' in the calculation of UK contributions. In future, revisions will only be made due to methodological improvements to the transition mechanism (see note 2).

The years 2002 onwards remain 'open' years, reflecting any revisions to National Accounts. From 2002, UK contributions are calculated under the ESA95 framework as shown in Table 1.2.

UK transactions with the institutions of the EU

Table 12.1 shows the UK contribution to the budget under the four categories of revenue raising ('own resources'), and payments flowing into the UK in the form of EU expenditure and the UK budgetary rebate. UK GNP/GNI forms the basis of the 'Fourth Resource' contributions.

Data to monitor government deficit and debt

The convergence criteria for Economic and Monetary Union (EMU) are set out in the 1992 Treaty on European Union (The Maastricht Treaty).[4] The Treaty, plus the Stability & Growth Pact, requires Member States to avoid excessive government deficits defined as general government net borrowing and

gross debt as a percentage of GDP. Member States report their planned and actual deficits, and the levels of their debt, to the European Commission. Data to monitor excessive deficits are supplied in accordance with EU legislation.[5]

The Treaty does not determine what constitutes 'excessive'. This is agreed by the Economic and Finance Council (ECOFIN). However, a Protocol to the Treaty does provide a reference value of 3 per cent of GDP for net borrowing and 60 per cent of GDP for gross debt.

The United Kingdom submitted the estimates in the following table to the European Commission in September 2008.[6]

	2004/5	2005/6	2006/7	2007/8
General government deficit				
net borrowing (£bn)	41.9	38.5	34.4	38.7
as a percentage of GDP[6]	3.5	3.0	2.6	2.7
General government debt				
debt at nominal value (£bn)[7]	483.8	531.5	574.2	614.4
as a percentage of GDP[6]	39.9	41.9	42.7	43.2

References

1 The harmonisation of gross national income at market prices (GNI regulation) was adopted in July 2003 under Council Regulation (EC) No. 1287/2003.

2 Commission Decision 97/178 set down a transition mechanism for deriving ESA79 GNP figures from ESA95 for the purposes of the EC budget. The mechanism was extended following Commission Decision 98/501 and the July 2001 meeting of the GNP Committee.

3 Council Directive 89/130/EEC.

4 Treaty on European Union (Luxembourg, Office for Official Publications of the European Communities, 1992).

5 Council Regulation (EC) No. 3605/93.

6 Data were also published in calendar years in the September 2008 *Government deficit and debt under the Maastricht Treaty* release.

7 At end year.

12.1 UK official transactions with institutions of the EU

UK transactions with ESA95 sector S.212

£ million

			1999	2000	2001	2002	2003	2004	2005	2006	2007
	UK resources										
P.62	Exports of services										
	UK charge for collecting duties and levies(net)[1,2]	QWUE	208	217	525	487	489	543	565	583	603
D.31	Subsidies on products, paid (negative resources)										
	Agricultural guarantee fund	EBGL	2 781	2 571	2 336	2 381	2 691	3 315	3 408	3 220	2 943
	European Coal & Steel Community grants	FJKP	–	–	1	–	–	2	–	–	–
D.75	Social assistance										
	European Social Fund	HDIZ	434	659	370	412	427	433	900	1 305	795
D.74	Current international co-operation										
	Fontainebleau abatement[2]	FKKL	3 171	2 084	4 560	3 099	3 560	3 592	3 655	3 570	3 523
	Grants to research councils and miscellaneous[2]	GCSD	5	–	8	13	10	12	13	24	4
D.92	Capital transfers, payable										
	Agricultural guidance fund	FJXL	47	82	26	–	2	49	80	50	150
	European regional development fund	HBZA	285	989	543	296	622	1 062	1 402	618	707
D.99	Agricultural compensation scheme payments[5]	EBGO	–	–	322	–	–	–	–	–	–
	Total identified UK resources	GCSL	6 931	6 602	8 691	6 688	7 801	9 008	10 023	9 370	8 725
	UK uses										
D.21	Taxes on products										
	EU traditional own resources										
D.212	Import duties	FJWD	2 024	2 086	2 069	1 919	1 937	2 145	2 237	2 329	2 412
D.214	Sugar levy	GTBA	46	44	31	25	18	25	24	–	–
D.214	European Coal & Steel Community levy	GTBB	–	–	–	–	–	–	–	–	–
	Third own resource contribution										
D.211	VAT contribution	HCML	3 920	4 104	3 624	2 720	2 775	1 764	1 980	2 165	2 293
D.211	Adjustment to VAT contribution	FSVL	–109	100	–49	88	–35	25	19	2	26
D.75	Miscellaneous current transfers										
	Fourth own resource contribution[3]										
	GNP fourth resource	HCSO	4 403	4 243	3 859	5 259	6 622	7 565	8 597	8 358	7 996
	GNP adjustment	HCSM	229	136	–1	76	150	–16	135	163	327
	Total GNP based fourth own resource	NMFH	4 632	4 379	3 858	5 335	6 772	7 549	8 732	8 521	8 323
D.74	Other current transfers										
	JET contributions and miscellaneous[3]	GVEG	11	6	24	10	18	–3	106	8	6
	Inter-government agreements[3]	HCBW	–	–	–	–	–	–	–	–	–
	EU non-budget (miscellaneous)[3]	HRTM	–	–	–	–	–	–	–	–	–
	Total identified UK uses	GCSM	10 524	10 719	9 557	10 097	11 485	11 505	13 098	13 025	13 060
	Balance, UK net contribution to the EU[4]	BLZS	–3 593	–4 117	–866	–3 409	–3 684	–2 497	–3 075	–3 655	–4 335

1 Before 1989 this is netted off the VAT contribution but cannot be identfified separately.
2 UK central government resources.
3 UK central government uses.
4 As defined in pre-ESA95 Blue Books.
5 Before 1999 these have been included in Agricultural guarantee fund payments (series EBGL).

UK Environmental Accounts

Part 5

Chapter 13

The UK Environmental Accounts at a glance

Oil and gas reserves

At the end of 2006, UK oil reserves were valued at £113.3 billion while gas reserves were estimated to be worth £85.2 billion.

The value of the UK's recoverable oil and gas reserves mainly depend upon the estimated physical amounts remaining, the rate of extraction and the assumed future price per unit of oil or gas, net of the cost of extraction. Since 1994, the estimated physical stock of reserves has fallen as a result of extraction, but the value of the reserves has generally risen, with values being sensitive to fluctuations in the price of oil and gas.

Value of oil and gas reserves, 1995–2006

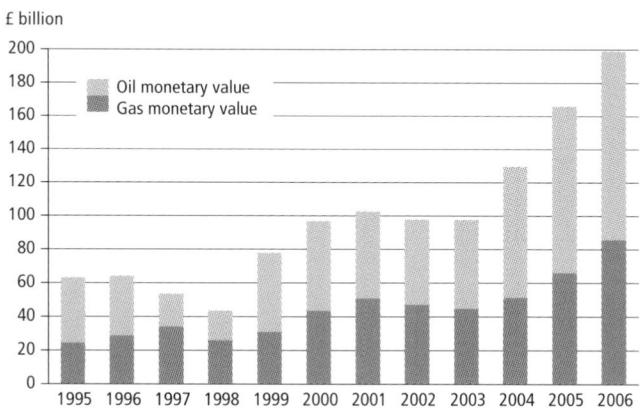

£ billion

Source: ONS

Energy consumption

Energy consumption, including electricity, by non-household sectors of the UK economy increased by 7.9 per cent between 1990 and 2006, while output (Gross Domestic Product) rose by 47.8 per cent in real terms. As a result, energy intensity (energy consumed per unit of output) has decreased by 27.0 per cent over the same period. The percentage of energy derived from renewable sources was 1.6 per cent in 2006 compared with 0.9 per cent in 1990.

Non-domestic energy consumption and output (Gross Domestic Product, CVM), 1990–2006

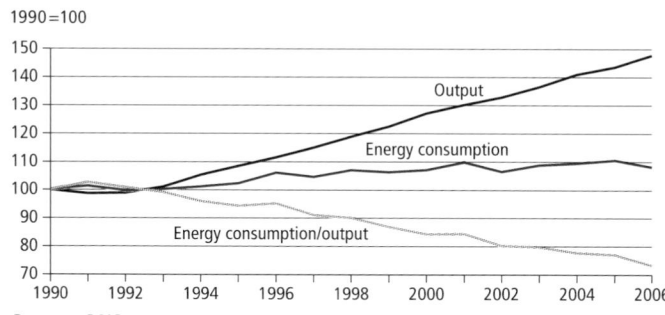

1990=100

Source: ONS

Atmospheric emissions

Total greenhouse gas emissions on a national accounts basis have fallen by 10.5 per cent since 1990, driven by a 14.2 per cent reduction in emissions from UK companies and the public sector. In contrast, emissions from the household sector have risen by 7.2 per cent, accounting for 20.9 per cent of emissions in 2006.

Between 1990 and 2006, the largest falls in greenhouse gas emissions occurred in other services (52.9 per cent). The largest increase was in transport and communications, up 47.0 per cent.

Emissions of the chemicals that cause acid rain have fallen by 58.6 per cent since 1990. Over this period there have been reductions in all industries. Emissions from households were 64.8 per cent lower in 2006 than in 1990, mainly reflecting falling emissions from the use of vehicles as a result of cleaner technology.

Atmospheric emissions of greenhouse gases and acid rain precursors, percentage change, 1990–2006

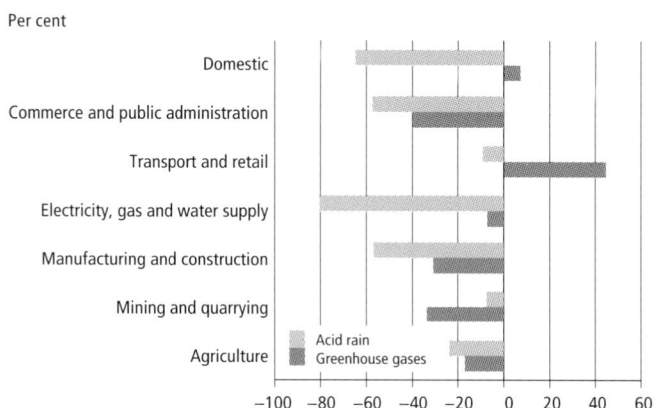

Per cent

Source: ONS

There were substantial improvements in the level of greenhouse gas emissions created per unit of output (emissions intensity), in most sectors of the economy between 1990 and 2006.

The largest fall in emissions intensity was in the commerce and public administration sector, falling by almost 66.1 per cent since 1990.

Emissions per unit of output from the transport and retail sector fell 9.1 per cent between 2005 and 2006 and are now 14.0 per cent lower than in 1990. The manufacturing and construction industries show a 4.5 per cent decrease in their emissions intensity in 2006, and reduced 37.3 per cent compared with 1990.

The emissions intensity from the non-household sector fell 5.6 per cent between 2005 and 2006 and is now 44.4 per cent below the 1990 level.

Material flow accounting

Material productivity has increased between 1990 and 2006.

This trend indicates that material use is falling in relation to the level of economic activity in the UK and supports evidence that domestic material use and economic growth have decoupled since 1990.

However, levels of imports have generally risen over the same period suggesting that some of the environmental impacts associated with consumption are being transferred abroad.

Environmental taxes

In 2007, environmental tax receipts amounted to £38.0 billion. By far the largest contributor to environmental taxes is duty on hydrocarbon oils such as petrol and diesel, which accounted for 64.5 per cent of the total in 2007, and where receipts increased by approximately £1.1 billion compared with the previous year. Receipts from Air Passenger Duty were the next largest increase, almost doubling in 2007, due mainly to increased tax rates.

Table 13.8 contains a breakdown of these taxes by 13 industries for 2004, consistent with Blue Book 2006. This shows that UK households pay £18.6 billion in environmental taxes, over half of all environmental taxes and three times the next highest contributor, the transport and communications industry. A revised industry breakdown consistent with latest National Accounts estimates published in Blue Book 2008 will be released in the autumn Environmental Accounts.

Greenhouse gas emissions per unit of output, (Gross value added CVM), 1990–2006

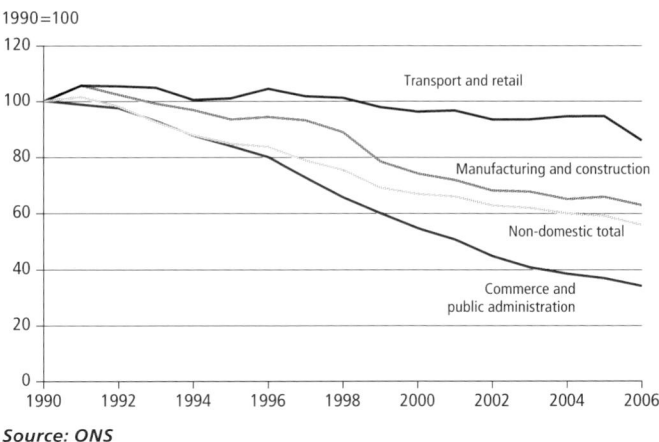

Source: ONS

Material flows in the UK

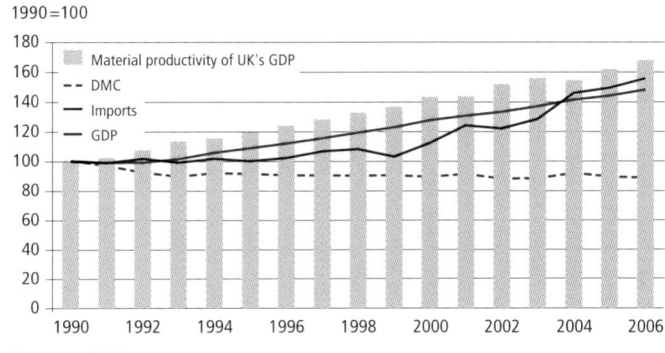

Source: ONS

Government receipts from environmental taxes, 1993–2007

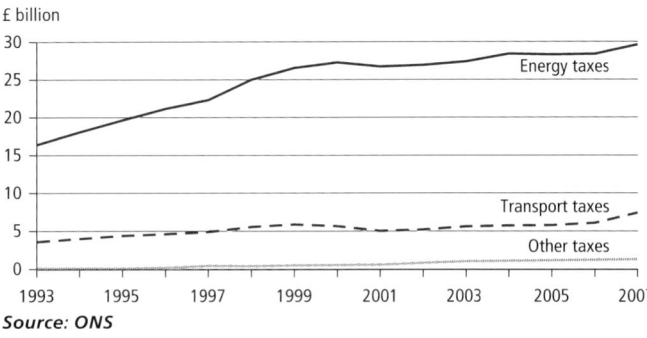

Source: ONS

Environmental protection expenditure

In 2004, public sector environmental protection expenditure was estimated at £5.9 billion with £3.5 billion spent on waste management and a further £0.7 billion on nature conservation, but only £0.3 billion directly on waste water management. Measures to protect air quality and the climate amounted to a further £0.3 billion.

Environmental protection expenditure data by industry for 2006, published by the Department for Environment, Food and Rural Affairs (Defra), is also included in this chapter.

Public sector environmental protection expenditure, 2001–2004

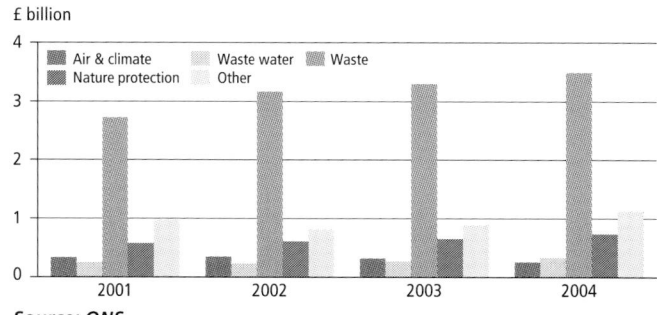

£ billion

Source: ONS

UK Environmental Accounts

Environmental accounts are 'satellite accounts' to the main National Accounts. Satellite accounts are extensions to the National Accounts, which facilitate analysis of the wider impact of economic change. Environmental accounts provide information on the environmental impact of economic activity (in particular on the emissions of pollutants) and on the importance of natural resources to the economy. Environmental accounts use similar concepts and classifications of industries to those employed in the National Accounts, and they reflect the recommended European Union and United Nations frameworks for developing such accounts.

The accounts are used to inform sustainable development policy, to model impacts of fiscal or monetary measures and to evaluate the environmental performance of different industrial sectors.

Most data are provided in units of physical measurement (volume or mass), although where appropriate some accounts are shown in monetary units.

This chapter includes information previously published in the spring 2008 edition of *Environmental Accounts*[1]. It updates information on environmental taxes and environmental protection expenditure. More detailed information on each of these accounts is available in *UK Environmental Accounts* on the National Statistics website:

www.statistics.gov.uk/statbase/Product.asp?vlnk=3698

The diagram below shows how the areas covered by environmental accounts relate to the economy as described by the National Accounts.

Environment and economy interactions

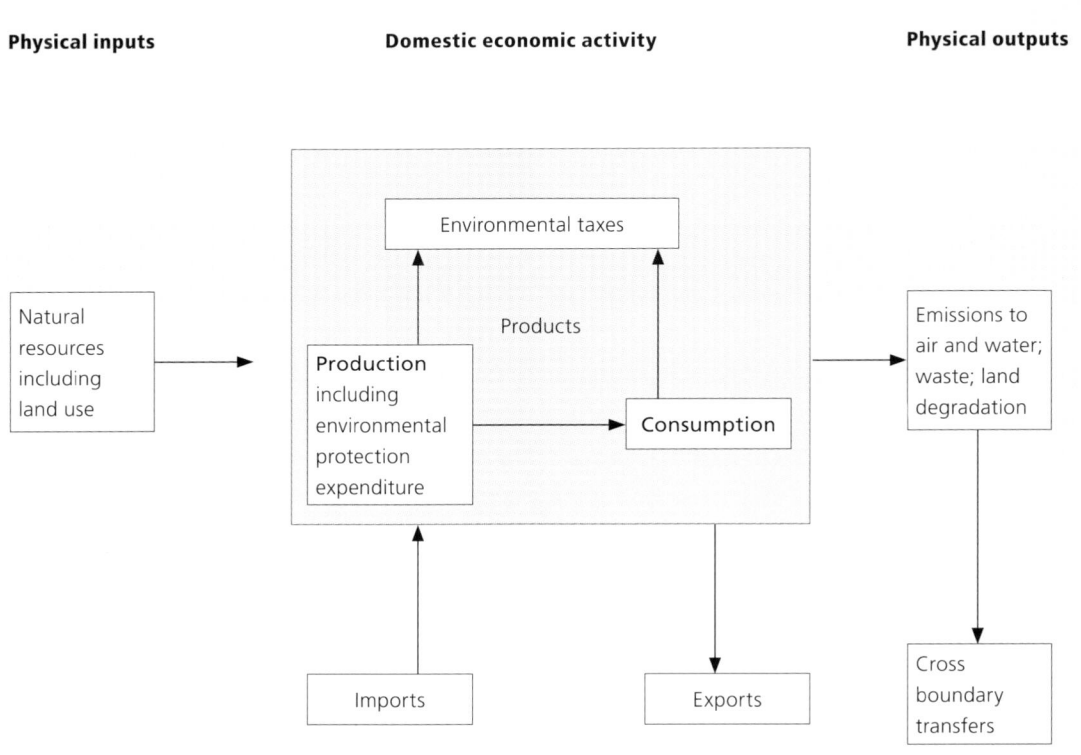

Oil and gas reserves (Tables 13.1 and 13.2)

Definition of oil and gas

Oil reserves include both oil and the liquids and liquefied products obtained from gas fields, gas-condensate fields and from the associated gas in oil fields. Gas reserves are the quantity of gas expected to be available for sale from dry gas fields, gas-condensate fields and oil fields with associated gas. Gas which is expected to be flared or used offshore is not included.

This publication uses new terminology introduced by the Department for Business Enterprise and Regulatory Reform (BERR) to describe UK reserves of oil and gas. Descriptions are now more closely aligned to those used by the oil and gas industry in order to improve general understanding and ensure consistency. Reserves are classified into the following categories: reserves, potential additional reserves and undiscovered resources. Undiscovered resources relate to those resources as yet undiscovered but potentially recoverable in mapped leads. Potential additional reserves are defined as discovered reserves that are not currently technically or economically producible. Reserves are classified as discovered, remaining reserves which are recoverable and commercial. These can be subdivided into proven, probable or possible depending on confidence level.

Simulation models using Monte Carlo techniques have been used each year by BERR to assess the likely existence and size of undiscovered oil and gas fields on the UK Continental Shelf (UKCS). The assessments are presented as ranges, but the limits of the ranges should not be regarded as maxima or minima. Estimates of the volume of undiscovered reserves have fluctuated considerably in recent years as new areas of UKCS have been subjected to statistical analysis and older areas have been re-assessed. Estimates are published annually by BERR and are taken from the BERR Brown Book.

The lower end of the range of total reserves shown in the table is the sum of estimated proven reserves and the lower end of the range of undiscovered resources for that year, net of cumulative production.

The upper end of the range of total reserves is the sum of estimated proven, possible and probable reserves, plus the upper end range of undiscovered resources, for that year, net of cumulative production.

The expected level of reserves is calculated as the sum of proven and probable reserves and the lower end of the range of undiscovered resources.

Other volume changes are calculated as the difference between the expected level of reserves at the start of the year, less production within that year, and the estimated level of reserves at the start of the following year.

Life expectancy is calculated as the expected level of reserves at the end of the year divided by the current level of annual extraction. This calculation gives an indication of the theoretical number of years for which extraction could be sustained at current levels. In practice, towards the end of that period, the rate of extraction is likely to decrease as individual oil and gas fields are exhausted, so the period of extraction will be longer than that implied by the life expectancy calculation.

Monetary valuation of oil and gas reserves

Expressing UK oil and gas reserves in monetary terms allows these subsoil assets to be compared with other economic entities. This provides a means for the commercial depletion of subsoil assets to be set against national income. Results are presented in Table 13.2 in the form of a balance sheet.

Since observed market values for transactions *in situ* in their original state are not widely available, the present value method is used to put a monetary value on the physical stocks of assets. This is an indirect valuation method measuring the current value of the asset's future streams of income by discounting the expected future rent, often referred to as the economic rent or resource rent. The method relies on information about the size of resource rent, the number of years for which the rent is to be received and the social discount rate to be applied.

The resource rent is the net income from extraction defined as total revenue from sales less all costs incurred in the extraction process that is, operating costs, depreciation of capital and an allowance for the return on capital. Decommissioning costs have not been included in these accounts. The rate of return on capital is estimated to be 8 per cent in real terms, in line with Eurostat recommendations[3], but it is worth noting that the resulting valuations are very sensitive to variations in this estimate. A three point centred moving average is used for the calculation of the unit resource rent.

The time span until the complete exhaustion of the reserves is the period over which resource rents are discounted, using the Eurostat recommended social discount rate of 4 per cent. Using these assumptions it is possible to calculate a present value of the stocks of oil and gas reserves at the start and end of each year. The accumulation account then breaks down the change between the start-of-year balance and the end-of-year balance. While physical stocks may change only as a result of extraction and other volume changes such as reassessments, monetary stocks can change for a number of other reasons.

Extraction is equal to the total resource rent for the year, effectively reducing the present value of the stocks by that amount. Positive values for extraction are a result of estimated negative resource rents. Revaluation due to time passing takes account of the fact that, as we move forward in time, the period over which the future rents are discounted is one year less, thereby reducing the effect of discounting future incomes. Other volume changes are reassessments which change the estimated physical stock of recoverable reserves.

The change in the extraction path sets out in monetary terms the addition or subtraction to the present value arising from a change in the amounts assumed to be extracted each year.

The change in unit rent gives the change in the future stream of income resulting from a change in the estimated unit resource rent. Any negative stock values result from estimated negative resource rents and have been left in the table in order to show the results of the assumptions made in the calculation.

Energy consumption (Table 13.3)

The Energy Consumption dataset gives estimates of total energy used by each industry and the proportion of total energy used from renewable resources. Detailed estimates of consumption of different fuel types by each sub-sector are given on the National Statistics website:

www.statistics.gov.uk/statbase/Product.asp?vlnk=3698

Unit of measurement

The unit of measurement is tonne of oil equivalent (toe), which enables different fuels to be compared and aggregated. It should be regarded as a measure of energy content rather than a physical quantity. Standard conversion factors for each type of fuel are given in the *Digest of UK Energy Statistics* (DUKES)[4].

Consumption of carbon fuels, energy used in transformation processes and losses in distribution

The consumption of carbon fuels, and the related consumption of energy, can be analysed from a number of different perspectives. In terms of atmospheric emissions, it may be helpful to identify which sectors are actually consuming the carbon fuels that give rise to emissions. From this perspective, fuels used by the electricity generation sector are attributed entirely to that sector, even though some of the energy is transformed into electricity. This analysis is shown in Part 1 of the table showing Energy Consumption.

In terms of energy consumption, it is possible to attribute energy used during the process of transformation into electricity, and the energy lost in distributing electricity to end users, either **directly** to the electricity generation sector, or **indirectly** to the consumers of energy. Parts 2 and 3 of the table in Energy Consumption consider energy consumption from both points of view. Part 2 allocates the consumption of energy directly to the immediate consumer of the energy, while Part 3 allocates these 'electricity overheads' of the major power producers to the user of the electricity.

Non-energy uses of fuels

Non-energy use of fuels includes, for example, chemical feedstocks, solvents, lubricants and road-making material. These uses have been excluded from the data.

Renewable energy sources

Renewable energy is defined to include solar power, energy from wind, wave and tide, hydroelectricity, and energy from wood, straw and sewage gas. Landfill gas and municipal solid waste combustion have been included with renewable energy for the purposes of defining energy sources in the context of sustainable development policy.

Sources and methods for estimating consumption of energy by industrial sector

Data for estimating fuel consumption by industrial sectors are collected by BERR and are published in DUKES. However, the figures shown in Energy Consumption differ from those given in DUKES in that:

- fuels used by the UK fishing fleet, UK international shipping and aircraft operators and ships and aircraft used for UK military purposes are included, whether or not they were purchased in the UK, whereas fuels purchased in the UK by non-resident operators are excluded

- purchases of petrol and diesel abroad by UK motorists and road hauliers are included

- non-energy uses of fuels for example, chemical feedstocks, solvents, lubricants and road-making material, are excluded. However, energy lost through gas leakage etc is included

- the classification of industrial sectors used in environmental accounts differs from that used in DUKES. In particular, the transport sector is defined to include only enterprises that provide transport services to other consumers (that is, public transport operators, freight haulage companies, etc.). The energy consumed by households' use of private cars is allocated to the domestic sector

The allocation of energy use to particular industries is primarily based on DUKES data. However, for certain industries better estimates are used as published by BERR in *Energy Trends*. Differences in publication times may result in minor reconciliation anomalies between ONS and BERR energy data.

Atmospheric emissions (Tables 13.4 and 13.5)

Tables 13.4 and 13.5 give estimates of pollutants directly emitted to the atmosphere by each sector. The figures are on a National Accounts basis and differ from the basis used to monitor progress against the Kyoto Protocol in that they include estimated emissions from fuels purchased abroad by UK residents[5], including those used by international shipping and aircraft on international flights. Emissions from fuels purchased in the UK by non-UK residents are excluded. Detailed estimates of pollutants from each sub-sector are given on the National Statistics website at:

www.statistics.gov.uk/statbase/Product.asp?vlnk=3698.

The website also gives details of emissions from acid rain precursors such as Sulphur Dioxide, other pollutants like Benzene and heavy metals including Lead and Zinc.

Pollutants and environmental themes

Atmospheric emissions can be aggregated according to their contribution to environmental themes such as greenhouse gases and acid rain. A description of the pollutants covered and the methodology used to calculate environmental themes is given in the annex to these notes.

Attributing emissions to industrial sectors

The disaggregation of national estimates of emissions to industrial sectors is based upon an initial disaggregation provided by the National Environmental Technology Centre (AEA Energy and Environment)[6] which maintains the National Atmospheric Emissions Inventory (NAEI)[7]. Emissions are estimated by multiplying fuel consumption by emissions factors and adding releases unrelated to fuel use such as methane arising from landfill.

The NAEI data is used to identify the main processes and industries responsible for the emissions, which are then allocated to individual sectors on the basis of information from a variety of sources. For example, emissions from diesel use by Heavy Goods Vehicles are allocated to sectors using vehicle mileage data from the Department for Transport. Expenditure information is also used, for example to allocate emissions arising from the use of various industrial coatings (for example, general industrial, heavy duty and vehicle refinishing) to relevant sectors in proportion to each sector's expenditure on paints, varnishes and similar coatings, printing ink and mastics, using the National Accounts supply-use tables as the main source. A full description of the methods and sources used in these accounts is available on request from the ONS Environmental Accounts branch.

There are a number of formats for the reporting and recording of atmospheric emissions data. These include the Intergovernmental Panel on Climate Change (IPCC) and United Nations Economic Commission for Europe (UNECE) measures both published by Defra and the National Accounts consistent measure published by the ONS. For further details please refer to *Environmental Accounts* on the National Statistics website.

Table 13.4, shows latest estimates of air pollutants directly emitted by each sector. Emissions generated by the electricity supply industry have not been reallocated to their customers in this analysis. Emissions from road haulage are given on an 'own account' basis, that is, attributed to the sector owning the transport rather than to the sector of the goods being transported. Similarly emissions from households' use of private cars are allocated to the domestic sector. Figures for total road transport emissions are provided separately.

Table 13.5 shows estimates of greenhouse gases and acid rain emissions by industrial sector.

Material flows (Table 13.6)

Material flow accounts record the total mass of natural resources and products that are used by the economy, either directly in the production and distribution of products and services, or indirectly through the movement of materials which are displaced in order for production to take place.

A material flow account balances the inputs (extraction of natural resources from the UK environment, and imports of goods) with the outputs (wastes, emissions to air and water, exports) and accumulation (in terms of new buildings etc) within the economy.

The direct input of materials into the economy derives primarily from domestic extraction, that is, from biomass (agricultural harvest, timber, fish and animal grazing), fossil fuel extraction (such as coal, crude oil and natural gas) and mineral extraction (metal ores, industrial minerals such as pottery clay, and construction material such as crushed rock, sand and gravel).

The direct input of materials from domestic sources is supplemented by the imports of products, which may be of raw materials such as unprocessed agricultural products, but can also be semi-manufactured or finished products. In a similar way the UK exports of raw materials, semi-manufactured and finished goods can be viewed as inputs to the production and consumption of overseas economies.

Water is used so widely and in such quantities that its inclusion in the accounts tends to obscure other resource use. For this reason, the accounts only include the water that is contained in products (for example, agricultural produce and imported beverages). Water for other consumptive uses (cleaning or irrigation) and *in situ* uses (such as hydroelectric power) is excluded from these accounts.

Hidden flows measure the quantity of material displaced by the process of extraction but not actually used in the production of goods and services. Indirect flows measure the quantity of material associated with imports of raw and semi-processed goods into the UK. Both hidden and indirect flows are measured indirectly by applying coefficients for particular materials and goods to the estimated levels of mass associated with domestic and overseas extraction. Therefore, there is a direct relationship between hidden flows and actual extraction. Levels are sensitive to assumptions embodied in the particular hidden or indirect flow coefficient used. Examples of hidden flows are unused extraction from mining and quarrying (also known as overburden), discarded material from harvesting (for example, wood harvesting losses such as timber felled but left in the forests), and soil and rock moved as a result of construction and dredging.

Indicators

There are a number of indicators which can be used to summarise the flows of materials into and out of the economy. Material flows show three of the main indicators used to measure inputs.

Direct Material Input (DMI) measures the input of materials directly used by the economy. It is the sum of domestic extraction and imports less exports.

Domestic material consumption (DMC) measures the total amount of material directly consumed by the economy. It is the sum of domestic extraction and imports less exports.

The **Total Material Requirement (TMR)** measures the total material basis of the economy, that is the total direct and indirect resource requirements of all the production and consumption activities. TMR includes the amount of used extraction in the UK, the imports into the UK and the resulting indirect or hidden flows associated with extraction in the UK and imports from other countries. Although TMR is widely favoured as a resource use indicator, the estimates of indirect flows are less reliable than those for materials directly used by the economy, and it can be argued that it double-counts trade flows, in that materials used both in the production of imports and in the production of exports are included. The indicator therefore needs to be considered alongside other indicators.

The **Physical Trade Balance (PTB)** measures the difference between the total mass of exports and the total mass of imports. This can be used to understand the internal relationship of material use in the UK.

Sources and methods

Data on the yields of agriculture, forestry and fishing come from the Food and Agriculture Organization (FAO)[8]. Mineral extraction data have been taken from the UK Minerals Yearbook[9] and information on the mass of imports and exports has been taken from trade information compiled by HM Revenue & Customs[10].

Factors applied to give estimates of the amounts of unused material moved for each tonne of used material have been taken from research carried out by the Wuppertal Institute on behalf of the Department for Environment, Food and Rural

Affairs (Defra)[11]. The methodology used to compile the account is also based upon the Wuppertal Institute's research.

Government revenues from environmental taxes (Table 13.7)

The environmental taxes table shows the level of revenues raised in environmental taxes in the United Kingdom.

Definition of an environmental tax

An environmental tax is defined as a tax whose base is a physical unit such as a litre of petrol, or a proxy for it, for instance a passenger flight, that has a proven specific negative impact on the environment. By convention, in addition to pollution related taxes, all energy and transport taxes are classified as environmental taxes. This definition has been agreed by international experts and adopted by the Statistical Office of the European Communities (Eurostat) and Organisation for Economic Co-operation and Development (OECD). It enables analysis to be based on the *effects* of taxes rather than the aims behind their introduction, that is, the aim of a tax for raising government revenue rather than reducing environmental degradation does not preclude it from being defined as an environmental tax.

Nevertheless, the interpretation and use of measures of environmental taxes need care. In particular, the levels of revenues from environmental taxes do not necessarily indicate the relative importance or the success of environmental policy. High environmental tax revenues can result either from high rates of taxes or from high levels of environmental problems (for example, pollution) leading to a large tax base. The broad measure of revenues can also fail to capture the effect of the differential rates that encourage a shift away from higher impact behaviour (such as the use of leaded petrol).

Taxes on energy products include duties on hydrocarbon oils used in road vehicles, the main ones being ultra low sulphur petrol and ultra low sulphur diesel. Taxes on energy products also include those used for non-transport purposes (such as industrial gas turbines and heating installations, with a reduced rate for energy saving materials) and the **fossil fuel levy**, which is levied on sales of electricity from fossil fuels and was used to compensate companies producing electricity from non-fossil fuel sources such as nuclear or renewable energy.

The **climate change levy**, which is a tax on non-domestic use of energy, was introduced in April 2001. The levy applies to the suppliers of the following energy types: electricity, natural gas as supplied by a gas utility, petroleum and hydrocarbon gas in a liquid state, coal and lignite, coke and seem-coke of coal or lignite, and petroleum coke. The rates of the levy are based on the type and quantity of fuel supplied, with a range of relief and exemptions available.

VAT on duty is calculated as a fixed proportion (in most cases 17.5 per cent) of the duty paid on hydrocarbon oils. In practice much of this VAT will be reclaimed by business, but it could be argued that the total will eventually be paid when the final product or service is purchased.

Taxes on road vehicles include Vehicle Excise Duty, which keepers of motor vehicles can pay on either a six monthly or annual basis. There have been various changes to this duty over recent years. Most recently, as from 1 May 2002, private cars, taxis and light goods vehicles registered before 1 March 2001 with an engine size up to and including 1549cc are subject to a lower tax than cars with engine sizes greater than 1549cc. The same vehicle types registered on or after 1 March 2001 are taxed according to the level of carbon dioxide emissions. This is now presented broken down by payments from businesses and households. Car tax was payable on purchases of new cars up until 1993 when it was discontinued.

Hydrobenefit was introduced in 1991 to protect energy consumers in remote areas, especially the Scottish Highlands and Islands, from excessive charges resulting from the increased costs involved in supplying those areas.

Air passenger duty was introduced on 1 November 1994. It applies to the carriage from a UK airport of chargeable passengers on chargeable aircraft at two different rates. The lower rate is charged where passengers are travelling to a UK destination or within the European Economic Area (EEA), and the higher rate applies in all other cases. On the year of introduction, the lower and higher rates of duty were £5 and £10 respectively. From 1 April 2001, standard rates of £10 for EEA destinations and £40 for other destinations have been applied. From 1 February 2007 these rates were doubled to £20 and £80 respectively. There are also reduced rates of duty for the lowest class of travel on any flights.

Landfill tax was introduced in October 1996 and aims to encourage waste producers to produce less waste, recover more value from waste, for example, through recycling or composting and to use more environmentally friendly methods of waste disposal. The tax applies to active and inactive (inert) waste disposed of at landfill sites. Generally when waste is committed to landfill it undergoes physical chemical or biological transformations which then react with surrounding matter. Known as leaching, this process can give rise to environmental damage and harm human health. Waste classified as inactive has insignificant levels of leachability, pollutant content and ecotoxicity. Types of waste excluded from this tax include dredgings, disposals from mines and quarries and also waste resulting from the clearance of contaminated land. A standard rate of tax is levied on active waste, this was introduced at the rate of £7.00 per tonnes and has since risen to £14.00 per tonne in 2003–04. This rate will

subsequently be increased each year until it reaches a medium to long term rate of £35.00 per tonne. A lower rate of tax is levied on inert waste, which has remained at £2.00 per tonne from the year of introduction.

The **aggregates levy** was introduced on 1 April 2002. The objective of this tax is to address the environmental costs associated with quarrying operations (noise, dust, visual intrusion, loss of amenity and loss to biodiversity), by reducing the demand for aggregate and encouraging the use of alternative materials where possible, for example, the use of waste glass and tyres in aggregate mixes. The tax applies to the commercial exploitation of sand, gravel and rock and includes aggregate dredged from the seabed within UK territorial waters. It is a specific tax, charged at £1.60 per tonne.

There is a wide range of exemptions for some quarried or mined products for example, coal, metal ores, industrial minerals and for minerals used in the production of lime and cement and for exports of aggregates. Imports of aggregates are taxed upon first sale or use in the UK.

Environmental taxes breakdown by 13 industries (Table 13.8)

The environmental taxes breakdown by 13 industries is based on general government environmental taxes data and unpublished Supply-Use data for taxes on products and production that are informed by latest available Supply-Use tables. From these sources it is possible to estimate allocations of environmental taxes to individual industries. A more detailed account of the methods used in this analysis is published in the August 2004 and October 2006 editions of *Economic Trends*[16].

Environmental protection expenditure (Tables 13.9 and 13.10)

Estimates of environmental protection expenditure should be regarded as approximate orders of magnitude only. Because of this qualification, the estimates shown fall outside the scope of National Statistics.

Comparisons with previous surveys

The information on spending by industries in 2006, which is summarised in environmental protection expenditure in specified industries, 2006 comes from a regular series of surveys conducted by the URS Corporation on behalf of Defra. The estimates from this survey and the earlier surveys should be regarded as very approximate and any comparisons between the results should be treated with care.

Definition of expenditure

Environmental protection expenditure is defined as capital and operational expenditure incurred because of, and which can be directly related to, the pursuit of an environmental objective. Spending on installations and processes which are environmentally beneficial, but which also produce revenue (or savings) exceeding expenditures, are excluded on the grounds that they are likely to have been carried out for commercial not environmental reasons. Also excluded are expenditures on natural resource management (for example, fisheries and water resources), on the prevention of natural hazards (for example, flood defence), on the provision of access and amenities to National Parks etc, and on the urban environment. The spending has been classified by the following groups of environmental concerns:

- Protection of ambient air and climate

- Waste water management

- Waste management

- Protection of biodiversity and landscapes

- Other abatement activities such as on the protection of soil and groundwater, protection against radiation, and noise and vibration abatement

- Other environmental expenditure, on research and development, education and administration

The spending shown in 2004 public sector environmental protection expenditure has also been classified by the following types of expenditure:

- current costs, including staff costs (compensation of employees), other on-going expenditure on purchases of goods and services and the estimated consumption of fixed capital

- capital expenditure or investment including outlays on land and on the additions of new durable goods to the stock of fixed assets for environmental protection

- income from sales, fees and charges for the provision of current or capital goods and services, such as fees for waste removal, but excluding taxes

- current and capital transfers to other sectors of the economy

- net transfers to and from the Rest of the World., in the form of aid or other grants, net of grants received from the EU.

There are five main categories of spending in environmental protection expenditure by specified industries:

- End-of-pipe=investment is defined as add-on installations and equipment which treats or controls emissions or reduces waste material generated by the plan, but which does not affect production processes.

- Integrated processes are adaptation or changes to production processes in order to generate fewer emissions or waste materials.

- In-house operating expenses cover operating costs necessary to run end-of=pipe or integrated facilities.

- Current payments made to others include all payments to third parties for environmental services, including payments for the treatment or removal of solid waste, water service company charges for sewage treatment, payments to contractors for the removal or treatment of waste waters, and payments made to environmental regulatory authorities.

- Research and development expenditure includes both in-house research and development and amounts paid to others such as trade associations and consultants.

Sources

Environmental protection expenditure in specified industries gives figures for spending by the extraction, manufacturing, energy production and water supply industries. They are drawn from a survey for 2006 carried out on behalf of the Department for Environment, Food and Rural Affairs (Defra) by URS Corporation Ltd.

Environmental protection expenditure by the public sector gives estimates for expenditures by the public sector and is based on information obtained from a variety of sources such as the public expenditure database and from various government departments, local authorities and the devolved administrations.

Data for industry and public sector environmental protection expenditure should not be added together as differing classification procedures make comparisons problematic.

Annex: Atmospheric pollutants and environmental themes

Greenhouse gases

There is a growing consensus that the rise in concentrations of greenhouse gases in the atmosphere has led to changes in the global climate system. The greenhouse gases included in the atmospheric emissions accounts are those covered by the Kyoto Protocol: carbon dioxide (CO_2), methane (CH_4), nitrous oxide (N_2O), hydrofluorocarbons (HFCs), perfluorocarbons (PFCs) and sulphur hexafluoride (SF_6).

Carbon dioxide (CO_2) emissions mainly come from the combustion of fossil fuels, but it is also produced in some industrial processes such as the manufacture of cement. Carbon dioxide is a long-lived gas remaining in the atmosphere for between 50 and 200 years. It is the main anthropogenic greenhouse gas.

Methane (CH_4) is produced when organic matter is broken down in the absence of oxygen. Large quantities are produced by enteric fermentation in cattle and sheep, by the spreading of animal manure and from organic waste deposited in landfill

265

sites. Methane is also emitted in coal mining, oil and gas extraction and gas distribution activities. Methane is a significant greenhouse gas.

Nitrous oxide (N_2O) is released in a few industrial processes and from the soil when nitrogenous fertilisers are applied in agriculture and horticulture. These are the main anthropogenic sources. It is a long-lived pollutant, lasting about 120 years in the atmosphere and is a potent greenhouse gas.

Hydrofluorocarbons (HFCs), perfluorocarbons (PFCs) and sulphur hexafluoride (SF_6) are artificial fluids that contain chlorine and/or fluorine. Because of their low reactivity and non-toxicity they were widely used as refrigerants, foam blowing agents, aerosol propellants and solvents.

To aggregate the greenhouse gases covered in the accounts, a weighting based on the relative global warming potential (GWP) of each of the gases is applied, using the effect of CO_2 over a 100 year period as a reference. This gives methane a weight of 21 relative to CO_2 and nitrous oxide a weight of 310 relative to CO_2. SF_6 has a GWP of 23,900 relative to CO_2. The GWP of the other fluorinated compounds varies according to the individual gas.

Greenhouse gas emissions are sometimes shown in terms of carbon equivalent rather than CO_2 equivalent. To convert from CO_2 equivalent to carbon equivalent it is necessary to multiply by 12/44.

Acid rain precursors

The term 'acid rain' describes the various chemical reactions which acidic gases and particles undergo in the atmosphere. The gases may be transported long distances before being deposited as wet or dry deposition. When deposited, hydrogen ions may be released, forming dilute acids, which damage ecosystems and buildings. The gases covered are sulphur dioxide (SO_2), nitrogen oxides (NO_x) and ammonia (NH_3).

The emissions are weighted together using their relative acidifying effects. The weights, given relative to SO_2, are 0.7 for NO_x and 1.9 for NH_3. This is a simplification of the chemistry involved, and there are a number of factors which can affect the eventual deposition and effect of acid rain. There may be an upward bias on the weights of the nitrogen-based compounds in terms of damage to ecosystems.

Sulphur dioxide (SO_2) is produced when coal and some petroleum products containing sulphur impurities are burnt. Sulphur dioxide is an acid gas that can cause respiratory irritation. It can damage ecosystems and buildings directly and is a major contributor to acid rain.

Nitrogen oxides (NO_x) arise when fossil fuels are burnt under certain conditions. High concentrations are harmful to health

and reduce plant growth. Like sulphur dioxide, nitrogen oxides contribute to acid rain; nitrogen dioxide (NO_2) also plays a part in the formation of ground ozone layer.

Ammonia (NH_3) is predominantly emitted from spreading animal manure and some fertilisers.

Other air pollutants

PM_{10}s are smoke particles whose diameter is less than 10 microns. They are regarded as responsible for some physiological damage and have been linked to premature mortality from respiratory diseases.

Carbon monoxide (CO) is produced in small quantities when fossil fuel is burnt with insufficient oxygen for complete combustion. At high concentrations carbon monoxide is toxic.

Non-methane volatile organic compounds (NMVOCs) cover a variety of chemicals, many of which are known carcinogens. Emissions of NMVOCs arise from the deliberate and incidental evaporation of solvents (for example, in paints and cleaning products), from accidental spillage and from non-combustion of petroleum products. The environmental accounts include natural emissions of NMVOCs from managed forests. NMVOCs play a role in the formation of ground level ozone, which can have an adverse effect on health. The NMVOC emissions include benzene and 1,3-butadiene.

Benzene is released largely from the distribution and combustion of petrol. It is a carcinogen which has also been found to cause bone-marrow depression and consequent leukopenia (depressed white blood cell count) on prolonged exposure.

1,3-Butadiene is a colourless, gaseous hydrocarbon. It is produced by dehydrogenation of butene, or of mixtures of butene and butane; it may also be made from ethanol. 1,3-butadiene is believed to be a carcinogen, for which the safe level is not known. Emissions of 1,3-butadiene arise from combustion of petroleum products and in its manufacture of synthetic rubber, nylon and latex paints in the chemical industry. 1,3-butadiene is not present in petrol but is formed as a by-product of combustion. The increasing use of catalytic converters through the 1990s has caused a significant reduction in emissions from the road transport sector.

Heavy Metals

Lead (Pb) is a heavy metal that is emitted from the combustion of petrol, coal combustion and metal works. Emissions of lead continued to fall in 2000, mainly as a result of the ban on the sale of leaded petrol from 1 January 2000. Lead has been found to inhibit the development of children's intelligence. If the levels of lead are sufficient, lead can cause degenerative processes such as osteoporosis, inhibit many enzyme reactions in the body and cause reproductive disorders such as sterility and miscarriages.

Cadmium (Cd) is a normal constituent of soil and water at low concentrations. Industrially, cadmium is used as an anti-friction agent, in alloys, semi-conductors, control rods for nuclear reactors and PVC and battery manufacture. The main sources of cadmium emissions are from waste incineration, and iron and steel manufacture. Emissions of cadmium have declined over recent years; this is mainly attributable to the decline in coal combustion.

Environmentally, cadmium is dangerous because many plants and some animals absorb it easily and concentrate it in tissues. Cadmium competes with calcium in the body, and if levels are sufficient, it will displace calcium, causing embrittlement of bones and painful deformations of the skeleton. Cadmium also competes with zinc in the body, and if levels of cadmium are high enough, cadmium will also displace zinc from enzymes in the body.

Mercury (Hg) emissions are generated by waste incineration, the manufacture of chlorine in mercury cells, non-ferrous metal production and coal combustion. Emissions of mercury have declined over recent years due to improved controls on mercury cells and their replacement by diaphragm cells and the decline of coal use. Due to the volatility of mercury, if levels are sufficiently high, compounds containing mercury attack and destroy various parts of the body, particularly teeth, lung tissues and intestines.

References

1 Office for National Statistics. *Environmental Accounts* Spring 2008 edition.

   www.statistics.gov.uk/statbase/Product.asp?vlnk=3698

2 Department of Business Enterprise and Regulatory Reform. *Development of UK Oil and Gas Resources* (the 'Brown Book'). Various issues (title has changed over the years). HMSO/TSO.

   www.og.berr.gov.uk/information/index.htm

3 European Commission (2000) *Accounts for subsoil assets: Results of pilot studies in European countries, 2000*. Office for Official Publication of the European Communities, Luxembourg.

4 Department of Business Enterprise and Regulatory Reform. *Digest of United Kingdom Energy Statistics*. Various issues. HMSO/TSO.

   www.berr.gov.uk/whatwedo/energy/statistics/publications/dukes/page45537.html

5 Office for National Statistics (2002) *Adjustments to the UK's atmospheric emissions and energy accounts to bring them on to a National Accounts 'Residents' basis*. Report to Eurostat, April 2002.

   www.statistics.gov.uk/downloads/theme_environment/Adjustments_UK_atmospheric_emissions_energy_accounts_national_accounts_residents_basis.pdf

6 AEA Energy and Environment.

   www.airquality.co.uk/archive/index.php

7 Department for Environment, Food and Rural Affairs.

   www.defra.gov.uk/environment/statistics/globatmos/gagccukem.htm

8 Food and Agricultural Organization (FAO), available at:

   www.fao.org/

9 British Geological Survey (2008) *UK Minerals Yearbook 2007*.

   www.bgs.ac.uk/mineralsuk/commodity/uk/ukmy.html

10 HM Revenue & Customs trade data, available at:

   www.uktradeinfo.com

11 Department for Environment, Food and Rural Affairs (Defra) *Resource Use and Efficiency of the UK Economy: A study by the Wuppertal Institute*.

12 Office for National Statistics (2003) UK Material Flows Review

   www.statistics.gov.uk/statbase/Product.asp?vlnk=3698

13 Office for National Statistics (2002) UK Material Flow Accounting. *Economic Trends* No. 583 (June 2002).

   www.statistics.gov.uk/CCI/article.asp?ID=140

14 Office for National Statistics (2005) Trends in UK Material Flows between 1970–2003. *Economic Trends* No. 619 (June 2005).

   www.statistics.gov.uk/cci/article.asp?ID=1174

15 Office for National Statistics (2006) UK environmental taxes: classification and recent trends. *Economic Trends* No. 635 (October 2006).

   www.statistics.gov.uk/CCI/article.asp?ID=1650&Pos=1&ColRank=1&Rank=224

16 Office for National Statistics (2004) An Industrial Analysis of Environmental Taxes. *Economic Trends* No. 609 (August 2004).

   www.statistics.gov.uk/cci/article.asp?ID=944

17 URS Dames and Moore (2007) *Environmental Protection Expenditure by Industry: 2006 UK Survey*. [June] 2008.

   www.defra.gov.uk/environment/statistics/envsurvey/index.htm

13.1 Estimates of remaining recoverable oil and gas reserves

		1995	1998	1999	2000	2001	2002	2003	2004	2005	2006
Oil (Million tonnes)											
Reserves											
Proven	JKOV	605	685	665	630	605	593	571	533	516	479
Probable	JKOW	765	575	455	380	350	327	286	283	300	298
Proven plus Probable	JKOX	1 370	1 260	1 120	1 010	955	920	857	816	816	776
Possible	JKOY	520	540	545	480	475	425	410	512	451	478
Maximum	JKOZ	1 890	1 800	1 665	1 490	1 430	1 344	1 267	1 328	1 267	1 254
Range of undiscovered resources											
Lower	JKNY	380	275	250	225	205	272	323	396	346	438
Upper	JKNZ	2 920	2 550	2 600	2 300	1 930	1 770	1 826	1 830	1 581	1 637
Range of total reserves											
Lower[1]	JKOA	985	960	915	855	810	865	894	929	862	917
Upper[2]	JKOB	4 810	4 350	4 265	3 790	3 360	3 115	3 093	3 158	2 848	2 892
Expected level of reserves[3]											
Opening stocks	JKOC	1 975	1 675	1 535	1 370	1 235	1 160	1 192	1 180	1 212	1 162
Extraction[5]	JKOD	−130	−132	−137	−126	−117	−117	−106	−95	−85	−77
Other volume changes	JKOE	−95	−8	−28	−9	42	149	94	127	35	130
Closing stocks	JKOF	1 750	1 535	1 370	1 235	1 160	1 192	1 180	1 212	1 162	1 215
Life expectancy[4] (years)	JKOG	13	12	10	10	10	10	11	13	14	16
Gas (billion cubic metres)											
Reserves											
Proven	JKOH	700	755	760	735	695	628	590	531	481	412
Probable	JKOI	780	585	500	460	445	369	315	296	247	272
Proven plus Probable	JKOJ	1 480	1 340	1 260	1 195	1 140	998	905	826	728	684
Possible	JKOK	435	455	490	430	395	331	336	343	278	283
Maximum	JKOL	1 915	1 795	1 750	1 630	1 535	1 329	1 241	1 169	1 006	967
Range of undiscovered resources											
Lower	JKOM	395	440	355	325	290	238	279	293	226	301
Upper	JKON	1 412	1 595	1 465	1 440	1 680	1 386	1 259	1 245	1 035	1 049
Range of total reserves											
Lower[1]	JKOO	1 095	1 195	1 115	1 060	985	866	869	824	707	713
Upper[2]	JKOP	3 327	3 390	3 215	3 065	3 215	2 714	2 500	2 415	2 041	2 016
Expected level of reserves[3]											
Opening stocks	JKOQ	1 945	1 885	1 780	1 615	1 520	1 430	1 235	1 184	1 120	954
Extraction[5]	JKOR	−70	−89	−99	−108	−104	−102	−102	−95	−86	−78
Other volume changes	JKOS	–	−16	−66	13	14	−93	51	31	−80	109
Closing stocks	JKOT	1 875	1 780	1 615	1 520	1 430	1 235	1 184	1 120	954	985
Life expectancy[4] (years)	JKOU	27	20	16	14	14	12	12	12	11	13

1 The lower end of the range of total reserves has been calculated as the sum of proven reserves and the lower end of the range of undiscovered reserves.

2 The upper end of the range of total reserves is the sum of proven, probable and possible reserves and the upper end of the range of undiscovered reserves.

3 Expected reserves are the sum of proven reserves, probable reserves and the lower end of the range of undiscovered reserves.

4 Based on expected level of reserves at year end and current extraction rates (source: ONS).

5 Negative extraction is shown here for the purposes of the calculation only. Of itself, extraction should be considered as a positive value.

Source: ONS and Department for Business Enterprise & Regulatory Reform

13.2 Oil and gas monetary balance sheet

£ million

		1995	1998	1999	2000	2001	2002	2003	2004	2005	2006
Oil											
Opening stocks[1]	JKPA	26 209	19 486	17 737	46 919	53 586	51 827	50 883	53 017	78 548	100 138
Extraction[2]	JKPB	−3 785	−2 001	−5 922	−6 875	−6 580	−6 326	−6 163	−8 261	−10 028	−10 293
Revaluation due to time passing	JKPC	1 700	898	2 415	2 734	2 558	2 333	2 523	3 658	4 921	5 258
Other volume changes	JKPD	−1 579	−64	−734	−295	1 467	5 051	3 237	6 103	2 133	8 362
Change in extraction	JKPE	276	175	448	−1 141	−961	−	−1 290	−2 253	−3 457	−3 454
Change in rent	JKPF	15 326	−1 273	32 576	11 625	594	−3 599	2 254	24 904	26 261	10 645
Nominal holding gains	C3OC	695	518	399	619	1 164	1 597	1 574	1 378	1 761	2 673
Closing stocks	JKPG	38 842	17 737	46 919	53 586	51 827	50 883	53 017	78 548	100 138	113 330
Gas											
Opening stocks	JKPH	15 370	33 632	25 416	30 483	42 985	50 458	46 566	44 229	50 763	65 364
Extraction[2]	JKPI	−1 479	−1 989	−2 704	−4 219	−5 049	−5 091	−4 977	−5 633	−7 618	−8 967
Revaluation due to time passing	JKPJ	978	1 259	1 554	2 141	2 514	2 466	2 163	2 511	3 497	3 871
Other volume changes	JKPK	3	−135	−803	256	359	−2 501	1 422	1 025	−4 020	7 052
Change in extraction	JKPL	943	409	1 288	1 334	−552	−355	−37	−1 072	−1 940	−1 541
Change in rent	JKPM	7 733	−8 653	5 159	12 588	9 269	34	−2 348	8 553	23 544	17 723
Nominal holding gains	C3OB	408	893	572	402	933	1 555	1 440	1 150	1 138	1 745
Closing stocks	JKPN	23 956	25 416	30 483	42 985	50 458	46 566	44 229	50 763	65 364	85 246

Source: ONS

1 The estimated opening and closing stock values are based on the present value method -see *Environmental Accounts* on the National Statistics website for more detailed descriptions of the methodology used. The estimates are extremely sensitive to the estimated return to capital and to assumptions about future unit resource rents.

2 Negative extraction is shown here for the purposes of the calculation only. Of itself, extraction should be considered as a positive value.

13.3 Energy consumption

Million tonnes of oil equivalent

		1990	1995	1996	1997	1998	1999	2000	2001	2002	2003	2004	2005	2006
Direct use of energy from carbon fuels														
Agriculture	JKPO	2.3	2.3	2.4	2.3	2.3	2.3	2.1	2.2	2.1	2.2	2.2	2.1	2.1
Mining and quarrying	JKPP	4.7	5.5	6.2	6.3	6.8	6.7	6.9	8.0	7.8	7.9	7.8	7.6	7.4
Manufacturing	JKPQ	42.3	41.6	42.9	42.9	41.9	41.8	41.0	39.8	37.7	38.2	37.4	37.7	35.7
Electricity, gas and water supply	JKPR	56.8	51.9	52.7	50.3	52.7	52.6	56.5	59.0	58.1	60.7	61.4	61.8	63.7
Construction	JKPS	2.9	3.1	3.3	3.3	3.4	3.4	3.4	3.5	3.5	3.6	3.7	4.0	4.0
Wholesale and retail trade	JKPT	5.5	6.1	6.3	6.1	6.2	6.5	6.6	6.3	6.0	6.2	6.5	6.3	6.3
Transport and communication	JKPU	22.3	24.8	26.9	27.4	28.7	28.6	29.6	30.9	31.1	32.2	33.8	34.9	32.7
Other business services	JKPV	2.6	2.8	2.9	2.7	2.8	2.9	2.9	3.0	2.6	2.6	2.6	2.6	2.6
Public administration	JKPW	3.8	4.0	4.0	3.9	3.6	3.5	3.3	3.5	3.6	3.4	3.5	3.4	3.3
Education, health and social work	JKPX	4.0	4.0	4.3	4.4	4.3	4.4	4.4	4.4	3.6	3.7	3.9	3.9	3.7
Other services	JKPY	2.5	2.4	2.5	2.1	2.1	2.1	2.0	2.2	1.9	2.0	2.0	1.9	2.0
Total non-household	IGJ9	149.8	148.5	154.2	151.7	154.7	154.8	158.7	162.6	158.0	162.5	164.7	166.2	163.6
Households	JKPZ	53.9	54.3	60.4	57.6	58.4	58.5	59.0	60.2	59.8	60.1	61.1	59.2	57.5
Total use of energy from carbon fuels	JKQA	**203.7**	**202.8**	**214.6**	**209.4**	**213.1**	**213.3**	**217.7**	**222.8**	**217.8**	**222.6**	**225.8**	**225.5**	**221.1**
Energy from other sources[1]	JKQB	17.7	23.1	24.0	23.8	25.0	24.0	21.4	22.1	21.3	20.6	19.4	19.8	18.5
Total energy consumption of primary fuels and equivalents	JKQC	**221.4**	**225.9**	**238.5**	**233.2**	**238.2**	**237.2**	**239.1**	**244.9**	**239.1**	**243.2**	**245.2**	**245.2**	**239.6**
Direct use of energy including electricity														
Agriculture	JKQD	2.6	2.6	2.7	2.7	2.6	2.6	2.5	2.5	2.5	2.6	2.5	2.5	2.5
Mining and quarrying	JKQE	4.9	5.7	6.4	6.5	7.0	6.9	7.1	8.2	8.0	8.1	8.0	7.8	7.6
Manufacturing	JKQF	49.7	48.7	50.4	50.3	49.3	49.2	48.3	46.8	45.2	45.9	44.8	45.3	43.2
Electricity, gas and water supply	JKQG	51.7	51.1	51.6	49.2	52.5	51.2	52.2	55.1	53.2	54.6	54.3	54.7	55.6
of which - transformation losses by major producers	JKQH	46.5	45.1	45.2	44.0	45.3	43.7	44.0	46.3	44.9	46.4	45.6	46.5	47.2
distribution losses of electricity supply	JKQI	2.1	2.5	2.4	2.5	2.4	2.4	2.5	2.7	2.6	2.6	2.6	2.6	2.7
Construction	JKQJ	3.0	3.3	3.4	3.5	3.5	3.5	3.5	3.6	3.7	3.7	3.8	4.1	4.2
Wholesale and retail trade	JKQK	7.4	8.3	8.6	8.7	8.8	9.2	9.3	9.1	8.9	9.1	9.4	9.4	9.4
Transport and communication	JKQL	23.0	25.7	27.8	28.4	29.7	29.6	30.6	32.0	32.1	33.3	34.9	36.0	33.8
Other business services	JKQM	4.3	4.7	4.8	4.8	4.9	5.1	5.2	5.4	4.9	5.0	4.9	5.0	4.9
Public administration	JKQN	4.7	4.6	4.5	4.3	3.9	3.8	3.6	3.8	3.8	3.7	3.8	3.7	3.5
Education, health and social work	JKQO	5.1	5.2	5.6	5.6	5.6	5.7	5.6	5.6	4.8	4.7	5.0	5.0	4.9
Other services	JKQP	3.1	3.0	3.0	2.6	2.6	2.6	2.5	2.7	2.4	2.6	2.6	2.5	2.6
Total non-household	IGK2	159.5	162.8	168.9	166.6	170.3	169.3	170.5	174.8	169.5	173.2	174.2	176.0	172.1
Households	JKQQ	61.9	63.1	69.6	66.6	67.8	68.0	68.6	70.2	69.7	70.0	71.0	69.3	67.5
Total energy consumption of primary fuels and equivalents	JKQR	**221.4**	**225.9**	**238.5**	**233.2**	**238.2**	**237.2**	**239.1**	**244.9**	**239.1**	**243.2**	**245.2**	**245.2**	**239.6**
Reallocated use of energy														
Energy industry electricity tranformation losses and distribution losses and allocated to final consumer														
Agriculture	JKQS	3.3	3.2	3.3	3.2	3.2	3.2	3.1	3.1	3.1	3.2	3.1	3.1	3.1
Mining and quarying	JKQT	5.2	6.0	6.7	6.8	7.3	7.1	7.5	8.5	8.3	8.4	8.4	8.3	8.1
Manufacturing	JKQU	64.1	61.8	63.6	63.0	62.2	61.8	60.5	59.0	57.6	59.0	57.3	58.1	56.0
Electricity, gas and water supply	JKQV	7.0	7.2	7.6	6.2	8.4	8.6	9.3	10.3	9.5	8.9	9.8	9.3	9.8
Construction	JKQW	3.2	3.6	3.7	3.7	3.7	3.7	3.7	3.8	3.9	4.0	4.1	4.4	4.4
Wholesale and retail trade	JKQX	11.2	12.3	12.7	13.2	13.2	13.5	13.9	13.9	13.7	14.1	14.3	14.5	14.7
Transport and communication	JKQY	24.2	27.4	29.5	30.1	31.4	31.2	32.2	33.8	33.8	35.2	36.8	37.9	35.7
Other business services	JKQZ	7.7	8.0	8.2	8.4	8.6	8.8	9.1	9.5	8.9	9.1	8.9	8.9	8.9
Public administration	JKRA	6.5	5.7	5.4	5.1	4.5	4.2	4.1	4.3	4.1	4.3	4.3	4.2	3.9
Education, health and social work	JKRB	7.3	7.3	7.9	7.8	7.9	7.8	7.6	7.7	6.8	6.5	6.8	6.9	6.8
Other services	JKRC	4.1	4.1	4.0	3.6	3.4	3.4	3.4	3.5	3.4	3.6	3.6	3.5	3.5
Total non-household	IGK3	143.7	146.7	152.7	151.1	153.8	153.4	154.4	157.7	153.1	156.1	157.4	159.0	154.9
Households	JKRD	77.7	79.2	85.9	82.1	84.3	83.8	84.6	87.2	86.1	87.1	87.8	86.2	84.7
Total energy consumption of primary fuels and equivalents	JKRE	**221.4**	**225.9**	**238.5**	**233.2**	**238.2**	**237.2**	**239.1**	**244.9**	**239.1**	**243.2**	**245.2**	**245.2**	**239.6**
Energy from renewable sources[2]	JKRF	1.9	2.6	2.5	2.4	2.7	2.8	2.8	2.8	3.0	3.1	3.4	3.5	3.7
Percentage from renewable sources	JKRG	0.9	1.1	1.0	1.0	1.1	1.2	1.2	1.2	1.3	1.3	1.4	1.4	1.6

1 Nuclear power, hydroelectric power and imports of electricty.
2 Renewable sources include solar power and energy from wind, wave and tide, hydroelectricity, wood, straw and sewage gas. Landfill gas and municipal solid waste combustion have also been included within this definition.

Source: AEA Energy & Environment, BERR, ONS

13.4 Atmospheric emissions, 2006

Thousand tonnes CO_2 equivalent

	Greenhouse gases[1]	Acid rain precursors[2]	Emissions affecting air quality								
			PM10[3]	CO[4]	NMVOC[5]	Benzene	Butadiene	Lead	Cadmium (tonnes)	Mercury (tonnes)
Agriculture	50 563	553	21.609	46.700	82.8	0.234	0.083	0.391	0.033	0.030
Mining and quarrying	26 759	92	13.236	35.400	95.8	0.437	0.015	0.294	0.074	0.022
Manufacturing	113 754	385	32.263	603.900	321.3	2.269	0.472	75.913	2.015	3.576
Electricity, gas and water supply	201 374	639	11.939	80.300	45.8	0.480	0.006	10.304	0.868	2.264
Construction	12 306	47	8.877	55.500	60.8	0.234	0.111	0.380	0.044	0.019
Wholesale and retail trade	19 810	53	6.191	70.700	55.0	0.262	0.168	12.286	0.095	0.034
Transport and communication	96 271	762	50.982	145.000	50.4	3.132	0.823	3.587	2.571	0.155
Other business services	7 300	14	1.898	46.100	4.3	0.105	0.040	0.114	0.037	0.003
Public administration	8 530	40	1.875	41.300	4.6	0.266	0.051	0.492	0.029	0.040
Education, health and social work	8 618	13	0.828	11.800	2.1	0.051	0.008	0.389	0.020	0.036
Other services	27 514	39	1.425	94.300	28.5	2.033	0.189	0.160	0.055	1.294
Households	151 658	256	37.829	1 098.900	247.1	7.082	0.630	4.574	0.344	0.156
Total	**724 455**	**2 892**	**188.953**	**2 330.000**	**998.5**	**16.586**	**2.595**	**108.883**	**6.184**	**7.600**
of which, emissions from road transport	128 533	391	32.979	998.500	104.400	2.623	1.450	2.1	0.418	0.004

1 Carbon dioxide, methane, nitrous oxide, hydro-fluorocarbons, perfluorocarbons and sulphur hexafluoride expressed as thousand tonnes of carbon dioxide equivalent.
2 Sulphur dioxide, nitrogen oxides and ammonia expressed as thousand tonnes of sulphur dioxide equivalent.
3 PM10 is particulate matter arising from various sources including fuel combustion quarrying and construction, and formation of 'secondary' particles in the atmosphere from reactions involving other pollutants sulphur dioxide, nitrogen oxides, ammonia and NMVOCs
4 Carbon monoxide.
5 Non-methane Volatile Compounds, including benzene and 1,3-butadiene.

Source: AEA Energy & Environment, ONS

13.5 Greenhouse gas and acid rain precursor emissions

Thousand tonnes CO_2 equivalent

		1990	1995	1999	2000	2001	2002	2003	2004	2005	2006
Greenhouse gases - CO2,CH4,N2O,HFC,PFCs and SF6[1]											
Agriculture	JKRH	60 959	58 796	58 021	55 753	52 817	53 145	52 801	52 579	51 581	50 563
Mining and quarrying	JKRJ	40 442	37 101	32 295	31 591	31 113	31 521	30 825	30 183	29 448	26 759
Manufacturing	JKRK	173 905	159 366	138 283	132 831	127 597	118 987	120 030	117 621	118 027	113 754
Electricity, gas and water supply	JKRL	216 921	177 721	162 342	174 831	186 729	181 730	189 710	190 045	192 638	201 374
Construction	JKRM	8 801	9 547	10 390	10 345	10 574	10 795	10 988	11 289	12 098	12 306
Wholesale and retail trade	JKRN	14 686	16 894	19 905	20 393	19 820	19 375	19 595	20 565	19 844	19 810
Transport and communication	JKRO	65 508	72 549	83 593	86 441	90 486	91 324	94 660	99 931	103 058	96 271
Other business services	JKRP	6 899	7 445	7 626	7 699	8 070	7 020	7 214	7 090	7 364	7 300
Public administration	JKRQ	10 617	10 573	9 179	8 722	9 162	9 306	8 648	8 819	8 813	8 530
Education, health and social work	JKRR	10 444	9 814	10 398	10 172	10 152	8 308	8 540	9 055	8 967	8 618
Other services	JKRS	58 402	52 683	40 984	38 787	35 253	32 089	29 205	27 805	27 533	27 514
Total non-household	IGK4	667 584	612 489	573 016	577 565	581 773	563 600	572 216	574 982	579 371	572 799
Households	JKRT	141 449	141 545	154 318	154 869	158 273	157 204	157 663	159 762	155 503	151 658
Total greenhouse gas emissions	JKRU	**809 034**	**754 034**	**727 332**	**732 433**	**740 044**	**720 803**	**729 880**	**734 743**	**734 875**	**724 455**
of which, emissions from road transport[2]	JKRV	111 934	114 711	123 951	123 399	123 495	126 182	126 202	127 451	127 989	128 533
of which, emissions from water transport[3]	F8ZP	17 016	17 016	16 629	16 132	20 551	22 290	23 796	27 449	27 286	19 388
of which, emissions from air transport[4]	F8ZQ	20 394	24 676	33 866	37 372	36 847	36 137	37 378	39 585	42 852	43 634
Acid rain precursor emissions - SO2,NOx,NH3[5]											
Agriculture	JKRW	726	662	662	603	593	583	568	576	556	553
Mining and quarrying	JKRX	100	83	80	80	74	76	91	87	87	92
Manufacturing	JKRY	933	759	519	457	439	395	387	394	397	385
Electricity, gas and water supply	JKRZ	3 277	1 937	1 001	1 072	1 006	929	947	765	652	639
Construction	JKSA	71	67	62	59	58	55	53	51	50	47
Wholesale and retail trade	JKSB	100	85	73	69	61	60	58	59	55	53
Transport and communication	JKSC	799	786	754	732	851	882	918	1 024	1 012	762
Other business services	JKSD	38	33	24	22	21	17	17	14	14	14
Public administration	JKSE	79	67	52	48	48	43	36	41	40	40
Education, health and social work	JKSF	61	43	27	21	19	14	14	14	14	13
Other services	JKSG	69	59	44	42	44	40	40	38	38	39
Total non household	IGK5	6 253	4 581	3 298	3 205	3 214	3 094	3 129	3 063	2 915	2 637
Households	JKUK	728	592	462	420	381	347	322	302	271	256
Total acid rain precursor emissions	JKUL	**6 981**	**5 174**	**3 760**	**3 627**	**3 596**	**3 441**	**3 450**	**3 365**	**3 186**	**2 892**
of which, emissions from road transport	JKUM	998	846	689	622	569	526	484	454	418	391

1 Carbon dioxide, methane, nitrous oxide, hydrofluorocarbons, perfluorocarbon and sulphur hexafluoride expressed as thousand tonnes of carbon dioxide equivalent.
2 Includes emissions from all road transport sources (eg HGVs, LGVs, cars and motorcycles) across all industries
3 Emissions from water transport industry (Environmental Accounts code 69)
4 Emissions from air transport industry (Environmental Accounts code 70)
5 Sulphur dioxide, nitrogen oxides and ammonia expressed as thousand tonnes of sulphur dioxide equivalent.

Source: AEA Energy & Environment, ONS

13.6 Material flows

Million tonnes

		1970	1975	1980	1985	1990	1995	1998	1999	2000	2001	2002	2003	2004	2005	2006
Domestic extraction																
Biomass																
Agricultural harvest	JKUN	42	38	47	47	46	47	51	52	51	45	51	48	48	47	45
Timber	JKUO	3	3	4	5	6	8	7	7	8	8	8	8	8	9	8
Animal grazing	JKUP	49	49	49	48	47	45	44	43	43	43	43	43	43	43	43
Fish	JKUQ	1	1	1	1	1	1	1	1	1	1	1	1	1	1	1
Total biomass	JKUR	96	92	101	100	101	100	103	104	102	97	102	100	101	100	98
Minerals																
Ores	JKUS	12	5	1	1	–	–	–	–	–	–	–	–	–	–	–
Clay	JKUT	38	33	25	23	21	18	16	15	15	14	14	14	15	14	13
Other industrial minerals	JKUU	14	11	11	11	11	10	8	8	8	9	8	9	8	8	8
Sand and gravel	JKUV	122	131	110	112	128	106	103	105	106	105	98	95	102	99	97
Crushed stone	JKUW	156	169	150	160	212	200	181	179	176	183	173	170	175	169	171
Total minerals	JKUX	342	349	298	307	373	334	309	308	305	311	293	288	300	290	289
Fossil fuels																
Coal	JKUY	149	129	130	94	94	53	41	37	31	32	30	28	25	20	19
Natural gas	JKUZ	11	37	39	37	43	71	90	102	109	106	104	103	96	88	80
Crude oil	JKVA	–	2	80	128	92	130	132	137	126	117	116	106	95	85	77
Total fossil fuels	JKVB	161	168	249	259	229	254	264	276	266	255	250	237	217	193	175
Total domestic extraction	JKVC	**598**	**608**	**648**	**666**	**702**	**688**	**676**	**687**	**673**	**663**	**645**	**626**	**618**	**583**	**562**
Imports																
Biomass	JKVD	38	33	30	31	38	40	42	42	42	46	47	49	50	50	50
Minerals	JKVE	30	32	24	34	41	50	54	50	51	54	55	55	60	58	59
Fossil fuels	JKVF	123	111	74	76	89	73	76	71	83	99	95	102	127	137	148
Other products	JKVG	6	7	14	15	19	23	31	30	34	34	32	34	36	35	35
Total imports	JKVH	**197**	**184**	**141**	**157**	**187**	**188**	**203**	**193**	**210**	**232**	**228**	**240**	**273**	**280**	**292**
Exports																
Biomass	JKVI	3	5	8	11	13	15	17	16	17	13	15	19	18	19	20
Minerals	JKVJ	17	20	26	22	25	39	46	42	44	43	42	44	48	48	50
Fossil fuels	JKVK	23	19	60	102	67	103	103	108	115	118	120	104	98	88	83
Other products	JKVL	5	7	8	11	12	17	20	21	21	21	20	21	21	21	21
Total exports	JKVM	**47**	**51**	**101**	**146**	**117**	**173**	**186**	**187**	**198**	**194**	**197**	**189**	**185**	**177**	**174**
Domestic Material Consumption (domestic extraction + imports - exports)	JKVU	**748**	**741**	**688**	**677**	**772**	**703**	**693**	**694**	**686**	**701**	**677**	**677**	**706**	**686**	**680**
of which																
Biomass	G9A8	131	119	123	120	125	126	128	129	127	130	134	130	133	131	128
Minerals	G9A9	355	361	296	319	389	346	318	316	312	322	307	298	312	300	298
Fossil fuels	G9AA	261	260	263	233	250	224	237	239	234	236	225	236	246	241	240
Indirect flows																
From domestic extraction (excl soil erosion)[1]	JKVN	576	575	633	627	693	634	589	620	567	572	564	549	547	519	487
Of which;																
Unused biomass	JKVO	25	23	32	35	37	37	40	40	40	35	40	38	38	37	36
Fossil fuels	JKVP	169	202	287	274	309	276	245	260	231	241	225	209	204	178	149
Minerals and ores	JKVQ	185	155	120	120	144	116	103	98	97	95	101	100	104	101	99
Soil excavation and dredging	JKVR	197	195	195	199	203	204	201	222	199	202	199	202	201	203	203
From production of raw materials and semi-natural products imported	JKVS	394	395	368	423	457	527	597	562	614	711	648	671	692	752	792
Other indicators																
Physical trade balance (exports - imports)[3]	DZ76	−150	−133	−40	−11	−70	−14	−17	−6	−13	−38	−32	−52	−88	−103	−117
Direct Material Input (domestic extraction + imports)	JKVT	796	792	789	822	889	876	879	881	884	896	874	866	891	863	855
Total Material Requirement (direct material input + indirect flows)	JKVV	1 765	1 762	1 790	1 872	2 039	2 036	2 065	2 063	2 064	2 179	2 086	2 086	2 130	2 134	2 134

1 Indirect flows from domestic extraction relate to unused material which is moved during extraction, such as overburden from mining and quarrying.
2 Components may not sum to totals due to rounding.
3 A negative physical trade balance indicates a net import of material into the UK.

Source: ONS

13.7 Government revenues from environmental taxes

£ million

		1993	1995	1999	2000	2001	2002	2003	2004	2005	2006	2007
Energy												
Duty on hydrocarbon oils	GTAP	12 497	15 360	22 391	23 041	22 046	22 070	22 476	23 412	23 346	23 448	24 512
including												
Unleaded petrol[1]	GBHE	4 242	5 901	11 952	11 527†	1 922	–	–	–	–	–	–
Leaded petrol/LRP[2]	GBHL	4 502	4 088	1 630	1 116†	655	102	70	67	20	15	13
Ultra low sulphur petrol	ZXTK	–	–	–	972†	10 198	12 548	12 025	12 086	11 645	11 274	11 213
Diesel[3]	GBHH	3 484	5 127	1 274	23	66	–	–	–	–	–	–
Ultra low sulphur diesel	GBHI	–	–	7 338	9 051†	8 560	9 129	9 562	10 281	10 802	11 203	12 017
VAT on duty	CMYA	2 187	2 688	3 918	4 032	3 858	3 862	3 933	4 097	4 086	4 103	4 290
Fossil fuel levy	CIQY	1 331	1 306	104	56	86	32	–	–	–	–	–
Gas levy	GTAZ	240	161	–	–	–	–	–	–	–	–	–
Climate change levy	LSNT	–	–	–	–	585	825	828	756	747	711	690
Hydro-benefit	LITN	22	27	35	42	46	44	44	40	10	–	–
Road vehicles												
Vehicle excise duty	CMXZ	3 482	3 954	4 873	4 606	4 102	4 294	4 720	4 763	4 762	5 010	5 384
Other environmental taxes												
Air passenger duty	CWAA	–	339	884	940	824	814	781	856	896	961†	1 883
Landfill tax	BKOF	–	–	430	461	502	541	607	672	733	804†	877
Aggregates levy	MDUQ	–	–	–	–	–	213	340	328	327	321†	339
Total environmental taxes	JKVW	**19 755**	**23 835**	**32 635**	**33 178**	**32 049**	**32 695**	**33 729**	**34 924**	**34 907**	**35 358**	**37 975**
Environmental taxes as a % of:												
Total taxes and social contributions	JKVX	9.0†	9.3	9.7†	9.3	8.6	8.7	8.5	8.3	7.7	7.2†	7.4
Gross domestic product	JKVY	3.0†	3.3	3.5†	3.4	3.1	3.0	3.0	2.9	2.8	2.7	2.7

1 Unleaded petrol includes superunleaded petrol.
2 Lead Replacement Petrol (the alternative to 4-Star leaded petrol introduced in 2000) is lead-free.
3 Duty incentives have concentrated production on ultra low sulphur varieties.

Source: ONS, Department for Business Enterprise & Regulatory Reform

13.8 Environmental taxes breakdown by 13 industries 2004

£ million

	Energy	Transport	Pollution	Resources	Total
Agriculture	95	64	1	–	160
Mining and quarrying	78	4	2	326	410
Manufacturing	2 439	82	71	–	2 592
Energy, gas and water supply	178	5	5	–	188
Construction	1 329	110	7	2	1 448
Wholesale and retail trade	2 151	232	54	–	2 437
Transport and communication	5 977	152	28	–	6 157
Other business services	820	187	60	–	1 068
Public administration	237	2	109	–	348
Education, health and social work	164	7	82	–	253
Other services	422	41	253	–	717
Households	14 065	4 490	–	–	18 555
Rest of the world	349	243	–	–	592
Total	**28 305**	**5 619**	**673**	**328**	**34 924**

Components may not sum to totals due to rounding

Source: ONS, Environmental Accounts

13.9 Environmental protection expenditure in specified industries 2006

£ million

	Protection of ambient air and climate	Waste water management	Waste management	Protection of bio-diversity and landscape	Other abatement activities	Research and development education and adminstration	Total environmental expenditure
Mining and quarrying	27	133	45	3	25	2	236
Food, beverages and tobacco products	14	280	158	2	64	7	525
Textiles, clothing and leather products	4	33	24	–	6	2	68
Wood and wood products	17	4	34	–	7	4	66
Pulp and paper products, printing and publishing	19	30	106	–	17	3	176
Coke, petroleum and nuclear fuel	27	19	6	–	53	1	106
Chemicals and man made fibres	54	100	93	1	30	15	293
Rubber and plastic products	20	21	67	–	36	3	146
Other non metallic mineral products	24	25	57	3	16	3	129
Basic metals and metal products	52	107	94	4	73	4	334
Machinery and equipment	14	33	80	2	53	4	187
Electrical, medical and optical equipment	4	13	24	–	9	5	55
Transport equipment	27	93	124	1	9	3	257
Other manufacturing	7	17	55	–	8	3	89
Energy production and water	518	26	22	32	940	24	1 562
Total expenditure in extraction, manufacturing, energy and water supply industries	**830**	**935**	**988**	**50**	**1 347**	**80**	**4 228**

1 The figures in these tables fall outside the scope of National Statistics.
2 Components may not sum to totals due to rounding.

Source: Department for environment, food and rural affairs

13.10 Environmental protection expenditure by public sector 2004

£ million

	Protection of ambient air and climate	Waste water management	Waste management	Protection of bio-diversity and landscape	Other abatement activities[1]	Research and development education and adminstration	Total environmental expenditure
Staff costs	89.8	152.6	656.0	328.0	39.9	159.7	1 426.1
Other running costs[2]	50.2	83.6	2 621.2	234.0	30.1	324.3	3 343.4
less							
Current income	−1.5	−3.7	−22.4	−1.4	0.3	−3.2	−32.5
Net operating costs	**138.5**	**232.5**	**3 254.8**	**560.6**	**69.7**	**480.9**	**4 737.0**
Capital payments[3]	43.4	28.6	238.0	145.2	435.5	96.8	987.4
less							
Capital receipts	–	–	−9.2	–	–	−1.1	−10.3
Net capital expenditure	**43.4**	**28.6**	**228.8**	**145.2**	**435.5**	**95.6**	**977.1**
Current grants and subsidies							
to industry	25.1	–	2.4	31.5	–	25.4	84.4
to households	–	–	–	–	–	8.2	8.2
Capital grants and subsidies							
to public corporations	–	70.8	–	–	–	–	70.8
to industry	0.2	–	–	–	3.4	0.4	4.1
to households	42.9	–	–	–	0.3	–	43.2
Net transfers to the rest of the world	–	–	–	1.1	0.2	–	1.3
Net expenditure[2]	**250.1**	**332.0**	**3 486.0**	**738.3**	**509.1**	**610.5**	**5 926.0**

1 Includes expenditure on the protection of soil and groundwater, on noise and vibration abatement, on protection against radiation and on other environmental protection activities.
2 Includes an allowance for the consumption of fixed capital.
3 Includes outlays on land.

Source: ONS, HM Treasury

Supplementary Information

Glossary

Above the line

Transactions in the production, current and capital accounts which are above the Net lending (+)/Net borrowing (financial surplus or deficit) line in the presentation used in the economic accounts. The financial transactions account is below the line in this presentation.

Accruals basis

A method of recording transactions to relate them to the period when the exchange of ownership of the goods, services or financial asset applies. (See also cash basis). For example, value added tax accrues when the expenditure to which it relates takes place, but Customs and Excise receive the cash some time later. The difference between accruals and cash results in the creation of an asset and liability in the financial accounts, shown as amounts receivable or payable (F7).

Actual final consumption

The value of goods consumed by a sector but not necessarily purchased by that sector. See also Final consumption expenditure, Intermediate consumption.

Advance and progress payments

Payments made for goods in advance of completion and delivery of the goods. Also referred to as stage payments.

Asset boundary

Boundary separating assets included in creating core economic accounts (such as plant and factories, also including non-produced assets such as land and water resources) and those excluded (such as natural assets not managed for an economic purpose).

Assets

Entities over which ownership rights are enforced by institutional units, individually or collectively; and from which economic benefits may be derived by their owners by holding them over a period of time.

Assurance

An equivalent term to insurance, commonly used in the life insurance business.

Balancing item

A balancing item is an accounting construct obtained by subtracting the total value of the entries on one side of an account from the total value for the other side. In the sector accounts in the former system of UK economic accounts the term referred to the difference between the Financial Surplus or Deficit for a sector and the sum of the financial transactions for that sector, currently designated the statistical discrepancy.

Balance of payments

A summary of the transactions between residents of a country and residents abroad in a given time period.

Balance of trade

The balance on trade in goods and services. The balance of trade is a summary of the imports and exports of goods and services across an economic boundary in a given period.

Balance sheet

A statement, drawn up at a particular point in time, of the value of assets owned and of the financial claims (liabilities) against the owner of these assets.

Banks (UK)

Strictly, all financial institutions located in the United Kingdom and recognised by the Bank of England as banks for statistical purposes up to late 1981 or as UK banks from then onwards. This category includes the UK offices of institutions authorised under the Banking Act (1987), the Bank of England, the National Girobank and the TSB Group plc. It may include branches of foreign banks where these are recognised as banks by the Bank of England, but not offices abroad of these or of any British-owned banks. An updated list of banks appears in each February's issue of the Bank of England Quarterly Bulletin. Institutions in the Channel Islands and the Isle of Man which have opted to adhere to the monetary control arrangements introduced in August 1981 were formerly included in the sector but are not considered to be residents of the United Kingdom under the ESA. Banks are included in the Monetary financial institutions (S.121/S.122) sector.

Bank of England

This comprises S.121, the central bank sub-sector of the financial corporations sector.

Bank of England – Issue Department

This part of the Bank of England deals with the issue of bank notes on behalf of central government and was formerly classified to central government though it is now part of the central bank sector. Its activities include, inter alia, market purchases of commercial bills from UK banks.

Basic prices

These prices are the preferred method of valuing gross value added and output. They reflect the amount received by the producer for a unit of goods or services minus any taxes payable plus any subsidy receivable on that unit as a consequence of production or sale (i.e. the cost of production including subsidies). As a result the only taxes included in the basic price are taxes on the production process – such as business rates and any vehicle excise duty paid by businesses – which are not specifically levied on the production of a unit of output. Basic prices exclude any transport charges invoiced separately by the producer.

Below the line

The financial transactions account which shows the financing of Net lending(+)/Net borrowing (–) (formerly financial surplus or deficit).

Bond

A financial instrument that usually pays interest to the holder, issued by governments as well as companies and other institutions, e.g. local authorities. Most bonds have a fixed date on which the borrower will repay the holder. Bonds are attractive to investors since they can be bought and sold easily in a secondary market. Special forms of bonds include deep discount bonds, equity warrant bonds, Eurobonds, and zero coupon bonds.

British government securities

See Gilts.

Building society

Those institutions as defined in the Building Society Acts (1962 and 1986). They offer housing finance largely to the households sector and fund this largely by taking short term deposits from the households sector. They are part of the monetary financial institutions sub-sector.

Capital

Capital assets are those which contribute to the productive process so as to produce an economic return. In other contexts the word can be taken to include tangible assets (e.g. buildings, plant and machinery), intangible assets and financial capital. See also fixed assets, inventories.

Capital formation

Acquisition less disposals of fixed assets, improvement of land, change in inventories and acquisition less disposals of valuables.

Capital Stock

Measure of the cost of replacing the capital assets of a country, held at a particular point in time.

Capital transfers

Transfers which are related to the acquisition or disposal of assets by the recipient or payer. They may be in cash or kind, and may be imputed to reflect the assumption or forgiveness of debt.

Cash basis

The recording of transactions when cash or other assets are actually transferred, rather than on an accruals basis.

Central monetary institutions (CMIs)

Institutions (usually central banks) which control the centralised monetary reserves and the supply of currency in accordance with government policies, and which act as their governments' bankers and agents. In the UK this is equivalent to the Bank of England. In many other countries maintenance of the exchange rate is undertaken in this sector. In the United Kingdom this function is undertaken by central government (part of the Treasury) by use of the Exchange Equalisation Account.

Certificate of deposit

A short term interest-paying instrument issued by deposit-taking institutions in return for money deposited for a fixed period. Interest is earned at a given rate. The instrument can be used as security for a loan if the depositor requires money before the repayment date.

Chained volume measures

Chained volume measures are time series which measure GDP in real terms (ie, excluding price effects).

C.i.f.

The basis of valuation of imports for Customs purposes, it includes the cost of insurance premiums and freight services. These need to be deducted to obtain the f.o.b. valuation consistent with the valuation of exports which is used in the economic accounts.

COICOP (Classification of Individual Consumption by Purpose)

An international classification which groups consumption according to its function or purpose. Thus the heading clothing, for example, includes expenditure on garments, clothing materials, laundry and repairs.

Combined use table

Table of the demand for products by each industry group or sector, whether from domestic production or imports, estimated at purchaser's prices. It displays the inputs used by each industry to produce their total output and separates out intermediate purchases of goods and services. This table shows which industries use which products. Columns represent the purchasing industries: rows represent the products purchased.

Commercial paper

This is an unsecured promissory note for a specific amount and maturing on a specific date. The commercial paper market allows companies to issue short term debt direct to financial institutions who then market this paper to investors or use it for their own investment purposes.

Compensation of employees

Total remuneration payable to employees in cash or in kind. Includes the value of social contributions payable by the employer.

Consolidated Fund

An account of central government into which most government revenue (excluding borrowing and certain payments to government departments) is paid, and from which most government expenditure (excluding loans and National Insurance benefits) is paid.

Consumption

See Final consumption, Intermediate consumption.

Consumption of fixed capital

The amount of capital resources used up in the process of production in any period. It is not an identifiable set of transactions but an imputed transaction which can only be measured by a system of conventions.

Corporations

All bodies recognised as independent legal entities which are producers of market output and whose principal activity is the production of goods and services.

Counterpart

In a double-entry system of accounting each transaction gives rise to two corresponding entries. These entries are the counterparts to each other. Thus the counterpart of a payment by one sector is the receipt by another.

Debenture

A long-term bond issued by a UK or foreign company and secured on fixed assets. A debenture entitles the holder to a fixed interest payment or a series of such payments.

Depreciation

See Consumption of fixed capital.

Derivatives (F.34)

Financial instruments whose value is linked to changes in the value of another financial instrument, an indicator or a commodity. In contrast to the holder of a primary financial instrument (e.g. a government bond or a bank deposit), who has an unqualified right to receive cash (or some other economic benefit) in the future, the holder of a derivative has only a qualified right to receive such a benefit. Examples of derivatives are options and swaps.

DIM (Dividend and Interest Matrix)

The Dividend and Interest Matrix represents property income flows related to holdings of financial transactions. The gross flows are now shown in D.4.

Direct investment

Net investment by UK/overseas companies in their overseas/UK branches, subsidiaries or associated companies. A direct investment in a company means that the investor has a significant influence on the operations of the company. Investment includes not only acquisition of fixed assets, stock building and stock appreciation but also all other financial transactions such as additions to, or payments of, working capital, other loans and trade credit and acquisitions of securities. Estimates of investment exclude depreciation.

Discount market

That part of the market dealing with short-term borrowing. It is called the discount market because the interest on loans is expressed as a percentage reduction (discount) on the amount paid to the borrower. For example, for a loan of £100 face value when the discount rate is 5% the borrower will receive £95 but will repay £100 at the end of the term.

Double deflation

Method for calculating value added by industry chained volume measures; which takes separate account of the differing price and volume movements of input and outputs in an industry's production process.

Dividend

A payment made to company shareholders from current or previously retained profits. See DIM.

ECGD

See Export Credit Guarantee Department.

Economically significant prices

These are prices whose level significantly affects the supply of the good or service concerned. Market output consists mainly of goods and services sold at 'economically significant' prices while non-market output comprises those provided free or at prices that are not economically significant.

Enterprise

An institutional unit producing market output. Enterprises are found mainly in the non-financial and financial corporations sectors but exist in all sectors. Each enterprise consists of one or more kind-of-activity units.

Environmental accounts

A satellite account describing the relationship between the environment and the economy.

Equity

Equity is ownership or potential ownership of a company. An entity's equity in a company will be evidenced by ordinary shares. They differ from other financial instruments in that they confer ownership of something more than a financial claim. Shareholders are owners of the company whereas bond holders are merely outside creditors.

ESA

European System of National and Regional Accounts. An integrated system of economic accounts which is the European version of the System of National Accounts (SNA).

European Investment Bank

This was set up to assist economic development within the European Union. Its members are the member states of the EU.

European Monetary Cooperation Fund

Central banks of member states of the European Monetary System deposit 20 per cent of their gold and foreign exchange reserves on a short-term basis with the European Monetary Cooperation Fund in exchange for ECUs. The Fund is the clearing house for central banks in the EMS.

Exchange Cover Scheme (ECS)

A scheme first introduced in 1969 whereby UK public bodies raise foreign currency from overseas residents, either directly or through UK banks, and surrender it to the Exchange Equalisation Account in exchange for sterling for use to finance expenditure in the United Kingdom. HM Treasury sells the borrower foreign currency to service and repay the loan at the exchange rate that applied when the loan was taken out.

Exchange Equalisation Account (EEA)

An account of central government held by the Bank of England in which transactions in the official reserves are recorded. It is the means by which the government, through the Bank of England, influences exchange rates.

Export credit

Credit extended overseas by UK institutions primarily in connection with UK exports but also including some credit in respect of third-country trade.

Export Credits Guarantee Department (ECGD)

A government department whose main function is to provide insurance cover for export credit transactions.

Factor cost

In the former system of national accounts this was the basis of valuation which excluded the effects of taxes on expenditure and subsidies.

Final consumption expenditure

The expenditure on goods and services that are used for the direct satisfaction of individual needs or the collective needs of members of the community as distinct from their purchase for use in the productive process. It may be contrasted with Actual final consumption, which is the value of goods consumed but not necessarily purchased by that sector. See also Intermediate consumption.

Finance houses

Financial corporations that specialise in the financing of hire purchase arrangements.

Financial auxiliaries

Auxiliary financial activities are ones closely related to financial intermediation but which are not financial intermediation themselves, such as the repackaging of funds. Financial auxiliaries include such activities as insurance broking and fund management.

Financial corporations

All bodies recognised as independent legal entities whose principal activity is financial intermediation and/or the production of auxiliary financial services. However, the United Kingdom currently treats financial auxiliaries as non-financial corporations.

Financial intermediation

Financial intermediation is the activity by which an institutional unit acquires financial assets and incurs liabilities on its own account by engaging in financial transactions on the market. The assets and liabilities of financial intermediaries have different characteristics so that the funds are transformed or repackaged with respect to maturity, scale, risk, etc, in the financial intermediation process.

Financial leasing

A form of leasing in which the lessee contracts to assume the rights and responsibilities of ownership of leased goods from the lessor (the legal owner) for the whole (or virtually the whole) of the economic life of the asset. In the economic accounts this is recorded as the sale of the assets to the lessee, financed by an imputed loan (F.42). The leasing payments are split into interest payments and repayments of principal.

Financial Services Adjustment

Now renamed FISIM (see below) this is a feature temporarily carried over from the previous system. The output of many financial intermediation services is paid for not by charges, but by an interest rate differential. The value added of these industries is shown including their interest receipts less payments, in effect imputing charges for their services. However, GDP in total takes no account of this, and an adjustment is necessary to reconcile the two. For the treatment in the new SNA (to be implemented fully in the EU at a later date) see FISIM. Since most output of these industries is intermediate consumption of other industries the difference between the two methods in their effect on total GDP is relatively small.

Financial surplus or deficit (FSD)

The former term for Net lending(+)/Net borrowing (–), the balance of all current and capital account transactions for an institutional sector or the economy as a whole.

FISIM

Financial Intermediation Services Indirectly Measured. The output of many financial intermediation services is paid for not by charges but by an interest rate differential. FISIM imputes charges for these services and corresponding offsets in property income. FISIM, an innovation of the 1993 SNA, has not yet been fully implemented in the UK economic accounts; the earnings are not yet allocated to the users of the services.

Fixed assets

Produced assets that are themselves used repeatedly or continuously in the production process for more than one year. They comprise buildings and other structures, vehicles and other plant and machinery and also plants and livestock which are used repeatedly or continuously in production, e.g. fruit trees or dairy cattle. They also include intangible assets such as computer software and artistic originals.

Flows

Economic flows reflect the creation, transformation, exchange, transfer or extinction of economic value. They involve changes in the volume, composition or value of an institutional unit's assets and liabilities. They are recorded in the production, distribution and use of income and accumulation accounts.

F.o.b.

Free on board, the valuation of imports and exports of goods used in the economic accounts, including all costs invoiced by the exporter up to the point of loading on to the ship or aircraft but excluding the cost of insurance and freight from the country of consignment.

Futures

Instruments which give the holder the right to purchase a commodity or a financial asset at a future date.

GFCF

See Gross fixed capital formation.

Gilts

Bonds issued or guaranteed by the UK government. Also known as gilt-edged securities or British government securities.

Gold

The SNA and the IMF (in the 5th Edition of its Balance of Payments Manual) recognise three types of gold:

- monetary gold, treated as a financial asset;
- gold held as a store of value, to be included in valuables;
- gold as an industrial material, to be included in intermediate consumption or inventories.

This is a significant change from previous UK practice and presents problems such that the United Kingdom has received from the European Union a derogation from applying this fully until the year 2005.

The present treatment is as follows:

- In the accounts a distinction is drawn between gold held as a financial asset (financial gold) and gold held like any other commodity (commodity gold). Commodity gold in the form of finished manufactures together with net domestic and overseas transactions in gold moving into or out of finished manufactured form (i.e. for jewellery, dentistry, electronic goods, medals and proof – but not bullion – coins) is recorded in exports and imports of goods.

- All other transactions in gold (i.e. those involving semi-manufactures such as rods, wire, etc, or bullion, bullion coins or banking-type assets and liabilities denominated in gold, including official reserve assets) are treated as financial gold transactions and included in the financial account of the Balance of Payments.

The United Kingdom has adopted different treatment to avoid distortion of its trade in goods account by the substantial transactions of the London bullion market.

Grants

Voluntary transfer payments. They may be current or capital in nature. Grants from government or the European Union to producers are subsidies.

Gross

Key economic series can be shown as gross (i.e. before deduction of the consumption of fixed capital or net (i.e. after deduction). Gross has this meaning throughout this book unless otherwise stated.

Gross domestic product (GDP)

The total value of output in the economic territory. It is the balancing item on the production account for the whole economy. Domestic product can be measured gross or net. It is presented in the accounts at market (or purchasers') prices.

Gross fixed capital formation (GFCF)

Acquisition less disposals of fixed assets and the improvement of land.

Gross national disposable income

The income available to the residents arising from GDP, and receipts from, less payments to, the rest of the world of employment income, property income and current transfers.

Gross value added (GVA)

The value generated by any unit engaged in production, and the contributions of individual sectors or industries to gross domestic product. It is measured at basic prices, excluding taxes less subsidies on products.

Hidden economy

Certain activities may be productive and also legal but are concealed from the authorities for various reasons – for example to evade taxes or regulation. In principle these, as well as economic production that is illegal, are to be included in the accounts but they are by their nature difficult to measure.

Holding gains or losses

Profit or loss obtained by virtue of the changing price of assets being held. Holding gains or losses may arise from either physical and financial assets.

Households (S.14)

Individuals or small groups of individuals as consumers and in some cases as entrepreneurs producing goods and market services (where such activities cannot be hived off and treated as those of a quasi corporation).

Imputation

The process of inventing a transaction where, although no money has changed hands, there has been a flow of goods or services. It is confined to a very small number of cases where a reasonably satisfactory basis for the assumed valuation is available.

Index-linked gilts

Gilts whose coupon and redemption value are linked to movements in the retail prices index.

Institutional unit

Institutional units are the individual bodies whose data is amalgamated to form the sectors of the economy. A body is regarded as an institutional unit if it has decision-making autonomy in respect of its principal function and either keeps a complete set of accounts or is in a position to compile, if required, a complete set of accounts which would be meaningful from both an economic and a legal viewpoint.

Institutional sector

See Sector.

Input–Output

A detailed analytical framework based on Supply and Use tables. These are matrices showing the composition of output of individual industries by types of product and how the domestic and imported supply of goods and services is allocated between various intermediate and final uses, including exports.

Intangible assets

Intangible fixed assets include mineral exploration, computer software and entertainment, literary or artistic originals. Expenditure on them is part of gross fixed capital formation. They exclude non-produced intangible assets such as patented entities, leases, transferable contracts and purchased goodwill, expenditure on which would be intermediate consumption.

Intermediate consumption

The consumption of goods and services in the production process. It may be contrasted with final consumption and capital formation.

International Monetary Fund (IMF)

A fund set up as a result of the Bretton Woods Conference in 1944 which began operations in 1947. It currently has about 180 member countries including most of the major countries of the world. The fund was set up to supervise the fixed exchange rate system agreed at Bretton Woods and to make available to its members a pool of foreign exchange resources to assist them when they have balance of payments difficulties. It is funded by member countries' subscriptions according to agreed quotas.

Inventories

Inventories (known as stocks in the former system) consist of finished goods (held by the producer prior to sale, further processing or other use) and products (materials and fuel) acquired from other producers to be used for intermediate consumption or resold without further processing.

Investment trust

An institution that invests its capital in a wide range of other companies' shares. Investment trusts issue shares which are listed on the London Stock Exchange and use this capital to invest in the shares of other companies. See also Unit trusts.

Kind-of-activity unit (KAU)

An enterprise, or part of an enterprise, which engages in only one kind of non-ancillary productive activity, or in which the principal productive activity accounts for most of the value added. Each enterprise consists of one or more kind-of-activity units.

Liability

A claim on an institutional unit by another body which gives rise to a payment or other transaction transferring assets to the other body. Conditional liabilities, i.e. where the transfer of assets only takes place under certain defined circumstances, are known as contingent liabilities.

Liquidity

The ease with which a financial instrument can be exchanged for goods and services. Cash is very liquid whereas a life assurance policy is less so.

Lloyd's of London

The international insurance and reinsurance market in London.

Marketable securities

Securities which can be sold on the open market.

Market output

Output of goods and services sold at economically significant prices.

Merchant banks

These are monetary financial institutions whose main business is primarily concerned with corporate finance and acquisitions.

Mixed income

The balancing item on the generation of income account for unincorporated businesses owned by households. The owner or members of the same household often provide unpaid labour inputs to the business. The surplus is therefore a mixture of remuneration for such labour and return to the owner as entrepreneur.

Money market

The market in which short-term loans are made and short -term securities traded. 'Short term' usually applies to periods under one year but can be longer in some instances.

NACE

The industrial classification used in the European Union. Revision 1 is the 'Statistical classification of economic activities in the European Community in accordance with Council Regulation No. 3037/90 of 9th October 1990'.

National income

See Gross national disposable income and Real national disposable income.

National Loans Fund

An account of HM Government set up under the National Loans Fund Act (1968) which handles all government borrowing and most domestic lending transactions.

Net

After deduction of the consumption of fixed capital. Also used in the context of financial accounts and balance sheets to denote, for example, assets less liabilities.

Non-market output

Output of own account production of goods and services provided free or at prices that are not economically significant. Non-market output is produced mainly by the general government and NPISH sectors.

NPISH

Non-profit institutions serving households (S.15). These include bodies such as charities, universities, churches, trade unions or member's clubs.

Operating surplus

The balance on the generation of income account. Households also have a mixed income balance. It may be seen as the surplus arising from the production of goods and services before taking into account flows of property income.

Operating leasing

The conventional form of leasing, in which the lessee makes use of the leased asset for a period in return for a rental while the asset remains on the balance sheet of the lessor. The leasing payments are part of the output of the lessor, and the intermediate consumption of the lessee. See also Financial leasing.

Ordinary share

The most common type of share in the ownership of a corporation. Holders of ordinary shares receive dividends. See also Equity.

Output for own final use

Production of output for final consumption or gross fixed capital formation by the producer. Also known as own-account production.

Own-account production

Production of output for final consumption or gross fixed capital formation by the producer. Also known as output for own final use.

Par value

A security's face or nominal value. Securities can be issued at a premium or discount to par.

Pension funds

The institutions that administer pension schemes. Pension schemes are significant investors in securities. Self-administered funds are classified in the financial accounts as pension funds. Those managed by insurance companies are treated as long-term business of insurance companies. They are part of S.125, the Insurance corporations and pension funds sub-sector.

Perpetual Inventory Model (or Method) (PIM)

A method for estimating the level of assets held at a particular point of time by accumulating the acquisitions of such assets over a period and subtracting the disposals of assets over that period. Adjustments are made for price changes over the period. The PIM is used in the UK accounts to estimate the stock of fixed capital, and hence the value of the consumption of fixed capital.

Portfolio

A list of the securities owned by a single investor. In the Balance of Payments statistics, portfolio investment is investment in securities that does not qualify as direct investment.

Preference share

This type of share guarantees its holder a prior claim on dividends. The dividend paid to preference share holders is normally more than that paid to holders of ordinary shares. Preference shares may give the holder a right to a share in the ownership of the company (participating preference shares). However in the UK they usually do not, and are therefore classified as bonds (F.3).

Prices

See economically significant prices, basic prices, producers' prices.

Principal

The lump sum that is lent under a loan or a bond.

Private sector

Private non-financial corporations, financial corporations other than the Bank of England (and Girobank when it was publicly owned), households and the NPISH sector.

Production boundary

Boundary between production included in creating core economic accounts (such as all economic activity by industry and commerce) and production which is excluded (such as production by households which is consumed within the household).

Promissory note

A security which entitles the bearer to receive cash. These may be issued by companies or other institutions. (See commercial paper).

Property income

Incomes that accrue from lending or renting financial or tangible non-produced assets, including land, to other units. See also Tangible assets.

Public corporations

These are public trading bodies which have a substantial degree of financial independence from the public authority which created them. A public corporation is publicly controlled to the extent that the public authority, i.e. central or local government, usually appoints the whole or a majority of the board of management. Such bodies comprise much the greater part of sub-sector S.11001, public non-financial corporations.

Public sector

Comprises general government plus public non-financial corporations.

Purchasers' prices

These are the prices paid by purchasers. They include transport costs, trade margins and taxes (unless the taxes are deductible by the purchasers from their own tax liabilities).

Quasi-corporations

Unincorporated enterprises that function as if they were corporations. For the purposes of allocation to sectors and sub-sectors they are treated as if they were corporations, i.e. separate units from those to which they legally belong. Three main types of quasi-corporation are recognised in the accounts: unincorporated enterprises owned by government which are engaged in market production, unincorporated enterprises (including partnerships) owned by households and unincorporated enterprises owned by foreign residents. The last group consists of permanent branches or offices of foreign enterprises and production units of foreign enterprises which engage in significant amounts of production in the territory over long or indefinite periods of time.

Real national disposable income (RNDI)

Gross national disposable income adjusted for changes in prices and in the terms of trade.

Related companies

Branches, subsidiaries, associates or parents.

Related import or export credit

Trade credit between related companies, included in direct investment.

Rental

The amount payable by the user of a fixed asset to its owner for the right to use that asset in production for a specified period of time. It is included in the output of the owner and the intermediate consumption of the user.

Rents (D.45)

The property income derived from land and sub-soil assets. It should be distinguished in the current system from rental income derived from buildings and other fixed assets, which is included in output (P.1).

Repurchase agreement (Repo)

A deal in which an institution lends or 'sells' another institution a security and agrees to buy it back at a future date. Legal ownership does not change under a 'repo' agreement. It was previously treated as a change of ownership in the UK financial account but under the SNA is treated as a collateralised deposit (F.22).

Reserve assets

The UK official holdings of gold, convertible currencies, Special Drawing Rights, changes in the UK reserve position with the IMF and European currency. They include units acquired from swaps with the European Monetary Co-operation Fund (EMCF).

Residents

These comprise general government, individuals, private non-profit-making bodies serving households and enterprises within the territory of a given economy.

Residual error

The term used in the former accounts for the difference between the measures of gross domestic product from the expenditure and income approaches.

Resources and Uses

The term *resources* refers to the side of the current accounts where transactions which add to the amount of economic value of a unit or sector appear. For example, wages and salaries are a resource for the unit or sector receiving them. Resources are by convention put on the right side, or at the top of tables arranged vertically. The left side (or bottom section) of the accounts, which relates to transactions that reduce the amount of economic value of a unit or sector, is termed *uses*. To continue the example, wages and salaries are a use for the unit or sector that must pay them.

Rest of the world

This sector records the counterpart of transactions of the whole economy with non-residents.

Satellite accounts

Satellite accounts describe areas or activities not dealt with by core economic accounts. These areas/activities are considered to require too much detail for inclusion in the core accounts or they operate with a different conceptual framework. Internal satellite accounts re-present information within the production boundary. External satellite accounts present new information not covered by the core accounts.

Saving

The balance on the use of income account. It is that part of disposable income which is not spent on final consumption, and may be positive or negative.

Sector

In the economic accounts the economy is split into different institutional sectors, i.e. groupings of units according broadly to their role in the economy. The main sectors are non-financial corporations, financial corporations, general government, households and non-profit institutions serving households (NPISH). The Rest of the world is also treated as a sector for many purposes within the accounts.

Secondary market

A market in which holders of financial instruments can re-sell all or part of their holding. The larger and more effective the secondary market for any particular financial instrument the more liquid that instrument is to the holder.

Securities

Tradeable or potentially tradeable financial instruments.

SIC

Standard Industrial Classification. The industrial classification applied to the collection and publication of a wide range of economic statistics. The current version, SIC92, is consistent with NACE, Rev.1.

SNA

System of National Accounts, the internationally agreed standard system for macroeconomic accounts. The latest version is described in System of National Accounts 1993.

Special Drawing Rights (SDRs)

These are reserve assets created and distributed by decision of the members of the IMF. Participants accept an obligation, when designated by the IMF to do so, to provide convertible currency to another participant in exchange for SDRs equivalent to three times their own allocation. Only countries with a sufficiently strong balance of payments are so designated. SDRs may also be used in certain direct payments between participants in the scheme and for payments of various kinds to the IMF.

Stage payments

See Advance and progress payments.

Stocks, stockbuilding

The terms used in the former system corresponding to inventories and changes in inventories.

Subsidiaries

Companies owned or controlled by another company. Under Section 736 of the Companies Act (1985) this means, broadly speaking, that another company either holds more than half the equity share capital or controls the composition of the board of directors. The category also includes subsidiaries of subsidiaries.

Subsidies (D.3)

Current unrequited payments made by general government or the European Union to enterprises. Those made on the basis of a quantity or value of goods or services are classified as 'subsidies on products' (D.31). Other subsidies based on levels of productive activity (e.g. numbers employed) are designated Other subsidies on production (D.39).

Suppliers' credit

Export credit extended overseas directly by UK firms other than to related concerns.

Supply table

Table of estimates of domestic industries' output by type of product. Compiled at basic prices and includes columns for imports of goods and services, for distributors' trading margins and for taxes less subsidies on products. The final column shows the value of the supply of goods and services at purchaser's prices. This table shows which industries make which products. Columns represent the supplying industries: rows represent the products supplied.

Tangible assets

These comprise produced fixed assets and non-produced assets. Tangible fixed assets, the acquisition and disposal of which are recorded in gross fixed capital formation (P.51), comprise buildings and other structures (including historic monuments), vehicles, other machinery and equipment and cultivated assets in the form of livestock and trees yielding repeat products (e.g. dairy cattle, orchards). Tangible non-produced assets are assets such as land and sub-soil resources that occur in nature over which ownership rights have been established. Similar assets to which ownership rights have not been established are excluded as they do not qualify as economic assets. The acquisition and disposal of non-produced assets in principle is recorded separately in the capital account (K.2). The distinction between produced and non-produced assets is not yet fully possible for the United Kingdom.

Taxes

Compulsory unrequited transfers to central or local government or the European Union. Taxation is classified in the following main groups: taxes on production and imports (D.2), current taxes on income wealth, etc (D.5) and capital taxes (D.91).

Technical reserves (of insurance companies)

These reserves consist of pre-paid premiums, reserves against outstanding claims, actuarial reserves for life insurance and reserves for with-profit insurance. They are treated in the economic accounts as the property of policy-holders.

Terms of trade

Ratio of the change in export prices to the change in import prices. An increase in the terms of trade implies that the receipts from the same quantity of exports will finance an increased volume of imports. Thus measurement of real national disposable income needs to take account of this factor.

Transfers

Unrequited payments made by one unit to another. They may be current transfers (D.5-7) or capital transfers (D.9). The most important types of transfers are taxes, social contributions and benefits.

Treasury bills

Short-term securities or promissory notes which are issued by government in return for funding from the money market. In the United Kingdom every week the Bank of England invites tenders for sterling Treasury bills from the financial institutions operating in the market. ECU-denominated bills are issued by tender each month. Treasury bills are an important form of short-term borrowing for the government, generally being issued for periods of 3 or 6 months.

Unit trusts

Institutions within sub-sector S.123 through which investors pool their funds to invest in a diversified portfolio of securities. Individual investors purchase units in the fund representing an ownership interest in the large pool of underlying assets, i.e. they have an equity stake. The selection of assets is made by professional fund managers. Unit trusts therefore give individual investors the opportunity to invest in a diversified and professionally managed portfolio of securities without the need for detailed knowledge of the individual companies issuing the stocks and bonds. They differ from investment trusts in that the latter are companies in which investors trade shares on the Stock Exchange, whereas unit trust units are issued and bought back on demand by the managers of the trust. The prices of unit trust units thus reflect the value of the underlying pool of securities, whereas the price of shares in investment trusts are affected by the usual market forces.

Uses

See Resources and Uses

Use Table

See Combined Use Table.

United Kingdom

Broadly, in the accounts, the United Kingdom comprises Great Britain plus Northern Ireland and that part of the continental shelf deemed by international convention to belong to the UK. It excludes the Channel Islands and the Isle of Man.

Valuables

Goods of considerable value that are not used primarily for production or consumption but are held as stores of value over time. They consist of precious metals, precious stones, jewellery, works of art, etc. As a new category in the accounts the estimates for them are currently fairly rudimentary, though transactions are likely to have been recorded elsewhere in the accounts.

Valuation

See Basic prices, Purchasers' prices, Factor cost.

Value added

The balance on the production account: output less intermediate consumption. Value added may be measured net or gross.

Value Added Tax (VAT) (D.211)

A tax paid by enterprises. In broad terms an enterprise is liable for VAT on the total of its taxable sales but may deduct tax already paid by suppliers on its inputs (intermediate consumption). Thus the tax is effectively on the value added by the enterprise. Where the enterprise cannot deduct tax on its inputs the tax is referred to as non-deductible. VAT is the main UK tax on products (D.21).

Index

Figures indicate Table numbers. The letter "G" indicates that the item appears in the Glossary. Where the item is discussed in the section introductions, the appropriate page number is given.

Key for this index

References are either to pages of text or to table numbers.

S – appears in sector tables which are numbered using the following system:

The table numbering system for the Blue Book shows the relationships between the UK, its sectors and the rest of the world. A 3-part numbering system (e.g. 1.7.2) has been adopted for the accounts drawn directly from the ESA95. The first two digits denotes the UK sector, the third digit denotes the ESA95 account. They are as follows:

0 Goods and services account

1 Production account

2 Generation of income account

3 Allocation of primary income account

4 Secondary distribution of income account

5 Redistribution of income in kind account

6 Use of income account

7 Accumulation account

8 Financial account

9 Financial balance sheet

ISBN 978-0-230-54566-3
ISSN 0267–8691

A National Statistics publication

National Statistics are produced to high professional standards as set out in the National Statistics Code of Practice. They are produced free from political influence.

About us

The Office for National Statistics

The Office for National Statistics (ONS) is the executive office of the UK Statistics Authority, a non-ministerial department which reports directly to Parliament. ONS is the UK government's single largest statistical producer. It compiles information about the UK's society and economy which provides evidence for policy and decision-making and in the allocation of resources.

The Director of ONS is also the National Statistician.

Palgrave Macmillan

This publication first published 2008 by Palgrave Macmillan, Houndmills, Basingstoke, Hampshire RG21 6XS and 175 Fifth Avenue, New York, NY 10010, USA

Companies and representatives throughout the world.

Palgrave Macmillan is the global academic imprint of the Palgrave Macmillan division of St. Martin's Press, LLC and of Palgrave Macmillan Ltd. Macmillan® is a registered trademark in the United States, United Kingdom and other countries. Palgrave is a registered trademark in the European Union and other countries.

A catalogue record for this book is available from the British Library.

10 9   8   7   6   5   4   3   2   1
17 16 15 14 13 12 11 10 09 08

Contacts

This publication

For information about the content of this publication, contact the Editor
Tel: 020 7014 2088
Email: john.dye@ons.gsi.gov.uk

Other customer and media enquiries

ONS Customer Contact Centre
Tel: 0845 601 3034
International: +44 (0)845 601 3034
Minicom: 01633 812399
Email: info@statistics.gsi.gov.uk
Fax: 01633 652747

Post: Room 1015, Government Buildings,
Cardiff Road, Newport, South Wales NP10 8XG
www.statistics.gov.uk

Publication orders

To obtain the print version of this publication, contact Palgrave Macmillan
Tel: 01256 302611
www.palgrave.com/ons

Copyright and reproduction

Printing

This book is printed on paper suitable for recycling and made from fully managed and sustained forest sources. Logging, pulping and manufacturing processes are expected to conform to the environmental regulations of the country of origin.

Printed and bound in Great Britain by Hobbs the Printer Ltd, Totton, Southampton

Typeset by Academic + Technical Typesetting, Bristol

for
.onal Statistics

United Kingdom
National Accounts:

The Blue Book

2008 Edition

Editors: John Dye
James Sosimi
Office for National Statistics

palgrave
macmillan